FOUNDATIONS OF EVIDENCE - BASED MEDICINE

FOUNDATIONS OF EVIDENCE - BASED MEDICINE

MILOS JENICEK, MD

Professor, McMaster University

Professor Emeritus, Université de Montréal
Adjunct Professor, McGill University

Hamilton, Ontario and Montréal, Québec
Canada

The Parthenon Publishing Group
International Publishers in Medicine, Science & Technology

A CRC PRESS COMPANY
BOCA RATON   LONDON   NEW YORK   WASHINGTON, D.C.

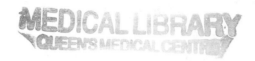
Library of Congress Cataloging-in-Publication Data
Jenicek, Milos, 1935-
   Foundations of evidence-based medicine / Milos Jenicek
     p : cm
   Includes bibliographical references and index
   ISBN 1-84214-193-7 (alk. paper)
   1. Evidence-based medicine. I. Title
   [DNLM: 1. Evidence-Based Medicine—methods.
     WB 102 J51f 2002]
   R723.J465 2002
616—dc21

British Library Cataloguing in Publication Data
   Jenicek, Milos, 1935–
   Foundations of evidence-based medicine
   1. Evidence-based medicine   2. Diagnosis   3. Epidemiology
   I. Title
   616

   ISBN 1-84214-193-7

Published in the USA by
The Parthenon Publishing Group Inc.
345 Park Avenue South
10th Floor
New York 10010, USA

Published in the UK and Europe by
The Parthenon Publishing Group Limited
23–25 Blades Court, Deodar Road,
London SW15 2NU, UK

Copyright © 2003 The Parthenon Publishing Group

ISBN 1-84214-193-7

Typeset by AMA DataSet Ltd., Preston, UK
Printed and bound in the USA

To three generations of the Jenicek clan:
Jana (my enduring wife), Tom, Andy, Chris,
Chantal, Janice, Lynn, Richard, Jared, Brooke
… and counting

Contents

Section II
How do we Do Things in Medicine
Gathering and evaluating evidence

Section III
Putting Experiences Together and Making Decisions in Medicine
Structured uses of evidence

Chapter 11

Analyzing and integrating a body of knowledge. Systematic reviews and meta-analysis of evidence

Chapter 12

Using evidence and logic in everyday clinical reasoning, communication, and legal and scientific argumentation

Chapter 13

Decision analysis and decision-making in medicine. Beyond intuition, guts, and flair

A Word From the Author

This book focuses mainly on reasoning, critical thinking and pragmatic decision-making in medicine.

Modern medicine does not revolve exclusively around new technologies such as magnetic resonance imaging, robotized microsurgery, genetic mapping or cloning of living organisms. Modern medicine also requires structured reasoning in an increasingly complex world of uncertainty and incomplete information of unequal quality. As such, this book outlines how to make the best possible crucial decisions in clinical care, disease prevention and health promotion.

Learning medicine not only involves memorizing a considerable volume of information, mastering sensory skills and communicating with patients and health professionals. It also requires excellent reasoning techniques, processing of information through sensory skills, judging the state of things, and decision-making. Classical textbooks of medicine or surgery examine mainly the former. This book covers the latter.

This book is intended primarily for young and less young physicians, as well as other health professionals from the fields of dentistry, veterinary medicine, nursing, clinical nutrition, psychology, and health administration who want to acquire the fundamental information needed to better understand and ultimately practice evidence-based medicine. It is also intended to help in the critical reading of medical literature and in the understanding of messages and reasoning of health professionals, planners and decision-makers. Experienced clinicians from various specialties who teach in-house staff with various levels of experience will want to refer to it to show their students how to reason and translate their experience into bedside decision-oriented research. Residents in specialty training programs around the world are becoming increasingly involved in medical research and want to understand its workings. Many of them learnt just enough epidemiology and other fundamentals years ago to pass their exams and their clinical guides did not always offer appropriate learning experiences. Hence, the fundamentals of epidemiology and other disciplines on which evidence-based medicine is based today are covered in this reading to the obvious benefit of medical undergraduates at exam time. However, the primary focus of this book is on medical and biological thinking and decisions endorsed only after the application of relevant quantitative methods and techniques.

Medical students will learn about evidence-based medicine at a later date and in greater detail. Before that, they must master the essentials of fundamental and clinical epidemiology and of logical thinking in medicine. Their final and licensure examinations will cover not only principles of evidence-based medicine, but also the basics of epidemiology and preventive or community medicine. This reading should help them succeed. Does this book follow current courses of epidemiology and other related disciplines? It does, but not entirely. In fact, it serves a kind of propaedeutics to reasoning and decision-making in health sciences practice and research. Many graduates and fully qualified health professionals wanting to refresh their knowledge of the foundations of evidence-based medicine such as epidemiology and clinical epidemiology will hopefully find this book a useful transition from the basic sciences of reasoning and measurement in medicine to their practice in today's evidence-based world. Most readers of this book will become family physicians or clinicians in various specialties. Some will even embrace epidemiology, community medicine or public health. Whatever career path is chosen, we all need the solid foundations of organized reasoning and the ability to make beneficial decisions for patients and communities, as discussed in this basic reading.

The most challenging endeavor for the author of this book was to write for the uninitiated, curious, intelligent, and doubtful, while making the message 'short and sweet'. The easiest thing to do is to reach the enthusiasts. An old academic adage says that Assistant Professors (Lecturers) teach more than they know, Associate Professors (Senior Lecturers) teach all they know, and Professors explain only what their students really need to know. The author has gone through all these stages only to realize that the last is the most difficult of all.

The reader will find that this book is organized according to the basic steps of clinical work with a patient and not according to some other scientific methodology, like descriptive, analytical or experimental techniques or designs. Specifically, this book is divided into three sections:

- The first section, '*How do we see things in medicine*', focuses on understanding how physicians think, reason and make decisions;
- The second section, '*How do we do things in medicine*', or '**Gathering and evaluating evidence**', explains how to obtain and evaluate good evidence at every step from risk assessment and diagnosis to final therapeutic or prevention decision-making. It offers essential definitions, formulae, outlines, flow charts and checklists useful in health measurement, case and occurrence studies, search for causes, clinical trials, and prognosis;
- The third section, '*Putting experiences together and making decisions in medicine. Structured uses of evidence*', shows how all the 'bricks' are integrated into the decision-making methodology and how medical evidence is assembled in view of obtaining the best possible answer to clinical questions. The emphasis here is on logical uses of evidence.

Readers will find two unusual chapters in this reading (Chapters 3 and 12) that examine logic and critical thinking. Acquiring good evidence is not enough. Good evidence must also be put to good use both logically and critically. Some essentials of reasoning, in other words thinking enlightened by logic,

are presented in these chapters. In the past, this was not taught at all. Student intelligence and remnants of logic picked up in college courses were expected to suffice. Hence, a more detailed explanation is justified. Moreover, the 'discussion' and 'conclusion' sections of medical articles are essentially logical discourses about evidence produced and presented in 'results' and all preceding sections. Valuable evidence may, in fact, be lost due to poor logical use or misuse.

The first and the third sections of the book present the necessary framework for the second section, which is primarily for busy medical students with exams in mind. Most of the chapters are introduced by an example of reasoning in practice, in the form of a logical syllogism. These argumentations are not necessarily all valid. They tend to reproduce reality and what may occur in real life with all its imperfections. Also, they underline the need for good evidence for the premises and conclusions of logical arguments. Many 'classics' are excluded from the bibliography. Instead, references cover a variety of information, which the reader might find in the literature when moving from more general topics to specific ones in health sciences. For example, diversity of definitions for such ordinary and ubiquitous terms as art, science, logic or reasoning shows how medical thinking is part of a wider domain of thought and human experience.

The references most often include basic expanded readings, practical applications or some key historical references or 'classics', mainly from major and easily accessible medical journals. If needed, it can be expanded through an electronic and manual literature search and retrieval.

The message should be as explicit as possible. Hence, some unavoidable computational examples are intentionally numerically oversimplified. For many, percentages are more understandable than much smaller proportions such as those seen in real-life cancer epidemiology. However, we should be aware of the real magnitude of health phenomena around us. More specific statistical techniques like standardization of rates, establishing life tables and survival curves, obtaining overall rates and ratios from stratified data or establishing confidence intervals for various observations belong to other programs and sources dealing with these methods and techniques. Some readers will find that notions and illustrative examples beyond the basics are only mentioned in passing. Both can be found, however, in the extensive bibliography that accompanies this overview of evidence-based medicine tools.

This book is conservatively written, in a manner similar to a literary essay. There are no exercises, but many, hopefully well-chosen, practical examples. This structure was selected for two major reasons: experienced lecturers who honor the author by referring to this book in their teachings almost always use their own exercises and problems in class. Also, they will correctly choose their own national health statistics, priorities, and clinical and public health experience to ensure relevance to the practice of medicine in their own countries, which may not necessarily be the author's.

In a state-of-the-art clinical practice, everything evolves: new medical technologies; normal values of clinical and paraclinical observations (reference data); diagnostic criteria; treatment indications; drug doses; treatment effectiveness; prognostic information given to the patient. Examples from these areas are quoted here to illustrate medical logic only and for didactic purposes. They should not be followed blindly in daily office work and bedside decision-making. Such information requires continuous updating and revision.

Friends, colleagues, and coworkers, who helped so much in the production of this book, are in no way responsible for potential errors – only the author is. Any monograph is not a true monograph. The author was privileged to have several remarkable critical readers: Professors Jean Lambert and Michèle Rivard (Université de Montréal – biostatistics), Geoffrey Norman (McMaster University – biostatistics), David Hitchcock (McMaster University – philosophy and logic), Marianne Xhignesse (Université de Sherbrooke – family medicine), Jim Bellamy (University of Price Edward Island – applications of fuzzy theory in medicine), Mrs. Gillian Mulvale (McMaster University – health economics). Illustrations were prepared by Mr. Jacques Cadieux (Université de Montréal – infographics), the language and style were reviewed by Mrs. Nicole Kinney (Linguamax Services Ltd.). The author remains indebted to all of them for guidance and for sparing himself and his readers from the worst in this reading, especially in places where we agree to disagree. A special appreciation goes to the Département de médecine sociale et préventive at the Université de Montréal for all the assistance and resources it provided for this project. Statistics Canada information is used with permission of the Ministry of Industry, as Minister responsible for Statistics Canada. Information on the availability of the wide range of data from Statistics Canada can be obtained from Statistics Canada's Regional Offices and its World Wide Web site.

Many textbooks are affected by globalization. They can be used successfully in different cultures, health systems, traditions, and values. In this respect, examples in this book, like major causes of death or patterns of morbidity, are drawn either from the author's North American experience or from countries which best illustrate the underlying message, such as the epidemiological transition of the Japanese society, or potentially extreme findings around the globe. They do not necessarily represent standards or ideal values to be adopted all around. The author would like to offer his readers a foundation on which to build their own specific experience, be it in family medicine, internal medicine, surgery, pediatrics, psychiatry, community medicine, or other specialties. Also, needless to say, dentistry, nursing, nutrition, medical records specialists or those in sanitary and environmental engineering share many common ways of thinking with what might now be called the 'logic of medicine', encompassing past and present experiences of epidemiology, clinical epidemiology, evidence-based medicine and other current streams of thought.

What makes a health professional? Not only perfect examination or surgical skills, but also sound reasoning and decision-making. Earlier generations were taught 'medical propaedeutics': the ability to learn and know before a 'real thing' occurs. This often involved the basic skills required of a clinical, laboratory, or community health clerk: interacting with patients; physical and paraclinical examinations; understanding and interpretation of basic findings. Today, other medical propaedeutics are also needed – how to think, reason, and make decisions in medicine in a logical, rational and organized manner.

This is the focus of the book. Even the title of this book is a word of convenience. Labels come and go, be they epidemiology, evidence-based medicine, or theory of medicine, but the common ground for all these paradigms remains: how to make medicine most beneficial for patients and communities.

The Hippocratic Oath tells us *primum non nocere* or 'first, do not harm'. The illogical, erratic and inefficient practice of medicine causes harm! In this respect, 'big heart, small brain' medicine must make room for 'big heart, big brain' medicine. In fact, is this not what we all want? Is this not what our patients and communities expect from us? Having said this, does the reader feel that about 400 pages on these topics is too much? Textbooks of medicine or surgery are usually five times more voluminous! They provide essential and vitally important ingredients for 'good medicine'. This book should help its readers understand what to do with such ingredients. If this book also enables its readers to learn how to think in medicine, its author will be delighted since when he was young, less experienced, yet eager to learn, his teachers often failed to touch upon these topics.

Milos Jenicek
Rockwood, January 2003

How do we See Things in Medicine

How do we see medicine, health and disease? A basic set of rules and fundamental paradigms

'. . . the art of medicine is the skilled application of medical science. In this sense, the art of medicine is no different from the art of engineering or architecture or any other applied science in which a large body of knowledge must be applied to everyday problems. Some engineers and architects are better than others: they are better 'artists'. . . . Clearly, it does little good for medical science and technology to make dramatic advances if these advances are going to be applied inefficiently and incorrectly.'
S. Schwartz and T. Griffin, 1986

Science may be described as the art of systematic oversimplification
Karl Popper, 1982

Logic is the technique by which we add conviction to truth
Jean de la Bruyère, 1688

INTRODUCTORY COMMENTS

Good physicians must successfully meet many challenges:

- The assimilation of a considerable volume of facts such as elements of anatomy, hundreds of syndromes for further pattern recognition, dosages of drugs and pieces of legislation or administrative rules governing medical practice.
- The acquisition of automatisms necessary for the execution of many clinical maneuvers such as those required to perform a physical examination or to practice emergency medicine.
- The ability to effectively communicate (listening and talking) with the patient, the patient's family, as well as members of the health team.
- The assessment of patient risks.
- The making of diagnosis and prognosis.
- The listing of problems and creation of a hierarchical classification.
- The making of decisions (choices).
- The mastery of exploratory and surgical procedures (performance).
- The management of patients after intervention (follow-up and care, control of disease course).
- The evaluation of the effectiveness and efficiency of cure and care.
- The respect of medical, cultural and social ethics as well as of patient values, preferences and expectations.
- Empathy.

Practicing medicine means not only applying our humanism, compassion, knowledge or skills, but also basing our actions on the fundamentals of philosophy, science, art and logic in their universal sense. Medicine is an integral part of such a universe and often, we do not realize the extent to which we follow its general rules. This book is about reasoning and making decisions when dealing with patients in a clinical setting or with groups of individuals in communities under our care. It also covers what we should know and the application of this knowledge.

Quantitative research (based on counting and measurement) and qualitative research methodology (based on understanding and interpretation) are both necessary to understand the workings of medicine today. In fact, there is no other way to evaluate and understand the expectations of both Canadian and American physicians and health professionals[1,2], namely:

- Placing patients' needs ahead of self-interest; commitment to scholarship; responsiveness to societal needs; working optimally with other health professionals.
- Integrity, respect, compassion, responsibility, courtesy, sensitivity to patient needs and to colleagues and other health care personnel.
- High standards of moral and ethical behavior.
- Recognition and management of physician impairment in peers and self.
- Concern for psychosocial aspects of care.
- Recognition of the importance of self-assessment, and willingness to teach.
- Understanding of the requirements for involvement of patients in research.
- Awareness of the effects of differences in gender, age, cultural, and social background.
- Honesty and dependability.

Many of these virtues reflect expectations for physicians already proposed at the time of Paracelsus (1493–1541), with some notable exceptions such as: '. . . *not to be married to the bigot, . . . not to be a runaway monk, . . . not practice a self-abuse, . . .* and *. . . not to have a red beard . . .*'[3]. Hence, health professionals require more than a discrete body of knowledge and skills. They are expected to value performance above reward, and are held to higher standards of behavior than are non-professionals[4].

To better understand the justification, uses and purposes of various methods and techniques of study, understanding, decision-making and evaluation in medicine, we must first define the context of medicine. This is because everything we do is based on the way we see things around us and on the values given to our actions and endeavors. For instance, the consideration and practice of euthanasia is heavily influenced by our understanding and interpretation of the commandment 'Thou shall not kill' in a given setting of faith, culture and societal values. The order *primum non nocere* ('first, do not harm') in the Hippocratic oath can be challenged in situations when some harm is necessary to heal and prevent the worst. Health promotion, screening for disease or treatment of complex health problems will depend not only on medical considerations of relevance or effectiveness, but also on economics, politics, administration and management in health sciences and society as a whole. Similarly, the value and justification of our reasoning, decisions, methods and techniques in medicine depend on the context of our practice. A lecturer who enters a classroom and tells his or her unprepared students that today they will learn about case–control studies in etiological research, should expect a 'what for?' question. Therefore, let us first define major paradigms in medicine, i.e. the ways we perceive major issues and characteristics of health, disease and care.

1.1 The art and science of medicine

Medicine is currently defined as '*the art and science of diagnosis, treatment, and prevention of disease, and the maintenance of good health*'[5]. To be a good physician, it is necessary to develop the art of medicine and to master medicine as a science in two areas. In **clinical medicine**, this art and science relate to a clinic or to the bedside in the actual observation and treatment of patients. In **community medicine**, they pertain to a body of individuals living in a defined area and having a common interest or organization[5] (or characteristics). Historically, medicine was learned mostly as an art.

Art, in general, has several pragmatic definitions:

- The employment of means to accomplish some desired end.
- A system of rules serving to facilitate the performance of certain actions.
- A system of principles and rules for attaining a desired end.
- A method of doing well some special work.
- The systematic application of knowledge or skill in effecting a desired result.
- An occupation or business requiring such a knowledge and skill[6].
- Skill as the result of knowledge and practice.
- A practical application of any science.
- A pursuit of occupation in which skill is directed towards the work of imagination, imitation, or design, or towards the gratification of the esthetic senses[7].
- Skill of expression in language, speech and reasoning[8].
- A system of principles and methods employed in the performance of a set of activities.
- A trade or craft that applies such a system of principles and methods. Example: the art of plastic surgery.
- Skill that is attained by study, practice, or observation: the art of the physician.
- Skill arising from the exercise of intuitive faculties. NB This being important in differential diagnosis or emergency medicine[9].
- Both skill and creative imagination[10].

These definitions all focus on art as a way of doing things. Other definitions, however, highlight the product of such endeavors, i.e. not only oil paintings, but also a successful rhinoplasty or facelift. This extensive list of even the most general definitions of art illustrates not only how differently we can approach things around us but also that art, evidence, science, philosophy or logic are not purely abstract terms. In fact, they have important practical meanings and implications, as will be shown throughout this reading.

The **art of medicine** requires:

- A clinician with an open mind and flexibility of reasoning.
- The ability to establish a good relationship with the patient.
- Manual and sensory skills.
- Clinical flair and intuition, i.e. an aptitude to infer from previous experience, without active and concrete recall, in order to make appropriate decisions.
- Clinical imagination.
- The capacity to persuade the patient to take responsibility for his or her own health and to convince the patient that the clinician will also share that responsibility.
- The aptitude to convert serendipity into insight of patient problems.
- The preservation and maintenance of human dignity (this is one difference between medicine and the advanced technical manipulation of human beings).

- The estheticism, elegance and style in the conceptualization, execution, evaluation, and communication of a clinical experience lived.

All these components of the art of medicine are of a highly subjective nature and are therefore hard to define and measure. But we also call medicine a science. Is it? **Science, in general,** is *the study of the material universe or physical reality in order to understand it*[6]. The **science of medicine,** on the contrary, is *organized reasoning.* Also, *science in medicine means discovery, implementation, uses and evaluation of evidence.* It is complementary to the art of medicine, since when they are combined, we obtain a better understanding of what good medicine, in the fullest sense of the term, should be.

As in other fields, both art and science in medicine require technical skills. Both focus on the creation of order from seemingly random and diverse experiences, on an understanding of the world and on conveying experience to others. The scientist, however, tends to use observations to discover universally true laws or concepts that may be invalidated later. By contrast, the artist creates some kind of permanently valid statement[11]. Therefore, medicine means the application of the fundamentals of art and science as defined above to the treatment and prevention of disease as well as to the promotion of health.

In Ancient Greece and throughout history, physicians were often outstanding philosophers first and only later became biologists. Avicenna or Averroes in the Arab world and Moses Maimonides or Solomon Ben Yehuda Ibn Gabirol in the realm of Judaic thought established links between antiquity, philosophy and their respective cultures. Medieval European thinkers who were non-physicians, like Albertus Magnus or Saint Thomas Aquinas in Germany or Roger Bacon in England, preceded modern western philosophers including the logical positivists of the twentieth century and beyond[10].

Historically, the science of medicine was focused on rigorous observation, measurement and interpretation. With the development of microbiology, biochemistry, histology, pathology, genetics and other basic sciences, the goal of medicine became a search for the **true** picture of a disease, the identification of **real** causes and a search for the **best** treatment. Such an approach was clearly deterministic: the absolute truth (as much as possible) was rigorously sought. Today, experimental medicine is often based on such an approach. Models are built, undesirable factors are controlled or excluded, and rigorous experimental conditions are sought in the search for an unequivocal result. Exact information, reality without error, is the ideal and the basis for the **deterministic paradigm of medicine.** However, the **deterministic paradigm of science and life is now progressively being replaced by a probabilistic approach.** From the latter point of view, any endeavor in the health sciences is subject to **random and systematic error,** even in the most controlled conditions. Moreover, **information** for decision-making is **almost never complete** and decision-makers always work with a considerable measure of **uncertainty.**

As in economics and finance, research and practice in medicine become probabilistic when faced with uncertainty and missing information as a ubiquitous reality. All subjects who smoke will not develop lung cancer and all subjects who abstain from drinking will not be absolutely free of the risk of hepatic cirrhosis. Just a few generations ago, a middle-aged man with a productive cough of abundant sputum and a loss of weight was supposed to have tuberculosis, especially if there was confirmation based on Koch's mycobacterium isolation at the laboratory. With our current knowledge of competing problems, such as bronchiectasies, silicosis, silico-tuberculosis, or neoplasms of the lung and bronchial tree, this diagnosis becomes probable, but not entirely certain (without the exclusion of other competing health problems). **Clinical uncertainty** is a reality today. It is caused by:

- Incomplete knowledge of the clinical problem (entity, etiology, controllability, prognosis, natural and clinical course of the disease);
- Incomplete information given by the patient;
- Incomplete information obtained by the physician;
- Erroneous information given by the patient (shame, lack of memory, lie);
- Erroneous recording of information by the physician;
- Erroneous interpretation of information by the physician;

- Missing observations (not sought);
- Information not recorded;
- Erratic reasoning and intellectual handling of information by health professionals.

All clinical decisions are and will be made with a variable degree of uncertainty leading to a variable probability of events and outcomes. In this context, rather than rigorous laboratory work, the **science of medicine** becomes also a structured and organized way of using probability, uncertainty, and facts in preventive medicine and clinical care to best benefit the patient and the community. It is a logical and systematic approach to the exploration, organization and interpretation of data from initial observations to clinical decisions and final conclusions concerning problems of interest. The latter are defined, measured, analyzed and interpreted with a satisfactory degree of reproducibility. Such a scientific approach to medicine should be applied to the entire scope of medical activities.

1.2 The goals of medicine and its ensuing strategies: Health protection, disease prevention, and health promotion

There are four main goals in medicine and public health today:

- To cure and heal what already exists (traditional).
- To prevent what doesn't exist yet but may come (also traditional).
- To maintain all that is already good.
- To change whatever is necessary to keep individuals and the community in the best possible state of health and fitness (health promotion).

These goals are as old as medicine itself, but the approaches, methods and techniques used to achieve them are quite new, refined, and improved in efficiency and effectiveness.

Three major strategies to reach these goals have been developed and are used in clinical medicine and public heath. Clinical medicine has benefited from the experience of public health in epidemiology, health economics, health programs and health services evaluation. Public health and health protection is now also benefiting to an increasing degree

from recent experience and methodological developments and innovations in clinical medicine and care. Medical care organization, decision analysis, medical meta-analysis, clinical epidemiology and clinimetrics, in particular, are increasingly useful in community approaches to health problems.

The scope of public health is becoming increasingly diverse. Initially, public health encompassed health protection, disease prevention and health promotion. These three fields are now distinct entities[11,12]. By contrast with medicine, **public health** ensures the protection, promotion and restoration of health *through* organized community action.

Health protection essentially includes environment-oriented (causal factor) activities such as occupational and environmental health, nuclear war prevention or environmental aspects of injury control.

Disease prevention is centered on problem-orientated activities as well as on the reduction of disease occurrence (primary prevention) and its course (secondary and tertiary prevention).

Health promotion is increasingly important in public health today. It can be defined as any activity that alters behavior, environment or heredity in a positive direction. Health promotion is individual-oriented and has the purpose of adopting or strengthening a healthy behavior and discontinuing an unhealthy one. To do this, factors such as knowledge, understanding, attitudes, motivation, rewards or penalties are taken into consideration[13].

Public health has powerful new tools. Just as medicine has antibiotics, new medical diagnostic technologies, immunosuppressive treatments and antineoplastic drugs, public health can now rely on 'hardware', such as genetically engineered vaccines and 'software', such as decision analysis, multivariate and multivariable analytical methods, meta-analysis and the whole interface between classical and clinical epidemiology. Public health policies and strategies have broadened. At times today, actors are more involved in health promotion and disease protection than health professionals. Old Virchow's adage that 'medicine is a social science and politics is not less than large-scale medicine' is increasingly becoming a reality.

1.3 How do we define and understand health and disease

Any diagnosis, understanding of causes, choice of treatment or prognosis in an individual patient or in the community requires an understanding of the nature of health problems and of their evolution. Good decision-making at all these levels must take into account several challenging paradigms (i.e. 'the way we see things'):

1. Health and disease can be defined in several ways[12–16] (See Table 1.1).
2. Diseases evolve in terms of their natural and clinical course in relation to co-morbidity and therapeutic intervention.
3. Several factors as 'webs of causes' reflect the etiology of disease (See Figure 1.1).
4. Exposure to causal factors varies in terms of duration and frequency.
5. Etiological factors interact when causing health problems (synergy and antagonism).
6. Biological responses to the action of causal factors are not uniform (reactions, adaptation, failure to adapt, paradoxical responses).
7. Etiological factors can be common to several health problems leading to 'webs of consequences'.
8. Demographical mobility of the population is a movable terrain for the spread of the disease in the community.
9. Information on disease or lived experience is fleeting. All subjects concerned do not provide it in a uniform manner. It also varies *per se* in terms of biological periodicity (chronobiology, chronopathology, chronopharmacology).
10. We cannot always avoid the occurrence of random and systematic errors (biases) when studying disease.
11. From a statistical point of view, our observations in medicine are subject to sampling theory. General characteristics of measured phenomena are not defined solely by the result of measurement in a specific study.
12. Facts (disease data, information) and their sense and meaning are almost never certain and complete (explanation and knowledge are limited).

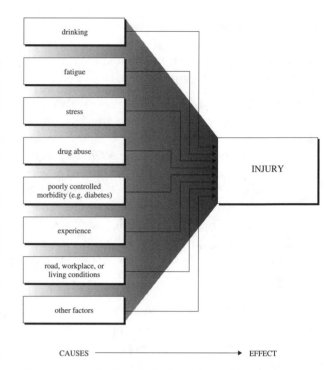

CAUSES   ⟶   EFFECT

Figure 1.1   Web of causes in the etiology of disease

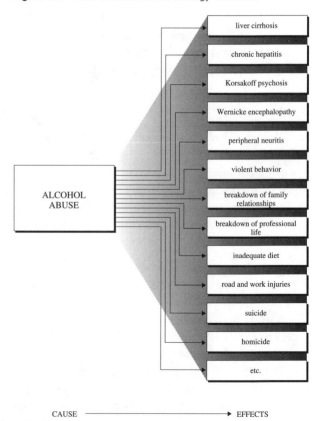

CAUSE   ⟶   EFFECTS

Figure 1.2   Web of disease consequences

Despite these paradigms, we must make the best clinical decisions possible. To this end, medical thinking, as well as methods of research and their interpretation and applications to health programs, are based on principles, methods and techniques which take into account all of the above. In a way, our clinical reasoning, its logic and architecture is dictated by the biological nature of health phenomena and by our often faulty and/or incomplete observations, their classification and interpretation (thinking). Subsequent chapters explain in greater detail most of these views and how they are used in practice and research. Now, however, let us attempt to define various health conditions and categories of attention such as health itself, disease, syndrome, impairment, disability and handicap.

1.3.1 Health

Numerous definitions of health and disease have been quoted in the literature[12]. Table 1.1 lists a few examples of how health can be defined. As we can see, no ideal definition is available. In practice, definitions which do not allow either measurement and/or count have mostly ethical and political values. They are difficult to use in health programs since they can't serve as a measure or gauge of the impact of a health program under study. For a considerable period of time, the World Health Organization's concept of health was a prevailing paradigm, an ideal to be achieved[13]. While excellent on a philosophical level, this definition is rather static since it is difficult to define in operational terms how healthy an individual is by simply excluding the presence of major diseases. In addition, the idea of physical capacity, fitness, mental abilities, and social integration or involvement is needed to complete the picture. Despite a great deal of effort[13–15], it is difficult to count health in people, to actually measure their health and to analyze how healthy the whole population is. Nevertheless, this must be done.

Table 1.1 Definition of health

Health is	Characteristic of definition	Source
'. . . a state of complete physical, mental, and social well-being, and not merely the absence of disease'.	Conceptual and static (Challenging to put in operational terms, to measure, and to merge.)	Ref. 12–14
'. . . a resource which gives people the ability to manage and even to change their surroundings. This view of health recognizes freedom of choice and emphasizes the role of individuals and communities in defining what health means to them. Viewed from this perspective, health ceases to be measurable strictly in terms of illness and death. It becomes a state that individuals and communities alike strive to achieve, maintain or regain, and not something that comes about merely as a result of treating and curing illnesses and injuries. It is a basic and dynamic force in our daily lives, influenced by our circumstances, our beliefs, our culture and our social, economic and physical environment . . .'	Philosophical (metaphysical) (Very difficult to translate in operational terms, especially in health promotion.)	Ref. 12,15
'. . . the state of an individual or of a group of individuals that allows them to adequately respond both biologically and socially to habitual environmental stimuli (climate, work, etc.) and to adequately adapt to new ones'.	Biological and dynamic (Challenging to define and to measure an adequate adaptation.)	Ours
'. . . the state of an individual or of a group in whom selected major health problems have been ruled out, according to well-defined criteria'.	Practical and pragmatic (Most often used in practice.)	Ours

1.3.2 Disease

Similarly, even greater problems arise if the magnitude of health problems in the community is assessed by counting 'unhealthy' subjects. An unhealthy subject can carry a:

1. **Disease**. This may be anything abnormal or unusual in objective terms and in the eyes of a health professional. For example, a critical narrowing of coronary arteries revealed by a coronary angiogram clearly indicates that the patient suffers from coronary heart disease.
2. **Illness**. An unhealthy state perceived by patients themselves. For example, a patient may suffer from a case of recurrent anxiety that is invisible to professionals or laymen around him. (The patient 'feels ill'.)
3. **Sickness**. In this case, patients look unhealthy to their family, coworkers or friends who perceive them as unhealthy. For example, an unresponsive catatonic schizophrenic 'looks sick' to his family. If a resident asks an intern to '. . . look after patient X, he is sick . . .', he has in mind a potentially threatening state, requiring surveillance and resolute care, if needed.

Sometimes, all three concepts corroborate such as in massive myocardial infarction, stroke, or tetanus. Sometimes, they all differ. An intoxicated drug abuser does not feel ill, but may look sick. Clinically asymptomatic incipient malignant melanoma of the skin may be ignored by the patient and his entourage, but is alarming to his physician. (The patient does not feel ill, does not look sick to others, but has a potentially fatal disease.)

Obviously, our counts of cases and assessment of disease occurrence in the community depend on how we define the health problems of interest. The concepts of disease, illness and sickness apply to a great variety of health problems since they have been defined on different bases during the development of medicine. As an example, the perception of gout as a disease in antiquity depended on its signs or symptoms. Later, with the development of anatomy and histology, a morphological description of gout was established. With the development of our knowledge of biochemistry and metabolism since the nineteenth century, gout is now considered a purine and pyrimidine metabolism disorder.

Even today, the physicians' compendium of disease sometimes includes morphologic entries such as appendicitis, right bundle branch block or otitis media, or other entries which may be biochemical (porphyria, Wilson's disease), physiological (flutter), or microbiological (salmonellosis) based on signs (measles, varicella, scarlet fever, before the discovery of their causes), symptoms (anxiety states, depression), behavior (drug dependency), or risk of disease ('candidates for other diseases', such as obese subjects, aggressive and compulsive-obsessive personalities, etc.). Hence, contemporary medicine must deal with the effects of a historical and heterogeneous perception of disease.

If we broadly define *disease* as **any state that has a distinct pattern, cause, prognosis (outcome), and which requires intervention**, several phenomena belong in this category:

- Purely **homeostatic actions**, such as non-suppurative inflammation;
- **'Actions to avoid actions'**, such as fainting or heat stroke;
- **Faulty adjustment** due to endogenous causes, such as agammaglobulinemia;
- Totally **anarchic responses** such as cancer or thyrotoxicosis[16].

Let us take this last example, thyrotoxicosis. It is just one of several identifications of an abnormality of the thyroid gland that can be analyzed and understood in different studies based on various perceptions, denominations and definitions. We could be interested in eponymic identification (Graves' disease), functional identification (hyperthyroidism), metabolic impact (thyrotoxicosis), manifestational identification (exophthalmic goiter), anatomic identification (thyroid hyperplasia) anatomopathologic identification (diffuse hyperplastic goiter, solitary hyperplastic nodule) or pathophysiologic and anatomic identification (toxic multinodular goiter – partly according to King[17]).

When taking into account the heterogeneousness of our perception of morbid state and its practical implications, disease can be broadly seen as a **clinical** entity in the form of a distinct pattern of symptoms and signs on which enough information has been collected to define and explain (causes, mechanisms of development, etc.) such a pattern, its outcome (prognosis), and the need for intervention (prevention and treatment). Such an entity is delineated by precise and well-defined inclusion and exclusion criteria. For the purpose of further reading, we can also define disease as any morphological and/or functional state which:

- Is unusual either for a given subject ('illness'), for a health professional ('disease' in proper terms), or for a patient's entourage ('sickness'); and
- Alters a patient's future (prognosis); and
- Requires some intervention (drugs, surgery, psychotherapy, follow-up, social support, etc.); and
- Is evident when intervention, cure, or preventive measures are available.

NB The fourth criterion of disease is obviously conditional, but it is also the most pragmatic. For example, a definition of anemia or malnutrition in a developed country may differ from that in a developing one, where adequate food and drug supply is available only for extreme cases.

1.3.3 Syndrome

The term syndrome means the occurrence of an identifiable set of clinical and paraclinical (laboratory) manifestations, either signs or symptoms appearing more often than by chance. Such a set of manifestations seemingly disparate at the beginning is uniform either by association or pathogenesis[18,19]. Its causes are multiple or unknown. Syndromes may occur in different diseases, but they have a common anatomical, physiological and pathological basis. Horner's syndrome (enophthalmos, myosis, ptosis of the upper eyelid, mydriasis, anhidrosis), Guillain-Barré syndrome (absence of fever, myalgia, motor weakness, abolition of tendon reflexes, elevated CSF protein without corresponding increase in cells) or nephrotic syndrome (edema, hypoalbuminemia, albuminuria) are good examples. Syndromes themselves are either not curable (although the underlying disease (if

known) is) or the subject of treatment themselves. For all of the above-mentioned reasons, it is not surprising that the number of syndromes in medicine is quite impressive[20].

1.3.4 Impairment, disability, handicap

Very often, disease is only the beginning of a longer process, extending into various impairments, disabilities or handicaps. These phenomena, of equal interest to the disease, require a similarly rigorous approach in their definition, counting and classification[11,21].

1. An **impairment** is noted whenever some function like sensation, movement, walking, speech, etc. is altered (i.e. when damage, weakness, etc. is noted).
2. A **disability** ensues if an impairment leads to an incapacity to work or if the subject is deprived of the power of acting.
3. A subject may thereafter develop a **dependency**, which is a certain degree of subordination, or living at some cost (because of an individual disability).
4. A person becomes **handicapped** if he is at a disadvantage due to the loss or reduction of functional ability.

For example, if one wishes to evaluate handicaps, it is necessary to go beyond the general, and often vague meaning of the term. A handicap is not just any perturbation of a body system or function. Several levels of observation can be made (Table 1.2). Obviously, there are many impaired subjects in the community, some of whom become disabled, some of whom become dependent, and some of whom are really handicapped.

If we do not specify what we are talking about, we could falsely label a patient or an individual in a health survey. Thus, the health of a community could be under- or overestimated. As an example, an elderly computer specialist has difficulty walking. He is impaired, but not disabled in relation to his work. His earnings and coverage of daily needs are not affected. Therefore, he is not dependent. Because he is not at any disadvantage due to his problem (such as loss of salary, job, chance of promotion, or involvement in fundamental social activities), he is not handicapped. A clear operational and meaningful

Table 1.2 Disease and its consequences

	DISEASE or DISORDER (Intrinsic situation)	IMPAIRMENT (Exteriorized)	DISABILITY (Objectified)	HANDICAP (Socialized)
Definition	Any state of an individual, defined according to precise inclusion and exclusion criteria, which alter his habitual state and expected future (outcome, prognosis) and which requires intervention (prevention and/or treatment). NB May be acute or chronic.	In the context of health experience, an impairment is any loss or abnormality in a psychological, physiological, or anatomical structure or function. (Note: 'Impairment' is more inclusive than 'disorder' in that it covers losses – e.g. the loss of a leg is an impairment, but not a disorder.)	In the context of health experience, a disability is any restriction or lack of ability (resulting from an impairment) to perform an activity within the range considered normal for a human being.	In the context of health experience, a handicap is a disadvantage for a given individual, resulting from an impairment or disability that limits or prevents the fulfillment of a role that is normal (depending on age, sex, social and cultural factors) for that individual.
Characterisics	Acute means 'ending in a sharp point' and implies a finite duration, which classically culminates in a crisis. 'Chronic', however, which is derived from a word meaning 'time', means 'long-continued'. A host of interrelated properties are associated with these contrasts in time scale, and they render unnecessary any precise formulation of the temporal boundary between acute and chronic processes.	Impairment is characterized by losses or abnormalities that may be temporary or permanent, and that include the existence or occurrence of an anomaly, defect, or loss of a limb, organ, tissue, or other structure of the body, including systems of mental functioning. Impairment represents the exteriorization of a pathological state, and it reflects disturbances at the level of the organ.	Disability is characterized by excesses or deficiencies of customarily expected activity performance and behavior, which may be temporary or permanent, reversible or irreversible, progressive or regressive. Disabilities may arise as a direct consequence of impairment or as a response by the individual, particularly psychologically, to a physical, sensory, or other impairment. Disability represents the objectification of an impairment and as such, it reflects disturbances at the level of the person.	Handicap is concerned with the value attached to an individual's situation or experience when it departs from the norm. It is characterized by a discordance between the individual's performance or status and the expectations of the individual himself or of the particular group of which he is a member. Handicap thus represents the socialization of an impairment or disability and as such, it reflects the consequences for the individual – cultural, social, economic, and environmental – that stem from the presence of impairment and disability.
Examples	Pre-senile dementia.	Memory loss, disturbance of conceptualization and abstraction.	Improper location in time and space, uncertain personal safety.	Impediment to orientation leading to the loss of employment.
	Obliterant thrombangeitis.	Intermittent claudication. Loss of a leg.	Abnormal walking.	Unemployment resulting from the disability to use both legs (e.g. stunt person, mail carrier).

Source: Modified from Ref. 21. Reproduced with permission of the WHO

definition of health and wellbeing gives meaning to whatever is done on and for the subject at hand.

1.4 Conclusions. Understanding the remaining chapters of this book

Medicine works as a closely interwoven web of art and science. Such an overused statement is, however, undeniably important because it is very concrete. King[17] gives an excellent practical example by quoting a physician examining a group of children with abdominal cramps while investigating a food poisoning outbreak. The physician's conclusion is that they all have food poisoning manifestations, **but one subject among them** has appendicitis. This

particular child who is transferred to surgery is the epitome of the art of medicine! The physician in question goes beyond the science of pre-test, post-test or revised probabilities of diagnosis and is serendipitous enough, i.e. 'artful' in reasoning, to go beyond the prevalent evidence. This text focuses primarily on the scientific aspects of medicine. The art of medicine must be perfected through practice, since thought is not a quality acquired by reading and memorizing books. In research and practice, all the above-mentioned concepts should be used in an integrated and logical manner. As the next chapter reveals, several fields of science contributed to the way we reason in medicine today. This information will help further our understanding of the underlying logic in medicine outlined in Chapter 3.

REFERENCES

1. *Project Professionalism*. Philadelphia: American Board of Medicine, 1998
2. Sugar LM, Catton PA, Tallet SE, Rothman AI. Assessment of residents' professional attitudes and behaviours. *Annals RCPSC*, 2000;**33**:305–9
3. Jacobi J (ed.). *Paracelsus. Selected Writings*. Translated by N Guterman. Princeton: Princeton University Press, Bollingen Series XXVIII, 1979
4. Cruess SR, Cruess RL. Professionalism must be taught. *BMJ*, 1997;**315**:1674–7
5. *Mosby's Medical Dictionary*. Revised 2nd Edition. St. Louis: The C.V. Mosby Co., 1987
6. Art. *On-line Medical Dictionary, www.graylab.ac.uk*
7. Brown L (ed.). *The New Shorter Oxford English Dictionary on Historical Principles*. Volume 1, 4th Edition. Oxford: Clarendon Press, 1993
8. *The New Encyclopaedia Britannica*. Volume 1. Micropedia. Chicago: Encyclopaedia Britannica, 1992
9. *The American Heritage© Dictionary of English Language*. Fourth Edition, 2000. Electronic edition: www.bartleby.com
10. Entries 'Art' and 'Philosophy, Western'. *Microsoft® Encarta® Encyclopedia*. ©1993–1997 Microsoft Corporation, electronic edition. See also: www.encarta.msn.com
11. Abelin T, Brzezinski ZJ, Carstairs VDL (eds). *Measurement in Health Promotion and Protection*. WHO Regional Publications, European Series No 22. Copenhagen: WHO Regional Office for Europe, 1987
12. Last JM (ed.). *A Dictionary of Epidemiology*. 4th Edition. New York: Oxford University Press, 2001
13. *Basic Documents*. 35th Edition. Geneva: World Health Organization, 1985
14. Office of the Assistant Secretary for Health. *Healthy People: The Surgeon General's Report on Health promotion and Disease Prevention*. Washington DC: Govt Printing Office, July 1979 (Stock No 017-001-0416-2)
15. Epp J. Achieving Health for All: A Framework for Health Promotion. *Can J Public Health*, 1986;**77**: 393–407
16. Murphy EA. The Normal. *Am J Epidemiol*, 1973;**98**: 403–11
17. King LS. *Medical Thinking. A Historical Preface*. Princeton: Princeton University Press, 1982
18. Manuila A, Manuila L, Nicole M, Lambert H (eds). Syndrome. In: *Dictionnaire français de médecine et de biologie en quatre volumes.(A French Dictionary of Medicine and Biology in Four Volumes.)* (Tome III) Paris: Masson, 1972:793-4
19. Warkany J. Syndromes. *Amer J Dis Child*, 1971;**121**: 365–70
20. Magalini S, Magalini SC. *Dictionary of Medical Syndromes*. 4th Edition. Philadelphia and New York: Lippincott-Raven, 1997
21. *International Classification of Impairments, Disabilities, and Handicaps. A Manual of Classification relating to the Consequences of Disease*. Geneva: World Health Organization, 1980

The work of physicians with individuals and communities. Epidemiology and other partners in evidence-based medicine

*Think what is feasible
and you will be amazed
what is probable.*
From the TV show 'Doc'

- *If it's green or wiggles, it's biology*
- *If it stinks, it's chemistry*
- *If it does not work, it's physics*
- *If it's people-gazing, it's epidemiology*
- *If it has nothing to do with those
nasty and pesky numbers, it's
qualitative research*
- *If it's all business, it's health economics*
- *If it justifies perpetuating other people's mistakes,
it's evidence-based medicine*
(Partly from a variety of sources)

In this chapter, we discuss the evolution of ideas underlying research and practice in medicine. To promote a better understanding of the subject, we also include definitions that go beyond the intuitive meaning[1,2] of the basic terms used in this chapter and in those that follow:

- **Models** are frameworks that establish how we look at particular subjects.
- **Concepts** are well-defined ideas drawn from a model.
- **Theories** are sets of concepts with an objective definition and explanation of a phenomenon of interest. A theory is a set of interrelated constructs (variables), definitions, and propositions that presents a systematic view of phenomena by specifying relations among variables, with the purpose of explaining natural phenomena[2].
- **Hypotheses** are propositions to be tested, accepted or rejected depending on the test result.
- **Methodologies** are ways of studying phenomena or topics that interest us.
- **Methods** or **techniques** are specific procedures used to improve and complete our understanding.

2.1 Common logic in dealing with individual patients and communities

A common intellectual path links the treatment of health problems in an individual or in groups of individuals. Let us take the example illustrated in Table 2.1. A general practitioner sees an overweight, middle-aged female patient in his office. She smells of alcohol, has yellow tobacco stained fingers, looks disheveled and has recently lost her job. He wants to know what possible health risks might affect such a patient (i.e. what diseases this patient may develop in the future). To this end, he will examine her to see what health problems she already has (i.e. making the diagnosis) and will verify which known causal factors she was exposed to in relation to her health problems (how much does she smoke, how much does she drink, what are her eating habits, her physical activity, etc.). In other words, he searches for causes. He will then choose an appropriate treatment (i.e. for respiratory and liver problems) and will check to see if such a treatment works (effectiveness of a clinical intervention). He must also foresee the outcome of problems in his patient (i.e. making a prognosis) and if he is a thorough practitioner, he will follow her over time to see if her condition improves or deteriorates and whether further intervention is necessary (follow-up or clinical surveillance of an individual).

At the same time, a physician involved in community medicine and public health notices a high occurrence of smoking, alcohol abuse and obesity in his community. He evaluates the risks of a future high occurrence of coronary disease, chronic obstructive lung disease, liver cirrhosis and other related problems in a community with a given lifestyle (i.e. he also

Table 2.1 Epidemiological components of clinical information given to patients

What physicians say to their patients	Clinical epidemiology components (what is needed)
'. . . you are at risk of developing coronary disease . . .'	Descriptive epidemiology, data on coronary disease incidence, risk evaluation.
'. . . eating animal fat means a heart attack . . .'	Etiological research.
'. . . in reality, you are not an easy case to deal with. You eat too much, you smoke too much, you don't exercise at all . . .'	Assessment and knowledge of risk factors (etiology).
'. . . you are obese, you have angina, diabetes and obliterated leg vessels (Buerger's disease) . . .'	Diagnosis.
'. . . do not eat too much fat, exercise more, stop smoking and drinking. This will make you healthier . . .'	Clinical trial.
'. . . you will live longer . . .'	Prognosis.
'. . . in fact, as you see, we must do several things . . .'	Clinical decision analysis.

assesses risks in the community). He then accounts for cases and states if disease occurrence has reached abnormal levels (i.e. an epidemiological diagnosis of an epidemic or endemic situation is made). Next, he will search for causes of such a high occurrence (determining causes of a high incidence of diseases of interest). After that, he will implement community health programs to control the occurrence of cases, and their outcome. A health education program of this type will aim to change lifestyles or screen for disease. He will then evaluate if such programs work. (Do they really change disease occurrence and the outcome of cases?) Finally, he will implement an epidemiological surveillance program to see if a better situation results or if there is further important exposure to risk factors which might lead to another high occurrence of disease in the future.

Table 2.2 shows that similar logical steps are needed for both clinical and community medicine. To understand disease as a community problem, individual cases must be uncovered, examined, treated and followed. A synthesis of individual cases is made to understand the same disease as a mass phenomenon (or a group problem). This is the basis of work in

Table 2.2 Epidemiology, clinical practice, and community health programs

Community		Individual	
Epidemiological methods and information needed	*Phases of a health program*	*Phases of clinical care*	*Epidemiological and other methods and facts needed*
Diagnosis and case identification	Identification of health problems and needs	Trigger of care (complaints etc.), history, review of systems, examination, diagnosis ('situation'– subjective and objective)	Medical care organization Clinimetrics Epidemiological data from the community (Bayes)
Health indicators and indexes Descriptive data	Establishing priorities for intervention (or study)	Creating a problem oriented medical record ('assessment')	Risk information Prognosis information Clinimetrics
Risk quantification	Statement of program objectives	Further exploration and treatment orders ('plan' what can be done to improve risk and prognosis)	Clinical decision analysis ('before') Clinical pharmacology Evaluation of chances of efficacy Effectiveness and efficiency Health economics Health ethics
Potential for control by implementing a selected intervention	Selection of activities to reach program objectives Putting human and material resources to work (program implementation)	Carrying out orders (putting therapeutic plans to work)	Health ethics Health care organization Process assessment
Assessment of intervention efficacy Control of random and systematic error (bias)	Evaluation Epidemiological surveillance and forecasting	Final assessment and follow-up	Impact evaluation (clinimetrics again) Clinical decision evaluation ('after') Prognosis Planning for the future

classical epidemiology as defined and explained below. The architecture of community health programs follows that of clinical medicine. Steps of health programs preparation, implementation and evaluation are similar in logic to those used in the handling individual patients. In the same way, each part of a health program work up requires both epidemiological information and methodology. Whether a physician works with individual patients or cares for the health of a community, he must fulfill several obligations in this order:

- Recognize any threats (risks),
- Identify health problem(s),
- React to them (prevention, treatment, etc.),
- Anticipate further developments of health problems under consideration (prognosis),
- Evaluate the outcome of his actions, and
- Follow up with patient(s) and/or the community.

To do this, several epidemiological methods, information, and techniques from other 'non-clinical' fields are needed. Patient charts and health programs in the community have a lot in common. Only their methods and information vary.

2.2 Patterns of reasoning in practice and research and key ways to decisions

There is more than one way to listen, examine and treat patients. Physicians can, in fact, choose several paths when reasoning and making decisions. For the purpose of the following comments, let us make a distinction between 'clinical reasoning' and 'clinical judgment'. **Clinical judgment** means the assigning of some value to something. **Clinical reasoning** refers to ways by which to arrive at judgments and any ensuing decisions and actions.

2.2.1 Key ways to make decisions

The work physicians perform is a mixed bag of reflex actions, blind actions, more refined thinking, and a structured approach to understanding and curing diseases. However, an emergency medicine specialist does not always have the luxury of taking time out to reflect, as do internists or psychiatrists. Some decision-making strategies[3], often labeled more or less

accurately as 'clinical reasoning'[4], and others are worthy of mention:

(a) **Pattern recognition** is a quick recollection of striking disease signs and symptoms that can be fitted into some learned or experienced sets of information representing diseases and syndromes. Such an arrangement of separate elements of observation and experience into a form, pattern or configuration representing a new unit of understanding beyond a simple summation of its components is termed *Gestalt* by psychiatrists and psychologists. Daily clinical practice, emergency medicine or simple observation of people in daily life is very often based on pattern recognition. Components of recollected patterns may be drawn either from direct observation of patients, medical literature, memory or shared ideas.

(b) At other times, in the sequenced reasoning used to make diagnosis or treatment decisions, **clues**[3] can give clinical thinking some direction. A **key clue** at the beginning of a clinical assessment or clues that appear during the 'work-up' of a case (**pivotal clues**) are used as a triggering element in branching and fitting into various disease pictures.

The use of clues is closely associated with the **suppression of information** in situations where a flood of data mask the essential. Some diseases, such as essential hypertension may be clinically mute in a patient consulting for some other manifest problem. Many abnormal paraclinical 'opportunistic' findings can lead to a clinical work-up of asymptomatic, and initially unsearched for manifestations. Further work relies on an **active search for lanthanic findings and situations,** as they are called[5].

(c) Clinical and paraclinical (laboratory) observations are used in **mathematical operations** such as the assessment of risks in the patient, the predictive value of a diagnostic test, the effectiveness of treatment or the making of a prognosis.

(d) A clinician may also proceed by **temporal–spatial organization** of findings and decisions to ensure a continuity of actions that are the most beneficial for the patient. Various flow charts like decision trees, clinical algorithms or other various dendrograms (branching of events and information from some triggering point like diagnostic hypothesis into an increasing web of elements under consideration) can serve as examples.

(e) A '**hunch**', '**hint**' or '**allusion**', i.e. indirect suggestion, premonition, suspicion or feeling is an 'educated guess' that is made almost subconsciously and falls somewhere between a simple guess and intuition in degree of certainty. A vague association can be made between clinical observation and some poorly recollected and learned, read or lived experience. It is used as a less scientific, but potentially valuable start to a more structured method of treating the patient.

(f) A **pragmatic, evidence-based approach** based on a better-defined use of the most important information in clinical decision-making is another advancement in the area of clinical work (*vide infra*). This is the focus of the present book.

These ways of reasoning and practice will always be part of medicine to various degrees although rationalism, pragmatism and logic will make up an increasing large segment of our thoughts and decisions.

(g) **Iterative problem solving, circles and loops** are, in some way, a translation of the scientific method into practice.

Let us remember that the **scientific method, in general,** refers to the gathering of information by careful observation, preliminary generalization or hypothesis formulation, '. . . *usually by inductive reasoning. This in turn leads by deductive logic to implications, which may be tested by further observations and experiments. If the conclusions drawn from the original hypothesis successfully meets these tests, the hypothesis becomes accepted as a scientific theory or law; if additional facts are in disagreement with the hypothesis, it may be discarded in favor of a new hypothesis, which is then subjected to further tests. Even an accepted theory may be overthrown if enough contradictory evidence is found . . .*[6]. There is no discovery of disease cause(s) or finding of new drugs or better surgery without an application and practice of the scientific method as defined above.

When dealing with disease in humans or in a group of humans, all aforementioned considerations must be put into a proper framework of thinking.

Johns[7], for example, considers diagnostic reasoning as a practical translation of the scientific method. However, it should be noted that this view applies not only to diagnosis, but also to any phase of clinical work. Figure 2.1 illustrates this paradigm.

The acquisition of clinical experience was summarized by Hamm[8] in various modes of inquiry, going from: Intuitive judgment, to peer aided judgment, system aided judgment, quasi-experiment, controlled trial, and finally to scientific experiment. In this progressive chain of experience, intuition decreases, analysis increases, the task becomes more structured and the mode of inquiry becomes more and more controlled. For Elstein and Bordage, clinical reasoning is a particular form of reasoning that is centered on a specific set of problems and governed by some principles common to all thinking[9]. According to Dreyfus and Dreyfus' theory, as quoted by Hamm[8], a novice proceeds from an analytical approach and reliance on others when dealing with clinical problems, perceptions, actions, orientation and decisions that are progressively more intuitive. During this process, he acquires competency, proficiency and himself becomes an expert. However, this point remains debatable, especially in light of decision analysis (see below).

(h) Our reasoning may go in one of two possible directions: **induction or deduction.**

The iterative process of scientific thinking involves three distinct phases: experimental (obtaining data), data analysis, and hypothesis formulation. This process can take place inductively or deductively. When data are initially collected and analyzed and a hypothesis is finally made (explanation is given), the sequence is called an **inductive method.** For example, an inexperienced clinical clerk examines a patient. He does not know what his patient's problem might be. He gathers as much information as possible from the patient's medical history, performs a detailed and complete physical examination and orders as many paraclinical tests as possible, including the most expensive ones. Once he has obtained all the results, he tries to figure out into which pattern these results might fit. He then proposes his diagnosis. In another example, general information is gathered in a national cancer or malformations registry. A

Iterative process of research

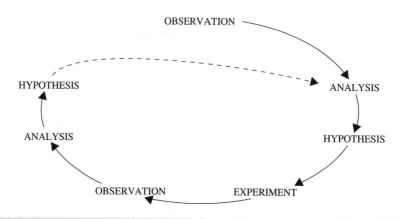

Iterative nature of clinical research

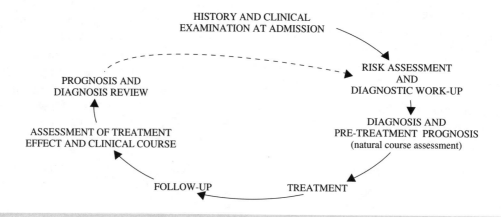

Iterative nature of medical practice

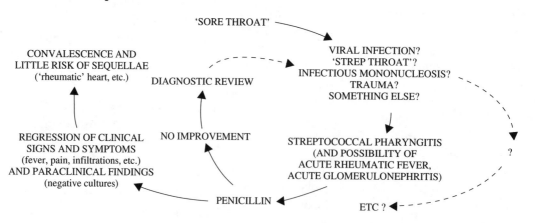

Figure 2.1 The scientific method and its translation into clinical practice and research. Source: Adapted from Ref. 7, expanded and modified

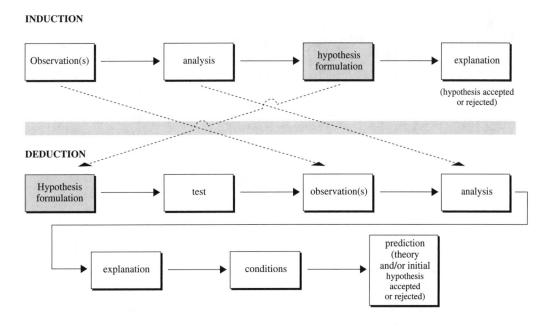

INDUCTION

N.B. Dotted lines indicate different positions of hypothesis in inductive and deductive research pathways.

Figure 2.2   Induction and deduction in medical practice and research

researcher compares disease occurrence according to the routinely noted marital status of subjects, and draws the conclusions that a particular cancer is related to being single. In both cases, data have been gathered first, without any previous hypothesis in mind, and subsequently analyzed to produce a final hypothesis (interpretation of data).

As a second alternative, another sequence may be chosen: A hypothesis is first formulated, then data collected (experiment) and organized in the best way to refute or accept the hypothesis in mind. Finally, an experiment is performed, and interpreted. This is a **deductive method.** Here is an example: An experienced clinician suspects lung cancer in an elderly man who smokes and complains of persistent cough and blood in his sputum. All examinations made and tests ordered are selected as to confirm the suspected problem or to identify other possible diseases (tuberculosis, etc.). In another example, a researcher questions whether congenital malformations are related to ionizing radiation to which individuals are exposed. To study this, he chooses a group of affected individuals and a control group of healthy subjects. He interviews parents of all the selected individuals to see whether or not they were exposed.

Having observed different rates of exposure in the groups under study, he raises the question as to whether these data confirm his hypothesis. (NB He could also study this by comparing the occurrence of a health problem in the exposed and unexposed groups; see Chapter 8.) Figure 2.2 compares these two basic approaches: induction and deduction.

Obviously, the use of a deductive method in research and clinical practice is intellectually much more powerful and satisfying since it brings more definitive results than an inductive approach, often unjustly termed 'milking' or 'dredging' of data. Both methods, however, are iterative and this is how wisdom is progressively built-up. If an inductive method were never used, most of the valuable information in routine data banks (e.g. demographic data, general surveys, etc.) and in research in general would be lost.

(i) Our reasoning is not often unidirectional, but it may be expanded by **arborization and ramification.**

Wherever good medicine is practiced, physicians go beyond the observation and analysis of a single case or event. This happens in clinical medicine and in

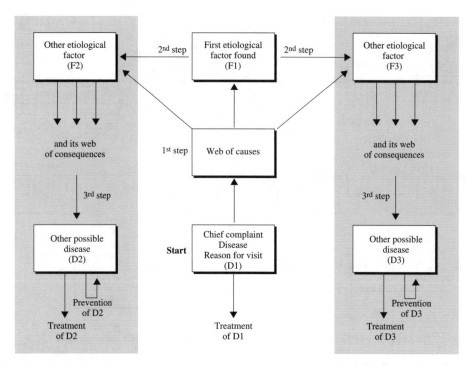

Figure 2.3 Exploration of causes and consequences in patients

public health as well. Let us examine Figure 2.3. In clinical practice, a family physician may notice depression in a patient (D1). The patient mentions that the problem occurred following a recent job loss. Further investigation uncovers heavy drinking (F2) and marital disruption (F3) in the patient's history. All three factors may be related to the patient's present problem (D1) in terms of a web of causes. Heavy drinking and marital disruption can, however, each have their own webs of consequences. When the physician properly assesses these factors, he may discover liver cirrhosis (D2) as an additional consequence of heavy drinking, and spousal abuse (D3) as a consequence of marital disruption (also due to F2 and other factors).

In public health, a similar approach is very useful. For example in Figure 2.4, the first case of a child suffering from whooping cough (index case) is found in the community (D1). The young patient is in his third week of disease. By including the incubation period, the field epidemiologist can go back six weeks to try to find the source (S) of the infection. (NB Other sources may be considered too.) From this source, other cases (D1, D2) may be detected. During approximately the same period as the index case

(D1), these other cases may have produced several additional contacts (Cs). If these contacts are detected as early as possible, earlier diagnosis and treatment (and prevention of additional contacts and cases as well) can take place.

2.3 Related fields in research and practice

To practice good medicine, generations of physicians have learned thousands of facts from books, lectures, and from personal communications with more experienced colleagues. They have also learned from personal experience, imitating others to develop clinical skills and reproducing the decisions and actions that have been successful in the past. However, the learning of facts and the acquisition of clinical skills are not sufficient for the practice of good medicine. A third component must be the mastery of objective reasoning and decision-making in medicine. In other words, our knowledge of what to do must be structured and organized based on facts we know (or ignore) and skills we can use so that an integration can take place allowing us to perform a particular action and evaluate its impact. Medicine has undergone several major stages of development:

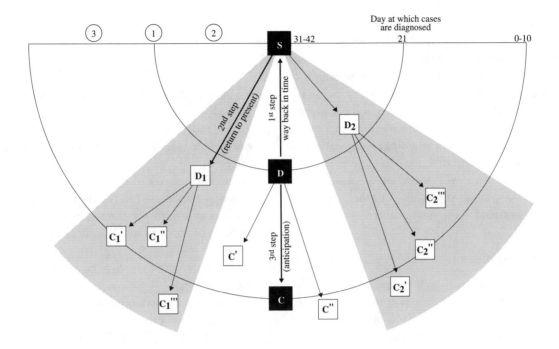

Figure 2.4 Going beyond an index case in field epidemiology and public health. Adapted and redrawn from Ref. 10

- Stage of **prevailing belief** in antiquity: religion, belief, superstition, conviction and experience guided ancient physicians in their practice.
- Stage of **sharing increasing experience** throughout the Middle Ages: travels, printed books, intercultural exchanges (however limited) became ways to share experience. Unsubstantiated convictions of effectiveness remained in practice, like bloodletting, scalding or purgatory.
- Stage of **understanding** until the twentieth century. There was nothing much to do besides an increasingly better diagnosis and discovery of infectious and non-infectious nature of disease. Anatomy, physiology and pathology established our understanding of cells, tissues, bodily fluids, organs, systems, their functioning and interacting.
- Stage of **organized reasoning, evaluation and decision-making** whose increasing importance characterizes the scientific component of medicine. Industrial revolution and advances in basic and applied sciences of physics, chemistry or bacterio-

logy. Advances in statistics and biostatistics enabled us to separate reality from randomness and fiction. Advances in informatics made possible handling large bodies of data by advanced and increasingly complex analytical methods, sophisticated samplings, or advanced medical data linkage.

Then, physician expectations were raised. Even about three generations ago, it was enough for a physician to improve himself as a diagnostician, an understanding interpreter of situation, and a skilful performer of clinical maneuvers. With increasingly effective surgical, antibacterial and other conservative treatments as well as with the refinement of diagnostic methods, an overload of rationalization and cost-effectiveness was created. Medicine now attempts to do more and better in an increasingly shorter period of time, often at the expense of the practice of 'human' medicine. Impressed by new technologies, some may underestimate the importance of physical examination or communication with the patient.

Our present patterns of reasoning are supported by various fields of experience, each contributing in its own way to obtaining evidence and incorporating it into contemporary medical reasoning. Principles, methods and techniques from these many fields of human experience are necessary for good medicine. Let us now define at least some of them including epidemiology, clinical epidemiology, biostatistics, health economics, qualitative research and evidence-based medicine. This will allow us to understand principles, uses, and relevance of the logic in medicine as outlined in the next chapter.

2.3.1 Epidemiology

Since antiquity, humans have been periodically plagued by deadly diseases which appeared either in unusual numbers at a given place and in a given period (epidemics), everywhere in great numbers (pandemics) or persisted in defined communities in high numbers for generations (endemics). These health problems (plague, cholera, parasitic diseases, small pox, child infections, etc.) needed to be properly counted, their causes identified and proper collective measures implemented. Besides quantitative methods, it was necessary to develop a philosophical, logical and epistemological framework for dealing with diseases, their occurrence, causes and interventions to control them. Such endeavors reflected a desire to build a structured thinking framework in disease understanding and control[11-14].

The term epidemiology comes etymologically from the Greek: 'epi' (upon), 'demos' (people) and 'logos' (study). Originally applied to the field of infectious diseases (study of epidemics), today it encompasses all health phenomena appearing as mass phenomena. **Epidemiology is defined** in the current edition of the Dictionary of Epidemiology[15] as '... *the study of the distribution and determinants of health-related states or events in specified populations, and the application of this study to the control of health problems*'. In operational terms, classical epidemiology may also be defined as *a way to study determinants of decisions in public health and community medicine and determinants of the impact of such decisions on individuals, groups of individuals,* *communities, diseases of interest, their treatment, and the health of those under scrutiny*[14,15 modified].

Classical epidemiology's **objectives** are:

1. To contribute to the best possible **identification of cases.**
2. To identify the importance of the **disease occurrence.** (Is it a priority in terms of health intervention?)
3. To identify **causes of disease(s)** – why they occur and why they persist in the community.
4. To **choose health programs** (which have the best chance of controlling the health problems of interest).
5. To evaluate how these programs work (**impact of interventions**).
6. To maintain **epidemiological surveillance** in terms of a dynamic evaluation of normalcy. In this way, **epidemiological forecasting** is possible and outbreaks and epidemics can be anticipated or prevented.

Based on the historical and contemporary contributions of epidemiology (such as an understanding of the natural history and the nidation of anthropozoonoses, the etiology of toxic shock syndrome or legionellosis, the discovery of slow infections, an explanation of the etiology of pellagra, etc.), its logic and methodology are now applied in fields of medicine and public health. Epidemiology can be applied to almost all mass phenomena, infectious or not, in health sciences and it has become a logical framework for objective reasoning in the health sciences with four distinct applications: classical (field) epidemiology, epidemiology as a research method, clinical epidemiology, and epidemiology in health planning and evaluation. In relation to epidemiology, medical research today is made up of four complementary categories:

1. Basic research, where 'parts' of patients are studied and where various methods and techniques of exploration are developed.
2. Research in classical or field epidemiology, where the magnitude of disease occurrence is explored, its causes identified, and interventions studied.
3. Research in clinical epidemiology, where the patient is studied as an entity (a sort of 'holistic

clinical research'), medical decisions are evaluated and their results, consequences and issues are clarified.

4. Health care and medical care organization research, where the **process** (besides of the impact) is studied. The focus most often is on non-medical factors such as health care organization, administration, fees and financial retributions.

The social, community and political roles of epidemiology are widening. For example, epidemiological evidence is increasingly considered (aside from its presumptive character) as one of the advanced stages (in addition to experimental research) in proofs of cause–effect relationships. Toxic tort litigation may serve as an example of a situation where epidemiology is used jointly by health professionals and by civil and criminal law professionals in judgments on the etiology of cases[16]. Toxicology, clinical opinion and micro-environmental studies are no longer sufficient fields of expertise in judicial cases where the health of individuals and communities is involved. This new civic and social dimension in epidemiology will undoubtedly continue.

2.3.2 *Clinical epidemiology*

Given the many focuses of epidemiology today, there are too many 'epidemiologies'. We apply this term to various independent variables (causes) under study such as occupational, social, genetic, or nutritional epidemiology as well as to different dependent variables (disease, consequence) when dealing with cancer, cardiovascular, injury or psychiatric epidemiologies. We relate it to place (field or 'shoe-leather' epidemiology, nosocomial or hospital epidemiology), to intrinsic characteristics of agents, to intra-individual spread (sero-epidemiology, molecular epidemiology[17], sub-clinical epidemiology[18]) and to particular phases of the natural or clinical course of disease (study of biological markers in addition to the latter). When we speak of epidemiology in the context of health science, we could mean veterinary epidemiology[19,20], dental epidemiology[21], etc.

There should be, in fact, only two epidemiologies today: good epidemiology and bad epidemiology. Good epidemiology is comprised of two distinct intellectual processes: classical and clinical epidemiology. In **classical epidemiology**, observations in

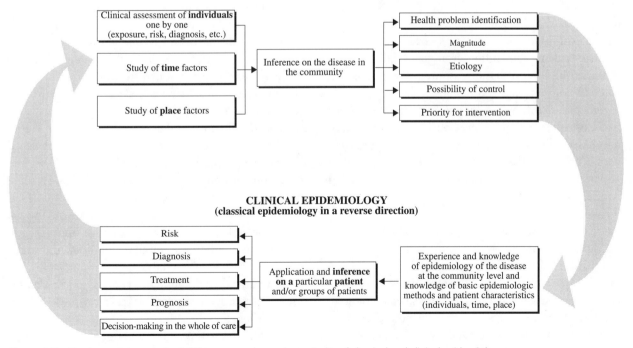

Figure 2.5 Fundamental conceptual differences and complementarity of classical and clinical epidemiology

individuals serve to make inferences on disease at the population level. However, in **clinical epidemiology**, we reverse the direction of medical reasoning when we use information acquired in groups of subjects to improve our decisions concerning individual patients and groups of patients. Figure 2.5 illustrates both directions of reasoning in epidemiology.

Clinical epidemiology is *the science and method of studying optimal decisions in clinical medicine, while taking into account the epidemiological characteristics of the patient and his outer clinical environment, the pathology concerned and the factors and maneuvers to which the patient is exposed in his clinical environment, especially medical actions.* Clinical epidemiology has three **practical objectives:**

1. To optimize daily clinical practice and its inherent decisions.
2. To organize, structure and rationalize better clinical research in its orientation towards clinical decision-making.
3. To better understand the quality, validity and relevance of medical experience as presented in medical papers, articles, rounds and other media.

The basic purpose of clinical epidemiology does not reside in the fact that denominators are often in the hospital or that clinical factors are the independent variables most often studied. As already mentioned, clinical epidemiology differs from 'classical' epidemiology at the level of basic reasoning. While classical epidemiology studies individuals, puts information together and infers for groups and disease on the basis of what was seen previously in cases and/or non-cases, clinical epidemiology works the opposite way. Clinical decisions about a patient or a group of patients are made by taking into consideration what is already known about the disease and population (groups). Such a procedure is applied to risk assessment, diagnosis, treatment, prognosis and medical decision analysis.

By studying clinical factors (such as medical decisions) rather than classical environmental factors (such as air or water pollution), clinical epidemiology reaches an important magnitude of new exposures and their consequences, and this for a reason: Many individuals undergo more blood tests, X-ray examinations and urine analyses than they have sexual partners or exposures to non-medical toxic agents during their lifetime! Obviously, there is an inherent interface between the classical and clinical epidemiological approaches. Both are necessary and both are complementary. They cannot exist without one another.

Traditionally, the logic of decisions in public health, health protection and preventive medicine has been more entrenched than in clinical settings where, incidentally, most of the gross national product allocated to health is placed. Clinical practice benefits from quantitative methodology and from the experience of fundamental epidemiology, while classical epidemiology improves considerably as a result of refining designs, analyses and interpretations of studies through clinical experience. In reality, it would be most regrettable to view classical epidemiology solely as an application of sophisticated quantitative methods. Several excellent monographs[22–25] offer more details about this important methodology for obtaining evidence in medicine.

2.3.3 Biostatistics

Students often ask if biostatistics and epidemiology are synonymous. They are not. **Statistics** is the science and art of collecting, summarizing, and analyzing data that are subject to random variation, whatever their field of application and subject might be. The term is also often applied to data themselves[15]. **Biostatistics** is currently defined as the application of statistics to biological problems which goes well beyond the field of medicine itself[15]. **Medical statistics** can therefore be considered a specific part of biostatistics. In fact, biostatistics focuses on the development and use of statistical methods to solve problems and to answer questions that arise in human biology and medicine[26]. Vital statistics, population growth studies and forecasting, multivariate analysis and other quantitative methods in causal research, design and analysis of randomized controlled clinical trials, human genetics and epidemiology or record linkage rely largely on biostatistical methodology.

Biostatistics is the vital backbone not only of epidemiology, but also of many other types of research in medicine. As for epidemiology, its ideas and ways of thinking are applied through and parallel to biostatistics. This explains why several basic concepts from the field of biostatistics are included in this reading. In research and practice, epidemiology and biostatistics are often so intertwined that their demarcation is a challenge in itself.

Many excellent books on biostatistics, complementary reading for this text, are currently available. Their sheer number alone excludes them from being quoted. Several leading medical journals have also or are publishing series of papers to keep health professionals updated and to help them understand this field. They include: *Mayo Clinic Proceedings* (1982), *Physiotherapy Canada* (1980–1981), *American Journal of Hospital Pharmacy* (1980–1981), *The Canadian Medical Association Journal* or *The Canadian Journal of Psychiatry,* to name just a few. In a remarkably skilful effort, these series help practicing clinicians and research novices move beyond their current scope of activities.

The role of biostatistics was and remains vital in many crucial fields of medicine: development and validation of diagnostic methods, search for causes of disease, evaluating effectiveness of treatment, making prognosis, obtaining an accurate picture of disease and other health phenomena occurring in the community, or in health services evaluation. From its mainly **descriptive role** in the nineteenth century, biostatistics expanded into the field of **inference**, i.e. the process of generalizing sample observations and drawing additional information from various sample comparisons (testing hypothesis). Hence, **descriptive statistics** and **inferential statistics** are currently used.

2.3.3.1 *Values beyond healing and cure. Health economics*

Health services are both similar and distinct from other economic goods and services, as first outlined in the nineteen sixties[27]. However, health economics today requires more than dealing with a demand for and supply of health care services. Economic evaluation focuses on the efficient use of scarce resources in monetary or human terms and the environment (the processes and interventions that guarantee the allocation of these scarce social and health resources). Medical decision-making requires not only a good knowledge of patients, but also of disease itself and its control. Such knowledge and its practice evolve in a functioning social environment that must be fully understood. Questions that interest health economists[28] reflect this reality:

- What factors other than health care influence health?
- What is the value of health?
- What are the demands for care?
- What is the supply of health care?
- How cost-effective and cost-beneficial is health care (microeconomics)?
- What is the equilibrium of the health market?
- How can all of the above be evaluated?
- How can a health system be planned, budgeted for and monitored?
- How do all the above-mentioned elements interact?

For Vale et al[29], economic evaluation is the comparative analysis of alternative courses of action in terms of both their costs (resource use) and effectiveness. Costs (money invested, human resources employed, clinical and paraclinical procedures), patient values and preferences, and effects (monetary gains or losses, health effects, patient perceptions, or quality of life) blur the limits between the health sciences and economics and neither can be ignored. Several types of evaluations characterize health economics[30,31, G. Mulvale, pers comm] :

- The identification of various types of costs and their measurement in monetary terms is similar across most economic evaluations.
- **Cost-identification or cost-minimization analysis**[32] simply compares costs of alternative ways to provide care, which results in the same type and volume of outcome of interest.
- **Cost-effectiveness analysis** (CEA) is used when the health effects (outcomes) differ between alternatives (not in type, but in the volume[31]) that are measured in the same units, such as life-years gained and others. It provides some form of ratio between costs and units of effect like year of life, etc. Net costs of providing services and specified health effects (outcomes) are determined and

cost-effectiveness ratios from competing interventions are compared. The lower the ratio, the more cost-effective the intervention[33].

- **Cost–benefit analysis** (CBA) or **cost–efficiency analysis** is used when there may be single or multiple outcomes, which are not common to the alternatives to choose from. The various outcomes are translated in monetary and other units to provide a common unit of measure. It examines whether a given health activity is worth paying for if those benefiting from it consider it worthwhile, even if they have to bear the full cost themselves[34]. The cost of the health program is subtracted from the benefit of the program, yielding a net benefit. If two or more mutually exclusive programs have positive net benefits, the one with the greatest net benefit is the intervention of choice[35].
- **Cost–utility analysis** (CUA) is used when the types of outcomes from alternative programs are not the same[31]. CUA takes into consideration the preferences individuals or society may have for a set of health outcomes. It allows for quality of life adjustments to a given set of treatment and outcomes. It also studies whether the quality of life reflects an outcome of interest and the cost of various outcomes are compared as well. The cost–utility ratio combines the quality and quantity of outcomes. Health care interventions with different effects can be compared using this method.
- **Incremental analysis** (IA) calculates additional costs in relation to the additional benefits of the competing strategies (programs).[34]
- **Sensitivity analysis** (SA) studies how the choice of preferred strategies changes if both costs and health outcomes are modified.

Excellent methodological guides on how to perform and understand studies in health economics have been published in the form of monographs[36], review articles[33–35,37–42] and guidelines[43–54]. Guides on how to evaluate such studies once they are published[32,39–41] have also been produced. The reader should search for additional information about this topic in the above-mentioned references since their scope extends well beyond that of this text. The health economics component is also progressively being introduced as a desirable part of decision-making in evidence-based medicine, particularly in clinical trials assessments[29,42].

2.3.4 *Qualitative research*

Contributors to probability-based quantitative research have been so successful that their achievements have overshadowed for some time the relevance of a deep understanding of patients facing disease and health care. Needless to say, this high 'quality' information fuels the gathering of multiple observations and of their quantitative analysis. How do patients perceive their disease? How do they value the diagnostic and therapeutic options that are offered to them? What happens exactly when a new health system reform is implemented? What is the clinical course with all its ramifications and consequences in a particular patient? Such opportunities for qualitative research abound.

Researchers in the qualitative area are interested in findings other than the precise quantitative results of laboratory tests or measurable findings obtained at the bedside or through surgery. These may be the patient's human and social experience, communication, thoughts, expectations, meaning, attitudes and processes related to interaction, relations, interpretation, activity, and other clinically important information[55]. All this information is most often much more difficult to define, obtain, and interpret than blood sugar or body weight. This is a challenge in the field of clinimetrics as outlined in Chapter 6 of this reading.

The quest for medical certainty through quantification began with Pierre Charles Alexandre Louis (1787–1872)[56,57,47]. At first, epidemiologists disregarded qualitative approaches to health problems because the objectives and methodology of this 'other research' were poorly developed, structured and defined. This is no longer the case. Moreover, the future of our understanding of health and disease relies on a proper and balanced marriage of qualitative and quantitative methods[48,49]. Contemporary medical research relies heavily on epidemiology and biostatistics. Observations are recorded, summarized, analyzed and interpreted with care to avoid bias, random error, or misrepresentation of events or target groups under study.

An impressive volume of concepts, methods, and thinking and their vocabulary[50] have been treated in *ad hoc* literature and reviewed elsewhere[51–54]. Many players in this original sector of the social sciences stress the equilibrium between what is found in *qualitative research,* i.e. an in-depth study of an individual or situation and in *quantitative research* i.e. a summary of sets of individual experiences. Qualitative research was simply, and perhaps best defined, by Strauss and Corbin[52] as '*any kind of research that produces findings not arrived at by means of statistical procedures or other means of quantification. . . . It can refer to research about person's lives, stories, behavior, but also about organizational, functional, social movements, or interactional relationships. . . . Some data may be quantified as with census data but the analysis itself is a qualitative one.*'

In **quantitative research**, series of observations are made and phenomena are quantified, counted, measured, described, displayed, and analyzed using statistical methods. We then infer on a problem as a whole, we see it through an overall experience. Biostatistics and epidemiology have been (and remain) pivotal in decision oriented medical research. Analyzing disease outbreaks, clinical trials, or systematic reviews (meta-analyses) of disease causes or of treatment effectiveness are examples of quantitative research. The primary objective of quantitative research is *to provide answers to questions that extend beyond a single observation.* In **qualitative research**, unique observations are the focus of interest. They are described, studied, and analyzed in depth. They are not considered a part of a given universe before being linked to other observations. The objective of this kind of research is primarily *to understand a case, a single observation itself.*

Research questions can be approached by induction or by deduction. **Inductive research** is centered on observations that serve as a basis for hypotheses and answers. **Deductive research** raises questions, gathers observations for the problem, and confirms or rejects hypotheses 'free from or independent of the subject under study'. Quantitative research is both inductive and deductive. Epidemiologists, for obvious reasons, prefer deductions. By definition, though, qualitative research is mostly inductive. In fact, qualitative research is driven not by hypotheses, but by questions, issues, and a search for patterns[47,54]. We agree with Pope and Mays[54] that '*a given observation (X, case)* 'is the focus of qualitative research with classification as its purpose'. By contrast, quantitative research enumerates *how many Xs.*

Let us remember that qualitative research principles are not unknown to medicine. Medical history, psychiatric interviews, or the study of index cases (i.e. those that lead to quantitative search) of disease outbreaks or of new phenomena (poisoning, infection, etc.) bear the characteristics of qualitative research. Obviously, an equilibrium between quantitative and qualitative research is both necessary and beneficial not only in social sciences, but in health sciences as well.

2.3.4.1 Qualitative research in general

The methodology of qualitative research as we know it today was developed beyond the health sciences by sociologists, anthropologists, psychologists and political scientists. It even quickly made its way into management[58], education[59,] evaluation[53] and evidence-based medicine[60,61]. The basic methodology was defined and practical experience was gathered and documented from many areas, as recounted in an ever-increasing number of *ad hoc* monographs[62–64]. Qualitative studies are based on five approaches[65]:

- **Biographical life histories** or 'telling the story of what happened to a single individual'.
- **A phenomenological study** summarizing lived experiences in several individuals.
- **A grounded theory study** or 'tell me as much as you can about this particular problem'. Its purpose is to generate or discover a theory.
- **Ethnography** describing and interpreting a cultural or social group or system.
- **A case study** exploring one or more cases over time through detailed data collection of rich in-context information from multiple sources.

The definition of a '*case*', which some[62] also call '*site*', still remains a bit vague[66]. It may be[64,67-modified]:

- ■ A person (in medicine and nursing),
- ■ An event or situation (marital discord, strike),

- An action (spousal abuse), and
- Its remedy (consulting and its result),
- A program (home care for chronic patients),
- A time period (baby boomer era),
- A critical incident (hostage taking),
- A small group (homeless people),
- A department (within an organization),
- An organization itself (company, political party),
- A community (people living on welfare, suburbanites, etc.).

One 'case' can be analyzed and presented in different ways. As an example, the Watergate scandal can be studied through the people behind the case, the event itself (a break-in at a political party's offices) or the attempts to cover it up[68]. For Rothe[64], '. . . *The term 'case study' comes from the tradition of legal, medical, and psychological research, where it refers to a detailed analysis of an individual case, and explains the dynamics and pathology of a given disease, crime, or disorder. The assumption underlying case studies is that we can properly acquire knowledge of a phenomenon from intense exploration of a single example . . .*'

A case study can be qualitative (search for a meaning) or quantitative (some kind of measurement). A clinical examination is both qualitative (history taking, psychiatric evaluation) and quantitative (anthropometry, examination of vital functions, etc.). A social worker focuses more on qualitative information through three types of case studies[69]:

1. In an *intrinsic case study*, a better understanding of a case is sought. Why did parents abandon their child?
2. In an *instrumental case study*, one seeks to better understand the problem represented by the case, or to refine the underlying theory of the problem (parental child neglect).
3. A *collective case study* is not an epidemiological case study (no target groups, no denominators, etc.), but rather the extension of an instrumental case study to several cases. Its concept closely resembles that of the 'case series reports', see Chapter 7.
4. Some researchers may study only selected phenomena that illustrate the case[70] well. Others may choose a '*monographic study*' that is as detailed and complete as possible. This research is inductive[71].

Case(s) researchers in medicine and social sciences agree that case studies do not permit generalizations. However, if a case study brings results contrary to a previous experience beyond case studies, generalizations from previous experiences should be reviewed. To improve the quality of findings, qualitative researchers use **triangulation**, i.e. the gathering of information from different sources, by different methods and by multiplying analyses and analysts. The term, which means 'looking at one thing from different angles', is derived from the field of navigation and military strategy.

In qualitative research, case studies are based on individuals or situations as 'cases'[66]. This explains their uses in policy, political science, public health administration research, community psychology and sociology, organizational and management studies, or city and regional planning[68]. Health institutions or agencies (such as Health Maintenance Organizations (HMOs), hospitals, neighborhood clinics[70]), their organization and functioning can also be studied as 'cases'.

For Rothe[64], the philosophy behind qualitative research includes:

- **Epistemology** or 'theory of knowledge'.
- **Ontology** or study of being, study of reality.
- **Axiology** or study of what is valuable.
- **Logical positivism** or validation of reality using scientific methods.
- **Hermeneutics** or interpretation and understanding in building contextual knowledge reflecting situational, cultural and social affairs. For Addison[63], it simply means 'the business of interpretation'.
- **Criticism**, which considers knowledge as a commodity related to ideologies, politics and economics.

2.3.4.2 *Qualitative research in medicine, nursing, and public health*

Qualitative research, like any other scientific concept, technique, and method does not escape the ebb and flow of developments from one field to another. Experience in the study of single individuals obtained from medicine, psychology, and nursing was used, modified and expanded in social sciences, business, finances, administration, law, military. In these other areas, the 'case' concept extended beyond an individual to situations, states, or events. The ensuing enriched methodology can now be found in health sciences.

For some time already, physicians have applied many elements of qualitative research in psychiatry (psychoanalysis in particular), in medicine and in surgery when taking up patients' histories or gathering clues in epidemiological inquiries. Nursing was also one of the health sciences that strongly supported qualitative research and structured and applied it to the science of care. In 1995, the *British Medical Journal* introduced its readers to qualitative research in health sciences and in medicine, in particular, by means of an excellent reader-friendly collection of articles that later appeared in book form[72]. Increasing pressure as to the content and form of medical papers is well known to medical authors and readers. This art of communication was brought to the forefront by papers based on quantitative research. Greenhalgh[73] suggests ways to read and understand '*papers that go beyond numbers*'. Hence, qualitative research has gradually joined the mainstream of findings in health sciences.

Family medicine[74] as well as nursing[75], as a health profession and area of health research, call for qualitative research. In health administration, medical care organization, and health services research, case studies are used in their expanded sense[76]. Incentives arising from de-insurance of *in vitro* fertilization, consequences of the introduction of public funding for midwifery, or patients' unmet expectations for care[77,78] can be quoted as examples. At the same time, qualitative research methodology, its relevance and fields of application were presented to physicians in several introductory articles[55,79–84], series of papers in *BMJ* in 1995,[85] and books[73,86]. Their focus is on patients as cases[73] and situations (services)[85,87]. Randomized clinical trials[88], clinical interviews[89], patients' unmet expectations for care[77] or cases of injury[90] can also be evaluated as cases in qualitative research. How do quantitative and qualitative research differ in their approach to a similar topic? This can be understood by examining Table 2.3. This table illustrates the problem of physical activity after

myocardial infarction. Research questions and objectives differ as do research designs. However, several common elements illustrate an increasingly comparable rigor in research and organization in both approaches.

2.3.4.3 Conclusions

The future certainly belongs to the interface between quantitative and qualitative research[91,92] in an equilibrium still to be established: Well-entrenched quantitative research and its fast developing qualitative equivalent have not yet reached similar levels of strength and experience, although both approaches to health problem solving are complementary. Qualitative research, in fact, must strive to be considered as trustworthy[92] as quantitative research. Dieppe[93] summarizes the situation: '. . . *Today, we are in the middle of a period of obsession with evidence-based medicine (EBM). At first sight, narrative-based medicine (NBM) might seem to be in direct conflict with EBM; after all, evidence for many people means objective data, not anecdote. These days numbers are everything . . . However, EBM and NBM need not be in conflict . . . There is a pressing need for synergy between these two approaches and there are no real barriers to such a development. . . .*'

Most of the information in the following chapters stems from the area of quantitative research since this reflects the current state of equilibrium in medicine today. Ultimately, physicians will learn more and more about qualitative research, but they must first accept clinical interviews and case histories as an important starting point of any qualitative inquiry[94,95,89].

2.3.5 Evidence-based medicine

In medicine and in all other health sciences, there is a constant search for the **best evidence** in an effort to prevent or cure physical, mental or social ailments and to promote the best possible health. This search focuses on the following questions: What method most easily diagnoses a problem? What is the most effective treatment? What will allow the development of the most accurate prognosis and the choice of an appropriate course of action for patient outcomes?

Table 2.3 Quantitative and qualitative research. Dissimilarities and common traits	
Components and organization of quantitative research	*Components and organization of qualitative research*
Title	**Title**
Hypothesis and research question to be answered by the study. Example: Does physical activity after myocardial infarction improve patients' survival and quality of life?	**Research question** (without hypothesis). Example: How do patients perceive physical activity after myocardial infarction? What is the relevance of this? How do patients value various outcomes of their disease?
Rationale (justification) for the topic or reason for selecting the topic based on the **literature review**.	**Rationale (justification) for the topic** based on the **literature review** allowing assessment of originality and complementarity of findings.
Research design. Example: Observational analytical study comparing groups of physically active and inactive myocardial infarction survivors.	**Research design.** Example: Longitudinal follow-up of a few individual patients in a hermeneutic grounded study.
Methodological issues (site selection, sampling and sample size, variables under study, data collection, analysis, and interpretation).	**Methodological issues** (site selection, selection of patients, repeated in-depth interviews, focus group discussions, triangulation of findings, recording of information, data analysis).
Running the research (timetable, human and material resources, tools, quality control, error management).	**Running the research** (timetable, human and material resources, quality control, tools, error management).
Expected results and significance of findings for research and/or practice.	**Expected results and significance of findings for research and/or practice.**

What should patients be told to help them lead as productive and happy a life as possible? In the past, religious faith was sufficient to give direction to individuals and communities. Today, more is needed.

Evidence of what is good for mankind shifted first from personal and collective experiences to **basic sciences**. Laboratories were supposed to provide all the answers. Pathology, physiology, biochemistry or genetics were the key to success. More recently, **new technologies** in diagnostic imagery, development of drugs, surgery, or information have lead to important advances. Such fundamental research has been enhanced by 'bedside clinical research'. Thus, a methodology of clinical and public health decisions based on evidence, probability, uncertainty, economic, social, cultural, political and ethical considerations was established based on 'evidence' coming from the other side of the laboratory door.

Epidemiology and biostatistics gave the health sciences reassuring definitions, **quantitative** information and their interpretation. In other fields, such as psychology, psychiatry and nursing, a desire to better understand what was 'behind and beside the numbers' led to the development and use of **qualitative research**. Today, clinical reporting reflects the new tendency to integrate both quantitative and qualitative research in our understanding of health and disease.

Observing and reporting clinical cases is a type of first line evidence seemingly as old as medicine itself. Other 'evidence' has also been gathered from occurrence studies, etiological research, clinical trials, field epidemiological intelligence and intervention, prognostic studies, risk and disease surveillance. The identification of the best evidence from among all these sources and the use of this evidence to make medical decisions has gradually become more structured and organized. The process has even been given an attractive new name: **evidence-based medicine** or EBM[96,97].

2.3.5.1 Historical context of evidence-based medicine

Until the mid-nineteenth century, personal and peer experience were practically the only sources of 'evidence', until 'evidence' was split into more clearly defined categories. One such source of evidence was laboratory studies and data leading to a better understanding of the anatomical-pathological mechanisms of disease, pharmacodynamics and body responses to risk factors, exposure and therapeutic interventions. French, German and Austrian medicine excelled in this area. A second source of evidence was derived from the increasingly rigorous definition, gathering, analysis, and interpretation of numerical information from demography, public health, and clinical medicine. British and North American contributions were considerable here. Such innovative works as Morris' *Uses of Epidemiology*[98] or MacMahon and Pugh's *Epidemiology*[99] impressed and influenced us at that time. In addition, the North American way of thinking in business, finances, military operations, social sciences, medicine and other health-related fields, brought with it the paradigm of working and making decisions based on probability, uncertainty, and incomplete information. The shift from deterministic to probabilistic medicine continued to gain strength. Chinese, Japanese and Korean medicines maintained and developed systems that combined the best of 'Western' and traditional Asian medicines, paving the way for a better understanding and evaluation of 'alternative' medicines.

The fundamental methodology of drawing information from the case itself about the disease, its etiology and ways to control it emerged from the public health field. This is also known as 'shoe leather' epidemiology. Clinical epidemiology[22–25], born in the 1970s and 80s, was somewhat the opposite of the classical approach[15,100]. It used epidemiological information obtained from the study of groups of patients and the community to make the best possible bedside decisions for an individual patient. Especially in the latter area, we rapidly came to realize that an acceptable quantity of data was usable only if the quality of data was satisfactory. Thus, clinimetrics[101,102] was created to establish the rules of 'quality production, use, and control' in medicine. Finally, we became more and more interested in the

efficaciousness (in model or ideal conditions), effectiveness (under current conditions) and efficiency (at what price) of our clinical and preventive practices. Ideally, evidence-based medicine should take into account all these historical sources of and needs for 'evidence' and in fact, if practiced properly, it does.

2.3.5.2 What is 'evidence'?

According to Webster's Dictionary[103], 'evidence' can be defined as follows:

- Any ground or reason for knowledge or certitude in knowledge.
- Proof, whether immediate or derived by inference.
- A fact or body of facts on which a proof, belief, or judgment is based.

In law: That by means of which a fact is established: distinguished from *proof*, which is the result of *evidence*, and *testimony*, which is evidence given orally. For Cress[104], evidence in law is information that tends to prove or disprove a fact in question. N.B. It is not a fact in itself.

Hence, for our purposes, 'evidence' can be: Any data or information, whether solid or weak, obtained through experience, observational research or experimental work (trials). This data or information must be relevant and convincing to some degree either to the understanding of the problem (case) or to the clinical decisions (diagnostic, therapeutic or care-oriented) made about the case. 'Evidence' is not automatically correct, complete, satisfactory and useful. It must first be evaluated, graded and used based on its own merit. This allows it to gradually become sufficiently convincing. For Auclair[105], '... *to qualify as a basis for medicine, evidence should have two characteristics that together are necessary and sufficient: it should consist of an observation that has been assessed as valid by experts knowledgeable in the field, and it should impart such a degree of probability on the (subjective) hypothesis that it is preferable that we act on it. ...*'

A randomized multiple blind controlled clinical trial may conceptually provide the best cause–effect (treatment–cure) evidence. However, this type of study may be unethical, unsuitable or unfeasible, in which case, other evidence must be considered better.

All practitioners quickly find that they must make decisions based on evidence of variable strength.

If EBM emphasizes working with the 'best' evidence, the concept of 'best' poses a great challenge. In molecular[17,106,107] or genetic[108] epidemiology, the best evidence may be sought in the subtle understanding of biological components, mechanisms, and interactions at the subcellular level or the interacting pathways of genetic and other factors pertaining to disease risk or prognosis. From a conceptual and methodological standpoint in clinical epidemiology, a randomized double blind controlled trial is better evidence that treatment works than a clinical case report or case series report. In fact, many[109,110] have established hierarchical classifications of evidence according to its strength. Usually, these systems propose five levels of evidence based on the capacity of different types of studies to establish a cause–effect link between treatment and cure or noxious agents and disease development:

Ref. 109	Ref. 110	
I	I	Randomized controlled clinical trials.
II–1	II	Well designed trials without randomization (II–1). Non-randomized trials or those with high alpha and beta errors (II).
II–2	III	Analytical observational studies.
II–3	IV	Multiple time series or place comparisons, uncontrolled ('natural') experiments.
III	V	Expert opinions, descriptive occurrence studies, case reports, case series reports.

Most concerns pertaining to this type of classification of evidence are generally centered on the indiscriminate application of 'best evidence' to particular subgroups of patients[111]. In reality, a good cohort or case control study may be better than a poorly designed, poorly executed and poorly interpreted randomized controlled clinical trial. Evidence from original studies is rarely homogeneous in the literature and contradictory results as evidence can be produced. By necessity then, the second source of evidence is a 'study of studies' (i.e. meta-analysis[112–114]), systematic reviews[115] and integration of available data on a given problem as originally presented in psychology and education. Medicine has adopted, adapted and further developed this search for evidence.

In medicine, we have defined meta-analysis as '. . . *a systematic, organized and structured evaluation and synthesis of a problem of interest based on the results of many independent studies of that problem (disease cause, treatment effect, diagnostic method, prognosis, etc.)*[112,113,100]. . .'. In the results of such an 'epidemiological study of studies', the quality of studies is assessed first (qualitative meta-analysis) and then numerical results are integrated statistically (quantitative meta-analysis) to determine if treatment works or if an agent is harmful to health. In EBM, the best evidence is combined with other components of clinical decision-making[116–118]. It can and should include individual clinical expertise, knowledge from basic sciences, and patient preferences and values. Presently, many questions related to this process remain only partially answered[117]: What clinical knowledge and experience is relevant? Which criteria allow experience and evidence to be combined? Which criteria favor experience over evidence or vice versa? How should experience and evidence be weighed? Are there any flow charts that organize in time and space the steps required to combine evidence and experience?

2.3.5.3 *What is evidence-based medicine?*

EBM brings organization and structure to medical decisions just as decision analysis or cost-effectiveness analysis already do, but in a different way. Table 2.4 summarizes two common definitions of EBM and shows how the concept fully applies to **evidence-based public health** (EBPH)[119]. It also indicates the steps required for both of these practices. EBM with its emphasis on evidence is the opposite of fringe medicines, alternative medicines, or complementary medicines, grouped by Cocker[120] into the teasing category of '**claims-based Medicine**', i.e. '. . . that's how it is because I'm telling you that that's how it is! . . . Evidence? Come on! It's obvious! . . .' One of the logical outgrowths of the EBM concept is **evidence-based health care**, that is '. . . a discipline centered upon evidence-based decision-making about

Table 2.4 Definition and steps of evidence-based medicine and evidence-based public health

Evidence-based medicine (EBM)	*Evidence-based public health (EBPH)*
Definition The process of systematically finding, appraising, and using contemporaneous research findings as the basis for clinical decisions	**Definition** The process of systematically finding, appraising, and using contemporaneous clinical and community research findings as the basis for decisions in public health
or: The conscientious, explicit, and judicious use of current best evidence in making decisions about the care of individual patients	*or:* The conscientious, explicit, and judicious use of current best evidence in making decisions about the care of communities and populations in the areas of health protection, disease prevention, and health maintenance and improvement (health promotion)
Steps for its practice Formulation of a clear question arising from a patient's problem which has to be answered Searching the literature for relevant articles and exploring other sources of information Critical appraisal of the evidence (information provided by original research or by research synthesis, i.e. systematic reviews and meta-analysis) Selection of the best evidence or useful findings for clinical decision Linking evidence with clinical experience, knowledge, and practice and with the patient's values and preferences Implementation of useful findings in clinical practice Evaluation of the implementation and overall performance of the EBM practitioner, and Teaching others how to practice EBM	**Steps for its practice** Formulation of a clear question arising from a public health problem Searching for evidence Appraisal of evidence Selection of the best evidence for a public health decision Linking evidence with public health experience, knowledge, and practice and with community values and preferences Implementation of useful evidences in public health practice (policies and programs) Evaluation of such implementations and of the overall performance of the EBPH practitioner, and Teaching others how to practice EBPH
Its goal: **The best possible management of health and disease in individual patient(s)**	*Its goal:* **The best possible management of health and disease and their determinants at the community level**

Source : References 116,117,119 – combined and modified.

individual patients, groups of patients or populations, which may be manifest as evidence-based purchasing or evidence-based management.'[121]. **Public health practice** follows a similar trend[122].

For health care decisions, Stevens[123] proposes more than an evidence-based approach through **knowledge-based health service**: '. . . *health care decisions (whether about a patient or a population) need to be focused on research-based evidence about the consequences of treatment **augmented** by the*

intelligent use of wider information on, for example, finance, patient flows and healthcare politics . . .'

EBM must be seen as a permanently evolving process in order to keep up with the pace of rapidly evolving experience and research production in health sciences. As an example, Aspirin may at first be considered the analgesic and/or antipyretic of choice for some patients. However, at a later time, because of Aspirin's adverse effects, the patients may be given Tylenol® instead.

EBM is approximately one decade 'young'. Since its inception[96,97], EBM has been the subject of series of articles in the *Journal of the American Medical Association (JAMA)*[124] and the *Medical Journal of Australia (MJA)*[125]. EBM theory and practice appear in a 'little red book'[126] (now becoming a 'little blue book'[127]) and other valuable monographs[128–130]. The search for evidence has also been outlined[131] and short introductory articles[132–134] have focused on it as well. Even related training programs have been created[135]. Several new journals have been launched such as *Evidence Based Medicine, Evidence-based Cardiovascular Medicine*, the *ACP Journal Club* (American College of Physicians' Journal Club), *Evidence-Based Nursing*, and *Evidence-Based Mental Health*. French-speaking readers have access to the *EBM Journal, Evidence-Based-Medicine. Relier la Recherche aux Pratiques. Édition française (Un journal de l'American College of Physicians et du BMJ Publishing Group)*.

The evidence-based approach has also expanded and been applied to many other major specialties and fields, such as health care in general[136,137], family medicine[138], clinical practice[139,140], pediatrics[141], critical care medicine[142], surgery[143], cardiology[144], psychiatry[145], laboratory medicine[146], health promotion[147], or public health[119,122,148–150], to name just a few. It has even permeated into dentistry, nursing, acupuncture, etc.

Views and opinions about EBM are still not unanimous. For example, the same introductory article[151] about EBM elicited the following Letters to the Editor: '*The article . . . could be the most important relevant scientific article I have ever read in my life . . .* '[152], as well as: '*. . . Quite frankly, this is the most specious and useless piece of garbage that I have encountered since I graduated from dental school.*'[153] As happens often, the truth lies somewhere in-between as supported by the literature and lived experience.

The growing acceptance of EBM as a novel way of reasoning and decision-making in medicine is inevitably accompanied by **critiques and calls for caution** that have already been reviewed elsewhere[119] and are still being produced. In essence, these critiques call for a non-dogmatic use of EBM as a replacement for everything else in medicine and its link and integration with the 'old arts' of medicine, basic sciences, patient or social (community) values. In reality, EBM should take into account clinical spectrum, gradient, clinimetric stratification and prognostic characteristics of disease[111]. Recommendations and guidelines can be made only when individual characteristics are compatible with those in research and synthesis. Linking 'group evidence' and the value of evidence for a specific patient remains a great challenge. In fact, EBM's application to the individual patient is a cornerstone of its further development.

Randomized controlled trials, considered among the best source of evidence of cause–effect relationships, cannot answer all clinical questions in medicine. For ethical and technical reasons, these studies are not always feasible. The scope of EBM is larger than EB treatment. Qualitative research, observational, descriptive and analytical studies, diagnosis, screening, prognosis, or ethics pose additional challenges in terms of relevance and justified use in EBM. These fields as well as treatment effectiveness research should be further developed and physicians should be properly trained in all these practices[154–156].

Why is EBM so challenging? We agree with Kernick[157] that '*. . . decisions in life are based on a cognitive continuum. Wired to the cardiological bed, heart disease succumbs to inferential statistics. But patients come and go: to the real world where attempts to impose a spurious rationality on an irrational process may not always succeed; where structures are highly complex and disease thresholds may not be met; where decisions are based on past experience, future expectations, and complex human inter-relationships; where doctors and patients have their own narratives* (and their own values and priorities!); *where time scales exceed those of the longest trial; and where the mechanisms of poverty are the greatest of dys-ease. . . .* '. Barriers overcome and bridges built[158,118], EBM remains a relevant and rewarding experience for patients, their physicians and their health planners and managers. **The philosophy and emerging practice of EBM** as well as its related clinical case reporting can be summarized as follows:

- 'Evidence' is based on real life observations.
- 'Evidence' is not a decision itself; however, good evidence is needed to make good decisions.
- **Obtaining the evidence is not using the evidence!**
- The evolution from practice and 'soft' experience to evidence-based experience has not yet been universally achieved.
- More evidence does not necessarily mean more EBM practice.
- Clinical research means *systematic* clinical observations.
- Clinical research evolved from an unsystematic gathering, analysis, interpretation, and use of data and information to a systematic and *integrated* approach.
- EBM is primarily about thinking. Computing and use of information technology are considered strictly supportive tools.
- EBM reflects a deterministic/probabilistic shift in today's paradigm of medicine dealing with uncertainty. EBM is more evolutionary than revolutionary.
- With EBM, clinical epidemiology is within the reach of all health professionals in today's information-based world.
- Changes in thinking, not textbooks, affect the way medicine is practiced.
- More cases where EBM is used are necessary. Several *ad hoc* seminars are not sufficient.
- EBM lends itself perfectly to problem and/or system-oriented teaching.
- EBM mastery does not replace clinical skills and experience. It organizes, expands, and completes them.
- Just as Flexnerian reform transformed medicine from erratic usage of experience and educated guesses to its modern scientific basis in North America, the EBM movement is considered another contemporary change in the way medicine is practiced.
- There must be an important trade-off between administrative, authoritative and authoritarian decisions on the one hand, and quality evidence-based judgments and their applications on the other.

As for **clinical case applications,**

- In case-based situations, there will be an increasing number of links between pattern recognition and a systematic evidence-based approach.
- The 'underdog' status of working with clinical cases must be overcome, as has already happened in more conclusive research based on single or multiple case observations.

Some **contrasts in the EBM concept** (i.e. 'one thing does not mean another') must be kept in mind:

- *Use of computers and databases* vs. *the way these tools are worked with*, and the way conclusions are drawn about problems.
- *Instinct and thinking* vs. *working with evidence* and making decisions based on the best evidence available.
- *'Primary' studies* on risk, diagnosis, treatment, prognosis, or decisions vs. *'integrative' studies* such as systematic reviews, clinical guidelines, algorithms and other clinician guides focusing on the most efficient, effective, and efficacious preventions and cures in the whole care and management of individual patients and groups of individuals.

2.3.5.4 *What does the future hold for EBM?*

EBM is a topic that many luminaries still love to hate. Nevertheless, EBM is here to stay because there will always be a need to find the elusive 'best evidence' in medicine. Any innovation like implementing EBM findings or findings from qualitative research must be seen as one of the tools to improve health. It should be and it will be evaluated for its effectiveness[159] like treatment already is in clinical trials, this time in a kind of 'evidence-based evaluation of EBM itself'. An astonishing ten years before the emergence of EBM, King[160] concluded that '*science has to do with evidence, a word that comes from the Latin* videre, *to see, with the added meaning of seeing clearly. . . . Evidence would thus be that which throws light on something conceptual, that permits us to see with the eye of reason. . . . Evidence permits inference, and thus indicates or suggests something beyond itself. Evidence always leads beyond itself, but where it leads will depend on the acuity of the eye of reason. . . .*' Can medicine afford not to be evidence-based?

2.4 Conclusions. Fulfilling the Hippocratic oath

For pragmatic reasons, **medicine** is often dichotomized as **'clinical'** (i.e. pertaining to a clinic or bedside, founded on actual observation and treatment of patients as opposed to the theoretical or basic sciences) or **'community-based'**, pertaining to the body of individuals living in a defined area or having a common interest or organization (or characteristics)[161]. However, all types of medicine must be ethical. They must make a distinction between right and wrong. To solidify this, physicians entering the profession must take the Hippocratic oath: A commitment to the ideals of medicine. Table 2.5 compares a classical Hippocratic oath[162] (from many of its versions) and its extension to cover other health professions[163]. Several components of the Oath are highlighted to indicate those commitments that are very difficult to meet without the contributions of the various fields described in this chapter.

The term **'clinical governance'** is increasingly given to the practice of Hippocratic ideals: It is currently defined and being further developed as an *'action to ensure that risks are avoided, adverse effects are rapidly detected, openly investigated and lessons learned, good practice is widely disseminated and systems are in place to ensure continuous improvements in clinical care'*[164]. It is hard to follow these types of commitments without the best possible evidence. Treatment must be effective and cause no harm (adverse reactions). The selected treatment must be the best among those that are available. Arguments for and against care options must be based on the best possible evidence. Such evidence must be explained and justified. Actions must be undertaken with the knowledge of limits of information available to the decision-maker and to the patient. Standards and bad practices must be identified, evaluated and the latter avoided. All actions must be performed with a fair and humane distribution of health resources. The following contribute each in its own way to our ideals:

- **Biostatistics** shows us the way to handle uncertainty and probability in medicine.

- **Fundamental epidemiology** enables us to infer on disease from the study of individual cases and the study of communities where they arise.
- **Clinical epidemiology** helps us make decisions when faced with one or more clinical cases on the basis of clinical epidemiology and other sources of acceptable evidence.
- **Evidence-based medicine and evidence-based public health** lead us to the best available evidence, knowledge, and experience and shows us how to apply them to clinical and community health problems in conjunction with patient and community preferences and values.
- **Health administration and economics** ensure that health policies and health care are correctly applied according to societal values and resources.
- **Medical logic** enables us to reason properly and to use evidence in our decisions in a non-fallacious way.

Biostatistics finds differences, epidemiology and EBM give them a meaning. Medicine will keep and strengthen its humanistic approach (art of medicine), but it also requires, particularly in its technological revolution, a solid logical basis with epidemiology as a fundamental reasoning and decision-making approach (science of medicine). Perhaps, we will not call it epidemiology in the future. However, at the moment, this term suits its purpose well especially given the historical contexts described above. As more facts become known, Reise[165] points out that:

> *'(1) the half-lives of 'facts' are decreasing all the time; (2) not all presently accepted 'facts' are worth knowing; (3) critical judgment rather than memory is the important faculty that should be fostered; and, most important of all, (4) whereas current knowledge is ephemeral and insecure; the process leading to new knowledge is well established and has an excellent track record . . .'.*

In this situation, medicine is based not only on the knowledge of facts, but also on the knowledge of what to do with them. The logic of medicine, objective clinical reasoning in medicine or the theory of medicine are just a few terms in the current medical literature denoting such a challenge.

Table 2.5 Role of epidemiology and evidence-based medicine in the pursuit of medical ideals

Classical Hippocratic oath[162]	*Draft revision of the Hippocratic oath*[163]
I swear by Apollo the physician, by Aesculapius Hygeia, and Panacea, and I take to witness all the gods, all the goddesses, to keep according to my ability and my judgment the following Oath:	'The practice of medicine is a privilege which carries important responsibilities. All doctors should observe the core values of the profession which center on the duty to **help sick people** and to **avoid harm**. I promise that my medical knowledge will be used to **benefit people's health**. They are my first concern. I will listen to them and provide **the best care I can.** I will be honest, respectful and compassionate towards patients. In emergencies, I will do my best to help anyone in medical need.

To consider dear to me as my parents, him who taught me this art; to live in common with him and if necessary to share my goods with him; to look upon his children as my own brothers, to teach them this art if they so desire without fee or written promise; to impart to my sons and the sons of the master who taught me and the disciples who have enrolled themselves and have agreed to the rules of the profession, but to these alone, the precepts and the instruction. I will **prescribe regimen for the good of my patients** according to my ability and my judgment and never do harm to anyone. **To please no one will I prescribe a deadly drug, nor give advice which may cause his death.** Nor will I give a woman a pessary to procure abortion. But I will preserve the purity of my life and my art. I will not cut for stone, even for patients in whom the disease is manifest; I will leave this operation to be performed by practitioners (specialists in this art). In every house where I come I will enter only for the good of my patients, keeping myself far from all intentional ill-doing and all seduction, and especially from the pleasures of love with women or with men be they free or slaves. All that may come to my knowledge in the exercise of my professional or outside my profession or in daily commerce with men which ought not to be spread abroad, I will keep secret and will never reveal. If I keep this oath faithfully, may I enjoy my life and practice my art, respected by all men and in all times, but if I swerve from it or violate it, may the reverse be my lot.

'I will make every effort to ensure that the rights of all patients are respected, including vulnerable groups who lack means of making their needs known, be it through immaturity, mental incapacity, imprisonment or detention or other circumstance.

'**My professional judgment will be exercised as independently as possible** and not be influenced by political pressures nor by factors such as the social standing of a patient. I will not put personal profit or advancement above my duty to patients.

'I recognize the special value of human life but I also know that the prolongation of human life is not the only aim of health care. Where abortion is permitted, I agree that it should take place only within an ethical and legal framework. I will not provide treatments which are pointless or harmful or which an informed and competent patient refuses.

'**I will ensure patients receive the information and support they want to make decisions about disease, prevention and improvement of their health.** I will answer as truthfully as I can and respect patients' decisions unless that puts others at risk of harm. If I cannot agree with their requests, **I will explain why.**

'If my patients have limited mental awareness, I will still encourage them to participate in decisions as much as they feel able to do so.

'I will do my best to maintain confidentiality about all patients. If there are overriding reasons which prevent my keeping a patient's confidentiality I will explain them.

'I will **recognize the limits of my knowledge** and seek advice from colleagues when necessary. I will **acknowledge my mistakes**. I will do my best to keep myself and colleagues **informed of new developments and ensure that poor standards or bad practices are exposed** to those who can improve them.

'I will show respect for all those with whom I work and be ready to share my knowledge by teaching others what I know.

'I will use my training and professional standing to improve the community in which I work. I will treat patients equitably and support a **fair and humane distribution of health resources**. I will try to influence positively authorities whose policies harm public health. I will oppose policies which breach internationally accepted standards of human rights. I will strive to change laws which are contrary to patients' interests or to my professional ethics.'

Reproduced with permission from the Oxford University Press (Ref. 162) and the BMJ Publishing Group (Ref. 163)

REFERENCES

1. Silverman D. *Doing Qualitative Research. A Practical Handbook*. London: SAGE Publications, 2000
2. Kerlinger FN. *Behavioural Research. A Conceptual Approach*. New York: Holt, Reinhart & Winston, 1979
3. Cutler P. *Problem Solving in Clinical Medicine. From Data to Diagnosis*. Second edition. Baltimore: Williams & Wilkins, 1985
4. Higgs J, Jones M (eds). Clinical reasoning in the health professions. In: *Clinical Reasoning in the Health Professions*. Oxford: Butterworth Heinemann, 2000; 3–14
5. Feinstein AR. Clinical biostatistics. LVII. A glossary of neologisms in quantitative clinical science. *Clin Pharmacol Ther*, 1981;**30**:564–77
6. *The Columbia Encyclopedia*. Sixth edition, 2001. Electronic edition: www.bartleby.com
7. Johns RJ. The collection and analysis of clinical information. In: McGhee H, Johns RJ, Owens AH, Ross RS eds. *The Principles and Practice of Medicine*. Nineteenth edition. New York: Appleton-Century-Crofts, 1976:2–6
8. Hamm RM. Clinical intuition and clinical analysis: Expertise and the cognitive continuum. In: Dowie J, Elstein AR eds. *Professional Judgement. A Reader in Clinical Decision Making*. Cambridge: Cambridge University Press, 1988:78–105
9. Elstein AR, Bordage G. Psychology of clinical reasoning. In: Dowie J, Elstein AR eds. *Professional Judgement: A Reader in Clinical Decision Making*. Cambridge: Cambridge University Press, 1988: 109–29
10. Raska K. *Epidemiologie*. Second edition. Prague: SZN Publishers, 1954
11. *Kawakita Y, Sakai S, Otsuka Y (eds). History of Hygiene. Proceedings of the 12th International Symposium on the Comparative History of Medicine – East and West, August 30–September 6, 1987, Susono-shi, Shizuoka, Japan*. Tokyo: Ishiyaku Euro-America, Inc., 1991
12. *Buck C, Lllopis A, Najera E, Terris M. The Challenge of Epidemiology. Issues and Selected Readings*. PAHO Scientific Publications No 505. Washington: Pan American Health Organization, 1988
13. *Greenland S (ed.). Evolution of Epidemiologic Ideas. Annotated Readings on Concepts and Methods*. Chestnut Hill, MA.: Epidemiology Resources Inc., 1987
14. *Rothman KJ (ed.). Causal Inference*. Chestnut Hill, MA: Epidemiology Resources Inc., 1988
15. *Last JM (ed.). A Dictionary of Epidemiology*. Fourth Edition. Oxford: Oxford University Press, 2001
16. Black B, Lilienfled DE. Epidemiologic proof in toxic tort litigation. *Fordham Law Review*, 1984;**52**: 541–95
17. Andre Thompson RC (ed.). *Molecular Epidemiology of Infectious Diseases*. London: Arnold, 2000
18. Evans AS. Subclinical epidemiology. The First Harry A Feldman Memorial Lecture. *Am J Epidemiol*, 1987;**125**:545–55
19. Thrusfield M. *Veterinary Epidemiology*. London: Butterworths, 1986
20. Schwabe CW. *Veterinary Medicine and Human Health*. Baltimore: Williams & Wilkins, 1984
21. Leske GS, Ripa LW, Leske MC, Schoen MH. Dental Public health. In: Last JM ed. *Maxcy-Rosenau Public Health and Preventive Medicine*. 12th edition. New York: Appleton-Century-Crofts, 1986:1473–513
22. Fletcher RH, Fletcher SW, Wagner EH. *Clinical Epidemiology – The essentials*. Baltimore and London: Williams & Wilkins, 1982
23. Sackett DL, Haynes RB, Tugwell PX. *Clinical Epidemiology: A Basic Science for Clinical Practice*. Boston: Little, Brown, 1984
24. Feinstein AR. *Clinical Epidemiology. The Architecture of Clincial Research*. Philadelphia: WB Saunders, 1985
25. Jenicek M, Cléroux R. *Épidémiologie clinique. Clinimétrie. (Clinical Epidemioloogy. Clinimetrics)*. St. Hyacinthe and Paris: EDISEM and Maloine, 1985
26. Brown Jr. BW. Biostatistics, overview. In: Armitage P, Colton T eds. *Encyclopedia of Biostatistics*. Volume 1. Chichester: John Wiley & Sons, 1998:389–98
27. Arrow K. Uncertainty and the welfare economics of medical care. *Am Econ Rev*, 1963;**53**:941–73
28. Maynard A, Kanavos P. Health economics: An evolving paradigm. *Health Econ*, 2000;**9**:183–90
29. Vale L, Donaldson C, Daly C, et al. Evidence-based medicine and health economics: A case study of end stage renal disease. *Health Econ*, 2000;**9**:337–51
30. Thornton JG. Health economics: a beginner's guide. *Br J Hosp Med*, 1997;**58**:1997
31. Appleby J, Brambleby P. Economic evaluation – the science of making choices. In: Pencheon D, Guest C, Melzer D, Muir Gray JA eds. *Oxford Handbook of Public Health Practice*. Oxford: Oxford University Press, 2001:102–10
32. Siegel JE, Weinstein MC, Russell LB et al. for the Panel on Cost-Effectiveness in Health and Medicine. Recommendations for reporting cost-effectiveness analyses. *JAMA*, 1996;**278**:1339–41
33. Provenzale D, Lipscomb J. A reader's guide to economic analysis in the GI literature. *Am J Gastroenterol*, 1996;**91**:2461–70

34. Neymark N. Techniques for health economics analysis in oncology: Part 1. *Crit Rev Oncol Hematol*, 1999;**30**:1–11. Part 2. *idem*:13–24

35. Eisenberg JM. Clinical economics. A guide to the economic analysis of clinical practices. *JAMA*, 1989;**262**:2879–86

36. Drummond MF, O'Brien B, Stoddart GL, et al. *Methods for the Economic Evaluation of Health Care Programs*. Second edition. Oxford: Oxford University Press, 1997 (1999 – reprinted with corrections)

37. Provenzale D, Lipscomb J. Cost-effectiveness: Definitions and use in the gastroenterology literature. *Am J Gastroenterol*, 1996;**91**:1488–93

38. Detsky AS, Naglie GI. A clinician's guide to cost-effectiveness analysis. *Ann Int Med*, 1990;**113**:147–54

39. Maniadakis N, Gray A. Health economics and orthopaedics. *J Bone Joint Surg (Br)*, 2000;**82-B**:2–8

40. Drummond MF, Richardson SW, O'Brien BJ, et al. for the Evidence-Based Medicine Working Group. Users' guides to the medical literature. XIII. How to use an article on economic analysis of clinical practice. A. Are the results of the study valid? *JAMA*, 1997;**277**:1552–7

41. O'Brien BJ, Heyland D, Richardson SW, et al. Users' guides to the medical literature. XIII. How to use an article on economic analysis of clinical practice. B. What are the results and will they help me in caring for my patients? *JAMA*, 1997;**277**:1802–6

42. Heyland D, Gafni A, Kernerman P, Keenan S, Chalfin D. How to use the results of an economic evaluation. *Crit Care Med*, 1999;**91**:1195–202

43. Laupacis A, Feeny D, Detsky A, Tugwell PX. How attractive does a new technology have to be to warrant adoption and utilization? Tentative guidelines for using clinical and economic evaluations. *Can Med Assoc J*, 1992;**146**:473–81

44. Naylor CD, Williams I, Basinski A, Goel V. Technology assessment and cost-effectiveness analysis: Misguided guidelines? *Can Med Assoc J*, 1993;**148**:921–4

45. Laupacis A, Feeny D, Detsky AS, Tugwell PX. Tentative guidelines for using clinical and economic evaluations revisited. *Can Med Assoc J*, 1993;**148**:927–9

46. Karnon J, Qizilbash N. Economic evaluation alongside *N*-of-1 trials: getting closer to the margin. *Health Econ*, 2001;**10**:79–82

47. Rosser Matthews J. *Quantification and the Quest for Medical Certainty*. Princeton: Princeton University Press, 1995

48. Goering PN, Streiner DL. Reconcilable differences: The marriage of qualitative and quantitative methods. *Can J Psychiatry*, 1996;**41**:491–7

49. Casebeer AL, Verhoef MJ. Combining qualitative and quantitative research methods: Considering the possibilities for enhancing the study of chronic diseases. *Chronic Dis Canada*, 1997;**18**:130–5

50. Schwandt TA. *Dictionary of Qualitative Inquiry*. Second Edition. Thousand Oaks: SAGE Publications, 2001

51. Jenicek M. *Clinical Case Reporting in Evidence-based Medicine*. Second edition. London: Arnold, 2001

52. Strauss A, Corbin J. *Basics of Qualitative Research. Grounded Theory Procedures and Techniques*. Newbury Park: SAGE Publications, 1990

53. Patton MQ. *How to Use Qualitative Methods in Evaluation*. Newbury Park: SAGE Publications, 1987

54. Pope C, Mays N. Reaching the parts others cannot reach: an introduction to qualitative methods in health and health services research. *Br Med J*, 1995;**311**:42–5

55. Malterud K. The art and science of clinical knowledge: evidence beyond measures and numbers. *Lancet*, 2001;**358**:397–400

56. Lilienfeld DE, Lilienfeld AM. The French influence on the development of epidemiology. In: Lilienfeld AM ed. *Times, Places and Persons*. Baltimore: The Johns Hopkins Press, 1980:28–38

57. Louis PCA. *Researches on the Effects of Bloodletting in some Inflammatory Diseases Together With Phtisis*. Birmingham: The Classics of Medicine Library, 1986. (re-edition. Boston: Hilliard, Gray Co., MDCCCXXXVI. From the 1844 French edition)

58. Hunt SD. On the rhetoric of qualitative methods. Toward historically informed argumentation in management inquiry. *J Manag Inquiry*, 1994;**3**:221–34

59. Merriam S. *Case Study Research in Education. A Qualitative Approach*. San Francisco: Jossey-Bass, 1988

60. Giacomini MK, Cook DJ for the Evidence-Based Medicine Working Group. Users' guides to the medical literature. XXIII. Qualitative research in health care. A. Are the results of the study valid? *JAMA*, 2000;**284**:357–62

61. Giacomini MK, Cook DJ for the Evidence-Based Medicine Working Group. Users' guides to the medical literature. XXIII. Qualitative research in health care. B. What are the results and how do they help me care for my patients? *JAMA*, 2000;**284**:478–82

62. Denzin NK, Lincoln YS (eds). *Handbook of Qualitative Research*. Thousand Oaks: Sage Publications, 1994

63. Crabtree BF, Miller WL. *Doing Qualitative Research*. Newbury Park: SAGE Publications, 1992

64. Rothe PJ. *Qualitative Research. A Practical Guide*. Heidelberg (Ont) and Toronto: RCI/PDE Publications, 1993

65. Creswell JW. *Research Design. Qualitative & Quantitative Approaches.* Thousand Oaks: SAGE Publications, 1994

66. Ragin CC, Becker HS (eds). *What is a Case? Exploring the Foundation of Social Inquiry.* Cambridge: Cambridge University Press, 1992

67. Miles M, Huberman AM. *Qualitative Data Analysis: A Sourcebook of New Methods.* Newbury Park: SAGE Publications, 1989

68. Yin RK. *Case Study Research. Design and Methods.* Newbury Park: SAGE Publications, 1988

69. Stake RE. Case studies. In: Strauss A, Corbin J. *Basics of Qualitative Research. Grounded Theory Procedures and Techniques.* Newbury Park: Sage Publications, 1990:236–47

70. Aday LA. *Designing and Conducting Health Surveys. A Comprehensive Guide.* San Francisco: Jossey-Bass, 1989.

71. Yin RK. *Applications of Case Studies Research.* Thousand Oaks: SAGE Publications, 1993

72. *Mays N, Pope C (eds). Qualitative Research in Health Care.* London: BMJ Publishing Group, 1996

73. Greenhalgh T. *How to Read a Paper. The Basics of Evidence Based Medicine.* Second Edition. London: BMJ Publishing Group, 2001:166–78

74. Burkett GL, Godkin MA. Qualitative research in family medicine. *J Family Practice,* 1983;**16**:625–6

75. Sandelowski M. One is the liveliest number: The case orientation of qualitative research. *Res Nurs Health,* 1996;**19**:525–9

76. Keen J, Packwood T. Case study evaluation. *Br Med J,* 1995;**311**:444–6

77. Kravitz RL, Callahan EJ, Paterniti D, et al. Prevalence and sources of patients' unmet expectations for care. *Ann Intern Med,* 1996;**125**:730–7

78. Inui TS. The virtue of qualitative *and* quantitative research. *Ann Intern Med,* 1996;**125**:770–1

79. Shafer A, Fish P. A call for narrative: The patient's story and anesthesia training. *Literature and Medicine,* 1994;**13**:124–42

80. Naess MH, Malterud K. Patients' stories: science, clinical facts or fairy tales? *Scand J Prim Health Care,* 1994;**12**:59–64 (quoted also as 1995;**13**)

81. Wright JG, McKeever P. Qualitative research: Its role in clinical research. *Annals RCPSC,* 2000;**33**:275–80

82. Poses RM, Isen AM. Qualitative research in medicine and health care. Questions and controversy. *J Gen Intern Med,* 1998;**13**:32–38, discussion: 64–72

83. Malterud K. Qualitative research: standards, challenges, and guidelines. *Lancet,* 2001;**358**:483–88

84. Powell AE, Davies HTO. Reading and assessing qualitative research. *Hospital Medicine,* 2001;**62**:360–3

85. Devers KJ, Sofaer S, Rundall TG. *Qualitative Methods in Health Services Research. Health Services Res,* 1999;**34**:1083–263

86. Gantley M, Harding G, Kumar S, Tissier J. *An Introduction to Qualitative Methods for Health Professionals.* London: Royal College of General Practitioners, 1999

87. Chard JA, Liliford RJ, Court BV. Qualitative medical sociology: what are its crowning achievements? *J Roy Soc Med,* 1997;**90**:604–9

88. Wilson S, Delaney BC, Roalfe A, et al. Randomised controlled trials in primary care: case study. *Br Med J,* 2000;**321**:24–7

89. Platt FW, McMath JC. Clinical hypocompetence: The interview. *Ann Int Med,* 1979;**91**:898–902

90. Rothe JP. *Undertaking Qualitative Research. Concepts and Cases in Injury, Health and Social Life.* Edmonton: The University of Alberta Press, 2000

91. Goodwin LD, Goodwin WL. Qualitative *vs.* Quantitative or qualitative *and* quantitative research? *Nurs Res,* 1984;**33**:378–80

92. Krefting L. Rigor in qualitative research: The assessment of trustworthiness. *Am J Occup Ther,* 1991;**45**:214–22

93. Dieppe P. Book of the month. Narrative Based Medicine. *J Roy Soc Med,* 1999;**92**:380–1

94. Donelly WJ. The language of medical case histories. *Ann Intern Med,* 1997;**127**:1045–8

95. Greenhalgh T, Hurwitz B (eds). *Narrative Based Medicine. Dialogue and discourse in clinical practice.* London: BMJ Books, 1998

96. Guyatt GH. Evidence-Based Medicine. *ACP Journal Club,* 1991 March–April;**114** (Suppl 2):A-16

97. Guyatt G, et al. Evidence-Based Medicine Working Group Evidence-Based Medicine. A new approach to teaching practice of medicine. *JAMA,* 1992;**268**:2420–5

98. Morris JN. *Uses of Epidemiology.* Edinburgh and London: Livingstone, 1967

99. MacMahon B, Pugh TF. *Epidemiology. Principles and Methods.* Boston: Little, Brown, 1970

100. Jenicek M. *Epidemiology. The Logic of Modern Medicine.* Montreal: EPIMED International, 1995

101. Feinstein AR. An additional science for clinical medicine: IV. The development of clinimetrics. *Ann Intern Med,* 1983;**99**:843–8

102. Feinstein AR. *Clinimetrics.* New Haven: Yale University Press, 1987

103. *New Illustrated Webster's Dictionary of the English Language.* New York: PAMCO Publishing Co., 1992

104. Cress JM. *Evidence.* In: *World Book* (CD version). Chicago: World Book Inc., 1999

105. Auclair F. On the nature of evidence. *Annals RCPSC,* 1999;**32**:453–5

106. Loomis D, Wing S. Is molecular epidemiology a germ theory for the end of the twentieth century? *Int J Epidemiol,* 1990;**19**:1–3

107. Perera FP, Weinstein BI. Molecular epidemiology and carcinogen-DNA adduct detection: New

approaches to studies of human cancer causation. *J Chronic Dis*, 1982;**35**:581–600

108. Schull WJ, Weiss KM. Genetic epidemiology: four strategies. *Epidemiol Rev*, 1980;**2**:1–18

109. The Canadian Task Force on the Periodic Health Examination. *The Canadian Guide to Clinical Preventive Health Care*. Ottawa: Health Canada, 1994

110. Sackett DL. Rules of evidence and clinical recommendations. *Can J Cardiol*, 1993;**9**:487–9

111. Feinstein AR, Horwitz RI. Problems in the « Evidence » of « Evidence-Based Medicine ». *Am J Med*, 1997;**103**:529 –35

112. Jenicek M. *Méta-analyse en médecine. Évaluation et synthèse de l'information clinique et épidémiologique. (Meta-analysis in Medicine. Evaluation and Synthesis of Clinical and Epidemiological Information.)* St. Hyacinthe and Paris: EDISEM and Maloine, 1987

113. Jenicek M. Meta-analysis in medicine. Where we are and where we want to go. *J Clin Epidemiol*, 1989;**42**: 35–44

114. Petitti DB. *Meta-analysis, Decision Analysis, and Cost-Effectiveness Analysis. Methods of Quantitative Synthesis in Medicine*. Monographs in Epidemiology and Biostatistics, Volume 24. New York and Oxford: Oxford University Press, 1994

115. Cook DJ, Mulrow CD, Haynes RB. Systematic reviews: Synthesis of best evidence for clinical decisions. *Ann Intern Med*, 1997;**126**:376–80

116. Rosenberg W, Donald A. Evidence based medicine: an approach to clinical problem solving. *Br Med J*, 1995;**310**:1122–6

117. 1.Sackett DL, Rosenberg WMC, Muir Gray JA, et al. Evidence-based medicine: what it is and what it isn't. *Br Med J*, 1996;**312**:71–2

118. Guyatt GH, Haynes RB, Jaeschke RZ, et al. for the Evidence-Based Medicine Working Group. User's guides to the medical literature. XXV. Evidence-Based Medicine: principles for applying the users' guides to patient care. *JAMA*, 2000;**284**:1290–6

119. Jenicek M. Epidemiology, Evidence-Based Medicine, and Evidence-Based Public Health. *J Epidemiol*, 1997;**7**:187–97

120. Cocker J. Henry VIII and I. *Stitches*, 1999, Number 92: 76–8

121. Muir Gray JA. *Evidence-based healthcare. How to Make Health Policy and Management Decisions*. New York: Churchill Livingstone, 1997

122. Pencheon D, Guest C, Melzer D, Muir Gray JA (eds). *Oxford Handbook of Public Health Practice*. Oxford: Oxford University Press, 2001

123. Stevens A. A knowledge-based health service: how do the new initiatives work? *J Roy Soc Med*, 1998;**91**(Suppl. 35):26–31

124. User's Guides to the Medical Literature. Series of articles in *JAMA*, starting in 1993;**270**:2093–5. In a book form: Guyatt G, Rennie D eds. *Users' Guides to the Medical Literature. A Manual for Evidence-Based Clinical Practice*. Chicago: American Medical Association Press, 2002

125. Rubin GL, Frommer MS (eds). EBM. Evidence. Experience. Series of articles. *MJA*, starting in 2001; **174**:248–53

126. Sackett DL, Richardson WS, Rosenberg W, Haynes RB. *Evidence-based Medicine. How to Practice and Teach EBM*. New York: Churchill Livingstone, 1997

127. Sackett DL, Straus SE, Richardson SW, et al. *Evidence-Based Medicine. How to Practice and Teach EBM*. Second Edition. Edinburgh and London: Churchill Livingstone, 2000

128. Dixon RA, Munro JF, Silcocks PB. *The Evidence Based Medicine Workbook. Critical Appraisal for Clinical Problem Solving*. Oxford: Butterworth Heinemann, 1997

129. Daves M, et al. (eds). *Evidence-Based Practice*. Edinburgh: Churchill Livingstone, 1999

130. Hamer S, Collinson G (eds). *Achieving Evidence Based Practice*. Edinburgh: Bailliére Tindall, 1999

131. McKibbon KA, Marks S, Eady A. *PDQ Evidence-Based Principles and Practice*. Hamilton: BC Decker Inc., 1999

132. Bigby M. Evidence-based medicine in a nutshell. A guide to finding and using the best evidence in caring for patients. *Arch Dermatol*, 1998;**134**:1609–18

133. Etminan M, Wright JM, Carleton BC. Evidence-based pharmacotherapy: review of basic concepts and applications in clinical practice. *Ann Pharmacother*, 1998;**32**:1193–200

134. Green L. Using evidence-based medicine in clinical practice. *Oncology*, 1998;**25**:391–400

135. Greenhalgh T, Donald A. *Evidence Based Health Care Workbook: Understanding research. For individual and group learning*. London: BMJ Books, 2000

136. Evidence-Based Care Resource Group (Oxman AD, principal coauthor). Evidence-based care: 1. Setting priorities: How important is the problem? *CMAJ*, 1994;**150**:1249–54. 2. Setting guidelines: How should we manage the problem? *Idem*:1417–23. 3. Measuring performance: How are we managing this problem? *Idem*:1575–9. 4. Improving performance: How can we improve the way we manage this problem? *Idem*:1793–6. 5. Lifelong learning: How can we learn to be more effective? *Idem*:1971–3

137. Reerink E, Walshe K. Evidence-based healthcare: a critical appraisal. *J Roy Soc Med*, 1998(Suppl. 35); **91**:1

138. Rosser WW, Shafir MS. *Evidence-Based Family Medicine*. Hamilton and London: BC Decker, 1998

139. Geyman JP, Deyo RA, Ramsey SD (eds). *Evidence-Based Clinical Practice: Concepts and Approaches*. Boston and Oxford: Butterworth Heinemann, 2000

140. Lee BW, Hsu SI, Stasior DS (eds). *Quick Consult Manual of Evidence-Based Medicine.* Philadelphia and New York: Lippincott-Raven, 1997

141. Feldman W (ed.). *Evidence-Based Pediatrics.* Hamilton: BC Decker, 2000

142. Marik PE. *Handbook of Evidence-Based Critical Care.* New York: Springer, 2001

143. Kreder HJ. Evidence-based surgical practice: What it is and do we need it? *World J Surg,* 1999;23:1232–5

144. Sharis PJ, Cannon CP. *Evidence-Based Cardiology.* Philadelphia: Lippincott Williams & Wilkins, 2000

145. Paris J. Canadian psychiatry across 5 decades: From clinical inference to evidence-based practice. *Can J Psychiatry,* 2000;45:34–9

146. Price CP. Evidence-based laboratory medicine: Supporting decision-making. *Clin Chemistry,* 2000; 46:1041–50

147. Perkins ER, Simnett I, Wright L (eds). *Evidence-Based Health Promotion.* Chichester and New York: J Wiley, 1999

148. Aveyard P. Evidence-based medicine and public health. *J Eval Clin Pract,* 1997;3:139–44

149. Glasziou P, Longbottom H. Evidence-based public health practice. *Aust N Z J Public Health,* 1999;23: 436–40

150. Brownson RC, et al. Evidence-based decision making in public health. *J Public Health Manag Pract,* 1999; 5:86–97

151. Raphael K, Marbach JJ. Evidence-based care of musculoskeletal facial pain: implications for the clinical science of dentistry. *JADA,* 1997;128:73–7

152. Niamtu J, III. Evidence-based care. Letter to The Editor. *JADA,* 1997;128:402–403

153. Cook TR III. A contrasting view. Letter to The Editor. *JADA,* 1997;128:403

154. Bordley DB, Fagan M, Theige D for the Association of Professors of Medicine. Evidence-based medicine: A powerful educational tool for clerkship education. *Am J Med,* 1997,102:427–32

155. Kenney AF, Hill JE, Mcray CL. Introducing evidence-based medicine into a community family medicine residency. *J Miss State Med Assoc,* 1998; 39:441–3

156. Green ML. Graduate medical education training in clinical epidemiology, critical appraisal, and evidence-based medicine: A critical review of curricula. *Acad Med,* 1999;74:686–94

157. Kernick DP Lies, damned lies, and evidence-based medicine. *Lancet,* 1998;351:1824

158. Haynes B, Haines A. Barriers and bridges to evidence based clinical practice. *Br Med J,* 1998;317:273–6

159. Christakis DA, Davis R, Rivara FP. Pediatric evidence-based medicine: Past, present, and future. *J Pediat,* 2000:136:383–9

160. King LS. *Medical Thinking. A Historical Preface.* Princeton: Princeton University Press, 1982

161. *Dorland's Illustrated Medical Dictionary.* 29th edition. Philadelphia: WB Saunders, 2000

162. Walton J, Beeson PB, Scott RB (eds). *The Oxford Companion to Medicine.* Volume 1. Oxford: Oxford University Press, 1986

163. Hurwitz B, Richardson R. Swearing to care: the resurgence in medical oaths. *Br Med J,* 1997;315: 1671–4

164. Earlam S, Brecker N, Vaughn B. *Cascading Evidence into Practice.* Brighton: Pavilion Publishing Ltd. and King's Fund, 2000

165. Reise E. In quest of certainty. *Am J Med,* 1984;77: 969–71

Chapter 3

The logic of modern medicine. Reasoning and underlying concepts

'There is one thing certain, namely, that we can have nothing certain; therefore, it is not certain that we can have nothing certain.
Samuel Butler (1612–1680)

'A doctor should never forget that he or she is a scientist. Every diagnostic and therapeutic decision should have a logical basis that can be clearly articulated to colleagues and patients . . . or in court.
J. Wroblewski, 1999

Logic is '. . . the art of going wrong, with confidence.'
S.W. Merrell and J.M. McGreevy, 1991
Definitely, if you are running short of solid evidence!

Ordo ab Chao (Order out of Chaos)
Masonic motto (undated)

In medical school, we were crammed full of fundamental facts including the anatomy of the abdominal wall and of the digestive tract, histopathology and clinical signs of inflammation of appendix, the clinical course of treated and untreated appendicitis, uses of antibiotics and surgery in the treatment of localized and generalized infection. Now, we need to know what information (evidence, clinical facts) is the most valuable for our clinical decisions, which include pushing the diagnostic process further, treating or not treating and informing the patient about outcomes of his or her disease. It is our correct and critical thinking which guides our mind and hand towards a properly executed tracheal intubation or lumbar puncture or which leads us to do something else or to do nothing. The chapters that follow (4–11) will introduce the rules according to which various types of evidence in medicine are obtained and evaluated. Once we have assimilated such essential information, we need to learn and understand how medical evidence should be used in our reasoning and decision-making.

From the previous chapter, we already understand some basic characteristics of the inner workings and components of medical practice. Every stage of clinical work or public health programming requires sound reasoning that 'makes sense'. In this chapter, we examine the classical paradigms of our thinking about medical problems in terms of classical logic and probability, as well as some modern competing theories in these two areas. More on the principles and rules of correct reasoning and decisions, as well as on the pitfalls to avoid will be given once a clearer picture of evidence (from Chapters 4–11) has been drawn. Chapter 12 will then tell us about the proper uses of evidence itself.

In the past, medical reasoning was considered just another example of the 'black box' of our understanding. The prevailing and rather defeatist attitude was that 'we know only what goes in and what goes out, but nothing in between'. We are now trying, however, to know more about medical reasoning and to understand its workings. Young members of the house-staff attending clinical rounds listen to the arguments and counter-arguments of their more experienced colleagues including the pros and cons of differential diagnosis, the choices between various treatments and the prognosis and balancing of risks and benefits for patient care. Are these exchanges understandable, do they sound 'logical' (and are they?) to the patient and are they based on sound evidence? How can students use the information learned from lectures and textbooks in such situations? Are there any general rules of the game?

3.1 Logic in medicine

We want medicine to be logical in order to better understand it and to use it effectively to the benefit of the patient. But are things that are 'logical' more easily understood than things that 'make sense'? Is logic part of our understanding of health and disease? The answer to these questions is a definite 'yes', since logic heavily underlies our epidemiological and biological thinking, interpretations and practical decisions. Let us now focus on the basic principles and applications of logic.

3.2 Logic around us

Many of us left school with the idea that philosophy is too abstract and theoretical, especially for our medical minds driven to the solution of concrete and practical problems in patient health. If **philosophy**, in general, is the study of ultimate reality, causes and principles underlying being and thinking[1], aren't we already putting it into practice in medicine through epidemiology and biostatistics?

A group of philosophers known as the *Vienna Circle* proposed, at the beginning of the twentieth century, that the object of philosophy is a logical clarification of thought; it is not a theory, but an activity. These first proponents of *logical positivism* advocated that logic, mathematics and experience could reduce the content of scientific theories to truth[1]. Their *verification* (or *verifiable*) *principle* stresses that a proposition (statement) is meaningful if, and only if, some sense experience would suffice to determine that it is true or false[1,2]. For medicine, in the light of its focus on evidence provided by experimental research, several views of logical positivists are worth quoting[2]:

- There are two sources of knowledge: logical reasoning and empirical experience.
- Logical experience includes mathematics, which is reducible to formal logic.
- Empirical knowledge includes physics, biology, psychology, etc.
- Experience is the only judge of scientific theories. However, scientific knowledge does not exclusively arise from experience: scientific theories are genuine hypotheses that go beyond experience.
- There is a distinction between observational and theoretical terms.
- There is a distinction between synthetic and analytic statements.
- There is a distinction between theoretical axioms and rules of correspondence
- Scientific theories are of a deductive nature.

Modern philosophers such as A. Comte, J.S. Mill, D. Hume, B. Russell, T. Kuhn and K. Popper contributed to the development of the **philosophy of science**. This domain was overviewed more recently by Salmon et al[3]. Induction, deduction and causality are examples of philosophical concepts, but with eminent and imminent practical implications of their topics within one particular science like biology or medicine and beyond one science (generalizability). From classical branches of philosophy[1], we are already most often interested in **logic** (laws of valid reasoning), **epistemology** (nature of knowledge and of process of knowing) and **ethics** (problems of right conduct). Let us now review definitions of some widely used and general terms. Such meanings apply to this reading.

3.2.1 *Philosophy in medicine is more than ethics. Some definitions of common terms in philosophy*

If asked about philosophy in medicine, many medical students will mention 'medical ethics'. However, philosophy is more than ethics. Philosophy differs from **science** in that science bases its theories wholly on established facts, whereas philosophy covers in addition to that, other areas of inquiry where no entirely satisfactory facts are available[1]. All these endeavors are necessarily based on **thinking**, which

itself, once verbalized is a matter of combining words in propositions[4]. For example, the premises and conclusion of an argument (*vide infra*) are propositions. Logic itself is part of a broader framework of **critical thinking**, i.e. '. . . a process, the goal of which is to make reasonable decisions about what we believe and what to do'[5]. **Reasoning** is thinking structured and objectified by logic, as defined above. Reasoning means directing thinking towards reaching a conclusion. Reasons are called premises, that which the reason supports is called the 'conclusion', and the whole piece of reasoning is called an 'argument'[6]. **Correct reasoning** is the practical skill of applying logical principles to particular cases[7]. Correct reasoning fuelled by satisfactory evidence produces knowledge. **Knowledge** may be defined as: A clear perception of fact, truth, or duty, that familiarity which is gained by actual experience, and a scope of information[5]. **Common knowledge** is shared knowledge between individuals. For example, human anatomy, allergy, coagulation or acid–base balance, belong to the realm of common knowledge in medicine. Understanding of common knowledge is one of the fundamental conditions of effective communication in medicine and anywhere else.

3.2.2 *Definitions of logic*

Definition making has its proper rules[7] and it is not always easy. The more definitions we have of a given subject, the more we are uncertain about its exact context and demarcations. In fact, the term 'logic' means different things to different people[6–16] and definitions of logic abound. Some of them are worth quoting in our context:

- The normative science, which investigates the principles of valid reasoning and correct inference[7], either dealing with conclusions, which follow necessarily from the reasons or premises (**deductive logic**) or with conclusions, which follow with some degree of probability from the reasons or premises (**inductive** logic).
- The basic principles of reasoning developed by and applicable to any field of knowledge; the **logic of science**[9].

- *Logic is not the science of Belief, but the Science of Proof, or Evidence* (John Stuart Mill)[6].

> If the principles of logic are applicable to any field of science, medicine should also be subjected to its general rules. The *logic of medicine* is a system of thought and reasoning that governs understanding and decisions in clinical and community care. It defines valid reasoning, which helps us understand the meaning of medical phenomena and leads us to the justification of the choice of clinical and paraclinical decisions about how to act upon such phenomena.

Logic, then, is a normative discipline, one that lays down standards of correct reasoning to which we ought to adhere if we want to reason successfully[6]. It focuses primarily on strengths and weaknesses (validity) of arguments and on how arguments are linked in their drive to the conclusion that should result from them. Let us first explain some basic elements and principles of logic. Their application to specific problems and challenges in medicine can be found in subsequent chapters.

3.2.3 Some basic elements and principles of logic

For those readers whose knowledge of the basic principles of logic has faded with time, this section briefly deals with the application of informal logic to medicine.

3.2.3.1 Arguments and syllogisms

We owe the fundamentals of logic to ancient Greek philosophers like Aristotle, Plato, Chrysippus of Soli or Socrates and to others such as Gottfried Wilhelm Leibniz, Francis Bacon and David Hume[17], George Boole[18], Bertrand Russell, or Karl Popper[6,19,20]. Several philosophers from the past, including René Descartes, even laid the foundations for our view of logic today.

Formally, logic concerns **arguments**. An **argument** is *an ensemble of discourse presenting some evidence.* It is made up of a conclusion in support of a given thesis and certain premises or considerations (sets of statements) related to the conclusion. An argument is deductively valid if its premises provide conclusive evidence for its conclusion. The contrary creates a deductively invalid argument. Logical argumentation is not about quarrelling or fighting. It is about **explaining, defending our reasons and having them endorsed by valuable evidence.** Argumentation and some logical discourse are ubiquitous in daily medical practice and in fundamental and bedside decision oriented research.

- At **clinical rounds,** we share our ideas with our colleagues and defend our conclusions about diagnosis, treatment or prognosis in a particular patient.
- We explain and defend our conclusions and recommendations in **patients' charts.**
- We explain the nature and origins of health problems and justify proposals for remedial action in **public health,** community medicine and health policies.
- We make clear our ideas and rationales for our conclusions in **medical articles** and **research papers.** Their 'discussion' and 'conclusions and recommendations' sections depend on solid logic.
- We defend our proposals in our **quest for grants in medical research.**
- We present and explain cases and give our opinion as health experts in **tort litigations** at courts of law, compensation boards, insurance and other social bodies.
- Last but not least, we need logic and arguments supporting our recommendations when **talking to the patient.**

As a matter of fact, '. . . *the critical standards of logic have application in any subject which employs inference and argument – in any field in which conclusions are supported by evidence*'.[21]

The basic model of our reasoning is a **logical argument or discourse.** For example, our assessment of risk or diagnosis or our decision to treat is a product of an argument. Each argument must be formulated as clearly as possible to give the correct meaning to whatever we do. Each of its components must be the best possible piece of sustainable evidence.

When discussing clinical cases during floor rounds, we are arguing (arguing), providing reasons for some statement or conclusion about the case. An **argument** is a set of statements, for some of which, the premises are offered as reasons for another statement, the conclusion. Michalos[22] defines an argument in other terms: '. . . *sequence of sentences divided in such a way that some of the sentences are supposed to be the reason, justification, guarantee, warrant, or support for some other sentence in the sequence. The sentences that provide the reason or warrant are called* **premises**. *The sentence that is supposed to be warranted by the premise is called the* **conclusion**.' It is not a verbal conflict! During clinical rounds, several colleagues may propose their sometimes contradictory, sometimes convergent views about the case (premises). Based on one, two or more than two such premises, some conclusion is reached about the diagnosis, treatment or prognosis of the patient. Often, more than one argument is needed to solve a clinical problem. There are several forms of argumentation. In this introduction, only an example of classical Aristotelian argumentation will be given.

The **categorical syllogism** is *a form of argument consisting of two premises (postulates, categorical statements) and a conclusion.* For example, we can state:

Premise A (p_1): Logic is common to all arts and sciences.
Premise B (p_2): Medicine is both art and science.
Conclusion (C): There must be logic in medicine.

- **Premises** are statements of evidence. Terms like *since, for* or *because* often signal a premise in a logical argument[21].
- **Conclusions** are statements that are supported by evidence. Terms like *therefore, hence, consequently, so,* or *it follows that* frequently introduce conclusions[21].
- **Inference** means 'path from premises to conclusion'.

Logical analysis is a study of relationships between a conclusion and the evidence to support it[21]. For example, if we concluded (C), that 'medicine **must** be logical', we might analyze the premises for the relatedness and completeness leading to such a conclusion. Such syllogisms follow the pattern:

A (alpha, p_1); **B** (beta, p_2); **therefore C** (gamma, c).

A **syllogism** was defined by Aristotle[6] as a '*discourse or argument in which certain things have been laid down (like A and B) and something other than what has been laid down (C), follows by necessity from their being so*'. For example: All clinically important aneurysms of the abdominal aorta are associated with a pulsating abdominal mass (p_1). A physician has detected such a pulsating abdominal mass in his or her patient (p_2). An aneurysm of abdominal aorta must be considered in this patient (C). Syllogisms, which are composed entirely of categorical statements, are called **categorical syllogisms**. Each categorical statement contains a **subject term** (a clinically important aneurysm) and a **predicate term** (associated with pulsating abdominal mass).

In mathematical logic, the symbol of inclusion '⊃' (i.e. 'if . . . then' or implication sign) is widely used in the literature. For example, C (the patient) is included to belong to the category of patients suffering from abdominal aortic aneurysm (A, p_1): $C \supset A$.

Symbolic or **formal logic** builds a formalized system of reasoning, using abstract symbols for the various aspects of natural language. Artificial intelligence is based on formal logic. Formal logic abstracts from the content propositions, statements, or deductive arguments structures or logical forms they embody. A symbolic notation is used to express these structures[1,7]. **Informal logic**[4,7,23] uses methods and techniques to analyze and interpret seemingly informal reasoning as it happens in the context of natural language used in everyday life, such as in an exchange of information between physicians on clinical rounds, in professional, administrative, or judiciary medical reports or in scientific papers. In the study of risk, treatment, prognosis, or any study of disease outcome, we may be interested in knowing whether ensuing conclusions, given premises which lead to them, are necessary, possible, probable, or impossible. Such properties are called *modal notions* and the logic associated with them is termed **modal logic**[7].

3.2.3.2 Deduction and induction in logic and medicine

Logic and medicine, in general, have assigned slightly different meanings to deduction and induction. **In**

formal logic, arguments may be **deductively valid** (a conclusion is definitely true if the premises are true) or **inductively strong,** when conclusions are probable if the premises are true (in the absence of further information). Deductive logic applies when premises can be secured from which a desired conclusion follows necessarily. Since certainty, however rare, is highly desirable in medicine, deductive logic is of primary interest for decisions in this field. Nonetheless, some conclusions may be inductive due to the nature of the problem under scrutiny. Hence, a **deductive argument** is an argument in which premises are intended to provide **absolute support** for a conclusion[24]. An **inductive argument** is an argument in which premises are intended to provide **some degree of support** for a conclusion[24].

As we have already seen in the preceding chapter, the terms deduction and induction are used **in medicine, in general,** not in a logical argument, but rather in the process of reasoning itself. For Cutler[25], deduction means going from established facts and general statements to an individual case. A conclusion is only as good (valid) as the propositions (general facts). Inductive reasoning often involves inference from a study of individual cases, leading to an established general principle from this study that is then applied to other cases.

In epidemiology (see Figure 2.3), *deductive reasoning* often involves using a general principle (or hypothesis) as a starting point for the collection, analysis and interpretation of data in order to confirm or refute this principle. *Inductive reasoning* typically involves the use of established facts (existing data and information) to draw a general conclusion or to confirm a hypothesis. Logic works in opposite directions for both deductive and inductive reasoning: Either from data to hypothesis formulation, acceptance or rejection or from *a priori* formulated hypotheses or propositions to the *ad hoc* gathering of data whose analysis and interpretation leads to the acceptance or rejection of the above. Debates on the preference of induction versus deduction continue. However, most research in this area is an iterative process centered on the flux between induction and deduction. As clinicians, we reason more or less successfully by induction (Francis Bacon, 1561–1626) rather than by deduction (René Descartes,

1596–1650). Let us look at an example of both inductive and deductive approaches to a clinical question. **By induction,** i.e. drawing a probable conclusion:

- This alcoholic patient who vomits fresh blood is known for having ruptured esophageal varices. (*Specific*)
- That alcoholic patient who vomits fresh blood is known for having ruptured esophageal varices. (*Specific*)
- Alcoholic patients who vomit fresh blood have ruptured esophageal varices. (*General*)

Often, clinicians try, successfully or not, to generalize beyond the basic argument: Alcoholic patients who vomit fresh blood bleed from ruptured esophageal varices. (Or, patients bleeding from ruptured esohpageal varices are alcoholics.) Such generalizations may not be always valid in the eyes of logicians.

Or:

- This delusional patient is schizophrenic. (*Specific*)
- That delusional patient is schizophrenic. (*Specific*)
- Delusional patients suffer from schizophrenia. (*General*)

By deduction, i.e. drawing a necessary conclusion:

- Alcoholic patients who vomit fresh blood have ruptured esophageal varices. (*General*)
- This patient who vomits fresh blood is an alcoholic. (*Specific*)
- Therefore, he has ruptured esophageal varices. (*Specific*)

Or:

- Delusional patients are schizophrenic (*General*)
- This patient is delusional (*Specific*)
- Therefore, he (she) must have schizophrenia (*Specific*). Let's check it out!

The validity of our concluding statements depend on the strength of evidence that **all** alcoholic patients who have ruptured esophageal varicose veins vomit fresh blood, or that **all** patients who bleed from esophageal varices are alcoholics or, for the second example, that **all** delusional patients suffer from schizophrenia, or that **all** schizophrenics are delusional. Everything depends on the question asked.

Let us return now to **induction and deduction in logic** and the specific meaning of these terms in this domain. Arguments may be fallacious because of their material content, their wording or an improper inference. Modern logicians like George Boole or Bertrand Russell have also developed ways to deal with deductive arguments other than categorical syllogisms[12]. For some, deduction ('leading forth', 'evolutionary', 'unfolding') means that once a set of axioms (uncontested facts) has been established, all their logical consequences are already fixed[25]. On the other hand, we can make other predictions, which follow inductively (with probability) from one's basis like in clinical prognosis at the hospital or weather forecasting outside. Formal logic focuses on propositions and deductive arguments, and it abstracts from their content and structures or logical forms. In fact, it is an a priori study. In this respect, there is a contrast with the natural sciences and all other disciplines that depend on observation for their data[7].

Both deductive and inductive logic are equally important for medicine. For example, we may particularly need deductive logic (deductively valid arguments) in making crucial therapeutic decisions and handling critical cases and situations in medicine and surgery. On the other hand, there is no meaningful prognosis without the best possible inductive logic and its inductively strong arguments.

3.2.3.3 *Implications of logic for medicine*

Don't we need the elements of logic when making a diagnosis, searching for causes or assessing the effect of treatment? If logic is a methodology of discussion and argument, don't we use it during clinical rounds, when making a differential diagnosis during consultations or when preparing research grant applications? Definitely! Diagnostic work-ups, choices of treatment and making prognosis are all, in fact, a sequence of arguments. Their premises and conclusions should be as solid as possible. Ideally, the premises should be the best evidence available, leading to an equally best evidence based conclusion. For example:

Premise A: Experience and clinical trials show that streptococcal throat infections are effectively cured and their complications prevented by antibiotics.

Premise B: My patient has a scarlet colored infiltration of the nasopharynx, hypertrophied tonsils covered by white patches and palpable submandibular lymph nodes. A laboratory exam of the throat swab confirms a streptococcal infection and its sensitivity to antibiotics.

Conclusion C: My patient can be cured effectively and the complications of her condition prevented by antibiotics.

There are two ways of researching in mathematics or in any other discipline (B. Russell)[7]: one aims at expansion, the other at exploring the foundations. However, uses of logic in medicine are not metaphysical. Instead, logic helps us better understand and make decisions in practice and research.

Many elements of general logic are already present in medicine. For example, epidemiologists or other clinical researchers refer to '**class**' or '**set theory**'[7,26,27] when forming groups to compare: sick or healthy, at risk individuals, employee categories, disease groups, etc. In reverse, some ideas originating in medicine expanded into the larger framework of logic. For example, the word '*semiotic*' was used by John Locke in the seventeenth century to describe the science of signs and significations[7] related to the medical theory of symptoms. **Semiotics** is now the general science of signs and languages. Patient/doctor communication in medicine is a field of semiotics[28]. In **applied logic**, one adapts elements from pure logic, like syllogisms, and applies them to beliefs or commands such as clinical orders or public health program choices and implementations. Pure logic is not interested in the persuasive power of arguments. The correct pathway of reasoning and link between premises and conclusions are of main interest. Salmon[21] stresses that '. . . *since the logical correctness or incorrectness of an argument depends solely upon the relation between the premises and the conclusion and is completely independent of the truth of the premises, we can analyze arguments without knowing whether the premises are true – indeed, we can do so even when they are known to be false.*' He is right. However, in health sciences and their practice, we need more. **In medical applications of logic, we cannot afford not to pay equal attention to the quality and solidity of evidence supporting conclusions, these being medical decisions and recommendations followed by actions. Acceptable medical reasoning relies on the combination of way of thinking and evidence(s) supporting it.**

Just as there is a *logic of understanding* (see above), is there a *logic of commands* when it comes to instructions or clinical orders? One can reason based on a set of commands: 'Do not give these gravely ill patients less than three drugs and do not give them more than four!' This might imply that the patients should receive three or four drugs. The logic of medical orders in practice still remains poorly understood and has not yet been studied enough. This should be remedied since illogical orders can obviously be detrimental to patient health. At this point, the reader might like to view floor rounds as a build-up of sequences of logical arguments in order to assess the fundamental quality of clinical reasoning and decisions. He or she might also like to look at the kind of evidence that is used to reach correct or incorrect conclusions.

So how should we view a connection between medical logic and evidence-based medicine? Until now, EBM focused mainly on the search, evaluation and application of evidence. Medical logic shows the gnostic mechanisms of how to use evidence by integrating it effectively into clinical and scientific reasoning in health sciences. Good medicine requires success in both evidence and logic, as well as in their uses. It is one of EBM's tasks to ensure the truthfulness of premises and conclusions. Physicians must see that the arguments respond to the common laws of formal logic <u>and</u> that both premises and conclusions are true, i.e. based on the best possible evidence be it an experimental proof, solid clinical experience or both. Why is this so? Because physicians may harm the patient under clinical care and entire communities in public health in three ways:

- If their conclusions do not follow from the information they have.
- If their premises are not true, i.e. based on weak and unacceptable evidence, which does not reflect the reality to which it is supposed to be applied.

- If both the reasoning and supporting evidence are bad.

For example, is our reasoning correct if we say:

Premise A: All physicians wear a white coat.
Premise B: Mary-Ann wears a white coat.
Conclusion C: Mary-Ann is a physician?

Certainly not! One may argue right away that other health professionals, laboratory technicians and many employees in the food or electronic industries wear white coats too. One may also state that all physicians do not necessarily wear white coats, since many psychiatrists don't. Hence, a logical argument may be formally or structurally correct, but not necessarily true and supported by satisfactory evidence of the full reality of the problem.

Similar discrepancies between reasoning, supporting evidence and the reality of the problem may occur anywhere in medical practice and research. We would certainly refute some clinical novice's argument that:

Premise A: Sore throats in younger sufferers are often caused by beta-hemolytic group A streptococci.
Premise B: Undesirable late complications of 'strep throats' like rheumatic fever may be prevented by antibiotics.
Conclusion C: All sore throat sufferers must receive penicillin.

In such an argument, cases, causes, differential diagnosis and treatment indications are poorly defined, based on poor criteria and all these considerations are not exhaustive of the reality of sore throats, their candidates, and the whole spectrum of clinical management of this problem. For example, are all cases of sore throat, 'strep throat'? (i.e. all caused by a bacterial infection treatable by antibiotics). If not, how many patients suffer from late complications when not treated by antibiotics? Is there enough evidence available on how many of these patients benefit from treatment by antibiotics? Our novice also extends what is true of younger sufferers from sore throats to all sore throat sufferers, whatever their age may be. Skilful execution of clinical maneuvers must be based on the mastery of reasoning which leads to their choice and real and expected performance.

3.3 Uncertainty and probability in medicine

Statements and conclusions in our logical discourses may be made either with certainty or with some lesser degree of probability. Essentially, there are three possible 'operating systems' of reasoning in medicine:

- Probability theory and its applications (well established).
- Chaos theory and its uses in clinical research (emerging).
- Fuzzy logic and fuzzy sets theory in handling imperfect or hard to interpret data (also emerging and increasingly attractive for many).

Are these tools contradictory or complementary?

3.3.1 *Determinism vs. uncertainty*

Past generations of physicians tried to make medicine 'as scientific as possible' by adopting a **deterministic paradigm of medicine**. This was accomplished by sending medicine to the laboratory and operating theatres. As an example, Pasteur's postulates defined infection and a surgeon could see, touch, and repair a ruptured organ. In the last century, medicine shifted towards the **probabilistic paradigm of medicine**. In medicine, we refer to probability more than we think. For example, a surgical resident admits a patient with an acute abdomen and concludes his or her report not by a definitive diagnosis, but by an 'impression': peritonitis, possibly ruptured appendix. Such a formulation can also be quantified in terms of probability.

Already in the 1980s, Bryant and Norman[29] paid attention to ways of translating natural clinical language into probabilities. In their spirit, one might ask: What does it means that an incipient sepsis is *probable* in this patient? What does it means that signs and symptoms in this young woman are *compatible* with extra-uterine pregnancy? These authors asked 16 clinicians to estimate the likelihood of presence of disease (from 0 to 1) associated with various frequent expressions in communication of

clinical findings. Figure 3.1 illustrates their findings. For example, for these 16 clinicians, a 'probable' disease or other event meant a 0.8 probability of patients having it. A 'doubtful' success of treatment meant a 0.2 probability of success of clinical intervention, and a 'moderate probability' indicated a 0.5 probability according to the clinicians. This is just one example of the importance of probability in the daily life of clinicians. The management of clinical problems by different physicians and its success may reflect meanings attributed to words used to reflect probability.

3.3.1.1 *'Classical' theory of probability*

The same surgical resident may know from experience and the literature that from 10 patients in similar conditions and at that stage of diagnostic work-up, 4 may have a ruptured appendix. Aside from an **absolute number** or **frequency** of such an event, i.e. 4, this experience may be quantified in three basic ways stemming from probability theory:

1. The **probability** of this event is quantified from 0 to 1.0. In this case, the probability is 4/10, four in 10 or 0.4 or the surgical resident can say that he is 40% sure that this patient has a ruptured appendix pending a more detailed evaluation of this case. Probability is a quantified expression or scale of the likelihood of an event, chance, or certainty.

2. **Odds** are the ratio of likelihood of the occurrence and non-occurrence of an event. For example:

$$4 : 6$$

Odds in terms of probability equal = $p/1 - p$

3. **Likelihood** is defined in the most general terms and very broadly as '*the probability of observed results (in a sample) given the estimates of the population parameters*' or as '*the conditional probability of observed frequencies given expected frequencies*'[30]. However, statisticians have more precise definitions for a 'likelihood function'[31].

We will see more about these expressions in Chapter 5 (health indicators) and Chapter 8 (search for causes of disease). Observations in medicine are often quantified in terms of probabilities and odds, which can then be considered **relative frequencies** (one

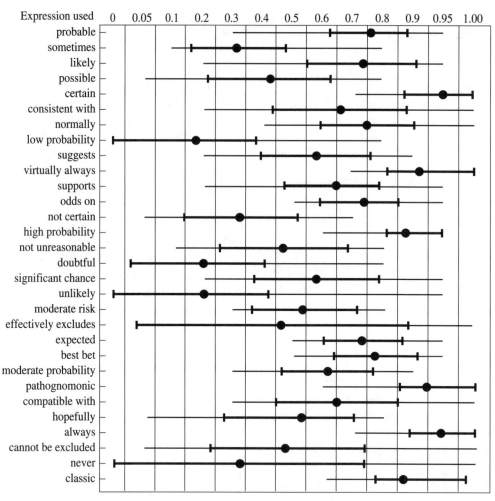

Figure 3.1 Subjective probability estimates of common terms used in routine clinical communication.
Source: Ref. 29. Reproduced with permission from the Massachusetts Medical Society

frequency plotted against something else, such as another frequency). Uncertainty and working with probabilities in a formal and colloquial sense is a ubiquitous and perennial attribute of medical practice[32,33] and research[34]. The most frequent question that practitioners hear from their patients is: 'Doctor, what are my chances?', whether the question relates to the probability of developing a disease (risk), of having it (diagnosis), of being cured (effective treatment) or of having good or bad outcomes (prognosis). An interest in games of chance led to John Graunt's application of ideas of relative frequency to plague mortality statistics in seventeenth century London. More fundamental contributions to probability theory were later made by Jakob

Bernouilli and Abraham de Moivre. Panufty Lvovich Chebyshev and Francis Galton also enhanced this field[35].

One of the basic ideas of probability theory is that under ideal conditions a repeated experiment could result in different outcomes in different trials. Such a set of outcomes is called a **sample space**. Our conclusions about possible outcomes depend on initial information or rules representing **conditional probabilities**. For example, our understanding of the spread of AIDS depends (is conditional) on our knowledge of its agent (a virus) and its mode of transmission from one person to another. Additional probabilities are produced by events themselves, such as a diagnostic process or a clinical trial.

According to probability theory, events are considered *a priori* as independent. Our search for causes of disease or an effective treatment seeks to disprove that events are independent, that they occur together **at random** only. The truth of any argument or proposition is uncertain. Such **uncertainty** can be partly, completely, or never elucidated by observational or experimental analytical research. This persisting variable degree of uncertainty led to the development of the theory and practice of decision-making in medicine as outlined later in this reading. What are the causes of this uncertainty?

- Our poor knowledge of the problem under study (etiology of essential hypertension or many cancers).
- Missing data for the complete understanding of a problem if all data are needed to solve the problem. However, 'there is never enough of data'.
- All available data are not correct because of poor measurement.
- Findings are poorly interpreted.
- Time, place and patients' demographic and clinical characteristics may vary.
- Conclusions are erroneously put into practice.
- Effectiveness of implemented decisions is not realistically determined.
- Poor distinctions are made between causes of disease cases and disease as an entity as well as between causes of disease itself (risk) and those of disease course and outcomes (prognosis).

This applies to research as well as to practice.

Most of our conclusions bear a certain degree of **randomness**. We are not always absolutely sure that the patient has the disease we diagnose. For example, we might be uncertain about the recurrence of cancer after the surgical removal of its primary lesion. Our conclusions are more or less **educated guesses**, based on our experience and our knowledge of **axioms** (uncontested facts), causes, gauging uncertainty, and uses of probability. A **stochastic process** is a process that incorporates some degree of randomness[36]. It is a search for truth that also accepts some degree of uncertainty. Those who use the technical term 'stochastic' want to circumvent the ambiguities of the term *random*[37] (governed by chance) or *statistical*

significance[38]. The Bayes theorem[39], formulated in the eighteenth century, was revolutionary for its probabilistic considerations that, in medicine, are mainly concentrated in the area of diagnosis (*vide infra*). However, it also applies to other kinds of evidence. For Murphy[37], two important conclusions can be drawn from Bayes' views:

1. In all but trivial cases, there is uncertainty. There are therefore always at least two conjectures or explanations under consideration.
2. The most rational assessment of evidence is that which combines the evidence included in it so far (*the prior evidence*) with the current further evidence (*the posterior evidence*) to produce a *revised evidence* (modified evidence).

One of the other important characteristics of our observations within the framework of probability theory is our 'black or white' (binary) categorization of events. Subjects are either male or female, young or old, healthy or sick (with a disease of interest). They are treated or not, they are exposed or not to noxious factors like carcinogens or poor diet. Hence, such characteristics and events, as well as their associations may be subjects of studies based on the probabilistic view of events.

Goodman's view aptly concludes this section: '. . . *Making clinical sense of a case means explaining its logic: why the patient exhibits certain symptoms, how this patient is similar to others, how various findings relate, and the mechanism by which interventions will affect the future outcome. In groups, individual details are averaged out, but these details may be critical to the causal explanation for an individual patient. Inevitably, however, a gap exists between what we understand in a given patient and what we are able to predict: this is where probability fits in . . .*'[33]. More about the fundamentals of probability theory[35,40] and its applications to medicine[41,42] can be found in the literature.

3.3.1.2 Chaos theory vs. probability theory. Beyond classical logic and probability

Chaos is another more recent paradigm of our ways of thinking. In the last half century, this theory was brought from its origins outside medicine to the attention of the general public[43] and to physicians in general medicine[44,45] as well. The history of chaos theory since its origins in the 1960s and its connection to medicine can be found in Theodorescu et al[46] and Barro and Jain's[47] reviews. For Lorenz et al[48], chaos or a chaotic process, is a combination of stochastic and deterministic events; stochastic behavior occurring in a deterministic system. Chaos theory explains small causes leading to disproportionately big consequences or irregular pathological–physiological phenomena such as fibrillation or shock. Colloquially, we define chaos as 'a state of utter confusion and disorder'[11]. According to chaos theory, 'chaos' is defined differently. It is seen as '*an aperiodic, seemingly random behavior in a deterministic system that exhibits sensitive dependence on initial conditions*'[49] or as '*apparently random or unpredictable behavior in systems governed by deterministic laws*'[6]. Hence, we can consider it a 'certain mess that can be explained, understood and used for the purpose of action'. The basic characteristics[49] of chaos are:

- It is both deterministic and aperiodic,
- It exhibits sensitive dependence on initial conditions,
- It is constrained to a relatively narrow range,
- It has a definite form (pattern),
- Small causes may lead to more important consequences,
- There is not necessarily a linear relationship between cause and effect,
- For proponents of chaos theory, the deterministic physical universe is nonetheless unpredictable because of the unavoidable uncertainties in our knowledge of initial conditions. The weather, organisms, road traffic and the stock market[50] are chaotic. If the physical universe is unpredictable (given our unavoidable uncertainties), how predictable are we or our health?

Various events act as **attractors** or point towards certain other events. An attractor is a non-chaotic fixed point where all motion eventually dies[50]. Cardiac arrest can be seen as a fixed-point attractor with the possibility of its reverse by resuscitation and other clinical means. According to Firth, various states (health, disease or death) can be considered

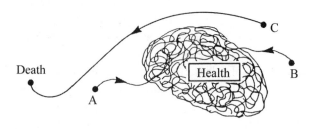

Figure 3.2 Health and death as coexisting attractors. Schema of 'health' and 'death' as two coexistent attractors. Unhealthy states A and B recover along the trajectories shown, but C is fatal. Source: Ref 50. Reproduced with permission of the BMJ Publishing Group

attractors[50] as illustrated in Figure 3.2. He speculates that medical treatment mainly affects the rate, rather than the fact of recovery. Return to health is a predictable path, even if the healthy state itself is chaotic.

Chaotic attractors may be **fractals**, or objects that have a similar structure according to many measurement scales like microbes under different magnification or branching of vessels. A bronchial tree such as in the branching of the trachea into smaller and smaller airways, the dendrite branching of nerve cells or blood vessels, and the branching pattern of certain cardiac muscles and in the His–Purkinje system all bear characteristics of fractals and their geometry[51,52]. Self-similarity of branching can be observed from one of its levels to another, from the biggest to the smallest. Chaos theory suggests that fractals, like seashores in nature or branching in various morphological and physiological systems, are a product of chaos. The more closely a fractal structure is observed, the more similar a pattern is observed. Fractals themselves are becoming bearers or substrates of chaotic behavior. Redundancy and irregularity in fractal structures make them robust and resistant to injury. Functions (and not just morphologies) also share fractal characteristics[51].

More refined measurements of physiological activities in the nervous system or of heart beats or white blood cell counts show that they are rather irregular ('chaotic') and that their 'regularization' precedes critical arrhythmia of a dying heart[53,54], epileptic or Parkinson's crisis or manic depression[51], stroke[55], tumor growth[56] and possibly other phenomena like aging[57] or Alzheimer's disease[58]. This does not hold, however, for all pathologies and functions. In epidemiology, the spread of some infectious diseases, especially in developing countries, can also be seen as 'chaotic'[59–61]. In health services evaluation[62], hospital emergency services can be considered 'chaotic' and remedies to improve their functioning might benefit from such an interpretation[63]. However, views about the role of chaos theory in organizational science and management are still not unanimous[64,65].

Usually, biological systems are thought of as *linear*[49], where one function depends on another. Such a relationship between a dependent and an independent variable can be plotted graphically. Chaotic behavior is *non-linear*. Small changes can lead to disproportionate effects[64]. An extreme sensitivity to initial conditions of chaotic behavior[51] might partly corroborate with older observations that the magnitude of biological responses can also depend on the initial value of a given physiological function. (See Chapter 1 for discussions on Heiby's *theory of reverse effect*[65] of drugs and other substances and Wilder's basimetric approach to the interpretation of biological responses based on his *law of initial value*[66].) Hence, in a sense, chaos theory flies in the face of the '*milieu intérieur stable*' (Claude Bernard's stable internal environment) and *homeostasis,* i.e. a natural trend of the organism to keep the internal (body) environment stable as understood by Walter Cannon[67,68]. Given this, is it healthy to be 'chaotic'[69,64]? We can also speculate that the *milieu intérieur stable* (i.e. stable internal environment) is 'chaotic' in the deterministic sense and that homeostasis, as an effort to keep the internal environment stable, is actually an effort to keep the internal environment 'chaotic'. However, any disruption of chaos in terms of reaching some stability or regularity must have its cause(s) and such a cause–effect relationship calls for explanations. Proponents of the chaos theory consider chaos as a deterministic phenomenon. It remains to be seen how deterministic 'cause' or 'effect' are in cause–effect relationships. This also challenges our traditional view that cause–effect relationships (like drinking and liver cirrhosis or smoking and cancer) in epidemiology are more or less linear. A better understanding and use of

chaos theory might explain and improve our persisting uncertainties in the fields of diagnosis, prognosis and elsewhere. Firth[50] gives an example of a heartbeat which is normally slightly irregular (no important attractor present) and which becomes more regular before a heart attack (a more important attractor present).

Chaos *per se* is seen as a non-linear process. Epidemic or pandemic spread of disease from seemingly less important index cases can also be viewed as 'chaotic', where the difference between two states that are initially closely similar grows exponentially over time[50]. In the future, we should therefore find other ways to analyze and interpret data in medicine. As usual, the path leading from theory to practical applications will not necessarily be short. It is not enough to compute and properly quantify differences in our observations. An equally challenging feat is the interpretation of one biological response after another, explaining their meaning as a whole and assessing how such information can be used for practical decisions in clinical action. Currently, chaos theory has important potential implications in epidemiology:

- A loss of chaos can be considered an independent variable and a possible cause closely preceding a critical morbid state (consequence).
- In reverse, a loss of chaos can be considered a consequence of some causal factors that remain to be identified.
- It can prove useful in elucidating prognosis of some diseases.
- It sets some limits for our complete understanding of causes or consequences of health and disease.
- It can suggest cause–effect relationships where none were previously suspected[69].
- As the paradigm of homeostasis, chaos theory remains for the moment a theory with an increasing number of experiences confirming its acceptability in several, but not all cases.
- Experiences with chaos theory may prove useful in diagnosis, as in the assessment of risks of heart attack from ECG or therapeutic-like reading oscillations of white blood cells in the treatment of chronic myelogenic leukemia, when setting a pacemaker, administering insulin, suppressing

tremors, treating epileptics or controlling out-of-sync circadian rhythms[70].

- It shows why a transfer of experience based on groups of individuals to an individual patient is often so challenging[71].

Crutchfield et al's statement[70] might, in fact, be the best conclusion for this discussion on chaos:

'The existence of chaos affects the science method itself. The classic approach to verifying a theory is to make predictions and test them against experimental data. If the phenomena are chaotic, however, long-term predictions are intrinsically impossible ... Chaos brings a new challenge to the reductionist view that a system can be understood by breaking it down and studying each piece. This view has been prevalent in science in part because there are so many systems for which the behavior of the whole is indeed a sum of its parts. Chaos demonstrates, however, that a system can have a complicated behavior that emerges as a consequence of a simple non-linear interaction of only a few components.'[70]

And what if chaos theory emerges just on the basis of more refined observation and measurement? Paradigms of chaos and homeostasis should then not be too mutually exclusive.

3.3.1.3 Fuzzy logic and fuzzy sets theory

Our observations are subject to random and systematic errors in measurement and interpretation as well. Different combinations of clinical and paraclinical manifestations occur in different patients and throughout the clinical course of disease. In addition, the biological nature of our observations and data in medicine makes them not only imperfect and incomplete, but also hard to interpret and explain. In daily life, we can remove sugar grain by grain from a spoon. However, when does this spoon cease to be a spoon of sugar? In medicine, our evaluation of low or high blood sugar can be difficult if values are assessed in small increments. Theoretically, a fasting glycemia of 3.7 mmol/l (668 mg/l) which is at the lower limit of the 95% normal range for adults, can be considered low, as well as that of 3.4, etc. At 5.18 (higher limit) and higher, we might consider glycemia still

normal but a bit high, then high, then definitely high and finally, we might assign it a diagnostic value as it becomes an indication for treatment. As glycemia increases, the degree of fit of its interpretation as a 'normal blood sugar level' decreases and vice versa. Figure 3.3 illustrates the qualification of blood pressure into sets using classical (probabilistic) and fuzzy logic by anesthetists[72]. For Steinmann[73], these 'sets of observations' are the subject of symbolic reasoning as a model of human thinking. Data are symbols to which we assign some meaning. Our meaning is imperfect because hypoglycemia or hyperglycemia, hypertension or hypotension can mean several values whose sets (or ensembles) are imprecise, overlapping or 'fuzzy'. Such vague concepts are the subject of **fuzzy sets theory**.

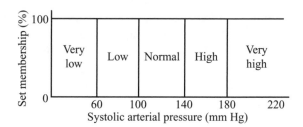

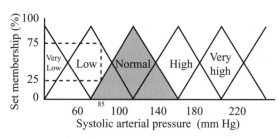

Figure 3.3 Classical and fuzzy categorization of systolic blood pressure. *Upper portion*: Sub-division of systolic arterial pressure into sets using classical logic. The boundaries of sets do not overlap. *Lower portion*: Sub-division of systolic arterial pressure into sets using fuzzy logic. The boundaries of each set form a triangle (e.g. the shaded area shows the extent of the 'normal' set) and overlap with neighboring sites. Dotted lines show the set membership for the value of 85 mm H_g. Source: Ref. 72. Reproduced with permission of the Board of Management and Trustees of the *British Journal of Anaesthesia* and Oxford University Press

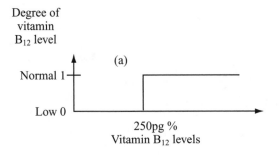

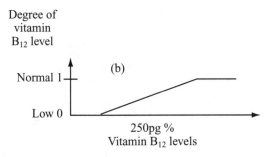

Figure 3.4 Classical and fuzzy representation of vitamin B$_{12}$ levels. (a) Classical logic representation of normal and low vitamin B$_{12}$ levels. (b) Fuzzy set for normal B$_{12}$ levels. Each possible level corresponds to a degree of normalcy. Source; Ref. 74. Reproduced with permission of the *Journal of Neurovascular Diseases* and Prime Publishing

In probability theory and applications, we simplify demarcations and limits of **sets**, i.e. collections of defined or distinct items. We clearly define who is healthy and who is ill, who smokes and who does not, who is treated and who is not. In fuzzy sets theory, such a binary system (yes or no, 'black' or 'white', 0 or 1) is replaced by a scale of values from 0 to 1, 'yes, perhaps, probably, definitely no', and different shades of gray between white and black. **Fuzzy sets** infuse the notion of continuity perhaps in both deductive and inductive thinking. Probabilities measure whether something will occur or not. Fuzziness measures the degree to which something occurs or some conditions exist[63]. It fills up Aristotle's 'excluded middle'. In an example dealing with B$_{12}$ levels, Dickerson and Helgason[74] show how such an 'excluded middle' is 'filled-up' in fuzzy sets theory (Figure 3.4).

If diagnostic, therapeutic or prognostic reasoning are based on the assessment of several variables that might be considered 'fuzzy sets', they require some kind of logic to deal effectively with such *multidimensional spaces* of vagueness, i.e. they need **fuzzy logic**. This logic is not fuzzy in itself since it is based on solid mathematical foundations[75]. However, the data to which it is applied are fuzzy. Different fuzzy sets can belong to other sets as well. From applications in industry, fuzzy theory moved into such disparate medical specialties as neurology[55,74], anesthesiology[72], nuclear medicine[76,77], oncology[78], biomedical engineering[79,80], psychiatry[81,82], clinical pharmacology[83], surgery[84–86], epidemiology of infectious disease[87], veterinary medicine[88,89] and nutrition[90], among others[91].

Bellamy[88] proposes that the multidimensional space depiction of a patient, combined with a fuzzy sets representation of the demographic, clinical and paraclinical variables characterizing the patient leads to a fuzzy systems model of the diagnostic process that can be implemented on a computer as a fuzzy decision system. Figure 3.5 illustrates that a web of observations having a potential diagnostic value can be linked to a web of diagnostic entities. Figure 3.6 shows that in a multidimensional analysis of several fuzzy systems (variables having potential diagnostic value), transitional diagnostic or prognostic corridors can be established between health and disease indicating an extension of membership to one or another of these categories. In human nutrition, Wirsam and Uthus[90] used the fuzzy theory to identify foods that should be a part of dietary recommendations. Figure 3.7 shows their evaluation of whole wheat bread and milk relative to values (Prerow's) indicating closeness to desirable recommended levels. Tri-(cubes) or multidimensional evaluations can be considered. Repeated evaluations in time should allow the assessment of the evolution of such diagnostic systems in relation to various attractors known from chaos theory.

Fuzzy diagnostic work-up methodology is basically common for medicine and veterinary medicine. For example, just as veterinarians are interested in the differential diagnosis of various problems in a postpartum cow[89], such as different forms of mastitis, or peritonitis, chronic infection, simple indigestion, vitamin D-like toxicity and other states[89], neurologists can be interested in the differential

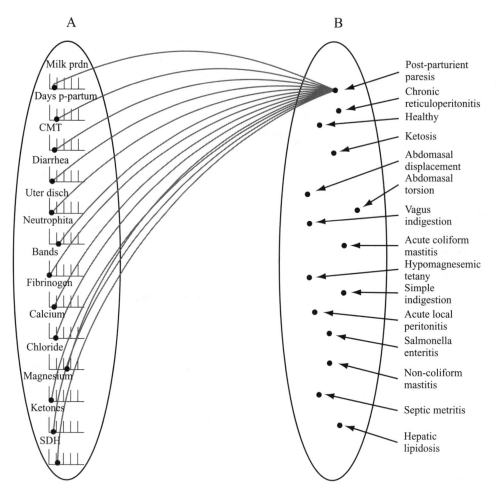

Figure 3.5 Webs of observations in fuzzy handling of differential diagnosis. The diagnostic process corresponds to a function of mapping between sets. In this example of a postpartum cow, the diagnosis is represented as a mapping from set A (values for properties of the cow) to set B (diagnostic categories for postpartum cows). The specific input values map the diagnosis 'postpartum paresis.' N.B. Non-veterinarians, read 'patient' instead of 'cow'. Source: Ref. 88. Reproduced with permission of the American Veterinary Medical Association

diagnosis of ischemic and hemorrhagic stroke, identification of underlying cerebral and subarachnoid hemorrhage. Cardioembolic, atherothromboembolic, lacunar and other ischemic strokes must also be differentiated[55]. Both examples have a similar fuzzy basis.

Even if fuzzy sets analysis provides a transitional opinion about a disease and better subsequent clinical decisions, some important questions remain unanswered. If the patient is diagnosed with a disease, he is treated. If the patient is probably sick, the decision to treat will depend on treatment effectiveness, cost, as well as on adverse effects noted in healthy, 'semi-ill' and definitely sick patients.

Treating healthy subjects is a malpractice carrying multiple risks for the 'healthy patient' who could also be called a misdiagnosed other disease sufferer. In many situations, a practitioner will require a clear identification of who is sick and who is not and who is a candidate for treatment.

Until now, medicine benefited most from probability theory and its applications. However, newer paradigms like chaos and fuzziness also make sense in many instances. Their use will require evaluation. Do they lead to a better diagnosis and consequently to a more effective treatment and better prognosis than probability theory? Does the patient benefit markedly from these new uses? In the near future,

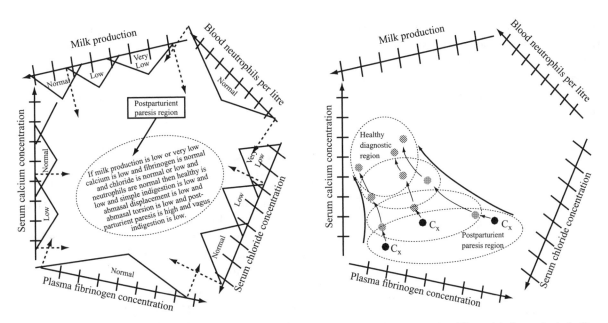

Figure 3.6 Multidimensional analysis and prognostic corridors in fuzzy sets applications to the differential diagnosis. *Left*: If each input variable or dimension of a diagnostic space is represented as a series of overlapping fuzzy subsets (e.g. normal, low, very low) certain combinations of fuzzy subsets correspond with particular diagnostic categories. *Right*: The diagnostic region for 'postparturient paresis' is equivalent to the fuzzy rule described in the right portion of the Figure (3.6). Source: Ref. 88. Reproduced with permission of the American Veterinary Medical Association

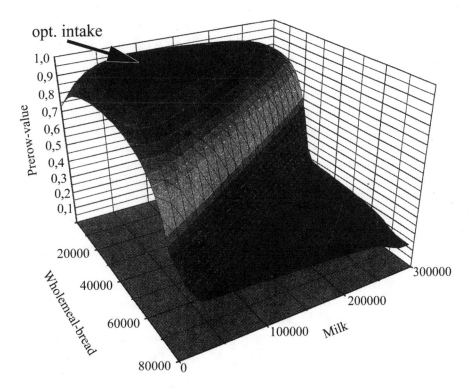

Figure 3.7 Response surface illustrating Prerow value linked to the variation of two dietary components. Source: Ref. 90. Reproduced with the Authors' permission

clinical trials including competing theories and strategies should provide answers to such pragmatic questions. If fuzzy systems act as universal approximators to handle complex, non-linear, imprecise and often conflicting relationships in multi-dimensional systems with a minimum of rules[88], an ensuing **fuzzy decision-making theory** and its application must still be perfected.

3.4 Conclusions

Reasoning is thinking enlightened by logic[92]. Rules of practice, basic and experimental research[37,93] as well as epidemiology, clinical epidemiology and EBM are based on such reasoning. In return, all these disciplines help better structure our reasoning for the benefit of the patient and mastering them, therefore, becomes a necessity. Obtaining valuable evidence is not enough. Its use must be logical too.

We are currently working within the framework of three complementary rather than competing theories: probability and uncertainty, chaos, fuzzy sets. Let us not make the mistake of pitting one against another. Griffiths and Byrne[94] state that '. . . *There are two current trends in general practice research that may appear contradictory: the promotion of evidence-based practice with a high value given to the numerical outcome research; and the increasing interest in qualitative research. The theories of chaos and complexity help us understand the link between qualitative research, where the results are categories of data and interpretation of meaning, and quantitative research, where outcome is measured.*'. All these old and new paradigms and theories may apply both to human biology and health care. Human heart activity as well as emergency services or walk-in clinics functioning may be 'chaotic'.

Probability theory served us well and continues to do so. Only the future and more experience with these approaches to health problems will show how chaotic and fuzzy the world is and how much is uncertain and probable. The impact of chaos on science and society

is, however, widening[95]. For the moment, a disproportionate volume of experience lies in the area of probability theory. To correct such imbalance between classical and fuzzy logic (see Chapter 12), fuzzy theory and fuzzy logic still must prove themselves as practical tools in daily medical thinking, practice and decisions. This is not an easy task.

What is medicine today from the point of view of formal thinking? It is many things:

- **Philosophy** (i.e. a formal inquiry into the structure of medical thought)[37,93]
- **Semiotics** (i.e. a study of the interpretation of signs, as a part of hermeneutics)[28]
- **Hermeneutics** (i.e. the art of interpretation in its broadest sense)[96]
- **Logic** (or flawless reasoning)[93,97,98]
- **Decision-making oriented** (i.e. showing how to translate all of the above into the best possible action)[99], and
- **Evidence-based.**

To be purposeful, evidence must be used logically and logic must be backed by evidence. Their joint use is a must. The patient can be harmed as much by the illogical use of evidence as by the use of a logical decision unsupported by evidence and even more, by the use of faulty logic without evidence.

Logic has made important inroads in everyday life and practice. If, for example, lawyers already have their own 'logic for lawyers'[100,101], should there not be some better, more complete and adapted 'logic for physicians'? The chapters that follow outline the essentials of acceptable evidence and its uses. They will show not only how important it is to support logical reasoning through evidence to make it relevant for interpretations and decisions in health sciences. They will also discuss how to obtain this evidence and how to judge its quality and acceptability. Basic principles will be outlined too on how to use it in a structured, focused and logical way within different fields of clinical and community health oriented activities that, on a lighter note, should be neither chaotic, nor fuzzy.

REFERENCES

1. *The Columbia Encyclopaedia*, Sixth Edition (electronic), 2001. www.bartleby.com

2. Murzi M. Logical positivism. In: *The Internet Encyclopedia of Philosophy*, 2001

3. Salmon MH, Earman J, Glymour C, et al. *Introduction to the Philosophy of Science. A Text by Members of the Department of the History and Philosophy of Science of the University of Pittsburgh.* Englewood Cliffs: Prentice-Hall, 1992

4. Engel SM. *The Chain of Logic.* Englewood Cliffs: Prentice-Hall, 1987

5. Ennis RH. *Critical Thinking.* Upper Saddle River: Prentice-Hall, 1996

6. Department of Philosophy, University of Guelph. *Logic Outline.* 7th edition, revised. Guelph: University of Guelph, November 2000. (22 pages, mimeographed)

7. Hughes GE, Wang H, Roscher N. The History and Kinds of Logic. In: McHenry R ed. *The New Encyclopaedia Britannica.* Macropedia/Knowledge in Depth. Volume 23. Chicago: Encyclopaedia Britannica Inc, 1992:226–82

8. *Websters Dictionary©, On-line Medical Dictionary*, 1998. www.graylab.ac.uk

9. *New Illustrated Webster's Dictionary of the English Language. Including Thesaurus of Synonyms & Antonyms.* New York: PAMCO Publishing Co., 1992

10. Neufeldt V, Guralnik DB (eds). *Webster's New World Dictionary of American English.* Third College Edition. Cleveland & New York: Webster's New World, 1988

11. Brown L (ed.). *The New Shorter Oxford English Dictionary on Historical Principles.* Volume 1 (A–M). Oxford: Clarendon Press, 1993

12. Barnhart CL, Barnhart RK (eds). *The World Book Dictionary.* Chicago: World Book, Inc., 1987

13. Schagrin ML. Logic. In: *The World Book Encyclopedia.* Chicago: World Book, Inc., 1992

14. *Encarta® World English Dictionary.* New York: St. Martin's Press, 1999

15. Logic and Argument. In: *The Guiness Encyclopedia.* Enfield: Guinness Publishing Ltd., 1990:494–6

16. *The New Encyclopaedia Britannica.* Vol.7. Micropaedia. Chicago: Encyclopaedia Britannica, Inc., 1992

17. Briskman L. Doctors and witchdoctors: Which doctors are which? – I. *Br Med J*, 1987;**295**:1033–6

18. George Boole and the mathematic of logic. Two chapters from Boole's *The Mathematical Analysis of Logic* (1847) and other excerpts reprinted in: *MD Computing*, 1992;**9**:165–74

19. Briskman L. Doctors and witchdoctors: Which doctors are which? – II. *Br Med J*, 1987;**295**:1108–10

20. Thornton S, Popper K. In: *Stanford Encyclopaedia of Philosophy.* Stanford: Stanford University, 2000. URL: http://plato.Stanford.edu

21. Salmon WC. *Logic.* Englewood Cliffs: Prentice Hall, Inc., 1963

22. Michalos AC. *Improving Your Reasoning.* Second edition. Englewood Cliffs: Pretnice-Hall, 1986

23. Copi IM. *Informal Logic.* New York: Macmillan, 1986

24. Klenk V. *Understanding Symbolic Logic.* Third edition. Englewood Cliffs: Prentice Hall, 1994

25. Cutler P. *Problem Solving in Clinical Medicine. From Data to Diagnosis.* 2nd edition. Baltimore: Williams & Wilkins, 1985

26. Lipschutz S. *Set Theory and Related Topics.* Second Edition. Schaum's Outline Series. New York: McGraw-Hill, 1998

27. Haight M. The logic of sets. In: *The Snake and the Fox. An Introduction to Logic.* London and New York: Routledge, 1999;**29–32**:193–218

28. Nessa J. About signs and symptoms: Can semiotics expand the view of clinical medicine? *Theor Med*, 1996;**17**:363–77

29. Bryant GD, Norman GR. Expressions of probability: Words and numbers. Letter to The Editor. *N Engl J Med*, 1980;**302**:411

30. Vogt WP. *Dictionary of Statistics and Methodology. A Nontechnical Guide for the Social Sciences.* Newbury Park: Sage Publications, 1993

31. Norman GR, Streiner DL. *Biostatistics. The Bare Essentials.* Second Edition. Hamilton and London: BC Decker Inc., 2000

32. Redelmeier DA, Koehler DJ, Liberman V, Tversky A. Probability judgment in medicine: Discounting unspecified possibilities. *Med Decis Making*, 1995; **15**:227–30

33. Goodman SN. Probability at the bedside: The knowing of chances or the chances of knowing? *Ann Intern Med*, 1999;**130**:604–6

34. Greenland S. Probability logic and probabilistic induction. *Epidemiology*, 1997;**9**:322–32

35. Siegmund DO/ Probability theory. In: McHenry R ed. *The New Encyclopaedia Britannica. Macropedia/ Knowledge in Depth.* Vol 26. Chicago: Encyclopaedia Britannica, 1992:135–48

36. *Last JM (ed.). A Dictionary of Epidemiology.* Fourth edition. New York: Oxford University Press, 2001

37. Murphy EA. *The Logic of Medicine.* Second Edition. Baltimore and London: The Johns Hopkins University Press, 1997

38. Feinstein AR. Clinical biostatistics. LVII. A glossary of neologisms in quantitative clinical science. *Clin Pharmacol Ther*, 1981;**30**:564–77

39. Bayes T. An essay towards solving a problem in the doctrine of chances. (read 23 December 1763). *Biometrika*, 1958;**45**:296–315

40. Steele JM. Probability theory. In: Armitage P Colton T eds. *Encyclopedia of Biostatistics*. Vol 5. Chichester and New York: J Wiley & Sons, 1998:3256–9

41. Probability: Quantifying uncertainty. In: Sox HC, Blatt MA, Higgins MC, Marton KI eds. *Medical Decision Making*. Boston and London: Butterworths, 1988:27–65

42. Dawson NV. Physician Judgments of Uncertainty. In: Chapman GB Sonnenberg FA eds. *Decision Making in Health Care. Theory, Psychology, and Applications*. Cambridge: Cambridge University Press, 2000:211–52

43. Gleick J. *Chaos. Making a New Science*. New York: Penguin Books, 1987

44. Pruessner HT, Hensel WA, Rasco TL. The scientific basis of generalist medicine. *Acad Med*, 1992;**67**:235–5

45. Griffiths F, Byrne D. General practice and the new science emerging from theories of 'chaos' and complexity. *Br J Gen Pract*, 1998;**48**:1697–9

46. Fuzzy logic and neuro-fuzzy systems in medicine and biomedical engineering. A historical perspective. In: Teodorescu HN, Kandel A, Jain LC eds. *Fuzzy and Neuro-Fuzzy Systems in Medicine*. Boca Raton: CRC Press, 1999;**1**:3–16

47. Barro S, Marin R. A call for a stronger role for fuzzy logic in medicine. In: Barro S, Marin R eds. *Fuzzy Logic in Medicine*. Heidelberg and New York: Physica-Verlag, 2002:1–17

48. Lorenz W, McKneally M, Troidl H, et al. Surgical research around the world. In: *Surgical Research. Basic Principles and Clinical Practice*. Third Edition. New York: Springer-Verlag, 1998:637–54

49. Denton TA, Diamond GA, Helfant RTH, et al. Fascinating rhythm: A primer on chaos theory and its application to cardiology. *Am Heart J*, 1990;**120**:1419–40

50. Firth WJ. Chaos – predicting the unpredictable. *Br Med J*, 1991;**303**:1565–8

51. Goldberger AL, West JB. Fractals in physiology and medicine. *Yale J Biol Med*, 1987;**60**:421–35

52. Goldberger AL, Rigney DR, West BJ. Chaos and fractals in human physiology. *Sci Am*, 1990;**262**:42–9

53. Kleiger RE, Miller JP, Bigger JT, Moss AR, Multicenter Post-Infarction Research Group. Decreased heart rate variability and its association with increased mortality after acute myocardial infarction. *Am J Cardiol*, 1987;**59**:256–62

54. Goldberger AL, West BJ. Applications of nonlinear dynamics to clinical cardiology. *Ann NY Acad Sci*, 1987;**504**:195–213

55. Helgason CM, Jobe TH. Causal interactions, fuzzy sets and cerebrovascular 'accident': The limits of Evidence-Based Medicine and the advent of Complexity-Based Medicine. *Neuroepidemiology*, 1989;**18**:64–74

56. Cross SS, Cotton DWK. Chaos and antichaos in pathology. *Hum Pathol*, 1994;**25**:630–7

57. Lipsitz LA, Goldberger AL. Loss of 'complexity' and aging. Potential applications of fractals and chaos theory to senescence. *JAMA*, 1992;**267**:1806–9

58. Rossor MN. Catastrophe, chaos and Alzheimer's disease. The FE Williams Lecture. *J Roy Coll Phys Lond*, 1995;**29**:412–8

59. May RM. Nonlinearities and complex behavior in simple ecological and epidemiological models. *Ann NY Acad Sci*, 1987;**504**:1–15

60. Philippe P. Chaos and public health. *Can J Public Health*, 1992;**83**:165–6

61. Philippe P, Mansi O. Nonlinearity in the epidemiology of complex health and disease processes. *Theor Med Bioethics*, 1998;**19**:591–607

62. Begun JW. Chaos and complexity: Frontiers of organizational science. *J Managt Inquiry*, 1994;**3**:329–35

63. Chinnis A, White KR. Challenging the dominant logic of emergency departments: Guidelines from chaos theory. *J Emerg Med*, 1999;**17**:1049–54

64. Goldberger AR. Non-linear dynamics for clinicians: chaos theory, fractals, and complexity at the bedside. *Lancet*, 1996;**347**:1312–4

65. Heiby WA. *Better Health and the Reverse Effect*. Deerfield, IL: MediScience Publishers, 1988

66. Wilder J. The law of initial value in neurology and psychiatry. Facts and problems. *J Nerv Ment Dis*, 1957;**125**:73–86

67. Cannon WB. *The Wisdom of the Body*. New York: WW Norton, 1932

68. Homeostasis and the sympatico-adrenal system. In: Wolfe EL, Clifford AC, Benison S eds. *Walter B Cannon, Science and Society*. Cambridge, MA: Boston Medical Library/Harvard University Press, 2000:144–65

69. Pool R. Is it healthy to be chaotic? *Science*, 1989;**243**:604–7

70. Crutchfield JP, Farmer JD, Packard NH, Shaw RS. Chaos. *Sci Amer*, 1986;**255**:46–57

71. Markham FW. A method for introducing the concepts of chaos to medical students. *Theor Med Bioethics*, 1998;**19**:1–4

72. Asbury AJ, Tzabar Y. Fuzzy logic: new ways of thinking in anaesthesia. Editorial. *Br J Anaesthesia*, 1995;**75**:1–2

73. Steinmann F. Fuzzy set theory in medicine. *Artif Intell Med*, 1997;**11**:1–7

74. Dickerson JA, Helgason CM. The characterization of stroke subtype and science of evidence-based

medicine using fuzzy logic. *J Neurovasc Dis*, 1997;2: 138–44

75. Kosko B, Isaka S. Fuzzy logic. *Sci Amer*, 1993; July:76–81

76. Simmons M, Parker JA. Fuzzy logic, sharp results. *J Nucl Med*, 1995;36:1415–6

77. Shiomi S, Kuroki T, Jomura H, et al. Diagnosis of chronic liver disease from liver scintiscans by fuzzy reasoning. *J Nucl Med*, 1995;36:593–8

78. Keller T, Bitterlich N, Hilfenhaus S, et al. Tumor markers in the diagnosis of bronchial carcinoma: new options using fuzzy logic-based tumor marker profiles. *J Cancer Res Clin Oncol*, 1998;124:565–74

79. Rau G, Becker K, Kaufman R, Zimmermann HJ. Fuzzy logic and control: principal approach and potential applications in medicine. *Artif Organs*, 1995;19:105–12

80. Ament C, Hofer EP. A fuzzy logic model of fracture healing. *J Biomech*, 2000;33:961–8

81. Ohayon MM. Improving decision-making processes with fuzzy logic approach in the epidemiology of sleep disorders. *J Psychosom Res*, 1999;47:297–311

82. Naranjo CA, Bremner KE, Bazoon M, Turksen IB. Using fuzzy logic to predict response to citalopram in alcohol dependence. *Clin Pharmacol Ther*, 1997;62:209–24

83. Sproule BA, Bazoon M, Shulman KI, et al. Fuzzy logic pharmacokinetic modelling: application to lithium concentration prediction. *Clin Pharmacol Ther*, 1997;62:29–40

84. Sawyer MD. Invited commentary: Fuzzy logic – an introduction. *Surgery*, 2000;127:254–6

85. Buchman T. Invited commentary: Fuzzy logic, clear reasoning. *Surgery*, 2000;127:257

86. Amin AP, Kulkarni HR. Improving the information content of the Glasgow Coma Scale for the prediction of full cognitive recovery after head injury using fuzzy logic. *Surgery*, 2000;127:245–53

87. Massad E, Burattini MN, Ortega NR. Fuzzy logic and measles vaccination: designing a control strategy. *Int J Epidemiol*, 1999;28:550–7

88. Bellamy JEC. Medical diagnosis, diagnostic spaces, and fuzzy systems. *J Am Vet Med Assoc*, 1997;210: 390–6

89. Bellamy JEC. Fuzzy systems approach to diagnosis in the postpartum cow. *J Am Vet Med Assoc*, 1997; 210:397–401

90. Wirsam B, Uthus EO. The use of fuzzy logic in nutrition. *J Nutr*, 1996;126:2337S–41S

91. Sadegh-Kazem K. Advances in fuzzy theory. *Artif Intell Med*, 1999;15;309–23

92. Johnson DM. Reasoning and logic. In: Sills DL ed. *International Encyclopedia of the Social Sciences*. New York and Toronto: Macmillan Co. & Free Press, 1968:344–9

93. Wulff HR, Pedersen SA, Rosenberg R, Introduction by A Storr. *Philosophy of Medicine. An Introduction*. Oxford, London, Edinburgh: Blackwell Scientific Publications, 1986

94. Griffiths F, Byrne D. General practice and the new science emerging from theories of 'chaos' and complexity. *Br J Gen Pract*, 1998;48:1697–9

95. *Grebogi C Yorke JA (eds). The Impact of Chaos on Science and Society*. Tokyo and New York: United Nations University Press, 1997

96. Cooper MW. Is medicine hermeneutics all the way down? *Theor Med*, 1994;15:149–80

97. Slaney JK. An outline of formal logic and its applications to medicine – I. *Br Med J*, 1987;295; 1195–7

98. Slaney JK. An outline of formal logic and its applications to medicine – II. *Br Med J*, 1987;295: 1261–3

99. Weinstein MC, Fineberg HV, Elstein AS, et al. *Clinical Decision Analysis*. Philadelphia: WB Saunders, 1980

100. Waller BN. *Critical Thinking. Consider the Verdict*. Englewood Cliffs: Prentice-Hall, 1988

101. Aldisert RJ. *Logic for Lawyers. A Guide to Clear Logical Thinking*. Third Edition. Notre Dame, Ind.: National Institute for Trial Advocacy, 1997

How do we Do Things in Medicine

Gathering and evaluating evidence

Chapter 4

Producing evidence.
Classification, objectives and
worthiness of medical research

*'Devising an experiment . . . is posing a question;
we never conceive a question without an idea which
invites an answer. I consider it, therefore, an absolute
principle that experiments must always be devised in
view of a preconceived idea, no matter if the idea be
not very clear nor well defined.*
Claude Bernard, 1865

*After all, the ultimate goal of research
is not objectivity, but truth.*
Helene Deutsch, 1945

Since the time of Claude Bernard, humanity has produced a good number of remarkable researchers and bright methodologists to answer conceived questions. It is astute discoverers and discerning users of their findings who still remain in short supply as well as good communication and understanding between all parties involved.

Research is a crucial source for the production of arguments, i.e. evidence for logical discourse, its premises and conclusions. Such evidence-fuelled logic is essential to make sound decisions in prevention, cure, and care. Several major categories of clinical research studies exist and as soon as physicians have the knowledge they need to count events (see Chapter 5) and identify them (see Chapter 6), they can start tackling three important problems:

- What is the clinical picture of cases, and what is the portrait of disease in the community? (When, where, and in whom does disease appear?)
- Why did a disease occur? What is its cause?
- What should be done about a disease, and does the chosen course of action work?

To answer these questions, two additional issues must be examined:

- How good are the tools (technologies) used in solving medical problems? This question focuses mainly on the quality of diagnostic and screening tests instruments and their output, measurement scales and classification, information collection techniques like clinical examinations, interviews and follow-ups as well as on the retrieval and review of information from the literature and other sources.
- What is the best way to solve a health problem once the required evidence is available? Decision pathways in problem solving, their organization and ensuing results must be understood.

4.1 Classification of studies of disease

4.1.1 *Descriptive, observational analytical, and experimental studies*

Descriptive studies give us a better understanding of how a problem looks. They answer the following questions: What's going on? How many, how much?

How important is the problem? What are its course, occurrence and severity? **Analytical studies** or **etiological research** deal with causes. Most often, they explain why a disease has occurred. **Experimental studies** expose subjects to preventive or therapeutic maneuvers in order to assess how these solutions work. **Clinical trials** are examples of such studies. The first two types of studies are most often **observational** since researchers do not have any influence on what happens. However, experimental studies are regarded as **interventional** because they allow clinicians to decide who will be treated and by what means.

Analytical studies can be observational as is the case of studies on smoking and health. People themselves choose to smoke (the researcher does not have control over their choice to smoke) and health risks such as lung cancer occurrence are studied and compared for smokers and non-smokers. Hence, this type of effort is an **observational analytical study**.

Another cause–effect relationship exists between drugs and their beneficial effect (alleviation or cure). The researcher decides who will be treated with a drug under study, and which drug will be used to treat a control group. This is termed an **experimental study**. For example: If a new disease appears in the community, such as toxic shock syndrome, AIDS or legionnellosis, the clinical picture of cases is established and a descriptive study of cases is established. Next, it is necessary to identify the disease occurrence (in terms of prevalence, incidence, mortality, case fatality, etc.) in different groups of people, at different time periods, and from one place to another. A descriptive study of disease spread between people is made. Further, disease in various groups of individuals or in different living environments is **compared** in terms of disease frequency. Causal relationships are assessed on the basis of comparisons of groups of subjects. An analytical (etiological) study is done in such a way as to search for causal factors of disease spread. However, we analyze these events 'as they occur', we do not interfere in the natural evolution of events or with people's choices as for their exposures and habits (smoking, occupation, etc.). We **observe** what is going on. Finally, we may consider a health program to change people's habits (IV drug use, unprotected sex) or test a new vaccine and we **decide** which individual or group will receive a protective intervention and which one will not. We test an **intervention** in a **clinical or field trial**. We 'control' or manipulate the situation. Our health habits modification program or the field trial of a vaccine are becoming a kind of **experimental study**.

As this sequence shows, noxious factors are studied for ethical reasons by observational analytical studies, whereas causal associations between beneficial factors (vaccine) are evaluated by clinical trials that are classical examples of experimental studies 'outside the laboratory'. Schematically, studies in medicine are classified as shown in Figure 4.1.

4.1.2 Longitudinal, cross-sectional, and semi-longitudinal studies

The following classification of studies based on time requires definitions and examples. Pediatricians can study growth (body, height and weight) in school age children from 6 to 14 years in three different ways: For a **longitudinal study**, a group of 6 year olds is re-examined yearly for nine years. Thus, **one group** of individuals is subject to **several consecutive examinations**. In a **cross-sectional study**, groups of different ages are chosen and **each group** is **examined once** at a given moment (year) yielding a composite picture of growth from age 6 to 14 in a one-year study. In a **semi-longitudinal study**, **several groups** are followed

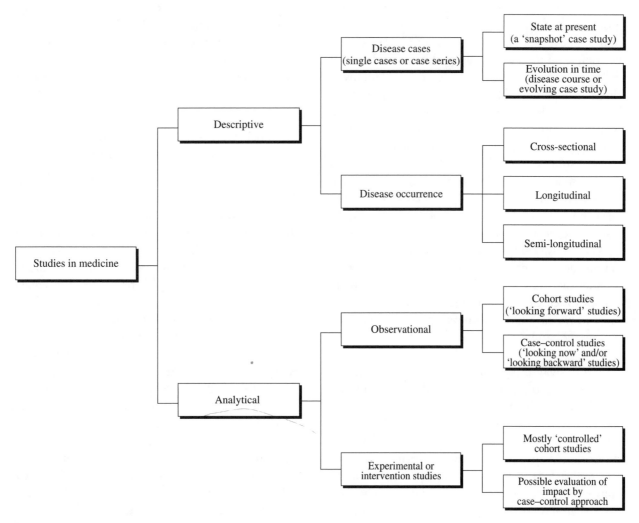

Figure 4.1 Classification of studies in medicine

Table 4.1	Schematic classification of studies in time	
Type of study	*Number of groups studied*	*Number of consecutive examinations in time*
Longitudinal	one	several
Cross-sectional	several	one
Semi-longitudinal	several	several

through **several examinations**. In the first year of study, three groups of children are measured (aged 6, 9, and 12 years). They are then re-examined the next year, at ages 7, 10, and 13 respectively. In the third year of study, they are 8, 11, and 14 years old. For reasons of feasibility, time, economy, and participation in the study, a semi-longitudinal study compromises on the number of study groups and the duration of study. In summary, a cross-sectional study can be completed in one year, using different subjects at different ages. A longitudinal study can follow a single group, but obtaining a desirable picture of height and weight in the children will take nine years. A semi-longitudinal study, however, requires only three years of follow-up. Table 4.1 summarizes these types of studies.

Sometimes in the literature, semi-longitudinal studies are called 'mixed longitudinal studies'. The term 'pure' longitudinal study should, however, be reserved for a study whose cohort (i.e. group of subjects entering a study at a given moment and followed in time) does not change in time: subjects do not leave or enter the study at any point. 'Mixed' longitudinal studies (often called 'open' longitudinal studies) are those in which subjects drop out at various moments during the study, with other subjects taking their place.

A three-way classification of studies in medicine better reflects the purposes of studies (exploratory, descriptive, analytic), their time directionality (prospective, cross-sectional, retrospective), and their observational or interventive nature. Each type of study should provide answers to specific questions and for each type of question, the methodological approaches are different, and the fields of application in clinical and community medicine are specific. As Table 4.2 shows, in descriptive studies, we simply

want to know **what happened, or what happens**. At this stage of dealing with clinical problems, we do not raise questions about causes (making hypotheses). Instead, we want to obtain an exact picture of events that might and should lead to the formulation of hypotheses about their causes.

The importance of descriptive studies that essentially produce a picture of disease occurrence should not be underestimated, despite the fact that some discount them because 'they do not provide answers to questions'. However, without a rigorous description and counting of events (disease cases, exposure to noxious factors, etc.), the ensuing analytical studies would be based on elements that nobody understands. Thus, descriptive studies must be undertaken as well as analytical studies or clinical trials. In fact, since each type of study offers answers to different questions, the studies should be considered complementary in the eventual decision-making process.

Any analytical study, be it observational or experimental, can be considered a three-step event as proposed by AR Feinstein[2] (see also Figure 8.1 in Chapter 8):

Initial state → action (intervention, clinical maneuver) → subsequent state

For example, in a study of noxious factors leading to disease such as smoking and cancer, a study of the initial state of individuals before they start to smoke is followed by a study of exposure (period and intensity of smoking, i.e. action). Finally, at a given moment, the development of cancer in some individuals under follow-up is determined (subsequent state). All three phases of such a process should be known and understood. The same should occur for non-smokers if the study is of an observational analytical nature. In clinical trials, the initial state of patients before treatment is determined, their treatment is followed as a 'clinical maneuver' and the treatment results are then evaluated (subsequent state). The same occurs for a control group (exposed to a placebo or alternative treatment). In a study of a diagnostic test, our knowledge of disease in patients before the test (initial state) is acquired, the test is applied (clinical maneuver) and its results are noted (subsequent state). The understanding and comparison of these steps allows us to understand the

Table 4.2   Epidemiological classification of studies in medicine

Topic	Question	Type of research	Example of fields of application and methods used in clinical medicine	Example of fields of application and methods used in community health
DIAGNOSIS	What is the problem?	Forming clinical entities.	Clinimetrics. Determination of internal and external validity of a test, etc.	Evaluation of screening tests.
	How important is the problem?	Measurement of severity of disease.	Clinimetric indexes.	Evaluation of screening programs.
	How did we arrive at diagnosis?	Study of diagnostic process.	Follow-up. Analysis of clinicians' practices.	Establishment of diagnostic criteria for disease surveillance.
OCCURRENCE	What happened? What happens? When, where, and in whom do problems appear? Risk of future problems. Probability of having a problem now.	Case(s) description. Disease description.	Cross-sectional or longitudinal case studies. Studies of natural and clinical course of cases.	Epidemiological portrait of disease. Epidemiological surveillance. Study of disease spread (epidemicity, pandemicity, endemicity). Disease clustering.
CAUSES	Why did it happen? What (who) is responsible?	Determination of causes. Etiological research.	Individual case(s) etiology. Identification of methods, subjects for further development. Extrapolations from disease etiology research. Meta-analysis.	Disease etiology research (comparative studies of exposure to various factors and disease occurrence (cohort and case–control studies). Meta-analysis. Elucidation of mechanisms of disease spread.
INTERVENTION (prevention and/or treatment)	Can we control case(s) or disease? Did we control case(s) or disease? Will it control (solve) the problem?	Efficacy, effectiveness, and efficiency evaluation.	Phase 1–4 clinical trials. Field trials. Pharmaco-epidemiological studies. Impact of secondary and tertiary prevention (mainly). Meta-analysis. Decision analysis.	Mainly impact of primary prevention. Meta-analysis. Decision analysis.
PROGNOSIS	What will happen? What might happen?	Study of disease outcome(s).	Survival or time-to-event studies. Descriptive and analytical studies of probabilities of events derived from case studies (disease course).	Epidemiological forecasting of exposures, disease occurrence and spread based on epidemiological surveillance.

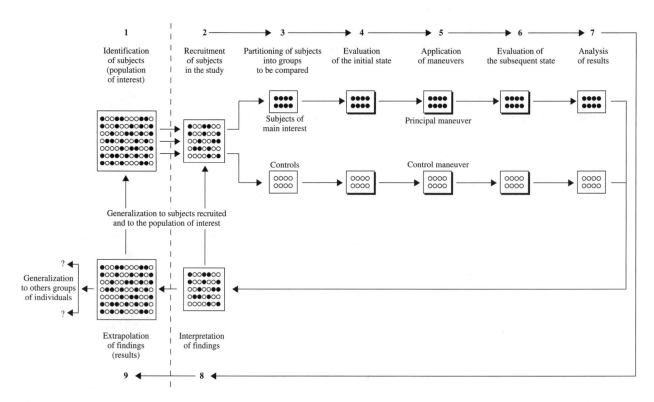

Figure 4.2 Nine stages of analytical studies

importance of the evidence produced by these studies. Subsequent chapters cover this topic in detail.

In addition to our understanding of the intrinsic organization and quality of a study, we want to know if its results can be applied to the entire group of individuals in the study and how the results can be extrapolated (generalized) to other individuals such as those with similar characteristics, the general population, etc. Figure 4.2 illustrates this. Strengths and weaknesses of these and other types of studies will be discussed in more detail in Chapters 5–11 and 13. They were also summarized recently by Hall and Kothari[3].

4.2 General scope and quality of evidence

Evidence in medicine comes from experience. Research studies are a written report of an organized experience. The usefulness of evidence is defined by four major questions and answers:

1. **How good are the study and the evidence itself?**

2. **Can I apply them to my patients and to a specific patient?**
3. **Is such an application feasible?**
4. **Can the usefulness (effectiveness) of such an application be evaluated?**

Until now, most of the experience has focused on the first two questions.

4.2.1 Worthiness of studies and the crucial role of the research question within a research protocol

The quality and scope of studies that produce evidence is inherent to their nature. Most often, we tend to expect more and better evidence than studies can deliver. An occurrence (descriptive) study will provide evidence about the spread of disease, but will not identify its causes. An observational analytical study does not have the same power of causal proof as a well-controlled experiment or clinical trial. A clinical trial focusing on the immediate effect of a drug does not provide evidence related to the

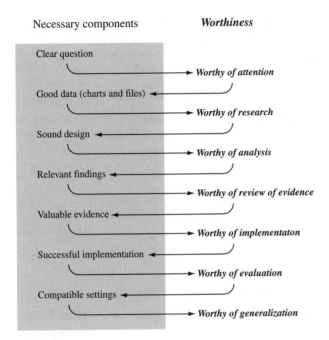

Necessary components   **Worthiness**

Clear question — Worthy of attention

Good data (charts and files) — Worthy of research

Sound design — Worthy of analysis

Relevant findings — Worthy of review of evidence

Valuable evidence — Worthy of implementaton

Successful implementation — Worthy of evaluation

Compatible settings — Worthy of generalization

Figure 4.3 Necessary components and worthiness of work in health sciences and practice

long-term prognosis and the full scope of outcomes of the disease under treatment. In addition, the worthiness of studies and evidence depends on the quality of the cascading characteristics of studies as illustrated in Figure 4.3. If the problem is poorly stated, all subsequent cascading steps will be compromised and could be rendered useless.

Any quest for new evidence relies on several clear formulations:

- The problem
- The background (relevance) of the problem
- The research question
- The general and specific objectives (expected results)
- The research design
- The methodological and technical aspects of the study of evidence

Questions are the cornerstone of the quest for evidence! Physicians can sometimes feel inadequate if they do not understand the purpose of a research paper. However, if the authors of the paper haven't clearly stated their question, the physicians are not necessarily at fault. The problem of treating arthritis

in the elderly serves as a good example. The nature of the quest for evidence will depend on the formulation of the question to be answered by the study:

- If we ask '**How frequently** is arthritis seen in the elderly and **how frequently** are non-prescription non-steroidal anti-inflammatory drugs (NSAIDs) used to treat it?', the answer calls for an **occurrence study** of arthritis in the elderly community. This will enable us to determine the prevailing manifestations (signs and symptoms) of arthritis and the number of people using NSAIDs to relieve their symptoms.

- A question such as '**What factors** lead elderly arthritis sufferers to use NSAIDs to relieve their suffering?' may require an **analytical observational study**, such as a case–control study comparing the characteristics of NSAID users and non-users.

- If the question asks '**How effective** are non-prescription NSAIDs in the long-term control of arthritis in the elderly?' the ensuing study can be either an **observational analytical study** comparing users and non-users of NSAIDs or a **clinical trial**, with a possible **systematic review of evidence** available across the medical literature.

- If we want to know '**What is the cost and usefulness** of over-the-counter NSAIDs in the control of arthritis in the elderly?' a **health economics study** might be in order.

- For those interested in knowing '**What are the best ways to choose** non-prescription drugs to improve the quality of life of elderly chronic arthritis sufferers and which of these drugs are the most appropriate?' **decision analysis** might be the study of choice.

- If a practitioner wants to find and identify appropriate candidates for non-prescription NSAID arthritis therapy in the elderly, a **study of a screening program** or a **validation of a diagnostic test** should be considered assuming a proper definition of arthritis at that age.

Unfortunately, clear questions are still not the norm in research or in practice and ambiguous questions lead to ambiguous answers. Most often, we ask and expect too much and since resources and opportunities for research are scarce, some researchers are tempted to discover more than actually exists.

Figure 4.4 shows that **a well formulated question should cover intervention, outcomes, population setting and condition of interest and that all these components should be defined and listed (if more than one) in operational terms**[4,5]. For Craig et al[6], a **comparator**, such as a control group, another disease, or an alternative treatment, a **best feasible primary study design** and a **best MEDLINE search term** are useful additional information related to and reflected in a good research question.

A clearly formulated question at the beginning of a study will determine the success of the study. If the question is not good, even a well-organized study based on good quality data will not provide acceptable evidence. Good evidence does not guarantee that the results of the study can be successfully put into the practice. Medicine is based on a mosaic of evidence related to specific topics. Each type of evidence is complementary in its global assessment and uses. Hence, the hierarchy of evidence and ensuing recommendations will be different for that of disease spread, its cases or chances of control.

4.2.2 Classification of evidence and ensuing recommendations

The most detailed classification of evidence and ensuing practical recommendations were elaborated in the assessment of therapeutic or prevention interventions and programs already briefly outlined in Chapter 2. The classification currently used throughout North America[7–9] is as follows:

Classification of evidence:

I. **Randomized** controlled clinical **trials** (at least one).

   I-a. Carrying **low** alpha and beta errors.

   I-b. Carrying **high** alpha or beta errors.

II-1. Evidence obtained from well designed controlled **trials without randomization**.

II-2. Evidence obtained from well designed **observational cohort** (non randomized concurrent cohort comparisons) **or case–control analytic studies**, preferably from more than one center or research group.

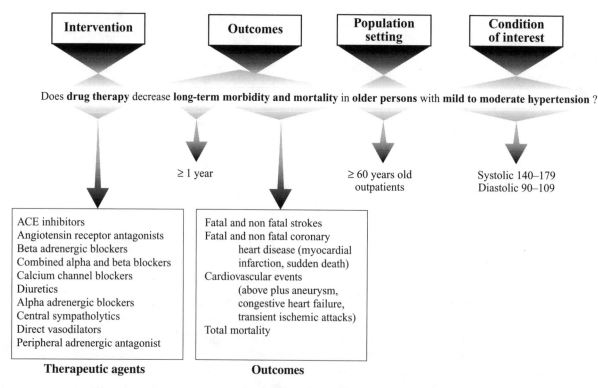

Figure 4.4 Desirable components of a good research question. Source: Ref. 5, reproduced with permission from the Author and Editor of *How to Conduct a Cochrane Systematic Review* (San Antonio Cochrane Center)

II-3. **Multiple time series or place comparisons** with or without interventions (including uncontrolled experiments) indicating a cause of a health problem or effectiveness of intervention against it.

III. **Opinions** of respected authorities, based on clinical experience, descriptive studies or reports of expert committees (e.g. guidelines based on consensus only).

Classification of recommendations:

A: There is **good evidence** to support the recommendation that the condition or activity be specifically **considered** in a health care or prevention program.

B: There is **fair evidence** to support the recommendation that the condition or activity be specifically **considered** in a health care or prevention program.

C: There is **poor evidence** regarding the **inclusion or exclusion** of the condition or activity in a health care or prevention program, but recommendations can be made on other grounds.

D: There is **fair evidence** to support the recommendation that the condition be **excluded from consideration** in a health care or prevention program.

E: There is **good evidence** to support the recommendation that the condition and activity be **excluded from consideration** in a health care or prevention program.

With this in mind, the US Preventive Services Task Force[10] evaluated the relevance of scoliosis screening. Figure 4.5 summarizes its experience and recommendations. Also, this example illustrates how to fracture (divide) a complex problem into more manageable and meaningful questions and topics. In other areas, evidence must be evaluated in ways that are different from an assessment of cause-effect relationships in different types of studies. These other assessments of evidence will be discussed in subsequent chapters.

4.2.3 *Does good evidence apply to my patient(s)?*

Readers of the *Users' Guides to the Medical Literature*[11] may notice that every assessment of evidence is followed by a discussion of its applicability to the individual patient[12], be it a problem of diagnosis, treatment, prognosis or other. However, some common rules can be considered for different topics and sources of evidence. A statistician would approach such a question by asking whether a given individual comes from a given population, i.e. the group of individuals used to establish the evidence or a target population of evidence-producing studies such as clinical trials. In this sense, we can also ask whether patients are eligible as subjects in the evidence-producing study(ies)? Similar characteristics such as age or gender are not sufficient. We want to define and find the best possible candidate for a treatment of interest.

A good match between the patient and evidence ideally relies on **comparable:**

- General demographic and social characteristics of the patient.
- Risks and *a priori* exposure to causal factors of disease (conditional).
- Diagnostic criteria of the health problem.
- Gradient (severity) and position in the spectrum of the disease (organ or system involvement).
- Co-morbidity (other disease from which patients suffer) and treatment for co-morbidity.
- Point in time in the disease course.
- Prognosis without intervention.
- Expected results (a non difference to be disproved).
- Accessibility to be diagnosed with disease.
- Accessibility to the spectrum of treatment, care and follow-up to those of the evidence-producing study(ies); including new technologies if those are of interest.
- Expected results (outcomes) of treatment in patients as opposed to those provided by the clinical trials generating the evidence.
- Health system, infrastructure and care offered to the patient.
- Patient values, preferences and choice that might be attributed to the individuals enrolled in the evidence-producing studies.

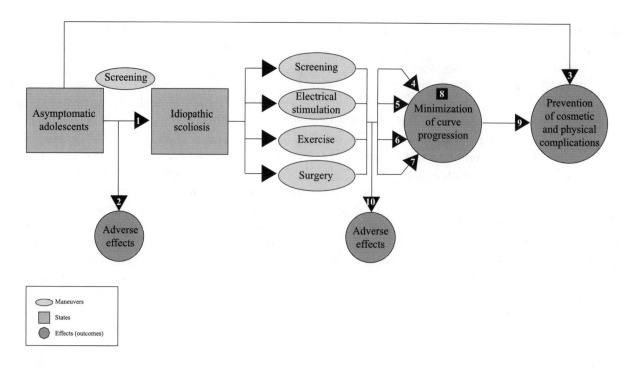

Linkage: Step in causal pathway	Evidence codes	Quality of evidence
1. Accuracy of screening tests: evidence that physical examination of back can detect curves	II-2	Fair: significant variation, poor reference standard, lack of evidence from physician screening
2. Adverse effects of screening: evidence that screening is associated with an increased risk of complications	III	Poor: most postulated adverse effects have not been evaluated in studies
3. Effectiveness of early detection: evidence that persons detected through screening have better outcomes that those who are not screened	II-3	Poor: uncontrolled studies based on trends after initiation of screening, failure to control for confounding temporal factors
4. Braces	II-2, II-3	Poor: selection bias, lack of internal control groups (most studies), inadequate follow-up, small sample sizes, lack of health outcome measures
5. Lateral electrical surface stimulation	II-2, II-3	
6. Exercise	I, II-3	
7. Surgery	II-2, II-3	
8. Curve progression: evidence that curves detected on screening are destined to progress to curves of clinical significance	II-3	Fair: significant number of patients unavailable for follow-up, variable measures of progression
9. Complications of curve progression: evidence that persons with scoliosis are more likely to experience back complaints, psychological effects, disability	II-3	Poor: studies generally lack control groups, have high attrition rates, include mixture of patients with different problems, and use variable measures to judge outcome
10. Adverse effects of treatment: evidence that treatment is associated with an increased risk of complications	III	Poor: most postulated adverse effects have not been evaluated in studies

Figure 4.5 Grading evidence for a health problem. Example of scoliosis. Screening. Source: Adapted from Ref. 10, public domain

- Patient and doctor compliance with the health care regimen.
- Absence of ethical constraints in choices to be treated or not.
- Physicians' and other health professionals' knowledge, experience and preferred practices.

Such a checklist might be useful as well when general strategies of care for specific group of patients are selected. **In essence, this checklist applies to all kinds of studies discussed in chapters on diagnostic methods and screening, disease causes (harm), treatment, prognosis, systematic review conclusions or decision analysis. The reader is advised to apply this checklist wherever appropriate and to refer back to it anytime. In addition to that, the reader of any medical paper will always ask whether it applies to the patient or patients under his or her care.**

Obtaining the best evidence from research is not enough and does not in itself make decisions either. Final decisions will depend on **clinical expertise** that combines and considers not only the quality of evidence, but also the clinical state and circumstances (patient's state, available care etc.) and patient values, actions and preferences[13,14]. Figure 4.6 illustrates such a situation. Clinical state and circumstances, patient preferences and actions, as well as research evidence are combined to various degrees across the practice of medicine. If we number the subsets in the Haynes et al diagram[14], Subset 1 appears to integrate all three elements that these authors consider as clinical expertise. Extremes are Subset 5 representing patient-pleasing practices, Subset 6 (going by reality and experience), Subset 7

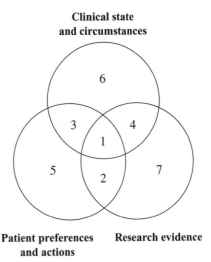

Clinical state and circumstances

Patient preferences and actions   **Research evidence**

Figure 4.6   Source: adapted from Refs. 13 and 14

(treating by the books) or some combination of the above (Subsets 2, 3, and 4). This is medicine in the real world.

4.3   Conclusion

With the above-mentioned general views in mind, we quickly realize that paradigms must be fuelled by specific methods and techniques. The chapters that follow will discuss this in greater detail. **Good research and its results do not necessarily lead to good clinical decisions! They are, however, the essential foundation of sound decisions that put research results within a context where the patient, the care provider and the conditions and circumstances of health services and care are brought together for optimal success.**

REFERENCES

1. Jenicek M. *Clinical Case Reporting in Evidence-Based Medicine.* Second Edition. London: Arnold, 2001
2. Feinstein AR. *Clinical Biostatistics.* St. Louis: CV Mosby Co., 1977
3. Hall KN, Kothari RU. Research fundamentals; IV. Choosing a research design. *Acad Emerg Med,* 1999;6:67–74
4. Counsell C. Formulating questions and locating primary studies for inclusion in systematic reviews. *Ann Intern Med,* 1997;127:380–7
5. Mulrow CM, Oxman A (eds). *How to Conduct a Cochrane Systematic Review.* Third Edition. San Antonio: San Antonio Cochrane Center, 1996
6. Craig JC, Irwig LM, Stockler MR. Evidence-based medicine: useful tools for decision-making. *MJA,* 2001;**174**:248–53
7. The Canadian Task Force on the Periodic Health Examination. *The Canadian Guide to Clinical Preventive Health Care.* Ottawa: Health Canada, 1994
8. US Preventive Services Task Force. *Guide to Clinical Preventive Services: Report of the US Preventive*

Services Task Force. Second Edition. Baltimore: Williams & Wilkins, 1996

9. Sackett DL. Rules of evidence and clinical recommendations. *Can J Cardiol*, 1993;9:487–9

10. US Preventive Services Task Force. Screening for adolescent idiopathic scoliosis. Policy statement. *JAMA*, 1993;**269**:2664–6

11. Guyatt G, Rennie D, The Evidence-Based Medicine Working Group. *Users' Guides to the Medical Literature*. Chicago: AMA Press, 2002. (See also series under the same title in *JAMA* since 1993)

12. McAlister FA, SE Straus, Guyatt GH, Haynes RB for the Evidence-Based Medicine Working Group. Users' Guides to the Medical Literature. XX. Integrating research evidence with the care of the individual patient. *JAMA*, 2000;**283**:2829–36

13. Haynes RB, Devereaux PJ, Guyatt GH. Clinical expertise in the era of evidence-based medicine and patient choice. (Editorial.) *ACP Journal Club*, 2002;**136**:A11 (8 pages, electronic edition)

14. Haynes RB, Devereaux PJ, Guyatt GH. Physicians' and patients' choices in evidence-based practice. Evidence does not make decisions, people do. *Br Med J*, 2002;**324**:1350

Assessing the health of individuals and communities. Health indicators, indexes, and scales

When treating an elderly arthritis sufferer, you should not expect him to measure his quality of life by how much it has improved on a scale of health and well being. He wants to climb stairs without pain, and your goal is to help him do that.

. . . He may also ask you about other risks to his health – his own risks, not those of his community, as seen through incidence studies. It is your job to give him a satisfactory answer. And, . . . by the way, you are paid for it!

5.1 General considerations

Evidence of good or ill health in an individual or community must be defined and quantified. Otherwise, further use of this evidence becomes meaningless. Health can be measured either directly or indirectly. **Direct measurement of health** in an individual implies not only the exclusion of disease, but also the assessment of biological functions (for example, in sports or occupational medicine), or the ability to adapt to new and/or extreme stimuli, such as in aerospace medicine. **Indirect measurement of health** relies on the assessment of disease or death frequency in the community to which an individual belongs. This individual's health is then evaluated according to the probability of his contracting or dying of a disease, based on the frequency of disease (or deaths) in his community in terms of existing or anticipated cases. Frequencies of **events** in the community (cases of disease, deaths, etc.) are studied not only in absolute terms, but also in relation to the whole community (rates) or by comparison with event frequency in other groups or communities, or with the frequency of other diseases (ratios). Event rates and ratios represent some of the basic tools used indirectly to assess the health of individuals and communities.

Another indirect measure of health is based on the assessment of **healthy behaviors** (physical activity, frugal but balanced food intake, personal hygiene, etc.) or **unhealthy habits** (smoking, alcohol abuse, overeating, physical inactivity) of an individual or community representing a probability of present or future health problems related to such behaviors[1]. Many large-scale surveys such as the Canada Health Survey used this approach in the assessment of health.

The number of health indicators, indexes and scales is ever increasing. From this wide array of measurements of health, the occurrence of disease and death in terms of their rates and ratios are the most widely used tools in the assessment of population health, in etiological research and in the assessment of the effectiveness of treatment and care as well as that of prognosis. These tools are ubiquitous in research, practice, and health policies.

5.2 Rates and ratios

Rates and ratios show the relationship between two frequencies of events such as causes of disease or deaths.

A **rate** is a demonstration of the relationship between an event's frequency and a population as a whole. It quantifies the occurrence of health events in a defined community. A rate is an expression of the frequency of a phenomenon. Thus, rates are computed as frequencies of events (numerators) related to the population from which they arise (denominators). They represent an event (frequency of cases as numerator) as a proportion of a total (denominator). This is usually done for a cohort (a group of subjects entering a study at a given time) and their susceptibility to health problems during a specific period (susceptible individuals). Elsewhere, availability of data permitting, rates take into account the duration of susceptibility (and exposure) of each individual (see the following section on incidence density). In the simplest cases, the mid-interval number of susceptible subjects is chosen as the denominator.

$$\text{Rate} = \frac{\text{numerator}}{\text{denominator}} \times \text{a power of 10}$$

$$= \frac{\text{number of events}}{\text{number of events} + \text{number of non-events}} \times \begin{array}{l} 1{,}000 \text{ or} \\ 10{,}000 \text{ or} \\ 100{,}000 \text{ etc.} \end{array}$$

Hence, observed frequencies represent numerators while an initial cohort or an average population during a period of interest represents denominators, all multiplied by a power of 10, which converts the rate from a fraction to a whole number[2]. For rare diseases, rates may be given per hundred thousand or per million. This is the case of incidence and mortality rates in studies where such data in denominators are available. Elsewhere, rates are reported in relation to the number of exposed persons to a given risk during a period of interest.

A national census is usually performed midway through the year, so denominators of demographic rates are already available for average populations during the period of interest. Wherever denominators are small and/or events are frequent, rates reported for the whole population at risk (a cohort at the beginning of the period) will differ more significantly from rates related to the average (or mid-period) population. For example, in one year, 25 deaths by injury are observed in a community of 1,000 subjects. The mortality rate is calculated as follows:

$$\frac{25 \text{ deaths}}{\substack{1,000 \text{ subjects (i. e. the 25} \\ \text{that died \textbf{and} 975 remaining} \\ \text{who were still alive or died} \\ \text{from other causes)}}} \quad \text{i. e. 25 deaths} \atop \text{per 1,000}$$

In this case, the figure found in the numerator (25 deaths) is also counted in the denominator (community of 1,000, including those 25 deaths and the remaining 9,975 who survived or died from other causes).

Using the previous example, the mortality rate related to a mid-year population would be:

$$\frac{25 \text{ deaths}}{\substack{1,000 \text{ subjects at the beginning} \\ 975 \text{ at the end of the period} \\ \text{hence } 987.5 \text{ subjects at mid-} \\ \text{year if deaths occur evenly} \\ \text{throughout this year}}} \times 1,000 = \frac{25.3 \text{ deaths}}{\text{per 1,000}}$$

*NB: This original concept of a rate is widely used in general medical literature. However, several research epidemiologists use this term only if disease occurrence is reported in relation to persons-period of time of exposure (or follow-up) in terms of 'incidence density' or 'true rate' (see section 5.3 for more information). In a given situation, a common term of prevalence, incidence, or mortality **level** might be acceptable. It might mean, depending on the case, either a **proportion** of prevalent cases (prevalence rate), cumulative incidence (incidence rate), incidence density ('true incidence rate'), or a proportion of individuals deceased (mortality rate or case fatality rate as defined in Section 5.2.2).*

Proportional rates – caution. No percentage is a true rate. Very often, especially in hospital-based studies, observed cases are presented as proportions of a total of all observations. For example, of all hospital

infections during one year, a hospital nurse epidemiologist reports that 40% of cases were coliform infections, 30% were caused by Staphylococci, and the remaining 30% were due to various other agents. This is valuable information, but it represents only cases with numerators of some unknown rates (i.e. how many infections in how many patients at risk). If another hospital were to report 25% coliform infections, 40% Staphylococcal cases and 35% other agent-related cases, it would be impossible to say if coliform infections were more prevalent in one hospital or another. Neither the absolute number of cases (numerators of a desired true rate), nor the frequency of patients at risk in each hospital (denominators) is known. These '**pie chart statistics**' or 'pizza slice data' do not allow comparisons of the magnitude of problems from an epidemiological point of view.

A **ratio** is a mathematical expression of a relationship between different entities in terms of numerators and denominators. A ratio may be a comparison of two rates. For example, in an urban community a mortality rate by traffic-related injury is found to be 25 per 1,000. In a rural community, a rate of 50 per 1,000 was observed. A rural/urban mortality ratio (or 'rate ratio') would be:

$$\frac{50 / 1,000 \text{ (rural)}}{25 / 1,000 \text{ (urban)}} \quad \text{i. e. } 2 / 1,000 \text{ (rural)}$$

This ratio indicates that the mortality rate in the country is double that of the city. It shows the numerator as a multiple of the denominator. By using ratios, two different entities are being compared in the numerator and denominator. Rural deaths represent the numerator, while urban deaths represent the denominator. In neonatology, fetal mortality rates are a frequency of fetal deaths related to all births (live and fetal deaths). Fetal mortality ratios, according to the same logic, are represented by fetal deaths (numerator) in relation to live births only (denominator).

This basic notion of rates and ratios has been considerably refined in epidemiological theory and research[3–6]. It may even be further adapted for a better understanding of measurements of health.

5.2.1 Rates and ratios applied to disease occurrence and deaths

It is clear that 10 deaths caused by injury during a one-year period in a community of 200 persons has a different meaning than the same number of deaths in a group of 400. Rates of cases in relation to the size of the community in which they occur allow for proper comparison, providing that the denominators are of comparable size. Hence, rates are multiplied by convenient coefficients, e.g. 100, 1,000, 10,000, etc. Twenty deaths from cancer occurring during the year in a community of 25,000 subjects represents a rate of 80 per 100,000, i.e.

$$\frac{20}{25,000} \times 100,000 \quad \text{or} \quad 20 \times \frac{100,000}{25,000}$$

The size of the denominator depends on the frequency of cases. If events are frequent, such as cases of measles during an epidemic, rates may be presented per 100 or per 1,000. Cancers are reported as rates per 100,000; post-vaccinal complications, even more rare than cancers, may be reported per 1,000,000 doses of vaccine. It is all a question of common sense and agreement.

5.2.2 Morbidity, mortality and case fatality

A dangerous chemical is released in a chemical plant. All 500 plant employees are exposed. During the year following the accident, 100 employees develop chemically induced pneumonia, and 50 die of it. Figure 5.1 illustrates this situation. A **morbidity rate** represents the frequency of cases occurring in the whole community, i.e. 100 per 500, or 20% in this example. A **mortality rate** (or death rate) represents the frequency of cases in the same community, i.e. 50 per 500, or 10%. It is defined as '*an estimate of the proportion of the population that dies during a specific period*'[2]. A **case fatality rate** represents deaths occurring only in subjects becoming ill, i.e. 50 per 100, or 50%. Hence, it is '*the proportion of cases of specific condition which are fatal within a specified time*'[2].

Mortality and case fatality rates are often confused in the literature, but they measure different things. Mortality rates express the impact of death on the whole community, while fatality rates are one measure of the severity of disease. Demographers are more interested in the former, clinicians in the latter. The distinction between deaths in all subjects and deaths in sufferers must always be made. AIDS is not as deadly in the general population where few subjects are at risk. Mortality rates are low. However, AIDS is deadly for infected subjects who develop the disease. The case fatality rate of AIDS at the moment of writing is absolute. Denominators for both rates are quite different.

NB: Technically, case fatality rates and mortality rates must be given with a specific period of time in mind. Mortality rates are usually given for current

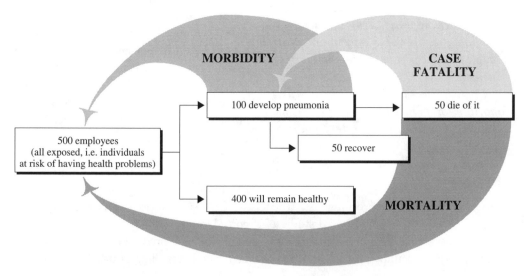

Figure 5.1 Morbidity, mortality, case fatality

years or for any other time period of interest. Case fatality rates use as denominators incident cases occurring in a well defined cohort. Deaths among these cases are expressed for a part of or for the whole natural or clinical course of disease, for the life expectancies of individuals (incurable disease), etc.

5.2.3 Crude rates and specific rates

Absolute or relative frequencies of all diseased or deceased persons, without further distinction, yield **crude rates** (overall or general, i.e. all causes and characteristics of the subjects combined). Diseases that cause cases or deaths, the characteristics of the persons involved, etc., are usually of more interest. Computations of event rates for particular diseases or persons yield **specific rates**. Disease-specific rates may be observed (for example, coronary disease incidence rate, or breast cancer mortality rate), age-specific rates (infant mortality rate), disease age-specific rates (trauma incidence rate in preschool age children), occupation-specific rates, area-specific rates, and so on. In such computations, the characteristics of subjects representing numerators must be the same as those in the denominators of given rates. For example, if an age-specific incidence rate of stroke during a year is to be computed in men aged 50–59 years old, the following frequencies should be related:

$$\frac{\text{Number of men aged 50–59 years suffering a new stroke during that year}}{\text{Total number of men aged 50–59 years susceptible to stroke during that year}} \times \begin{array}{l}\text{a convenient} \\ \text{coefficient of} \\ 10^n\end{array}$$

5.3 Prevalence and incidence as measures of morbidity

When studying morbidity, one must distinguish between the measurement of an instant occurrence and the spread of disease in time. Measurements of prevalence and incidence allow this distinction.

A disease's **prevalence** is indicated by a frequency of cases at any given moment (or at any moment during a period of interest). Related to a precise denominator, it becomes a **prevalence rate**, i.e. 'The total number of all individuals who have an attribute or disease at a particular time (or during a particular period) divided by the population at risk of having the attribute or disease at this point in time or midway through the period'[2]. (*NB: However, to be more precise, prevalence is more a proportion than a rate in the dynamic terms of the latter.*) A disease's **incidence** represents the frequency of new cases **only** during a given period of time. Related to a denominator of subjects susceptible to illness during that period, it becomes an **incidence rate**[2]. Figure 5.2 serves as a numerical example. Several measures of morbidity can be drawn from this picture. The **incidence rate of cases** (i.e. cumulative incidence) is 4 per 994 (*NB Cases 2, 3, 4, and 9 are new cases, cases 1, 5, 6, 7, 8 and 10 were already ill before the year under study*). The **point prevalence rate** (or proportion) at the beginning of the year is 4 per 1,000 (*NB: Cases 5 and 6 are in remission and they cannot be detected at that time*). The **incidence of spells** (attacks) of disease (first attacks plus all relapses) is 11, i.e. case 2(1), case 3(3), case 4(1), case 5(1), case 6(1), case 8(2), case 9(1), and case 10(1) = 11. As rates, they may be reported for all cases, all individuals or for susceptible individuals only (to 10, 994, or 1,000 depending on what information is needed). Spells of disease in all cases only study disease history (course) and eventually its severity. Spells related to the whole community are of interest in the planning of health care and services.

NB: For the sake of terminological and nosological purity, several epidemiologists prefer to call the above 'simple' rates rather than 'proportions' (in the case of prevalence) or 'cumulative incidence' (during follow-up visits, how many susceptible persons from an original cohort will fall ill in a given period of time), the latter being a measure of average risk or cumulative incidence. When further studying risk, the use of 'true' rates is recommended in terms of 'force of morbidity' or 'incidence density'. (See section 5.4). However, such 'simple' rates as defined above are strongly rooted in current medical literature. As a matter of fact, they may reflect 'true' rates if it is given that on average, routine national health statistics) are exposed during a comparable period of time to some etiological factor under study. For

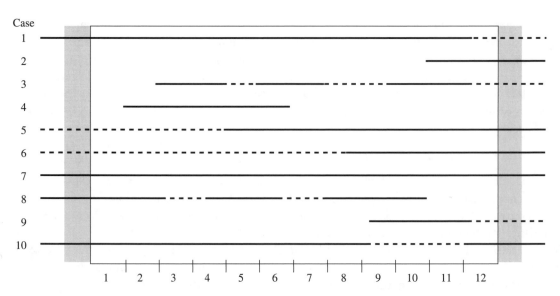

Figure 5.2 Prevalent and incident cases, spells, first attacks and relapses of disease occurring in the community of 1,000 individuals. Continuous lines indicate all types of spells (attacks) of disease. Interrupted (dotted) lines indicate periods of remission. Continuous lines preceded by interrupted lines indicate relapses of disease, i.e. attacks subsequent to the first attack or to any relapse

example, this is one reason why yearly 'rates' of health events are reported in the population (number of subjects) at the mid-year period.

In practice, if the health of individuals is evaluated **only once** during a given period, usually only the prevalence of disease can be established from such an instant study. An overview of disease incidence in the community requires **at least two examinations** of this community in time, one at the beginning and one at the end of a given period, allowing new cases to be recognized. *NB The concept of prevalence as above is also called **point prevalence**. It is a 'snapshot' of an epidemiological situation. Other measures of prevalence, such as **period prevalence**, which also includes old cases, beginning before the period under study, are used less and less. In our example, period prevalence would be 10 per 1,000, i.e. any case might be detected at least once during the year under study.*

Hence, prevalence and incidence are frequencies of cases, prevalence and incidence rates in most health statistics and reports are related to specific denominators. In everyday epidemiological jargon, absolute and relative frequencies are confused; when writing about prevalence, authors sometimes mean prevalence rates, etc. Readers must be vigilant about authors' intended meaning. For practical purposes, prevalence gives an idea of the importance of disease

at a given time and incidence measures disease propagation. Health planners often refer to prevalence.

5.3.1 Incidence density or force of morbidity

For many epidemiologists and statisticians, incidence density is the 'true' measure of disease occurrence rate and its dynamics[6] or 'true rate'. Hence, in epidemiological research, the general term of 'rate' is often restricted to the following: In many situations, such as the study of occupational diseases in relation to exposure to dangerous causal factors in the workplace, workers are exposed to these factors for varying periods of time. When such groups of subjects are compared, calculation of rates of disease should take into account not only the number of subjects concerned, but also the duration of time for which each subject was exposed to a particular risk. In this situation, rate denominators are not simply numbers of workers, but the product of persons **and** time (year, month, hour, shift, etc.) involved in the process for each of them. Incidence of events is indicated in such cases as **incidence density** or **force of morbidity**. Consequently, one person who works one shift contributes by one person-shift to the denominator. One person who has worked three shifts or three persons working one shift only each produce three persons-shifts.

For example, the risk of needle-stick injuries to nursing staff at two hospitals is being compared[7]. The measure of risk will be the occurrence of accidents in a defined group of nurses during a defined period (one year). Full-time employees, part-time nurses or nurses on call all work different numbers of shifts in a year. Given considerable differences in time worked in both hospitals (one hospital relying much more on part-time and on-call workers than the other), comparing the risk of needle-stick injuries is made simpler by using denominators that reflect the total number of persons and the time they spent at work. *NB Other denominators may also more closely reflect 'density', such as rates of needle-stick injuries per 100,000 syringes purchased by the hospital, per 1,000 nurses-shifts of work, etc.*

The use of simple incidence rates and incidence density rates depends on the information required. Incidence density rates eliminate the relationship between the duration of exposure and the occurrence of cases. If the relationship between the rate of cases and duration of exposure were analyzed, simple rates might be compared for different strata reflecting different exposures, or correlations might be evaluated between the duration of exposure and the frequency of cases by more refined quantitative methods. When basic rates are defined, it is noted that mid-period population is often selected as a denominator. This is another method of estimating incidence density when more information on exposure is not available.

5.4 Using observed rates as probabilities of health concerns

Incidence, prevalence, fatality or mortality rates (or proportions) as seen in the community can be used as probabilities when assessing individual patients. Existing or future problems can be evaluated this way.

5.4.1 Probabilities of pre-existing health concerns – diagnostic guess (estimate)

The prevalence rate can be used to express the probability of an individual having a disease when the individual belongs to a community where the disease is prevalent at a given rate. If an elderly patient belongs to a community in which the prevalence of atherosclerosis is as high as 60%, it may be said that the patient has a 6 to 4 chance of having atherosclerosis. It is more probable than not that the patient has atherosclerosis, and an examination should be carried out so that atherosclerosis can be ruled out or treated accordingly. If a male retiree lives in a community in which 10% of individuals have high blood pressure (prevalence rate of hypertension in the community), his *a priori* probability of having this condition is 0.1. Before examining this patient, a physician may reasonably assume that this patient is hypertensive.

5.4.2 Probability and risk of future health concerns in healthy individuals

The probability of an individual developing a disease (or dying) in a defined time, given the characteristics of the individual and his community, represents an **individual risk**. This means that the subject does not have the problem yet, but may (not will) get it in the future. The next few pages will explain incidence and mortality rates in the assessment of individual risk. If 333 individuals in a community of 1,000 subjects are injured during a year, their individual risk of injury is 0.333, 33.3%, or one in three.

5.4.3 Probability and prognosis of additional health concerns (or of deterioration in health) in already sick individuals

The probability of an individual developing complications (or dying) of an already existing disease does not represent an assessment of individual risk, but rather an assessment of **prognosis**. Chapter 10 is entirely devoted to the area of prognosis.

5.5 Relationship between various measures of morbidity and mortality

Many health problems occur in the community in a relatively steady pattern over time. The clinical course is rather uniform in terms of the duration of individual cases. Outbreaks are exceptional, as are rapidly increasing or decreasing trends. In these cases, the following two relationships may help in better understanding the disease spread, occurrence and impact.

5.5.1 Prevalence, incidence and disease duration

In the above-mentioned situation, the following formula applies:

$$P = I_d \times \bar{d}$$

where P is prevalence, I_d incidence density, and $\bar{d}$ average duration of cases. For example, the point prevalence of brain tumors, P, in a given year is 69 per 100,000, their annual incidence rate (simplest density incidence rate, I_d, by assuming equal time of susceptibility for all) is 17.3 per 100,000 (fictitious data), and the average duration, $\bar{d}$, of cases is about four years.

Many chronic diseases will fall within this category as well, such as Parkinson's disease, hypertension, several cancers, multiple sclerosis, diabetes, etc. More frequent and uniform cases of disease might also be the subject of analysis, such as influenza cases complicated by pneumonia, etc. Using another example, in a given year, a high occurrence of influenza and influenza-like infections is expected in a community of elderly citizens. It may be expected that about 20% of cases will be complicated by pneumonia requiring hospitalization. Attending staff may be interested in knowing how many hospital beds will be needed to accommodate pneumonia cases. It is known that 2,500 new cases of influenza and influenza-like infections (I) were noticed during the previous year (incidence of the disease). Twenty percent, i.e. 500 cases, yielded pneumonia, requiring an average hospitalization of 7 days (average duration of pneumonia or $\bar{d}$). Number of beds occupied at any day of the period by pneumonia cases (P) is then:

Number of beds (i.e. prevalent pneumonia cases at a given moment or point prevalence)		New pneumonia cases during the period		Average duration of hospitalization for pneumonia
P	=	I_d	×	$\bar{d}$
10	=	500	×	0.02

NB 7 days, i.e. 1 week, represents 1/50 or 0.02 of the year under study.

In another situation, emergency room staff might be interested in how efficiently patients are transferred from the emergency ward to other hospital wards. During a one-month period, 200 emergency patients used emergency room beds (incidence of the use of emergency beds). A morning round at the emergency department shows that 10 beds are occupied by patients waiting for transfer to other wards (point prevalence of occupied beds). According to the same formula, ($\bar{d} = P/I_d$), i.e. 10/200 = 0.05 of the month, i.e. one day and half. This delay could be worse, but emergency staff might want to further shorten patient stays by obtaining more rapid transfers to the wards.

Figure 5.3 shows the estimated prevalence and incidence of leading cancers in Canadian men and women. The authors[8] correctly point out that prevalence reflects both incidence and survival (i.e. duration). The prevalence of prostate cancer in men or breast cancer in women is higher than their incidence. On the other hand, the incidence of pancreatic cancer in both sexes is higher than its prevalence. These data show in terms of duration ($P = I_d \times \bar{d}$) that survival is longer in prostate or breast cancer cases than it is in individuals suffering from pancreatic cancer, which is in accordance with clinical experience itself.

5.5.2 Mortality, incidence and case fatality

In situations similar to those above, a mortality rate (M) for a given health problem can be estimated as a product of incidence rate (I) and case fatality rate (CFR).

$$M = I \times CFR$$

Recently, Fowler et al[9] reported incidence and fatality rates of adult respiratory distress syndrome in patients suffering from various conditions or complications. For example, if the mortality rate due to adult respiratory distress syndrome in severely burned patients was 25% (or 0.25 as a decimal) and its incidence rate 50% or 0.5 (fictitious data), its case fatality rate must be 50% or 0.5, i.e. 25%/50% or 0.25/0.5. Obviously, the higher the fatality rate, such as in the case of pulmonary aspiration, the closer the

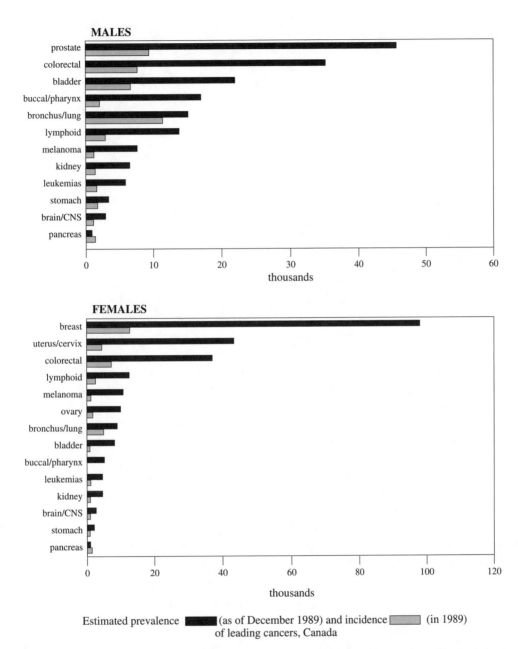

Figure 5.3 Incidence and prevalence of cancer in Canadian men and women. Reproduced from Ref. 8, with permission from the *Canadian Journal of Public Health*

mortality rate to the incidence rate (almost all patients suffering from pulmonary aspiration die from the syndrome in this study).

The two above-mentioned concepts were formulated in textbooks by MacMahon and Pugh[10] and further refined by Kleinbaum, Kupper and Morgenstern[6] and Freeman and Hutchison[11,12].

5.6 Using health indexes in describing disease spread

If disease occurrence rises above the expected (i.e. usual or habitual) level, three situations can occur. An **epidemic** represents an unusual incidence rate at a given moment and a given place. If no cases exist in the community, even two new cases (transmission

Table 5.1	Criteria for modes of disease occurrence			
		Time and place limitations of disease occurrence		
		Time	*Place*	*Example*
Type of occurrence	*Epidemic*	Limited	Limited	Food poisoning following a community gathering
	Pandemic	Limited	Unlimited	Multicontinental spread of influenza
	Endemic	Unlimited	Limited	Coronary heart disease, stroke, or obesity in North America. Protozoal diseases in the tropics

from one case to the other must be demonstrated) represent an epidemic. Wherever cases already exist in the community, usual incidence rates must be known in terms of their point estimates and their confidence intervals. New rates beyond the upper limits of such intervals indicate an epidemic situation (Figure 5.4). A **pandemic** represents an unusual incidence rate of disease in a given time period, but unlimited in space. Usually if disease spreads beyond one continent, a pandemic can be considered. Influenza pandemics are a classical example of such situations. The disease becomes **endemic** whenever a high occurrence rate is noted without any restriction as to a precise period (for example, from one decade to another). If several subsequent generations are affected, the disease may be considered endemic. For example, malaria is endemic (i.e. unlimited in time) in many countries with warm climates, and coronary

disease and obesity are endemic in North America. Table 5.1 summarizes these three situations.

The term **hyperendemic** is used in cases where disease is present in terms of high incidence and/or prevalence rate in a given community over a protracted time period ('constantly present'), appearing equally in all groups following selected characteristics (e.g. all age groups are affected). Malnutrition, bilharzias or malaria are often hyperendemic in several regions in the tropics.

Obviously, incidence rates represent the basic measure of the disease's spread. Unusually high incidence rates indicate epidemics and pandemics, and high prevalence rates over time suggest endemicity. If both measures are elevated over time, hyperendemicity should be considered. Figure 5.5 shows fictitious data regarding disease occurrence, leading to long-lasting cases. A sudden increase in incidence

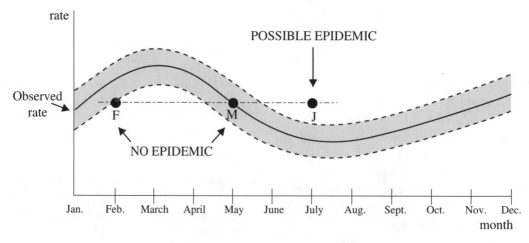

Figure 5.4 Example in which the same incidence rate does not always mean an epidemic

and its slower regression suggests a common source epidemic in unvaccinated and/or susceptible communities. (Most subjects are exposed at the same time to a common source, such as gastroenteritis outbreaks after social gatherings at which the same foods are consumed.) A more symmetrical increase and decrease of incidence tends to reflect person to person spread of disease, such as in many respiratory diseases or childhood infections (mumps, scarlet fever, etc.). Provided that the disease's incubation period is known, the incidence rate peak indicates the moment when the maximum number of subjects end their incubation period by developing the disease. By going back in time, the most probable moment of exposure and the source of infection may be identified.

5.6.1 Attack rates and secondary attack rates

The overall incidence rate possible during a period in which disease may occur, given its exposure to a common source and its incubation period, represents an **attack rate** of that disease. If a group of people at a banquet consumes mayonnaise prepared from duck eggs that were contaminated with salmonella, all persons subsequently suffering from salmonella and becoming ill as soon as 6 hours after the meal (including even those becoming ill after 36 hours) would represent the attack rate of salmonella related to the banquet. Attack rates of an irradiation disease after a nuclear accident should include all late cases given the degree of exposure.

A **secondary attack rate** is defined as an incidence rate when primary case(s) (often called the index case or cases), i.e. the first ones to be found, are excluded from the numerator and denominator. For example, a primary school opens in a partially immunized community. Fifty children out of 200 are immunized against diphtheria. The next day, two children are diagnosed with diphtheria, and 18 more fall ill before the end of the new school year's first week. Given diphtheria's incubation period of two to six days, the first two cases must have carried the disease from outside the community, and the subsequent 18 cases might have been transmitted by the above-mentioned primary (or index) cases. The overall attack rate for the first week of school would be 20 per 150 (50 are immunized or already had the disease). The secondary attack rate would be 18 per 148 (i.e. 150 less two index cases).

$$\text{Secondary attack rate} = \frac{\text{all incident cases} - \text{index cases}}{\text{all subjects} - \text{non susceptible individuals} - \text{index cases}} \times 10^x$$

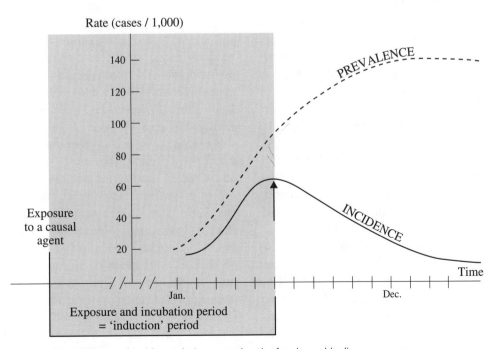

Figure 5.5 Example of prevalence and incidence during an outbreak of an incurable disease

Secondary attack rates allow for a better understanding of the seriousness of the spread of disease in this community. On the contrary, if 18 cases had been discovered on the second day of school and only two cases at a later date, the overall attack rate would also be 20 per 150. However, the secondary attack rate would be 2 per 132, indicating a much less serious spread of disease in this community.

5.6.2 Point estimates and interval estimates of rates[13]

Various studies evaluate community health by studying samples of individuals in a defined community. Rates of events are established by observation of these samples. For example, if an influenza epidemic is anticipated, it may be relevant to know how many senior citizens in a community are immunized against this disease. If a prevalence rate of vaccination (which may represent a so-called **herd immunity**) is found to be low, this rate could be increased to prevent seniors from contracting the disease, as well as its serious complications such as pneumonia or death. A sample of 600 subjects was obtained from a total of 20,000 seniors (65 years and over) in a given area. Two hundred and forty of these subjects had recently been immunized against the expected variant of influenza virus threatening the community during the current epidemic period (winter–spring). The point estimate of the vaccine coverage (immunization rate) would then be 240 per 600, or 40%. It might be worthwhile to know the best estimate of such a rate in the whole community from which the 600 subjects were obtained – the rate might be different.

Following the reasoning described in Chapters 1 and 2, it is reasonable to assume that if 100 studies based on 100 different samples were drawn successively from this same community, a true rate would be found somewhere in a range of values (point estimates in these 100 studies) into which 95% of these studies would fall (99% or 90% might be also considered, depending on the precision desired). This would be an interval estimate of the immunization rate being studied. Let us say that a confidence interval for this immunization rate of 40% would be 0.40 ± 0.0392. It is reasonable to conclude that the

herd immunity (vaccine coverage) in this community of 20,000 may be as low as 36% or as high as 44%. An immunization rate of 36% would not be enough to prevent the spread of influenza in this community and given the risks (serious cases of pneumonia, etc.), an appropriate catch-up immunization program in this age group might be considered. For example, if 80% of all non-immunized subjects were to contract influenza (80% of 7,200, i.e. 36% of 20,000), 5,760 cases are at stake. If 5% of these cases were to develop serious or fatal pneumonia, 288 pneumonia cases represent a warning that all possible measures should be taken to prevent an epidemic of influenza in this community.

Compare Community A with two other communities (B and C). In Community B, an interval estimate (95 or 99%) of immunization rate was found as 54% to 66%, and an estimate of 42% to 58% was found in Community C. Before further statistical considerations and computations, the overlap of these confidence intervals may be compared. Where overlap occurs, it is reasonable to conclude that observed differences in point estimates may be due mainly to chance, as would be the case in Communities A and C. Where these estimates do not overlap (Communities A and B), the differences in immunization rates in these communities are not due to chance only. Being 'statistically significant', the relevance and importance of these immunization rates should be examined from the epidemiological and clinical points of view. If another study yielded a point estimate of 12 with a confidence interval of 11 to 13 per 1,000, both studies would yield statistically significant results. (*NB However, from an epidemiological and practical viewpoint, given the spread of measles, a difference of three cases per 1,000 when comparing attack rates would not be considered important. From a medical standpoint, decisions such as whether or not to immunize, isolate, etc. would not change from one community to another.*) This example gives an application of the basic principles of interval estimations to an incidence rate (attack rate in this study). Any other disease occurrence measures, such as mortality rate, prevalence rate, fatality rate, etc., are computed and interpreted in a similar way. The use of confidence intervals was recently recommended along with classical inferential statistical analysis. More information on this subject can be found in Altman et al[13].

5.6.3 Crude rates and standardized rates

Disease or deaths as they occur in the community are reported as crude rates. However, if communities differ in age, and if disease or death were related to this difference (such as heart disease, injuries, or cancers), crude rates comparing young and old populations would be misleading. This procedure, which defines rates in communities with comparable characteristics of interest (usually age, sex, race, ethnic group, etc.), is called **standardization**. Its products are standardized rates.

Two methods of standardization exist. Direct standardization is used whenever large denominators are available and event frequencies are not too small, giving 'unstable' or 'floating' rates (in computational language). Indirect standardization is used whenever a risk of unstable rates occurs. The following examples illustrate these situations. The principle of **direct standardization** is that rates observed in one community are applied to a 'standard' or 'reference' population and its denominators. Such a newly computed rate 'as if the original population had denominators of the reference population' represents a **standardized rate**. In **indirect standardization**, original data in different groups are also compared. However, the purpose of indirect standardization is not to obtain another standardized rate, but rather a ratio of rates on the same population before and after standardization.

In indirect standardization, the procedure is, in a way, the reverse of direct standardization. Rates observed in a reference population are applied to denominators in a study population. The resulting numbers of cases in all age groups are added, and this newly obtained rate is compared to the crude one, resulting in a ratio called the **standardized mortality** or **morbidity ratio**. Indirectly standardized rates are usually used when studying small populations in whom rare events occur, for example leukemia deaths related to agricultural chemicals used in small, rural communities. When studying time trends in morbidity or mortality, rates in a given year (for example, the last available year or any other year)

can be used as the reference rate. Thus, standardized mortality (morbidity) ratios can be computed for a sequence of years of interest. Evolution of disease in time can be made more explicit in that manner than comparing crude rates for years concerned.

Caution on the limited use of standardized morbidity (mortality) ratios: Standardized mortality ratios can be compared in different communities if, and only if, they are based on comparable reference rates.

5.7 The most important health indicators and indexes

A good deal of theoretical work is being done to find the best assessment of health for an individual or a community. Presently, two approaches are commonly used. Either indirect measures are followed, such as the aforementioned assessment through the frequency of health problems, or direct measurements, such as the assessment of an individual's fitness, are used.

Health is usually measured with health indexes and indicators. A **health indicator** represents an individual's characteristics that can be defined qualitatively. For example, abnormal (elevated) blood pressure is an indicator of hypertension, and elevated blood sugar is an indicator of diabetes. A **health index** is a quantitative expression of an indicator. Blood pressure of 160/100 is an index of hypertension, and a fasting blood sugar of 300mg/dl is an index of diabetes. Poor pre- and postnatal survival of fetuses and infants is an indicator of mother/child health and of the quality of obstetrical/pediatric care during that time. A perinatal mortality rate is an index of that care. These distinctions are not common and the term **indicator** is used in general literature. Most information on health is seen throughout the literature and practice as health indexes. These may be classified and understood in several ways. Table 5.2 illustrates such a classification according to the source of data, directness of measurement, and various aspects of health.

For practical purposes, all health measurements must be:
- Easily obtained without sacrificing the quality of data;

Table 5.2 Classification of Selected Health Indexes and Indicators

Indexes based on routine demographic data
- Life expectancy
- Life expectancy 'in good health'
- Potential years of life lost
- Distribution of population according to its characteristics

Indicators based on hospital and community counting of cases of disease and deaths and their causes
- Mortality
- Morbidity
- Case fatality

Indicators based on assessment of the disease's impact
- Absenteeism
- Hospital and other services admissions
- Use of primary care facilities
- Deficiencies, impairments and handicaps
- Periods (days) of restricted activity
- Quality of life

Indicators of well-being
- Physical well-being
- Mental well-being
- Social well-being
- Spiritual well-being
- General well-being (all of the above)

Indicators and indexes based on way of life
- Exposure to factors that produce undesirable effects (past or present)
- Exposure to noxious agents in the environment
- Self-exposure to noxious agents (tobacco, alcohol, other drugs)
- Non-exposure to beneficial factors such as physical activity or healthy food intake (i.e. being inactive and eating poorly)
- Stressful life events
- Exposure to factors having beneficial effects (past or present)
- Herd immunity through immunization
- Proper living conditions and daily living habits
- Harmonious social environment

Indicators of level of good health
- Physical fitness
- Adaptability

Composite indicators and indexes
- Combinations from above-mentioned categories

- Available at a reasonable cost;
- 'User friendly', i.e. easy to use, analyze and interpret;
- Sensitive enough to reflect changes in health in relation to the impact of noxious and beneficial factors and of medical and sanitary interventions.

Basic measurements of health, such as morbidity and mortality data derived from hospital sources, from demographic registries and from special surveillance programs and sources, are usually more satisfactory (and they are most often used in the literature and as professional information) than other composite indexes. **The more complex health indexes are, the more they encompass a large spectrum of health care, and the less operational they are.** The following comments and illustrations cover only the most important and relevant elements of the above.

5.7.1 *The most important health indicators*

Some health indicators are used routinely on the basis of national and local health statistics and demographic data, others are used for specific and well-focused epidemiologic studies, and the rest are used for individual assessment. The most frequent indicators, their practical meaning and some typical values are defined below. Let us stress right away that it is not enough to correctly calculate rates, ratios or health indexes. Their **interpretation** is equally important. For example, if two or more mortality rates are to be analyzed and interpreted:

- **Look first at their numerators.** What causes their differences? Consider higher incidence (or the interplay of disease prevalence, incidence and duration), higher case fatality rate, or both (remember $M = I \times CFR$), better detection, reading errors, different medical care (records), failure to treat successfully, etc.
- **Then look at their denominators.** Were these populations stable? Consider people moving in and out, people moving between various health services, one population aging faster than the other, different health, social and demographic characteristics, different exposures to various risk factors, etc.

5.7.2 *Indicators from the field of demographics and routine vital health*

Each community routinely tracks its live births, stillbirths, deaths and marriages (to a variable extent). Periodic population censuses (i.e. every four years) give additional data that yield various indirect measures of the community's health as a whole. These definitions closely match those in the current edition of the *Dictionary of Epidemiology*[2] and the *International Classification of Diseases*[14] *(see also References 23, and 24.) However, minor national differences can exist depending on the availability (or non-availability) of data.*

Life expectancy (expectation of life) is the average number of years an individual at a given age is expected to live if current mortality rates continue to apply[5].

Disability-free life expectancy. Wherever hospital and other routine data allow the identification of chronic and/or incapacitating conditions, the number of years from the onset of disease may be withdrawn, giving life expectancy in good health, i.e. until the first chronic condition appears as a modifier of the quality of life for the remaining years left to live. At birth, disability-free life expectancy in comparison to overall life expectancy is 10 years shorter in Canadian men and 16 years in Canadian women[15].

Quality-adjusted life expectancy Wherever different conditions arise which may alter quality of life, such as institutionalization or disabilities, years lived under these conditions may be given different values (weight). By weighting (multiplying by a certain value) various periods of life, another form of life expectancy may be obtained which reflects both the number of years lived and under which conditions. Computational methods and their applications to Canadian data are available in the literature[15].

The measurement of **quality of life** as one possible weighting factor is getting increasing attention, as evidenced in introductory articles[16], new methods of scaling such as Spitzer et al[17] or EuroQol[18] proposals, and *ad hoc* overviews[19–21]. Weighting of years by quality of life may be quite arbitrary, or may be based on a more structured assessment of the individual's physical, mental and/or social functioning. For example, a weighting factor of 0.4 may be assigned to years of institutionalized disability, 0.5 to a period of inability to perform major activities, 0.6 to a period of restricted major activity, 0.7 to one of minor activity, 0.5 to a period of short-term disability, and weighting factor of 1.0 may be assigned to a period of no disability whatsoever[15]. According to overall life expectancy at birth in 1978, Canadians can expect to be affected by disability for fewer than 15 years. However, about half of Canadian life expectancy after age 65 will be marked by various limitations[15].

However important the complex measurements, composite indexes and scores of quality of life are for research purposes and health policies and planning, their components are more important for the practice of and decisions in medicine. An incapacitated patient wants to walk again or eat without assistance and not to improve his quality of life score from 0.2 to 0.4 on some scale based on 30 aspects of living.

Potential years of life lost represent the years of normal life expectancy lost by persons dying of a particular cause[2]. This concept is now widely applied to Canadian data[22]. For example, a 20-year-old man who dies in a traffic accident can be said to have lost 50 years of life, using the combined life expectancies in Canada for men and women. Statistics of years lost by cause stress the limitations of this indicator of health. Any health condition fatal at an early age has an obviously greater impact on years lost. If used for comparative purposes, this indicator is most efficient when comparing various causes of death in persons of a comparable age. It makes more sense to compare years lost to chronic diseases, injuries or mental disorders at age 20, 40, or 60 than to combine all ages, since deaths by injury in young persons will also have

a noticeable impact on any condition, even common conditions manifesting later in life.

A population pyramid is a graphic representation of different groups of a population according to sex (men represent the left side of the figure, women the right) and age (usually five-year intervals are superimposed, younger ages at the base, the older on the top) in absolute numbers or as a proportional representation. A large population pyramid base indicates a high fertility rate. If the pyramid becomes more of a 'column', such as in many developed countries today, it reflects a low fertility rate, higher life expectancy (higher pyramid) and more aged individuals 'on the top of the pyramid' (higher age strata as in Canada today[23], Figure 5.6). Indented age groups reflect low fertility rates and/or high mortality rates, such as occur during famines, wars, deep economic recessions or epidemics of highly fatal diseases affecting specific groups. An 'asymmetry' of the pyramid's left side (men) and right side (women) may reflect, in some countries, the impact of loss of life during wars and social upheavals. The shape of the Canadian pyramid in the past century is seen today in many Third World countries, which have a fertility and

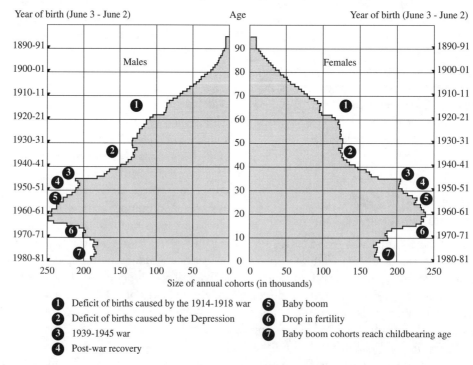

Year of birth (June 3 - June 2)   Age   Year of birth (June 3 - June 2)

| | Males | | Females | |

Size of annual cohorts (in thousands)

① Deficit of births caused by the 1914-1918 war   **⑤** Baby boom
② Deficit of births caused by the Depression   **⑥** Drop in fertility
③ 1939-1945 war   **⑦** Baby boom cohorts reach childbearing age
④ Post-war recovery

Figure 5.6 Population pyramid, Canada, June 3, 1981. Source: Ref. 23, reproduced with permission of the Minister of Industry as Minister responsible for Statistics Canada

mortality rate and other conditions comparable to Canada generations ago.

5.7.3 Indicators based on births

Frequency of births (live or stillborn) in relation to the population indicates the health of the community as a species and its potential for long-term survival and evolution. Table 5.3 gives current definitions of birth, fertility, and low birth weight rates[24]. High birth rates and fertility rates are necessary for survival of the species. As indicators of the community's good health, they must be associated with low morbidity and mortality at young ages, long life expectancy and favorable socio-economic indicators such as food production, revenue or gross national product per capita, etc. The opposite is true in many of the world's poor countries. In these circumstances, high birth and fertility rates in conjunction with poor economic indicators often show a dramatic worsening of the nation's health. At the beginning of this century, the fertility rate in Canada was comparable to the current rate in many developing countries. It has now fallen during three generations to one-third of its value.

5.7.4 Indicators based on frequencies of disease cases and deaths

Causes of disease and death are not the same throughout life. This variation is most important at early and advanced ages. Indicators must thus reflect these facts in monitoring a child's pre- and postnatal development, as well as that of the mother. Figure 5.7 illustrates phases of follow-up of health during the prenatal (fetal morbidity and mortality) and postnatal periods of development. Prenatal and postnatal periods and events accounted for in health indicators are defined below.

Fetal and infant health indicators and definitions for corresponding rates and ratios can be found in references[14,23–25]. It must be understood that the same definitions apply to morbidity rates (ratios) as defined in terms of mortality. As already specified, rates include numerator events in their denominators, ratios do not (Table 5.4). Why are so many indicators necessary? During the rapid evolution of ontogenesis, numerous factors intervene and act upon the health of an individual. The exact hierarchy of similar and other factors causing fetal losses still remains to be better understood. Infant, neonatal and post-neonatal mortality rates in Canada and the United States show that the first 24 hours of life are crucial and responsible for the greatest proportion of deaths during the neonatal period[26]. Congenital anomalies, anoxic and hypoxic conditions, and immaturity (in decreasing order) are the major causes of neonatal mortality in North America[26].

In the history of developed countries such as Japan, the decrease in infant mortality rates is due mostly to better control of perinatal causes and infant infections[27]. During infancy, perinatal health

Table 5.3 Health status indicators used for describing natality

Indicator	Numerator	Denominator	Expressed per number of individuals (to the denominator below)
NATALITY			
Birth rate	Number of live births reported during a given time interval	Estimated mid-interval population	1,000
Fertility rate	Number of live births reported during a given time interval	Estimated number of women in age group 15–44 years at mid-interval	1,000
Low birth weight rate	Number of live births under 2,500 grams (or 5½ lbs) during a given time interval	Number of live births reported during the same time interval	100

Source: Adapted from Ref. 24. Public domain

Table 5.4   Fetal and infant health indicators

Health indicator	Numerator	Denominator
Early fetal death rate	Number of fetal deaths during early fetal period	Number of fetal deaths during early fetal period plus the number of live births occurring during a given time interval
Intermediate fetal death rate	Number of fetal deaths during intermediate fetal period	Number of fetal deaths occurring during an intermediate fetal period plus the number of live births occurring during a given interval (usually one year)
Late fetal death rate	Number of fetal deaths (late fetal period)	Number of fetal deaths occurring during late fetal period plus the number of live births occurring during a given time interval (usually one year)
Fetal death ratio	Number of fetal deaths reported during a given time interval	Number of live births reported during a given time interval
Neonatal mortality rate	Number of deaths under 28 days of age reported during a given time interval	Number of liveborn children during the same time interval
Early neonatal mortality rate	Number of liveborn children deceased during their first 168 hours of life (7 days), i.e. neonatal period I and II	Number of liveborn children during a given time interval (usually one year)
Late neonatal mortality rate	Number of liveborn children deceased after their first 168 hours of life until the end of the first lunar month of their life (< 28 days completed) i.e. neonatal period III	Number of liveborn children during a given period (usually one year)
Post–neonatal mortality rate	Number of deaths from 28 days of age up to, but not including, one year of age, reported during a given time interval	Number of fetal deaths of 28 weeks or more gestation reported during the same time interval plus the number of live births occurring during the same time interval*
Perinatal mortality rate I	Number of fetal deaths of 28 weeks or more gestation reported during a given time interval plus the reported number of infant deaths under 7 days of life during the same time interval	Number of fetal deaths of 28 weeks or more gestation reported during the same time interval plus the number of live births occurring during the same time interval*
Perinatal mortality rate II	Number of fetal deaths of 20 weeks or more gestation reported during a given time interval plus the reported number of infant deaths under 28 days of life during the same time interval	Number of fetal deaths of 20 weeks or more gestation reported during the same time interval plus the number of live births reported during the same time interval*

*Some statistics reporting perinatal mortality only in children weighing over 100 g at birth will obviously give lower perinatality rates than those based on all live births irrespective of birth weight.

problems (ICDA), certain causes of mortality in early infancy, congenital anomalies, and other symptoms or ill defined conditions cause most of the deaths under one year of age in North America[28].

Maternal morbidity and mortality are usually studied in relation to pregnancy, delivery and the puerperium (approx. 6 weeks after birth). An expectant mother may die during pregnancy (i.e. due to

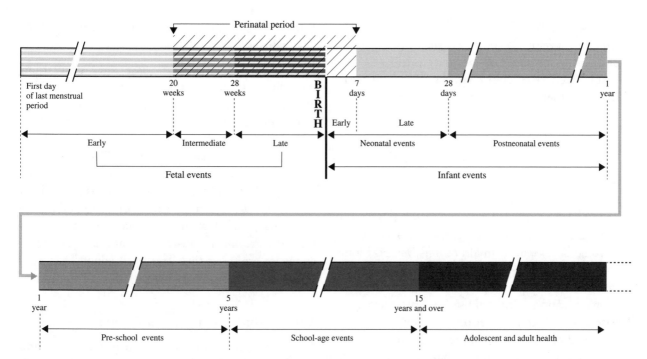

Figure 5.7 Periods of follow-up for health indexes in early life. Events of interest are most often cases of disease (morbidity) or cases of death (mortality)

missed extrauterine pregnancy and its consequences), delivery (uncontrolled uterine atonia, hemorrhage and embolus), or after the birth (puerperal sepsis). Deaths not due to maternal conditions during such periods are not included (such as the death of a pregnant woman in a traffic accident). **Maternal death** is the death of any woman, from any cause, while pregnant or within 42 days of termination of pregnancy, irrespective of the duration and the site of pregnancy[25].

Direct maternal death is an obstetrical death resulting from obstetrical complications of the pregnancy state, labor, or puerperium, due to interventions, omissions, incorrect treatment, or a chain of events resulting from any of the above. **Indirect maternal death** is an obstetrical death resulting from previously existing disease, or disease that developed during pregnancy, labor, or the puerperium; it is not directly due to obstetrical causes, but aggravated by the physiologic effects of pregnancy. **Non-maternal death** is an obstetrical death resulting from accidental or incidental causes not related to the pregnancy or its management. **Maternal death rate** is the number of maternal deaths (direct, indirect or non-maternal) per 100,000 terminated pregnancies for any specified period[25]. Contributions to the numerator and denominator must be within the same time period. In current national statistics the formula is:

Numerator: Maternal deaths due to pregnancy, delivery or puerperal conditions

Denominator: Live births during a given period

$\times$ Expressed per 10,000 or 100,000 of individuals in denominator

It can be observed that maternal mortality rate is not a true rate because the number of pregnancies in the denominator is replaced by live births. This is a purely practical concession, given the availability of live birth figures compared to an almost impossible accounting of the number of pregnancies in a community. Wherever maternal mortality is very low (less than one maternal death per 10,000 live births), every death counts in health statistics. Maternal deaths are declared individually and are the subject of analysis whether or not they are related to the pregnancy. If maternal mortality is studied in population subgroups (i.e. socio-economic strata), rates may be even lower in some instances. In these studies, rates are reported per 100,000 live births instead of 1,000.

This must be taken into account when data is compared. In developed countries such as Japan[27], improvements in maternal mortality rates are most probably due to the better control of direct obstetrical causes rather than the control of indirect ones.

5.7.5 *Indicators for the child and adolescent periods*

During fetal development, early losses are due to the basic incompatibility between ovum and sperm and the genetic material they carry, gross errors of embryonic development (malrotations, malpositions of organs, agenesis, etc.), and as unfavorable intra-uterine conditions due to poor health of the mother (i.e. malnutrition, drug abuse, injury, metabolic diseases, etc.). Late fetal period and neonatal health also depend on the quality of prenatal care, obstetrical care during delivery and perinatal care delivered by physicians, nurses or midwives, and the mother herself. During post-neonatal life, family factors such as nutrition, personal hygiene and morbidity of the family nucleus, have a great impact on the health of the infant. Additional conditions (social, environmental and others) outside the family nucleus contribute to the child's health from pre-school age. For the above-mentioned conditions, perinatal morbidity (mortality) rates are a sensible indicator of the quality of health care when comparing countries, where more direct information on health care is lacking. Similarly, infant mortality (morbidity) rates reflect more upon the socio-economic conditions of the countries or communities being compared.

From a technical standpoint, notions of rates and ratios may be confused, so readers must follow the definitions used for the national statistics of each country. Also, intervals defining the perinatal period are not necessarily those given in Table 5.4 or Figure 5.7. This must also be taken into account. As for deaths in children, the predominant role of accidents as the major cause of death in pre-school and school age children is evident in most countries. In persons aged 15 years and over, cardiovascular diseases, neoplasms, accidents, poisonings, and violence represent the five major causes of death in Canada and the US[26].

5.8 Mortality in the general population and its causes

In developed countries, the last three generations have lived through dramatic changes in morbidity and mortality. At the beginning of this century, the four major causes of death in the United States[29] (as well as in many other countries) were tuberculosis, pneumonia, diarrhea and enteritis. Today, none of these infectious diseases appears among the ten major causes of death in North America. Tables 5.5 and 5.6 summarize the five major causes of death and potential years of life lost in Canadian men and women today[30]. Prevalent causes of death in developing countries are those that developed countries experienced about three generations ago[31].

5.9 Morbidity in the general population

Morbidity data is obtained from primary care and hospital statistics or from special surveys such as the Canada Health Survey and others[33], or the National Health Survey in the United States (see current issues of the Vital and Health Statistics Series). Whereas current upper respiratory and other infections appear as the major cause for office visits, leading causes of hospitalization differ. After pregnancy and childbirth, circulatory, digestive and respiratory problems are the most frequent cause of hospitalization and discharge[34]. Special surveys are needed to assess the prevalence of health problems and to picture morbidity in the community at large. Arthritis and rheumatism, limb and joint diseases, hay fever and other allergies are the problems most apt to occur in the Canadian community[23]. As for chronic conditions, sinusitis, heart disease, thyroid condition, diabetes, and bronchitis/emphysema prevail[34]. (NB Discrepancies between statistics are usually the result of different survey methodologies, data collection or disease or health problem definitions, among others.)

5.10 Occurrence of common signs and symptoms in medical outpatients

Assessing the frequency of disease manifestations in patients[35–37] is also of interest. Symptoms and signs of disease bringing patients to medical care generate

Table 5.5   Major causes of death, Canada, 1998, Males

Cause of death	Deaths	% of total deaths	PYLL[1]	ASMR[2]
1. Circulatory disease	39,948	35.3	192,463	297.2
- Coronary heart disease	24,353	21.5	125,700	178.9
- Stroke	6,488	5.7	22,561	49.5
2. All cancers	32,958	29.2	241,679	234.0
- Lung cancer	10,018	8.9	69,122	70.1
- Colorectal	4,021	3.6	24,930	28.9
- Prostate	3,664	3.2	8,558	27.9
- Lymphoma and leukemia	3,134	2.8	31,494	22.1
3. Respiratory disease	11,380	10.1	33,023	88.0
- Chronic obstructive lung disease	5,765	5.1	13,681	44.1
4. Accidents/Poisonings/Violence	8,886	7.9	262,198	61.0
- Suicide	2,925	2.6	95,785	19.4
- Motor vehicle accidents	2,006	1.8	71,439	13.8
5. Diabetes	2,885	2.6	16,288	21.0

[1]Potential years of life lost (Ages 0–75)
[2]Age-standardized mortality rates per 100,000 population (Ages 0–85+)

Male Canadian Population in 1998: 14,981,500
(Postcensal estimation to July 1, 1998 – Statistics Canada – Demographic Statistics 2000)

Table 5.6   Major causes of death, Canada, 1998, Females

Cause of death	Deaths	% of total deaths	PYLL[1]	ASMR[2]
1. Circulatory disease	39,450	37.5	81,081	182.2
- Coronary heart disease	19,814	18.9	36,157	92.0
- Stroke	9,147	8.7	19,654	41.9
2. All cancers	28,775	27.4	226,612	153.9
- Lung cancer	6,250	5.9	49,668	34.5
- Breast	4,873	4.6	50,393	26.4
- Colorectal	3,769	3.6	20,350	19.2
- Lymphoma and leukemia	2,476	2.4	19,142	13.2
3. Respiratory disease	10,454	9.9	24,670	48.6
- Chronic obstructive lung disease	4,094	3.9	10,595	20.0
4. Accidents/Poisonings/Violence	4,381	4.2	85,130	24.4
- Suicide	774	0.7	24,575	4.9
- Motor vehicle accidents	929	0.9	28,900	5.9
5. Diabetes	2,871	2.7	10,097	14.1

[1]Potential years of life lost (Ages 0–75)
[2]Age-standardized mortality rates per 100,000 population (Ages 0–85+)

Female Canadian Population in 1998: 15,266,500
(Postcensal estimation to July 1, 1998 – Statistics Canada – Demographic Statistics 2000)

considerable workload and costs to elucidate organic etiology which occurs in only a minority of cases. Chest pain, fatigue, dizziness, headache, edema, or back pain most often bring patients to the attention of their primary care physician. These health indicators are interesting from the point of view of medical care organization and health economics. Patients do not visit their physicians because their hemoglobin levels are low, but because they feel tired.

5.11 Other health indicators

5.11.1 Assessing well-being in the general population – composite indicators

In the past 25 years, much has been accomplished to diversify measurements of health. To improve upon data from routine vital and health statistics, various scales were developed to assess physical[38], mental[39] or social[40] well-being or some combination of the above in an overall assessment of the health status of individuals. From a practical point of view, these indicators present several concerns and limitations. They attempt to encompass several, if not all, health conditions which might exist in the community independent of medical diagnoses or specific problems. **The more these indicators are global, the less they are operational.** The second concern deals with the manner in which various levels of health are scored. Third, it is still unknown how sensitive these indicators are to active changes in health status. The use of these indicators in the community will show where problems exist, but researchers must return to the community to assess specific problems using more precise methods. It is therefore difficult to conceive of health programs that would improve 'overall health' in realistic terms.

5.11.2 Assessing wellness in patients

Patients recovering from acute conditions (such as injuries) or chronic-care patients (arthritis sufferers, cancer patients, etc.) should be evaluated for their ability to function and consequently for their quality of life[4,42–44]. Again, scores are given to various aspects of the patient's ability to function in daily activities, subject to the patient's own perceptions and attitudes[45]. Considerable individual[16,17] and collective[18–21] initiatives resulted in the methodology of the assessment of quality of life. For example, in the EuroQol descriptive classification[18], mobility, self-care, main activity, social relationships, pain and mood are evaluated. Most often, various aspects of daily life, health, and care are graded and scored more objectively as in the Spitzer et al[17] quality of life index. In their SF-36 (social functioning) system, Keller et al[45] categorize various aspects of life into groups reflecting physical functioning, general well-being, and mental functioning in the assessment of overall health. Most of these methods of evaluating quality of life suit health planners very well. However, clinicians must never forget that an elderly patient suffering from arthritis does not want to be treated with the goal of improving his quality of life score by points on a scale; rather, the patient wants to climb a flight of stairs without assistance, or does not want to be in pain. From a clinical point of view, parts of the quality of life may be more important than the whole. Some of these indexes already represent quantitative and qualitative clinical measurements of a patient's status and will be discussed as examples in the next chapter on clinimetrics. Readers concerned with assessing individuals' health status will be interested in other sources that update and summarize this subject[19,20,46,47]. A clinician reading a paper on the health-related quality of life must be aware not only of the relevance, validity, and completeness of various aspects of life measured, but must also decide:

- If the information from the study will help inform patients, and
- If the study design simulates clinical practice.

Much more emphasis has been placed on the methodological quality of various measurements of the quality of life[19] than on the evaluation of their use and relevance in routine clinical practice and for patients themselves. Rules of applicability of the quality of life assessment studies to clinical practice[48] generally reflect those listed in Chapter 4 of this text.

5.11.3 Health assessment of individuals according to beneficial and harmful habits and exposure to various factors

Sometimes, only exposure to certain factors can be determined in the community. If it is known how many subjects exposed to a given factor are ill (i.e. proportion of smokers with chronic bronchitis), the prevalence of disease can be estimated. If it is known how many subjects will develop a disease if exposed to a certain factor, the incidence of disease can be estimated (i.e. incidence rate of violent and criminal behavior in drug users). If a disease has multiple causes (as it most often does), etiological research (see later in this text) explains the proportion of cases due to exposure to a given factor among others (the so-called etiological fraction). To do this, the proportion of individuals exposed to various factors should be known in the community of interest. Similarly, the proportion of individuals exposed to beneficial and protective factors helps assess the health of individuals and communities[49–52]. In another example, exposure to positive factors such as immunization can be evaluated. **Herd immunity** (in its simplest expression, a proportion of the community immunized against a given disease) can also reflect the health status of individuals and the community.

5.12 Conclusions

A vast array of health indicators is available today[19,20,46,47,53]. However, the most useful, and the most often used, are the oldest and the simplest ones, such as different expressions of mortality and morbidity with each serving a particular purpose. Besides these traditional indicators, new methods of assessment of physical, mental and social well-being are multiplying at a considerable rate. Rather than properly validating existing indicators by using them widely in practice, authors are often inventing new ones. (A new indicator bearing the name of its author is a better warrant of immortality than using existing indicators). The correct utilization of a given health indicator relies primarily on its ability to give the necessary information and answers to precise questions: How many persons are bedridden at a given moment? How many subject fall ill? How many will die? It is essential that both authors and readers understand this.

REFERENCES

1. Health and Welfare Canada and Statistics Canada. *The Health of Canadians: Report of the Canada Health Survey*. Ottawa: Supply and Services Canada, 1981

2. Last JM (ed.). *A Dictionary of Epidemiology*. 4th Edition. New York: Oxford University Press, 2001

3. Elandt-Johnson RC. Definition of rates: Some remarks on their use and misuse. *Am J Epidemiol*, 1975; 102:267–71

4. Kind P. The Development of Health Indices. In: Teeling Smith G ed. *Measuring Health: A Practical Approach*. New York: J Wiley, 1988:23–43

5. Rothman KJ, Greenland S. *Modern Epidemiology*. 2nd Edition. Philadelphia: Lippincott Williams & Wilkins, 1998

6. Kleinbaum DG, Kupper LL, Morgenstern H. *Epidemiologic Research. Principles and Quantitative Methods*. London: Lifetime Learning Publications, 1982

7. Jagger J, Hunt EH, Brand-Elnaggar J, Pearson RD. Rates of needle-stick injury caused by various devices in a university hospital. *N Engl J Med*, 1988;319:284–8

8. Mao Y, Morrison H, Semenciw R, et al. The prevalence of cancer in Canada. *Can J Public Health*, 1991;82:61–2

9. Fowler AA, Hamman RF, Good JT, et al. Adult respiratory distress syndrome: Risk with common predispositions. *Ann Intern Med*, 1983;98:593–7

10. MacMahon B, Pugh TF. *Epidemiology. Principles and Methods*. Boston: Little, Brown, 1970

11. Freeman J, Hutchison GB. Prevalence, incidence and duration. *Am J Epidemiol*, 1980;112:707–23

12. Freeman J, Hutchison GB. Duration of disease, duration indicators, and estimation of the risk ratio. *Am J Epidemiol*, 1986;124:134–49

13. Altman DG, Machin D, Bryant TN, Gardner MJ (eds). *Statistics with Confidence – Confidence Intervals and Statistical Guidelines*. London: BMJ Books, 2000

14. World Health Organization. *International Classification of Diseases Injuries and Causes of Death* (Vol. I). Geneva: WHO, 1977

15. Wilkins R, Adams OB. *Healthfulness of life. A Unified View of Mortality, Institutionalization, and*

Non-Institutionalized Disability in Canada, 1978. Montreal: Institute for Research on Public Policy, 1983

16. Guyatt HGH, Feeny DH, Patrick DL. Measuring health-related quality of life. *Ann Intern Med,* 1993;**118**:622–9

17. Spitzer WO, Dobson AJ, Hall J, Chesterman E, et al. Measuring the quality of life of cancer patients. A concise QL-index for use by physicians. *J Chronic Dis,* 1981;**34**:585–97

18. The EuroQol Group. EuroQol – a new facility for the measurement of health-related quality of life. *Health Policy,* 1990;**16**:199–208

19. McDowell I, Newell C. *Measuring Health. A Guide to Rating Scales and Questionnaires.* 2nd Edition. New York and Oxford: Oxford University Press, 1996

20. Staquet MJ, Hays RD, Fayers PM (eds). *Quality of Life Assessment in Clinical Trials. Methods and Practice.* Oxford: Oxford University Press, 1998

21. Gandek B, Ware JE Jr. (eds). Translating Functional Health and Well-Being: International Quality of Life Assessment (IQOLA) Project Studies of the SF-36 Health Survey. *J Clin Epidemiol,* 1998;**51**:891–1214

22. Romeder J-M, McWhinnie Jr. Potential years of life lost between ages 1 and 70: An indicator of premature mortality for health planning. *Int J Epidemiol,* 1977;**6**:143–51

23. Péron Y, Strohmenger C. *Demographic and Health Indicators. Presentation and Interpretation.* Ottawa: Supply and Services Canada (Statistics Canada), 1985

24. *Descriptive Statistics. Rates, ratios, proportions, and indices.* Atlanta: Center for Disease Control, US DHEW PHS, (pp.3–8), Doc. No 00–1886 (undated)

25. American Medical Record Association. *Glossary of Hospital Terms.* Chicago: American Medical Record Association (Now: American Health Information Management Association), 1976

26. Vital & Health Statistics. Hospital Use by Children in the United States and Canada. *Comparative International Vital and Health Statistics Reports.* Series 5, No 1, Hyattsville: US Dept Health Hum Serv, DHHS Publ. No (PHS) 84 –1477, August 1984

27. *1989 Health and Welfare Statistics in Japan.* Tokyo: Health and Welfare Statistics Association, 1990

28. Pan American Health Organization. *Health Conditions in the Americas, 1980–1984.* Volume I. Washington: Pan Am Health Org, Ac. Publ. No 500, 1986

29. *Health United States 1987.* Hyattsville: US Dept Health Hum Serv, DHHS Publ. No (PHS) 88–1232, 1988

30. Wilkins K, Mark E. Potential years of life lost, Canada, 1990. *Chron Dis Canada,* 1989;**13**:111–5

31. Preliminary data. Ottawa: Statistics Canada (R Semenciw), Personal communication, 2001

32. WHO. *World Health Statistics Annual 1990.* Geneva: World Health Organization, 1991

33. Kendall O, Lipskie T, MacEachern S. Canadian health surveys, 1950–1997. *Chron Dis Canada,* 1997;**18**: 70–92

34. Health Canada, Statistics Canada, CIHI. *Statistical Report on the Health of Canadians.* Prepared by the Federal, Provincial and Territorial Advisory Committee on Population Health for the Meeting of Ministers of Health, Charlottetown, PEI, September 16–17,1999. Ottawa: Health Canada, 1999

35. Kroenke K, Mangelsdorff AD. Common symptoms in ambulatory care: Incidence, evaluation, therapy, and outcome. *Am J Med,* 1989;**86**:262–6

36. Kroenke K, Arrington ME, Mangelsdorff AD. The prevalence of symptoms in medical outpatients and the adequacy of therapy. *Arch Intern Med,* 1990; **150**:1685–9

37. Ingham JG, McC Miller P. Symptom prevalence and severity in a general practice population. *J Epidemiol Community Health,* 1979;**33**:191–8

38. Belloc NB, Breslow L, Hochstim JR. Measurement of physical health in a general population survey. *Am J Epidemiol,*1971;**93**:328–36

39. Berkman PL. Measurement of mental health in a general population survey. *Am J Epidemiol,* 1971; **94**:105–11

40. Renne DS. Measurement of social health in a general population survey. *Social Sci Res,* 1974;**3**:25–44

41. Grogono AW, Woodgate DJ. Index for measuring health. *Lancet,* 1971; **II**,7732:1024–6

42. Katz S (ed.). The Portugal Conference: Measuring Quality of Life and Functional Status in Clinical and Epidemiological Research. *J Chronic Dis* 1987;**40**(6)

43. Linn MS. A rapid disability rating scale. *J Am Geriatr Soc,* 1967;**15**:211–4

44. Akhtar AJ, Broe GA, Crombie A et al. Disability and dependence in the elderly at home. *Age Ageing,* 1973;**2**:102–11

45. Keller SD, Ware JE Jr, Bentler PM, et al. Use of structural equation modeling to test the construct validity of the SF-36 Health Survey in ten countries: results from the IQOLA Project. *J Clin Epidemiol,* 1998;**51**: 1179–88

46. Berg RL. *Health Status Indexes.* Chicago: Hospital Research and Educational Trust, 1973

47. Health-Status Indicators and Indexes. In: Dever GEA ed. *Community Health Analysis. A Holistic Approach.* Germantown and London: Aspen Systems Corp., 1980:169–225

48. Guyatt GH, Naylor DC, Juniper E, et al. for the Evidence-Based Medicine Working Group. Users' guides to the medical literature. XII. How to use articles about health-related quality of life. *JAMA,* 1997; 277:1232–7

49. *Canada Fitness Survey: Canada's Fitness. Preliminary Findings of the 1981 Survey.* Ottawa: Fitness Canada

(Government of Canada, Fitness and Amateur Sport), 1982

50. *Standardized Test of Fitness, Operations Manual*. 2nd Edition. Ottawa: Government of Canada, Fitness and Amateur Sport, 1981

51. Adult Health Practices in the United States and Canada. *Comparative and International Vital and Health Statistics Reports*, Series 5, No 3. Hyattsville: US Dept.

Health Hum Serv, DHHS Publ. No (PHS) 88–1479, 1988

52. *Health United States 1986 and Prevention Profile.* Hyattsville: PHS, National Center for Health Statistics, DHHS Publ. No. (PHS) 87–1232, 1986

53. Chevalier S, Choinière R, Bernier L, et al. *User's Guide to 40 Community Health Indicators.* Cat. No H39-238 1992 E. Ottawa: Supply and Services Canada, 1992

Chapter 6

Identifying cases of disease. Clinimetrics and diagnosis

I had . . . come to an entirely erroneous conclusion which shows, my dear Watson, how dangerous it always is to reason from insufficient data.
Arthur Conan Doyle, 1859–1930

Before ordering a test, decide what you will do if it is (1) positive or (2) negative; if the answers are the same, don't do the test.
Archibald Leman Cochrane, 1972

At the end of a patient visit, review once more (1) the working diagnosis and (2) the proposed plan to deal with it. Then ask, 'Is there anything else?'. You will be amazed (and patients will be gratified) at how often a less obvious reason for the visit is revealed.
Christopher D. Stanton, 1999

Depression is not a Prozac® deficiency.
Christine Northrop in *The Toronto Star*, 2001

During an emergency medicine call, you are asked to evaluate a patient brought to the emergency department for abdominal pain of unknown origin. On admission, the patient is nauseous. She has already vomited once before arriving at the hospital. You notice, on palpation, a tenderness in the right lower abdominal quadrant and a right-sided palpation pain during a rectal examination. The hematology laboratory draws your attention to mild leucocytosis. You establish a 'working diagnosis' of appendicitis. Because the patient is an otherwise healthy nulliparous woman of childbearing age, you will also consider a differential diagnosis because you do not want to miss an ectopic pregnancy, endometriosis or other problem associated with abdominal pain as an index manifestation on admission. You now find yourself in the middle of medicine's logical discourse:

Clinical practice	Logical discourse	Evidence
You have just recorded history and clinical and paraclinical data	The patient has a history and manifestations of acute abdomen **(Premise A)**	Qualitative evidence from interview, quantitative evidence from exams. **Evidence gathered** (based on soft and hard data)
You have established a working diagnosis	The patient probably has appendicitis **(Premise B)**	**Evidence defined**
You have written orders	Frequent follow-up and and surgery without delay if the working diagnosis is confirmed or another final diagnosis implies surgery **(Conclusion C)**	**Additional evidence gathered and used in decision-making**

To solve this clinical problem, you need well-formulated arguments and a string of best possible evidences on which your postulates and conclusion (decisions and clinical orders) are based. The best possible evidence from a good clinimetric evaluation of abdominal and rectal pain and the information from the patient's history are necessary for Postulate A. Your pattern recognition of the patient's manifestations will probably be the fastest available evidence for your working diagnosis (Postulate B). Your knowledge of inclusion and exclusion criteria for competing diagnoses as well as that of overlapping and additional manifestations of competing diseases will help you order further tests to exclude competing diagnoses in such a differential diagnostic process or will help you follow the patient and perform surgery in case your working diagnosis is confirmed (Conclusion C).

Your success will depend on the best evidence from the literature, clinical experience, patient preferences (in this case, the patient does not have much choice) and clinical circumstances which you will integrate through your clinical expertise. To know if arguments or postulates and their supporting evidence are valid, it is first necessary to master the basic rules of a clinimetric and diagnostic process and their results as outlined in this chapter.

Evidence in medicine is only as good as a physician's senses, quality of observation, interpretation and recording of clinical experience. Risks, rates, and ratios, and their uses in causal research, clinical trials, prognostic studies, reviews of evidence or decision-making, are only as meaningful as the information by which they are fuelled. This chapter will help the reader understand and assess the value of such a 'fuel'.

New technologies are rapidly producing an increasing number of measuring tools, storing devices, and diagnostic and screening methods. However, their validity and usefulness must be established. As an example, how does magnetic resonance work, and does it aid the diagnostic process more than other imaging technologies? In addition to these challenges, a vast array of diagnostic and screening methods have became a part of medical culture, often without a similarly rigorous evaluation. How effective is a clinical examination in the diagnostic work-up of a streptococcal sore throat? Is screening for occult blood in stools in the elderly better than a colonoscopy in the search for colorectal cancer and competing pathologies of the rectosigmoid part of the digestive tract? The evidence produced by both old and new diagnostic processes and the associated simple or complex technological devices is subject to the same method of quality evaluation. Logic dictates that current literature focus equally on both new and old processes.

6.1 From clinical observation to diagnosis: Clinimetrics

Modern medicine requires that attention be paid to highly sophisticated data provided by modern technologies. Lengths, angles, degrees, densities, rads, or titers represent **hard data**, on which the 'science of medicine' relies. Likewise, joy, sorrow, pain, discomfort, malaise, anxiety, solitude, fear, withdrawal, delusions, or tangential thinking represent important **soft data**, on which the 'art of medicine' is based. Both categories are equally important, and both must be carefully identified, evaluated and classified in order to form the basis for identifying patients with a particular problem needing treatment, support or comfort.

Relating to biometrics, econometrics or sociometrics, etc., Feinstein coined the term **'clinimetrics'** in the medical field. He originally defined it as *'the measurement of clinical phenomena'* or *'the domain concerned with indices, rating scales, and other expressions that are used to describe or measure symptoms, physical signs, and other distinctly clinical phenomena in clinical medicine'*[1]. Basic definitions and their applications have already been widely discussed in the literature[2-4].

Over the past two centuries, medicine has become more 'scientific' by its increasing reliance on fundamental data provided by laboratories (biochemistry, hematology, pathology, radiology, etc.). But all these data are preceded by the physician's work at the bedside; patient complaints must be recorded, history taken and observations made, recorded, and assembled in such a way as to represent the patient's problems and the disease requiring care and cure. Production of such raw individual data as a blood cell count or identification of an individual's marital status is called **mensuration**[1]. Further processing of raw data (classification etc.) represent **measurement** in terms of assigning quantitative as well as qualitative (classification, group formation, scaling) attributes to clinical observations in individual patients and in groups of patients or other subjects. In these terms, the original concept (which applies essentially to the procedure leading to diagnosis) may be extended and applied to all mensuration and measurement of health phenomena in a patient and in a community.

Good diagnoses depend primarily on high-quality clinical work with patients. The patient's life and well-being also depend on it. Moreover, it is essential, if disease is to be studied in a community setting, to assess its occurrence in terms of prevalence or incidence, to compare risks, to elucidate its cause(s) or to evaluate the success of interventions. This is just one of many reasons for an interface and interdependence between often artificially dichotomized clinical and community medicine and public health. If clinical work is poorly done, any artistry in epidemiology and biostatistics will not solve the problem (exacting methods applied to poor data).

In routine work, the patient's problems are identified. Then, supported by a clinical examination, a careful 'impression' is made of one or (more often) several problems, which is the basis for a differential diagnosis ('which one of these?'). The final diagnosis is then supported by additional examinations, paraclinical testing (laboratory), etc. Brief diagnoses are the exception rather than the rule. For example, when a soldier or civilian sustains a severe abdominal injury in wartime, a diagnosis of penetrating abdominal trauma is not difficult. More often, however, the procedure takes more time. A poorly communicating, fatigued patient will trigger a more detailed clinical work-up, which may eventually identify anemia, nutritional deficiency, endocrinopathy (hypothyroidism), or catatonic schizophrenia (exaggerated for the sake of explicitness).

Diagnosis is *'the process of determining health status and the factors responsible for producing it'*. It can be applied to an individual, family group, or community. The term is applied both to the **process** of determination and to its findings[3], i.e. to the **endpoint** of such a clinimetric process. From a practical point of view, the following are of interest:

- Good organization and structure of the diagnostic **process** (bedside clinimetrics);
- The quality and explicitness of the formulation of a diagnostic **entity** (clinical identity);
- The validity of methods leading to the diagnosis (**end product**);

- How diagnostic procedures (diagnosis making) and their endpoint (diagnosis itself) are used in a larger clinical framework, i.e. how diagnoses are used in decisions to treat etc. (practical use).

6.1.1 Bedside clinimetrics

The clinimetric pathway begins with the examination of the patient and ends with the categorization into a defined clinical entity. As Figure 6.1 (exaggerated for the sake of explicitness) shows, observations first lead to the acquisition of **clinical data**, which are subsequently evaluated and worked into distinct entities (diagnosis) in terms of **clinical information**. Each of the following six steps must be performed properly. Errors, omissions, or incompetent clinical reasoning have a compounding effect, resulting in poor clinical decisions and/or a poor study of disease frequency and causes in the community.

1. Patients should not be rushed into speedy examinations. Sufficient time must be given to **global observation**.
2. The **isolation** of manifestations of interest should be as complete, detailed, and well recorded as possible. In particular cases, 'negative' observations should also be recorded (no cutaneous lesions indicating skin neoplasia, etc.)
3. When **describing** clinical observations, exhaustive attention should be given to all important manifestations, such as dermatologists describing configuration, extension, color, spatial distribution, texture, and other characteristics of skin lesions. If technical equipment is needed (e.g. a sphygmomanometer), it must be in a good working order, appropriate for a given individual (e.g. different cuffs for different ages), and mensuration (the act of taking blood pressure) should be properly carried out by a well-trained clinician.

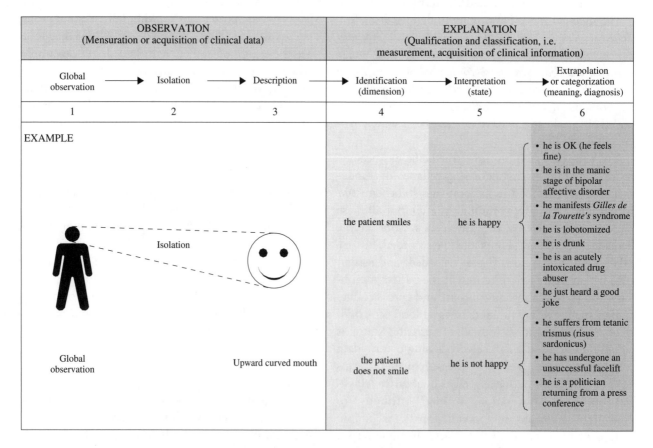

Figure 6.1 Clinimetric pathway: From clinical observation to diagnosis

4. **Identification** means making sense of an isolated observation previously described. Very often, clinical records of a physician's observations start only by identifying what was seen before. Primary observations disappear, remaining unknown. Returning to basic information would be impossible should it ever be necessary. A proper compromise between the requirements of speedy clinical work with economy and efficiency of mind and adequately detailed clinical charts is a considerable challenge, if both sides are to be satisfied.

5. **Interpretation** is an associative process linking previously observed elements with additional perceptions and clinical observations. This second step in explanation requires an increasing degree of clinical competence.

6. A **final inference** is made on a patient's state by classification into a diagnostic category as an end point of the clinimetric process. The patient should be classified according to precise criteria from a mutually exclusive and exhaustive set of categories.

A major practical problem remains a constant substitution of clinical observations (data) by clinical information. Expiratory wheezes are replaced by 'asthmatic breathing', 'prostatic dysuria' replaces difficult, delayed and forceful voiding, etc. A 'normal size uterus' on physical examination is recorded by a clinical clerk instead of 'the size of the uterus palpated is 7–9 cm', etc.

Clinical observations are of primary importance in bedside research. They contain less of a 'clinician's soul' (correct and incorrect decisions) than clinical information. There is no way to revert to clinical data from a sole piece of clinical information retained in records.

6.1.2 *Hard and soft data in clinimetrics*

Hard data in medicine are those which may be defined as qualitatively as possible to avoid misclassification, e.g. between an ill subject (specific disease), a healthy subject or a subject suffering from another problem (another disease). For example, a finding of trisomy-21 indicates Down's syndrome. Such a chromosomal abnormality is considered hard data. A clear quantitative dimension, in terms of count or measurement (discrete and continuous variables), is also hard information. Blood cell counts, blood pressure, gastric acidity, and stroke volume are all hard data. Clinical signs as manifestations perceivable by the physician are often hard data. Laceration, bleeding, heart murmurs, wheezes, or degree of dilatation of the cervix during labor obtained by an experienced clinician fall into this category.

However, many clinical data are so-called **soft data**. Symptoms as manifestations perceived and reported by the patient, as well as some clinical signs, are mostly soft data. Poor demarcation often exists between normal and abnormal subjects or manifestations, such that measurement and quantifications are difficult if not impossible. What is a 'massive' expectoration or hemoptysis? An overnight full or half-full spittoon? How many practitioners bother measuring the cubic centimeter content of a spittoon, or note sputum production in milliliter quantities in the patient's chart? Many clinical observations are soft. The extent (spectrum, gradient) of the disease, stress and distress, some data obtained at emergency and intensive care wards (time, rush), interpersonal relationships, or coping fall in this category. All clinical symptoms (not perceived by a person other than the patient) are soft data. Pain, well-being, anxiety, delusions, love or hate are some examples of this. Some, if not many, data in nursing and social care are soft by nature: being relaxed, looking comfortable, having adequate psychological or social support, being reintegrated socially and professionally, etc.

We have progressively realized that soft data are as important in many situations as hard data. The former were often discounted from clinical research as being part of the 'art of medicine' and without relevance for 'serious' clinical research and practical work. However, the opposite is true. Not only do many specialties depend greatly on soft data, such as psychiatry, and, to a great extent, pediatrics and geriatrics, etc., but also soft data are important for many clinical decisions in many other fields. Patients are discharged not only because their blood electrolytes are normal, but also when clinicians are confident that they have the psychological and social skills necessary to cope with convalescence and a return to normal life. The term 'hardening of soft data' was coined to describe the process of making soft data more usable in research and practice. As Figure 6.2 shows, it puts soft data on a more equal footing with the hard ones by providing soft data with:

- More rigorous **definitions**;
- More complete **specifications** (such as site, nature, spread or character in the measurement of pain[6]);

- A reasonable **dimension** (scale of pain);
- Better and more complete **record-keeping** in medical charts;
- A **parallel meaning** in better-known dimensional hard data;
- A degree of **exposure** when dose–effect relationships exist; or
- The use of special **statistical methods**, such as probit[7] or ridit[8] analysis.

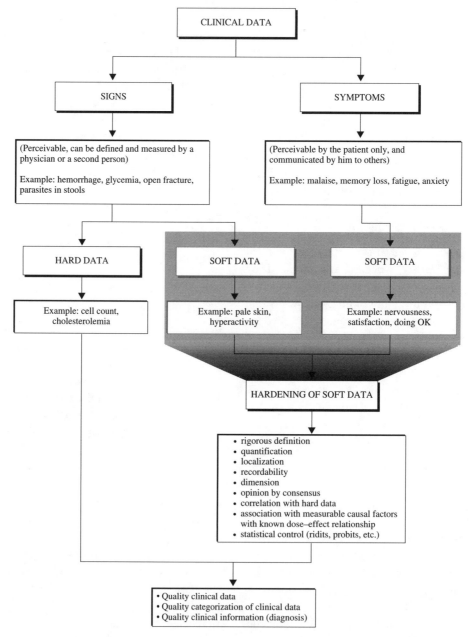

Figure 6.2   Clinical data and clinical information

For example, to obtain harder data on the median age at menarche in girls, when retrospective data are unreliable (poor recall), probit analysis (based on frequency of menstruating and non-menstruating girls at a given age) allows for a more precise estimation of such statistical parameters as median age at menarche, standard deviation of this age, etc[9].

Description, classification and analysis in terms of ridits (related to independent distribution unit) was proposed by Bross[8] to minimize, for example, the misclassification and further comparison of subjects, categorized according to softer criteria such as the severity of injury or measurement of well-being[10,11]. In oncology, the hardening of soft data was successfully applied to such clinical data as mood, affect, depression, cognitive functions, pain and analgesia, nausea and vomiting as well as sexual dysfunction, quality of life, social environment of the patient, and perceptions of care[12]. The presence of soft clinical conditions also influences how soft data is obtained. The psychological effect of a physician's authority (iatrotherapy[13]), interchange of nonverbal messages between clinician and patient, their perception and preservation (psychiatric interview), proper environment and setting for interview and examination are important. It is only recently that more attention has been paid to the clinimetric process, leading to good diagnosis and effective treatment. The clinimetric procedure is initiated by various motives to[14]:

- Complete the medical **history**;
- Assess potential **future disturbances** (risk and prognosis);
- Detect unsuspected **additional problems** (screening);
- Help **management of care** (monitoring function).

In addition, obtaining clinical data depends on the patient. Denial[15], or a reaction to the clinical environment and to persons in the area, may either facilitate or hinder acquisition of data. Physicians also affect the clinimetric process in a number of ways that have only recently been brought to our attention and understanding through increasingly structured and more rigorous qualitative research:

1. Do we perceive health problems as breakdowns to be fixed (North America) or as altered states of equilibrium (psychological, metabolic, etc.) to be re-established[16]?
2. Do we let the patient speak enough[17]?
3. Do we hear the patient or do we listen to the patient[18]?
4. How do we make patients more communicative by our appearance[19]?
5. Do we break barriers of dialect[20], of metaphors[21]?
6. Does our empathy help[22,23]?
7. Do we not ignore such non-specific information (and its role) as laughter[24] or other components of behavior or affective states associated with disease and/or health?
8. How do we proceed logically from data to information, such as in the assessment of somatization and the disorders in comparison with organic problems[25]?
9. What are our perceptions of the patient's disease and our beliefs about it[26].
10. At what stage of clinical measurement are we making errors? Can they be detected[27]?

It is easy to see that jumping to conclusions has a snowball effect: the final diagnosis may ultimately be incorrect, and the patient may be poorly treated. The problem is important not only from a clinical but also from and epidemiological point of view: cases and disease occurrence are poorly assessed, risks and exposures are poorly defined, incorrect causes can be considered. Epidemiological assessment of interventions may be hampered by an erroneous identification of the frequency of intervention, disease exposure, or other phenomena of interest. Demography or medical geography has at times taken medical information for granted, as if it were solid or 'written in stone'. This, however, is not always the case. The interface between field epidemiology and clinical epidemiology is also evident for the reasons discussed above.

6.2 Assembling a diagnostic entity (category)

Assembling a diagnostic entity is not a haphazard process that follows some kind of inspiration. It has a methodology of its own.

6.2.1 *Diagnosis based on one variable only*

In many instances, a diagnosis is made by finding an 'abnormal' value of a physiological function. If blood hemoglobin levels are low (under 12 mg% in an adult woman), anemia is diagnosed. If blood pressure levels are high (a diastolic pressure above 90 or 95 mmHg), hypertension is considered. However, critical levels separating 'normal' from 'abnormal' subjects (i.e. those with disease) may be defined differently[28]. The less satisfactory diagnostic classification is based on a simple statistical distribution of observed values in a group of subjects. If mean hemoglobin values in women are 14 mg% with a standard deviation (SD) of 1 mg%, it is purely arbitrary to say that values lower than two standard deviations, i.e. levels lower than 12 mg%, indicate anemia. This statement only means that such a value belongs to a category into which fall 2.5% of subjects in the community under study (mean values ± 2 SD indicate 2.5% of subjects on each side of the normal distribution in descriptive statistics). Similarly, an abnormal zone might be defined as being below three standard deviations, etc.

An additional problem arises by applying statistical criteria of abnormality when several independent tests are used. According to Cebul and Beck[29], the probability that a completely normal subject will have normal results on all $\underline{n}$ tests is $(0.95)^n$. If 5% of subjects are considered abnormal (mean plus or minus two standard deviations), subjects submitted to 12 independent tests would be considered normal with a probability of only 54%. In other terms, the number of 'abnormal' subjects will increase with the number of independent tests performed:

1 test $1.0-(0.95)$ 5.00% abnormal subjects
2 tests $1.0-(0.95 \times 0.95)$ 9.75% abnormal subjects
3 tests $1.0-(0.95 \times 0.95 \times 0.95)$ 14.26% abnormal subjects etc.

If **any value is found to be abnormal** in relation to what is usually observed in the community, this value **should have a distinct clinical meaning**:

- It should **affect** the **well-being** of the individual (e.g. low hemoglobin levels are associated with fatigue, etc.);
- It should indicate the **need for treatment**;

- The treatment should **improve the function** under scrutiny and the clinical manifestations associated with it;
- The treatment should be **more beneficial than harmful**;
- The patient's **prognosis should improve** with treatment;
- Diagnostic values should identify subjects that society can still **afford to treat**.

6.2.2 *Diagnostic entity based on several manifestations (variables)*

The same pragmatic considerations as discussed above apply in the case of an entity identifying a disease sufferer. Many diagnostic entities have been established intuitively (by recognizing patterns) throughout extensive clinical experience. Often becoming 'classics', these entities work well in practice. Examples include Horner's syndrome (ipsilateral miosis, ptosis, enophthalmus, hidrosis and flushing of the face) related to paralysis of the cervical sympathetic nerves, or the diagnostic criteria such as 'four Ds' for pellagra, representing a tetrad of 'dermatitis – diarrhea – dementia – death'. At present, more refined statistical methods such as hierarchical Boolean clustering[30–32] can be used to determine a diagnostic category and its criteria. For example, this was applied to the classification of systemic lupus erythematosus[33].

6.2.3 *Syndrome versus disease as diagnostic entities*

Clinical and paraclinical manifestations of abnormal states are grouped into two distinct entities: syndromes and diseases. A **syndrome** is a *cluster of signs and symptoms of morphological and/or functional manifestations, appearing disparate a priori, but which may be considered as an entity. This entity represents a clinical but not necessarily an etiological entity*[34–36]. An extrapyramidal or posterior cord syndrome may be caused by trauma, inflammation, tumor, etc. A nephrotic syndrome may be related to renal amyloïdosis, membranous glomerulonephritis, renal vein thrombosis, etc. A syndrome is identified as such if such a clustering of manifestations cannot be attributed to random causes, and if it has a common biological basis. It must be biologically plausible. The above-mentioned examples are plausible as syndromes since a hereditary mechanism (autosomal dominant transmission) causes Marfan's syndrome, and spinal lesions cause extrapyramidal syndrome, etc.

Such a definition of syndrome is recent. Throughout the history of medicine, different characteristics of new or old phenomena of unknown etiology were assembled on the basis of experience and pattern recognition in the observation of many cases. Names of syndromes may reflect[34,37,38] etiology (abused child syndrome), pathogenensis (dumping syndrome), striking feature (whistling face syndrome), an eponym (Goodpasture syndrome), patient's name (Crowden syndrome), compound designation (Hurler syndrome = alpha-L-iduronidase deficiency), mythical nomenclature (gargoyle syndrome), animal nomenclature (cat-cry syndrome), or anything else. These entities, however, often retain their names as syndromes despite later discovery of their etiology. Down's syndrome or toxic shock syndrome may be good examples of this. Many syndromes have been established for purely gnostic reasons; they explain what happens, such as extrapyramidal syndrome. Not all syndromes, however, are indications for treatment.

In contrast to a syndrome, a **diagnostic category of disease** is *a cluster of signs and symptoms delineated by stringent operational definitions, given an entity having a specific etiology, clinical impact on the patient, specific prognosis and outcome, indicative of and susceptible to treatment (intervention).*

Unfortunately, both terms are still used interchangeably. As a result, readers must be attentive when reading the literature. For example, before understanding its etiology, the term toxic shock syndrome was used. Even after its etiology was better understood (as 'staphylococcal scarlet fever' or as a staphylococcal septicemia with specific manifestations), its name persisted despite the fact that the syndrome became a distinct diagnostic category. Should the same be said about AIDS? Any diagnostic entity may be defined according to **conceptual criteria**, such as acute hypovolemic shock with cutaneous and mucosal manifestations as well as fever, or

according to **operational criteria**, i.e. in numerical terms: temperature above 38.5°C, systolic or diastolic blood pressure less than fifth percentile for age, orthostatic hypotension 30 mmHg fall and more in systolic blood pressure, 20 mmHg of the diastolic one, syncope, etc.[39], fall in systolic pressure, 20 mmHg. Operational criteria should be used wherever they are available and wherever possible. In any case, there is no single way to determine an 'abnormal value'. The best method is probably to find the level associated with undesirable signs and symptoms affecting the patient that, if untreated, result in a poor prognosis but may be medically controlled if treatment is provided. Such a stringent set of criteria for clinical abnormality have, however, not been routinely applied in the literature.

6.3 Intellectual process involved in making a diagnosis

Making a **qualitative diagnosis** means identifying the existence of a clinical problem. Making a **quantitative diagnosis** means identifying the seriousness of a clinical problem once it is identified (severity etc.). Section 6.5 will discuss this distinction. During the last decade, considerable progress has been made in understanding the pathways that lead physicians, by a process of diagnosis, to the diagnosis itself[40,41]. There are several ways to arrive at a valid diagnosis[28,42–47].

6.3.1 Diagnosis by pattern recognition

Observations made are instantly fitted into previously learned patterns. For example, if a physician finds a patient lying in opisthotonos, with eyes wide open, laryngospasm, 'risus sardonicus', salivation, and in a non-communicative state, suffering from spasms which can be easily elicited by various stimuli such as light or sound, a diagnosis of tetanus will likely be made. Defense spasms on palpation of the abdomen associated with right hypogastric pain on rectal examination and mild leucocytosis in a nauseated patient in an emergency room will suggest appendicitis. Pattern recognition may be made on a visual (exanthema), tactile (palpation), auditory, or olfactory (smell of breath or urine) basis, or on a

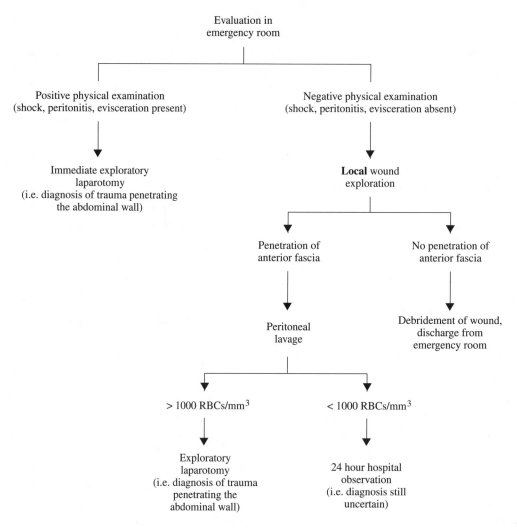

Figure 6.3 Management of a stab wound of the anterior abdomen: an algorithm. Source: Ref. 48, reproduced with permission from Lippincott, Williams and Wilkins

combination of all of the above[44]. Some clinical situations, however, require other processes of diagnosis. Pattern recognition and image processing are also used in computer-assisted medical diagnosis[45].

6.3.2 Diagnosis by arborization (multiple branching)

In this procedure, the diagnostic process advances by logical steps from one decision to another. Such strategies are based on a sequence of steps, where each step depends irrevocably on the result of the previous one until the complete solution to the diagnostic problem is reached and presented as flow charts. With the input of other clinical information,

such as treatment and its result or the performance of other tests, clinical algorithms are established[43]. In such situations, physicians dispose of unequivocal directions in time, that is, how to proceed while accumulating progressively clinical and paraclinical data and information. More information on this subject can be found in the chapter on clinical decision analysis and how clinical decisions are made. Figure 6.3 represents a simple clinical algorithm[48].

6.3.3 Diagnosis by exhaustive exploration of data. Inductive diagnosis

If a patient suffers from an abnormal mass with pain, why not start with a simple X-ray of the abdomen, then an ultrasound, CAT scan and magnetic resonance, and see what all these results mean? This is a kind of diagnostic dredging in which a maximum of clinical and paraclinical information is introduced. By induction, the clinician proceeds to various hypotheses, which can be formulated on the basis of the sequence and combination of clinical data available. This procedure is often favored by inexperienced clinicians (clerks or interns) or by practitioners of defensive medicine, in which nothing is left to chance either to appease a staff member or to avoid legal pursuits and malpractice litigations. This procedure is expensive and slow. Deductive reasoning and clinical flair progressively replace the inductive approach to diagnosis when clinical experience is acquired. The process of inductive diagnosis is a hidden generator of wasteful medicine and must be limited as much as possible.

6.3.4 Hypothetico-deductive diagnosis

'Reported blood in stools, with a history of weight loss, pain, and a palpated mass suggest a possible colorectal cancer. Rectosigmoidoscopy, biopsy and a full radiological work-up will be needed to rule out or to confirm this working diagnosis . . .' In such an approach, index manifestations and data lead to a hypothesis (working diagnosis). Subsequent examinations are chosen. They should confirm the hypothesis or lead to another differential diagnosis. A young person complains of nausea and vomiting. At an office examination, epigastric and periumbilical palpation pain were elicited. Further work-ups are ordered to rule out appendicitis. Attention will be paid to the possibility (and confirmation) of a mesenteric lymphadenitis of viral origin, nephrolithiasis, gastro-enteritis, and/or extrauterine pregnancy. The art of an experienced clinician will be characterized by a judicious choice of a restricted set of hypotheses relevant to patient characteristics and information obtained. Such a **method of 'steepest ascent'**[45] is characteristic of a more experienced physician.

A seasoned clinician will also proceed deductively, but in a more refined manner, based on **probabilistic reasoning**. The clinician will assess the meaning of clinical observations (signs or symptoms) in terms of their sensitivity, specificity and predictive value. If the patient comes from a well-known community, the clinician will evaluate the occurrence of disease in that community, which might be considered the patient's (prevalence). An *a priori* diagnostic (prevalence) will then be combined with conditional probabilities (occurrence of positive or negative results, sensitivity, specificity, etc.) to obtain *a posterior* or revised probability of suspected disease. Such a diagnostic process based on Bayes' theorem is further illustrated in the following section (4.3).

In **causal reasoning**[45], etiological pattern recognition is made first. Persistent cough, bloody sputum and recent rapid weight loss, associated with Horner's syndrome in a heavy smoker for 30 years, will suggest lung cancer given the known causal link between smoking and respiratory tumors.

In **deterministic reasoning**[45] (also called categorical reasoning), unambiguous rules are followed on the basis of compiled knowledge: **if** a throat culture reveals the presence of streptococci (clinically this may manifest as tonsillitis, palpable regional lymphadenitis, strawberry-red injected nasopharynx, etc.), **then** (a **certain action is appropriate**) antibiotics must be given to treat a bacterial infection of the throat. The above-mentioned procedure of following clinical algorithms is an extension or sequence of deterministic or categorical reasoning in diagnosis.

6.3.5 Computer-assisted diagnosis

Based on artificial intelligence theory, **'if . . . then'** categorical and deterministic reasoning[49], various programs have been proposed to aid diagnosis, such as Internist[50] or others[51–53]. Abdominal pain, dyspepsia, or other index manifestations (signs and/or symptoms) represent entries in computer analysis of data based on 'if . . . then' reasoning and Bayesian theory. Limits of practical use are still discussed[45] and further improvements are stressed[54]. Computer-assisted diagnosis requires more extensive validation in practice at the moment of writing. For the moment, computer-assisted diagnosis will not replace physicians, but it may be useful to better structure and complement the diagnostic process in institutions where these facilities are available.

6.4 Qualitative diagnosis and its validity – 'Does the patient have the disease?'

Making a diagnosis does not invariably lead to perfect results. Errors almost always occur. If a laboratory test for occult bleeding or streptococcal infection is developed, it is used by different people with differing knowledge of these procedures, and with different skills and capacities to evaluate the results. Tests are applied to different patients at different stages in disease history and course, and in subjects suffering from one or several diseases that may or may not be treated. Sometimes, procedures done to avoid erroneous results are complex and cumbersome and not followed scrupulously, yielding false positive or false negative results. For example, in the past, patients undergoing fecal occult blood testing in the search for colorectal cancer were instructed not to consume the following for 48 hours before the test[55]:

- Vitamin C supplements;
- Oral iron supplements (false positive results);
- Foods with a high peroxidase activity;
- Red meat;
- Aspirin or nonsteroidal anti-inflammatory drugs (may induce gastrointestinal bleeding).

The more complex the procedure, the less compliance (adherence) can be expected from patients and occasionally, physicians as well. The two most important aspects of the validity of diagnostic methods are:

1. The **internal validity** of a diagnostic method, i.e. its ability to identify disease such as a clinical entity (a case) separate from non-cases.
2. The **external validity** of a diagnostic method (test), i.e. its ability to yield comparable results if used in different environments by different health professionals, using different instruments and working in various conditions.

Two types of tests must be taken into consideration:

1. **Diagnostic tests** are tests pointing unequivocally to a disease. A positive result for a diagnostic test is an indication for treatment of the disease. The inference standard used is the true presence or absence of disease.

2. **Screening tests** are tests that[56]:
   - Should identify a possible health problem in otherwise healthy subjects;
   - Should point to a problem that may have escaped a physician's attention during routine practice;
   - Do not confirm a diagnosis, but do identify possible disease sufferers who should be submitted to diagnostic procedures confirming the disease;
   - Are quick, inexpensive, and widely acceptable for the public and professionals;
   - Are not *per se* indicative of treatment (only re-testing).

For example, if occult blood in stools is suspected as a result of a single Greegor's test, the patient is not immediately scheduled for bowel resection. More testing is needed. Fecal occult blood testing is thus a screening procedure. A single blood pressure measurement giving elevated systolic and diastolic pressure requires repetitive measurements as well as clinical and paraclinical work-ups to exclude renal and/or endocrine causes of hypertension, etc., before the diagnosis of essential hypertension is made and appropriate treatment prescribed. A single random blood pressure measurement is a screening test for hypertension, just as an isolated finding of a low blood hemoglobin level is a screening test for iron-deficiency anemia. Both diagnostic and screening tests must have their internal and external validities known and evaluated by the following methods.

6.4.1 Internal validity of a diagnostic test

The term **diagnostic test** may include one or more clinical observations leading to diagnosis (such as blood pressure measurement), as well as a set of findings from the case history and clinical examination (leading to the suspicion of acute appendicitis) or any paraclinical procedure (such as enzyme testing in the diagnostic work-up of alcohol abuse and dependency). The result of a diagnostic test when compared to some reference method (biopsy, finding during operation or at autopsy, etc.) must correctly identify cases and non-cases of disease. Nonetheless, positive test results are obtained in some healthy subjects,

Table 6.1 Basic contingency table to evaluate the internal validity of a diagnostic test

		Result of a reference diagnostic method or a true state of health		
		Diseased persons	*Persons without disease*	
Result of diagnostic clinical procedure or laboratory test	Positive	True positive results or TP (disease confirmed)	False positive or FP (health not confirmed) absence of disease	Total of positive results for a test (TP+FP)
	Negative	False negative or FN (cases of disease missed)	True negative or TN (absence of disease confirmed)	Total of negative results for a test (TN+FN)
		Total of diseased persons targeted by the test (TP+FN)	Total of healthy subjects who are candidates for a diagnostic procedure (TN+FP)	

while some cases of disease are missed because of false negative results. Table 6.1 summarizes this situation and provides multiple information on the worthiness of a diagnostic test.

Goulston et al[57] evaluated the validity of procedures in general practice to diagnose bowel tumors. They found the most accurate procedure to be clinical history, followed by physical examination and proctoscopy made by general practitioners (GP). Some patients were re-examined by a histopathologist as a reference procedure. The following table (Table 6.2) corresponds to the theoretical categories in the previous table. (NB What if there is no standard as can occur in psychiatry and elsewhere? Schulzer et al[58] recommended replacing the standard with results of repeated observations, such as in the diagnosis of glaucoma in ophthalmology.)

6.4.1.1 Sensitivity of a test

Test sensitivity answers the following:

- Theoretical questions:
  - How does the test perform for sick individuals?
  - How many positive results are obtained in diseased individuals?
- Practical question:
  - How many cases (from total cases in a given community, target population or group) may be identified by a positive test result?

Table 6.2 GP's assessment of likelihood of colorectal cancer

Determined by investigations (histopathology)

Assessed by GP	Determined by investigations (histopathology		Total
	Cancer	*Not cancer*	*Total*
Cancer	12 (TP)	46 (FP)	58
Not cancer	4 (FN)	83 (TN)	87
Total	16	129	145

*GP = general practitioner. Symbols as in Table 6.1. Source: Ref. 57 Reproduced with permission from Elsevier Science (*The Lancet*)

- Who is primarily interested?
  - Field epidemiologists, community physicians, and public health professionals who want to control the prevalence and further spread of disease by primary and secondary prevention programs.
- Major problem:
  - Low sensitivity leads to the loss of patients or candidates for treatment. This is especially serious in situations where the patient will die if untreated. Low sensitivity also leaves diseased subjects in the community as a source of infection for others.

- Example:

$$\text{Sensitivity} = \frac{\text{TP}}{\text{TP} + \text{FN}} \times 100 = \frac{12}{12 + 4} \times 100 = 75\%$$

- Comments:
  - There is no certain level of sensitivity that makes a test acceptable (many practitioners believe in the 'magic' number of 80% or better, for no specific reason). If the search for colorectal cancer was limited only to those methods available to physicians in general practice, a sensitivity of 75% would mean that 25% of cases (or every fourth case) would be missed, diagnosed at a later date, or unsuccessfully treated at a time when the disease had progressed to its terminal stages. However, a sensitivity of 50% also means that a simple 'flip of a coin' would detect (at a lower cost than any other screening or diagnostic method) 50% of existing patients. Only another 50% would be detected compared to the diagnostic method under study. The same applies for specificity (see further).

Visually speaking, sensitivity evaluates the left portion of the 2 × 2 table (Table 6.1).

In clinical uses, Sackett et al[59] propose a mnemonic **SnNout**, i.e. when a test or sign has a high **sensitivity**, a **n**egative result rules **out** the diagnosis. This may be true in clinical practice if used only for patients in which the disease is suspected and if the specificity (*vide infra*) of the test/sign is equally high. A highly sensitive test may have a low specificity (see section 6.4.1.3).

A highly sensitive test yields many true positive results, but negative results may be either true or false negative. The predictive value of a negative test result should be known if possible.

6.4.1.2 *Specificity of a test*
- Theoretical question:
  - How many negative results are obtained in non-diseased individuals?
- Practical questions:
  - How does the test perform in healthy (non-diseased) individuals?
  - How many healthy subjects will be confirmed by a negative test result?
- Who is primarily interested?
  - Health economists and administrators, alarmed by the high cost of reassessment of a large number of false positive results by expensive and sophisticated reference methods (to exclude healthy subjects as candidates for treatment).
  - If treatment is risky for the patient (secondary effects as a trade-off for effectiveness), clinicians want to avoid treating patients for nothing.
- Major problem:
  - Iatrogenic production of undesirable drug effects and elevated cost of reference testing of non-diseased individuals.
- Example:

$$\text{Specificity} = \frac{\text{TN}}{\text{TN} + \text{FP}} \times 100 = \frac{83}{83 + 46} \times 100 = 64.3\%$$

- Comments:
  - About one-third of non-diseased subjects would be reassessed by expensive and time-consuming reference methods to eliminate non-candidates for treatment. Even in a community of aged subjects, where the prevalence rate of colorectal cancer would be as high as 1% in 1,000 subjects under investigation, over 330 subjects would be re-examined at the high cost of a full-scale diagnostic work-up to rule out a nonexistent cancer (by advanced imagery, histopathology). In general, the establishment of rate and absolute numbers of false positive results will depend on what a given community can afford.

Visually speaking, specificity evaluates the right portion of the 2 × 2 table (Table 6.1 and 6.2).

Sackett et al[59] propose a mnemonic **SpPin**: when a sign or test has a high **sp**ecificity, a **p**ositive result rules **in** the diagnosis. Again, this is most effective in situations where the test/sign also has a high sensitivity and if it is used in individuals in which the disease is not suspected in the first place.

A highly specific test yields many true negative results. Again, positive results may be either true or false positive. A predictive value of a positive test result should also be known if possible.

6.4.1.3 *Relation between sensitivity and specificity*
Many screening tests and diagnostic methods have high sensitivity and specificity as well. For example, the ELISA test for AIDS has a high sensitivity (93.4–99.6%) and specificity (99.2–99.8%)[55]. In

many other cases, high sensitivity is obtained at the price of low specificity and vice versa. This occurs in situations where the probability of disease depends on the level of a measured physiological function. For example, the higher the blood pressure, the more probable the existence of hypertensive disease. If a diagnostic or screening level for hypertension is set, for example, at a diastolic of 85 mmHg, most hypertensive patients would be detected (high sensitivity). However, many subjects would have a blood pressure higher than 85 mmHg without having hypertensive disease (physiological variability of blood pressure, stress, fright or anxiety state, error made by an examiner). If the screening level for hypertensive disease is set at 110 mmHg for diastolic pressure, non-diseased subjects would be excluded from further attention (high specificity), but many hypertensive patients (all having lower diastolic pressures than 110 mmHg) would be missed (low sensitivity).

For functions of indirect correlation with disease (the lower the blood hemoglobin, the greater the probability of iron deficiency anemia), the opposite is true. A 12 g% of blood hemoglobin as an indicator of anemia is a fairly sensitive but non-specific diagnostic level. A 10 g% will give a more specific but less sensitive test.

Any diagnostic level must be justified. There is always a trade-off between 'good' (true) and 'bad' (false) results for a test. (NB Fuzzy theory and its applications partly address this problem.)

6.4.1.4 Serial and parallel testing
To identify a health problem, several screening or diagnostic tests are often used. They can be organized in two ways.

Serial testing means that a first test is performed, and if the result is positive, the second test is carried out, and so on. This is a historical example of the use of diagnostic tests for syphilis or AIDS[60], as stated in 1985. In the first case, a VDRL slide test may be performed, and if positive, a TPI (treponema immobilization) test confirms or refutes the results of VDRL. In searching for AIDS, an ELISA test may be performed first, followed by a Western blot test if ELISA is positive. Serial testing improves specificity of diagnosis. The second test refines the positive results of

the first one, and rejects false positive results. It does not discover additional cases. In practice, if high serial testing sensitivity is desirable, the most sensitive test should be performed first. However, a 'paradox of dollars and good sense' exists. Very often, the **cheapest** test, not the most sensitive, is performed first for economic reasons. The economically viable sequence of tests must be considered. The second test does not mitigate the deficiencies of the first.

Parallel testing means that two or more tests are performed. Any positive test result identifies a case. For example, in a screening program for breast cancer, some women are encouraged to perform self-examination of their breasts, others are evaluated by clinical examination at various office visits in general practice, while the remainder are examined by their gynecologists or other specialists. Any positive results from these examinations will lead to a complete assessment (xeromammography, biopsy, etc). Thus, parallel testing improves the sensitivity of a screening program. **Either** test result counts. If the same test is used repetitively, it does not automatically mean that serial testing has been carried out (e.g. repetitive blood pressure measurement). It must always be specified whether the **last** positive test in the sequence (serial testing) or **any** positive test, regardless of order (parallel testing), is indicative of diagnosis. While sensitivity and specificity are important in public health and community medicine, the predictive value of a test result has important implications for clinical practice.

6.4.1.5 Predictive value of a positive test result
In current jargon, the term 'positive predictive value' is also used.
- Theoretical question:
  - From all positive results, how many have been found in disease sufferers?
- Practical question:
  - What is the probability, in the case of a positive test result, that the patient has the disease?
- Who is primarily interested?
  - Any clinician wants to know with some certainty that the patient has the disease if the tests are positive. Since diagnosis leads to treatment, a clinician must have as much **certitude** as possible **before taking action**.

- Major problem:
  - This criterion is particularly valued in action- (or intervention-) oriented medicine such as practiced in North America. However, there is no ideal predictive value. A higher value is more likely to be valid. If the predictive value of a positive result is 50%, the patient may or may not have the disease. If this value is less than 50%, it is more probable that the patient does not have the disease, and this test is worthless for clinical decisions.
- Example:
  - Predictive value of a positive result

$$= \frac{TP}{TP+FN} \times 100 = \frac{12}{12+46} \times 100 = 20.7\%$$

- Comments:
  - This indicates that diagnostic procedures for colorectal cancer based solely on general medicine practices are not indicative of disease or of the need for treatment. A physician cannot be sure that the patient has cancer. A referral and a more complete diagnostic work-up are necessary.
  - Visually speaking, the predictive value of a positive test result evaluates the upper portion of the 2 × 2 table.
  - On the contrary, if we look at how many false positive results are produced out of all positive results, i.e. FP/TP + FP, we obtain a sort of **false worry (false alarm)** rate which gives us the proportion of all positive test results according to which we are telling the patient that more testing is needed when this is not the case.

6.4.1.6 *Predictive value of a negative test result*
This is also known as a negative predictive value.
- Theoretical question:
  - What proportion of all negative results is found in people who do not have the disease?
- Practical question:
  - What is the probability, in the case of a negative result, that the patient does not have the disease? How sure can a clinician be that a decision **not to treat the patient** is right? The clinician wants **to be sure before deciding not to take action**.
- Who is primarily interested?
  - Any clinician who wants to be sure that a decision not to treat the patient is correct.

- Major problem:
  - To treat patients not needing treatment increases the cost of medical care.
- Example:
  - Predictive value of a negative test result

$$= \frac{TN}{TN+FN} \times 100 = \frac{83}{83+4} \times 100 = 95.4\%$$

- Comments:
  - 'When ruling out cancer in general office practice, a physician is more than 95% sure that the patient does not have cancer. The patient does not need to see a gastroenterologist for a more complete assessment. The predictive value of a negative test result should be known to any physician practicing conservative, 'primum no nocere' medicine. Useless and costly treatment with important side effects should obviously be avoided in non-diseased subjects.
  - Visually speaking, the predictive value of a negative test result evaluates the lower portion of the 2 × 2 table.
  - NB If, on the contrary, we look at how many false negative results are produced out of all negative results, i.e. FN /FN + TN, we obtain a sort of **missed opportunity or false reassurance rate**, on the basis of which we can focus on how many patients from among those who produced a negative test result might actually have the disease in question.

The assessment of internal validity doesn't only apply to laboratory diagnostic tests. Clinical bedside diagnostic maneuvers can also be evaluated this way[61]. It shows, for example, that the Valsalva maneuver has a better predictive value of a positive test result for hypertrophic cardiomyopathy than a decreased handgrip. A transient arterial occlusion increase appears perfect to detect mitral regurgitation and ventricular septal defect. However, some healthy subjects may show false positive results[61].

6.4.1.7 *Variability of predictive values of diagnostic and screening tests*
The internal validity of a test is most often determined by taking a group of diseased and non-diseased subjects, and performing both tests on each individual (test and reference assessment). The sensitivity and

specificity of the test is given. This information is usually provided by companies producing diagnostic test equipment (machines, kits, chemicals, etc.). When using such a test, a physician must realize that predictive values will vary according to the different populations tested. For example, if a very sensitive and specific test such as ELISA were used in screening for AIDS in a community where the prevalence of seropositivity is very low (e.g. a suburban shopping center, where there would probably only be a few intravenous drug users, hemophiliacs, or homosexual males relative to the rest of the population), the following would happen: many healthy (seronegative) subjects would be examined, yielding several false positive results. A few seropositive subjects would show false negative results. When calculating predictive values, the predictive value of a negative result would increase with the decrease of prevalence, while the predictive value of a positive result would decrease. If the same test were to be performed in a large group of intravenous drug-using prostitutes, where the prevalence of seropositivity is very high, more false negative and fewer false positive results would be found.

It may be noted that the probability of disease according to the result of the test (called posterior probability) also depends on the prevalence of the disease (prior probability), i.e. before testing. This relationship was quantified in medicine based on theoretical principles, proposed in the general field of chance by Reverend Thomas Bayes in the late 1700s[62]. The following terminology is used in this reading:

- An *a priori* probability of disease is the probability of having a given health problem before a diagnostic maneuver (test) is performed. The prevalence rate of this disease in the community to which a patient belongs according to his or her characteristics is often used to estimate such a probability.
- An *a posteriori* probability of disease is given by the predictive value of a positive test result.
- A **revised** probability is the probability of disease based on the consideration of both *a priori* and *a posteriori* probabilities. (Bayes' theorem specifies this.)

In this approach (the development of which may be found in an informative book by Sox et al[63]), the

following are considered in the computation of predictive values:

Prior probabilities (before the test is performed):
(a) Prevalence rate of the disease in the community from which the patient comes (i.e. the probability of having the disease if one belongs to this community, sharing common characteristics of person, time, and place).
(b) 1 – Prevalence, or the probability of not having the disease (rate of healthy subjects in the community).

Post-test probabilities (given by the test performed):
(a) Sensitivity, or probability of having a positive test result if diseased.
(b) 1 – Sensitivity, i.e. rate (or probability) of false negative results in diseased subjects.
(c) Specificity, or probability (rate) of true negative results in healthy (non-diseased) subjects.
(d) 1 – Specificity, i.e. rate (or probability) of false positive results in non-diseased subjects.

On the basis of this information, the following predictive values in terms of **revised probabilities** may be computed, combining prior and posterior probabilities as quoted above:

Predictive value of a positive test result

$$= \frac{(\text{prevalence})(\text{sensitivity})}{(\text{prevalence})(\text{sensitivity}) + (1 - \text{prevalence})(1 - \text{specificity})}$$

Predictive value of a negative test result

$$= \frac{(1 - \text{prevalence})(\text{specificity})}{(1 - \text{prevalence})(\text{specificity}) + (\text{prevalence})(1 - \text{sensitivity})}$$

If an ELISA test with 95% sensitivity and 99% specificity were performed in a community 'at low risk' where the prevalence of AIDS seropositivity is 1 per 1,000 (0.001), the predictive value of a positive test result would be:

$$\frac{0.001 \times 0.95}{(0.001 \times 0.95) + (0.999 \times 0.01)} = \frac{0.00095}{0.01094} = 0.0868$$

(or about 9%)

In a Central African community where heterosexual spread and other factors lead to a 40% prevalence rate of seropositivity, the predictive value of a positive test result would be:

$$\frac{0.4 \times 0.95}{(0.4 \times 0.95) + (0.6 \times 0.01)} = \frac{0.38}{0.389} = 0.976 \quad \text{(or about 98\%)}$$

Therefore, if a positive result is found in a suburban shopping center crowd, it is more improbable than probable that the subject is HIV-positive. If the same result is found in Central Africa, it is almost certain that the subject is HIV-positive.

Generally speaking, the lower the prevalence of disease in a target community (i.e. the community in which the test is performed), the lower the predictive value of a positive test result, and the higher the value of a negative result. The higher the prevalence, the higher the predictive value of a positive test result and the lower the value of a negative result. In practice, if a diagnostic or screening test is provided with sensitivity and specificity values, the physician using it must realize that predictive values will be dependent on the community to which the patients belong.

Predictive values of test results based on Bayes' theorem may be overestimated in evolving (longitudinal) screening programs. Once a population or cohort is initially screened (i.e. in a cross-sectional program), most of the prevalent cases are detected, treated, and then excluded from a subsequent additional search in time. The remaining cases are either those missed as false negative or not reached by the program, or forthcoming incident cases. If the cohort under study is an open one, additional prevalent and incident cases arrive and depart from the outside world through migration. In such cases, predictive values of positive test results may be lower, and those of negative test results higher, than initially thought. An influx of high-risk groups in the community may work in the opposite way if disease occurrence in the community rises sharply.

6.4.1.8 *Validity as reflected by true and false positive results*

Besides sensitivity, field specificity and predictive values of diagnoses, it is desirable to find tests that give as many true positive results as possible, with a minimum of false positives. The same applies to negative results. Two methods clarify this problem: likelihood ratio and the receiver-operating characteristics curve.

Likelihood ratios[64–66] are appropriately named. The likelihood ratio of a positive test result is the probability of a particular positive test result given disease divided by the probability of the same result given no disease, i.e.

$$\text{Likelihood ratio (positive test result)} = \frac{\text{sensitivity}}{1 - \text{specificity}}$$

It is a ratio of 'good' and 'bad' positive test results rates.

The higher the likelihood ratio, the more accurate the test. For example[67], an abdominal CT scan for diagnosing splenic injury has a 95% sensitivity and 96% specificity rating. The likelihood ratio of its positive result is 23.8.

On the other hand, thermograms for screening breast cancer in women have a 61% sensitivity and 74% specificity[68]. The likelihood ratio is:

$$\frac{0.61}{1 - 0.74} = 2.35 \quad \text{a very poor ratio indeed!}$$

The creative use of likelihood ratios often helps in practical decision-making. For example[76], radiologists may wish to know the validity of a chest CT in the detection of possible mediastinal lymph node metastases in lung cancer. Table 6.3 illustrates likelihood ratios if CT scanning is used in the evaluation of lymph nodes of various sizes. Results indicate that this method should not be used when evaluating small nodes with a short-axis diameter less than 15 mm. (CT scan would yield more false positive than true positive results.)

The likelihood ratio of a negative test result is:

$$\text{Likelihood ratio (negative test result)} = \frac{1 - \text{sensitivity}}{\text{specificity}}$$

Once again, very few false negative results should be obtained (1 − sensitivity). Therefore, a negative result is more likely to be a true negative result (specificity). The smaller the likelihood ratio for a negative result, the more accurate the test from this point of view.

Table 6.3 Likelihood ratios of mediastinal lymph nodes in lung cancer patients

Node short-axis diameter (mm)	Likelihood ratios*
0–9	0.16
10–14	0.23
15–19	3.3
20–29	13.3
30–infinity	Infinity

*Derived from sensitivities and 1 – specificities plotted on receiver-operating characteristics curve by Glazer et al: diameter greater than or equal to 10 mm, sensitivity 0.95, specificity 0.30; diameter greater than or equal to 15 mm, sensitivity 0.80, specificity 0.94; diameter greater than or equal to 10 mm, sensitivity 0.70, specificity 0.97; diameter greater than or equal to 30 mm, sensitivity 0.30, specificity 1.0.

Source: Ref 64. Reproduced with permission from the American Roentgen Ray Society

NB One would expect this ratio to be based on the logic of the likelihood ratio of a positive test result, i.e. 'specificity/1-sensitivity', or 'good' negative results/'bad' negative results, but the above-mentioned formula has so far been customarily accepted across the literature.

Appendix 1 in Sox et al[63] gives an extensive list of likelihood ratios for a vast array of clinical and paraclinical tests. Within the framework of a Bayesian approach to diagnosis, the likelihood ratio may be used in relation to the prevalence of disease to determine the predictive value of a positive test result. To do this, Fagan[69] proposed a nomogram on the basis of which any of three composing variables may be estimated if two others are known.

Receiver operating characteristic curves (ROC curves)

Very often, a quantitative variable serves as an indicator (i.e. diagnostic tool) of disease. A cut-off point is fixed, and above this point disease is considered. For example, diastolic blood pressure levels lead to a diagnosis of hypertension, high levels of creatinine phosphokinase indicate myocardial infarction or another fresh tissue lesion, elevated glycemia indicates diabetes, etc. What is the best cut-off point? At almost any level, false positive and false negative results will occur. If, at any point under

consideration, likelihood ratios can be determined (which is possible if a group of diseased and non-diseased persons is evaluated by one criterion under consideration and by a reference examination or test), a graph can be plotted between two axes, one representing sensitivity (i.e. proportion of true positive results in subjects with a disease, meaning 'good' positive results), another specificity (or 1 – specificity, meaning the proportion of false positive results in non-diseased subjects, meaning 'bad' positive results). Such a string of likelihood ratios gives a 'receiver operating characteristic curve'.

Figure 6.4 gives an example of ROC curves. Cherian et al[70] studied the possibility of respiratory rates measured during physical examinations of children being used as an indicator of lower respiratory infection, and at what age this method might give the best results. Such a picture may be analyzed several ways:

What is the overall validity of the test given its positive results? First, visually speaking, the configuration of an ROC curve may be best observed if it is 'bulging', 'domed' or curved as much as possible towards the upper left corner of the graph. The overall discriminating power of the test is better than if the curve were to approach a straight line between the left lower and upper right corners of the graph, indicating that the likelihood ratio at any position of the line would be 1.0 (as many true positive as false positive results). In this sense, Figure 6.4 shows that the respiratory rate will better indicate the presence of lower respiratory infections in infants under 35 months of age than in children over 35 months of age. (Statistical note: This visual assessment is strengthened in research by calculating and comparing surfaces under ROC curves by the Hanley and McNeil methods[71,72].)

At what level should the best cut-off point be set? Visually speaking, the cut-off point closest to the upper left corner of the graph (if sensitivity counts when accepting a reasonable minimum of false positive results) represents the highest likelihood ratio of a positive test result in situations where true positive and false positive results are equally important. In other situations, where a clinician wants to detect as many cases as possible and can afford it for the price of a higher proportion of correctable false

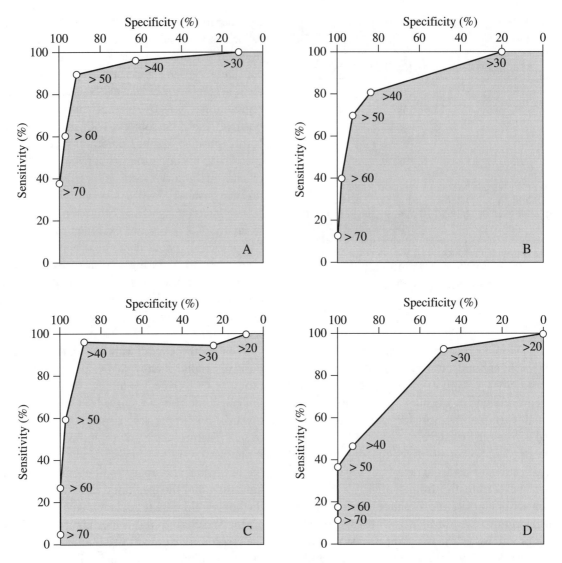

A : less than 12 mo.; B : 12 to 23 mo.; C : 24 to 35 mo.; D : > 35 mo.

Figure 6.4 ROC curves for respiratory rates as indicators of lower respiratory infection in infants and children. Source: Ref. 70, reproduced with permission from Elsevier Science (*The Lancet*)

positive results, a higher demarcation point on the sensibility scale may be considered.

Inventive approaches to various diagnostic questions using recent clinico-epidemiological methods strengthen clinical strategies and decisions. These are based on several complementary considerations and not on a single quantitative method. From this chapter alone, it is evident that information on various aspects of internal validity can be complementary. Each approach answers different questions.

In general, sensitive tests will be selected whenever cases should not be missed (where patients would die without early treatment). As an example, it is imperative to screen for phenylketonuria. Screening for incurable diseases such as AIDS (at the moment of writing) does more to protect possible contacts than to save the patient. Specific tests are selected when false positive results might lead to costly examinations, expensive treatment and interventions that have risky side effects. It would be unwise to do a lobectomy for lung cancer on the basis of a non-specific test whose false positive result would be frequent in healthy subjects. Efficient tests (having both high sensitivity and specificity) are selected when treatment of false positive results or neglect of false negative results would be catastrophic. All treatments based on invasive and aggressive surgical and other techniques for otherwise incurable diseases (i.e. some cancers) should be decided on the basis of the most efficient tests available. Galen and Gambino studied the appropriateness of tests in more detail in their practical monograph[73]. In the above-mentioned situations, predictive values of positive and negative test results should be as high as possible, depending on the best internal validity of tests and the prevalence of disease as mentioned above.

6.4.1.9 *Differential diagnosis*

As early as their first clinical experience, physicians have to face the challenge of dealing with signs and symptoms in the patient that may be common to several diseases. Nevertheless, a proper diagnosis must be made: what disease, from an array of diseases sharing similar clinical and/or paraclinical manifestations, does the patient have? Or, does the patient have more than one disease from the above-mentioned array? A differential diagnosis is mandatory. Beyond an exclusionary process by successive pattern recognition, more structured methodological approaches to differential diagnosis must be developed. Several directions have, in fact, been explored and although they are still not always explicit for a practicing physician, they increasingly complete an intuitive differential diagnosis.

6.4.2 *External validity of a diagnostic test*

A test's external validity relies on its ability to yield comparable results, if used by different teams, in different environments, on different patients, or if repeated (test retest). The external validity of a study, on the contrary, is the ability to generalize its result beyond the sample under study. The following example illustrates the challenge of reproducibility (syn. repeatability, agreement). A new and more accurate test for occult blood in stools was developed to detect cancer. A test result may be negative (0), slightly positive (+) or strongly positive (++). The test was carried out by two physicians (A and B) on 100

patients. Both obtained the same number of readings as follows:

	Blood in stools			
	0	+	++	Total
Physician A:				
Number of readings in patients	60	28	12	100
Physician B:				
Number of readings in patients	60	28	12	100

The test appears perfectly reproducible. However, it is not known how readings corroborated from one patient to another. When this is done, the following cross-tabulation gives these frequencies:

		Physician A			
		0	+	++	Total
	0	40	20	0	60
Physician B	+	14	6	8	28
	++	6	2	4	12
	Total	60	28	12	100

It may be noted that the true reproducibility of the test is only 50%, i.e. 40 + 6 + 4/100 = 50%.

An even better idea on this matter may be obtained by computation of the Kappa coefficient[74,3], which is a ratio of all observed and expected concordant readings. The Kappa coefficient may vary from -1.0 (no reproducibility at all) through 0.0 (random reproducibility) to 1.0 (perfect concordance given results, test, or persons). Fleiss gives more basic information on such a study of agreement between raters, tests, etc.[74]. The Kappa coefficient may also be weighted if a different importance is given to different agreements or disagreements.

Qualitative attributes of diagnostic tests may be somewhat esoteric for novices. Statements such as 'this test was validated' project a sense of approval. Validity does not have a universal meaning. Table 6.4 summarizes its components in terms of questions that it tries to answer. If a test is valid in one sense, it does not automatically mean that it is valid for other considerations. Very often, a great discrepancy exists in our knowledge of the internal and external validity of diagnostic methods. Sometimes, much more is known about internal validity, such as for diagnostic

---

Table 6.4 Validation and validity of a diagnostic method (test)

External validity (reproducibility)
- Repetition of the test (test-retest)
- Users (different people)
- Tools (instruments, machines)
- Setting (laboratory, field, hospital floors, clinics)

Internal validity
- How does the test separate diseased (abnormal) individuals from healthy (normal) individuals?
- How does the test separate this disease from other diseases (differential diagnostic power)?
- How does the test work compared to other tests?
  - o Does it yield the same results?
  - o Does it yield complementary results?
  - o Does it yield a new result (other?)
- Representivity
  - o Clinical gradient
  - o Clinical spectrum
  - o Type or kind of patients

Feasibility
- Requirements for training
- User friendliness (learning, fatigue, stress, attention, etc.)
- Patient friendliness (pain, etc.)
- Load (time, cost, etc.)

---

methods of breast cancer. Elsewhere, validation of diagnostic methods stops by determining external validity assessment. In psychiatry, where reference assessment is often delicate, assessment of reproducibility prevails and unfortunately ends there, because there are no reference tests available in many situations.

What must be done in the absence of an 'external golden standard'? Schulzer et al[58] recently proposed using the results of repeated (replicated) measurements of the test under study as a reference point. Even though it originates in ophthalmology, it might be worth studying and developing further in psychiatry, or in any other field where it is hard to rely on some reference diagnostic method (no biopsy or autopsy is yet unequivocal evidence of schizophrenia). Both internal and external validities are separate and complementary components. A diagnostic method may have excellent internal validity but be hardly reproducible, such as in the case of new technologies. On the other hand, a poor method from the point of view of internal validity (poor criteria, unclear description of its architecture, etc.) may be reproducible yielding perfectly comparable but worthless results everywhere. In this sense, good internal validity is a prerequisite for the assessment of the external validity of tests. Table 6.5 reviews some practical questions pertaining to the quality of diagnosis. Its quantitative guidelines may be found in Chmura-Kraemer's monograph[75].

Table 6.5 Validity of diagnoses

Problem	What is the quality of the diagnosis as a process and end product?
Practical question	What was found? Was it found using reliable techniques?
Specific questions	Does the diagnostic method separate diseased subjects from non-diseased ones? Is the diagnosis based on methods that can be used by anyone, anywhere, and in different patients? How does this method work in practice?
What clinical epidemiology does	Evaluation of internal and external validity of a diagnostic or screening test. Effectiveness of diagnosis when coupled with appropriate treatment.
Sources of failures, reasons for high costs, useless work	Excessive attention to external validity without good knowledge of internal validity. Poor assessment disregarding the clinical course of disease and comorbidity(ies). Method does not reflect changes in patients' health status. Under-use of knowledge of validity in practice (it is not used and translated into practical decisions, e.g. Bayes).

6.5 Quantitative diagnosis and its clinimetric indexes. 'How severe is this case?'

To properly assess disease severity, valid clinimetric tools such as clinimetric indexes are necessary. **Clinimetric indexes** are aggregates (sets) of qualitative and/or quantitative characteristics to describe in precise and operational terms a patient's health status. Clinimetric indexes fall into two broad categories. The previous part of this chapter discussed one type of clinimetric index, i.e. ensembles of various variables and criteria, to best identify the presence or absence of disease. Hence, numerous **qualitative (i.e. non-directional) clinimetric indexes** were developed to identify disease (i.e. to make a qualitative diagnosis) and are in current use. The previously mentioned criteria for diagnosis of toxic shock syndrome[39], or Jones' criteria to diagnose rheumatic fever[76], are good examples of a qualitative clinimetric index. Second, once a disease is identified, a quantitative assessment must often be performed. **How serious is the disease? Quantitative** diagnosis using appropriate (i.e. directional) **clinimetric indexes** serves this purpose. The following examples illustrate some of the most important properties of clinimetric indexes in this area.

As with any diagnostic tool, a valid clinimetric index should adequately describe the degree of disease evolution and impact (in terms of disease gradient and spectrum). Patients are often classified in different categories, representing ordinal scales. Each category should:

- Reflect a different prognosis;
- Be indicative of a particular treatment, different from one category to the next;
- Be clearly demarcated.

In fact, the movement of patients from one category to another should sensibly reflect improvement or worsening of the patient's status (evolution of disease). Measuring (and reflecting) the impact of treatment should also be useful. The same criteria apply if scores or numerical values replace categories in some clinimetric indexes.

From a practical point of view, clinimetric indexes as tools of quantitative diagnosis must be simple, understandable, easy to measure and classify in order to be successful. They must be 'clinician-friendly'. In addition to different aspects of internal and external validity, clinimetric indexes must also be validated as tools for qualitative diagnosis. The current edition of the Dictionary of Epidemiology[3] quotes construct, content, and criterion validity as follows:

Construct validity: The extent to which the measurement corresponds to theoretical concepts (constructs) concerning the phenomenon under study. Theoretically, if the phenomenon should change with age, a measurement with construct validity would reflect such a change.

Criterion validity: The extent to which the measurement correlates with an external criterion of the phenomenon under study. Two aspects of criterion validity can be distinguished:

1. *Concurrent validity:* The measurement and the criterion refer to the same point in time. An example would be a visual inspection of a wound for evidence of infection validated against the bacteriological examination of a specimen taken at the same time.
2. *Predictive validity:* The measurement's validity is expressed in terms of its ability to predict the criterion. An example would be an academic aptitude test that was validated against subsequent academic performance.

There are two types of quantitative clinimetric index. The first category is represented by **indexes measuring one disease**, i.e. working 'inside a qualitative diagnosis' (e.g. staging of cancer[77,78]). Killip and Kimball's functional classification of myocardial infarction[79] or the classification of gestational diabetes[80] are good examples of this category of index. The second category is represented by **indexes that apply to a wider variety of health problems**. Various methods for scoring trauma[81–85], Glasgow assessment of coma[86], Nelson's index of severity for acute pediatric illness[87], APACHE scoring for follow up of patients in intensive care units[88,89], or Apgar score for the evaluation of the newborn[90,91] belong to this category. Some of these indexes are based on clinical assessment, such as the Canadian Neurological Scale[92–94], some rely considerably on paraclinical evaluation[89], while others are based mainly on data focusing on the assessment of the quality of life, such as the Barthel index in stroke[95]. Not all currently used indexes have been completely validated nor do they fulfil all desirable criteria and aspects of validity. All have their advantages and disadvantages, which must be known to clinicians who use them in clinical decision-making.

6.5.1 Indexes for one disease entity. Examples

In the first category of clinimetric indexes, Killip and Kimball's classification of myocardial infarction[79] accurately reflects the prognosis of these patients, which varies from one category to another. For example, the incidence of cardiac arrest in functional class I (no heart failure) is 5%, in class II (heart failure) 15%, in class III (severe heart failure) 46%, and in class IV (cardiogenic shock) 77%. Elsewhere, the classification of gestational diabetes also reflects different levels of perinatal morbidity and mortality, the risk of congenital malformations, or differentials in birth weight[80].

6.5.2 Indexes covering several diagnostic entities. Examples

In the second category, the Apgar Score[90,91] (Table 6.6) is a classic example of a 'clinician-friendly index'. This index, however, does not meet all desirable criteria of validity (e.g. different prognostic values and indications to treat). An obstetrician or neonatologist will try to resuscitate (intubation, suction, cardiac massage, etc.) any newborn, whether the Apgar score is 1 or 3, or give oxygen and ventilate whether the score is 4, 5 or 6[96,97]. The Glasgow coma scale[86] (Figure 6.5) is a good reflection of the evolution of general anesthesia and recovery, while Nelson's score for severity of pediatric illnesses can be related to the probability of hospitalisation[87]. The Canadian Neurological Scale was recently devised to monitor mentation and motor functions in stroke patients[92]. It was extensively validated according to the criteria mentioned earlier[93,94].

Trends toward increasingly composite clinimetric indexes have been noted. The combination of several basic indexes is expected to complement and compensate for deficient characteristics of various

Table 6.6 Apgar score – original presentation – Method of scoring the evaluation of a newborn infant*

| Sign | *Score** * | | |
	0	1	2
• Heart rate/min	Absent	Slow (<100)	>100
• Respiratory effort	Absent	Weak cry: hypoventilation	Good: strong cry
• Muscle tone	Limp	Some flexion of extremities	Well flexed
• Reflex irritability (response of skin stimulation to feet)	No response	Some motion	Cry
• Color	Blue: pale	Body pink: extremities blue	Completely pink

*Evaluation 60 sec after complete birth of infant (disregarding cord and placenta).
**Score of 10 indicates infant in best possible condition.
Source: Ref 91. Redrawn and reproduced with permission of the American Medical Association (*JAMA*)

components. When choosing a **clinimetric index**, a clinician should look for the following **desirable characteristics**:

- A solid biological basis (content);
- A clear directionality and quantitative dimension (correlation of numerical values with the severity of the health problem or state);
- Numerical expressions (values) must reflect the clinical reality (i.e. a doubling of the score should correspond to a doubling of care, or a double risk of poor prognosis, etc.);
- A good prognostic value;
- Sensitivity to treatment effects (improvements or worsening of health status);
- Usefulness for clinical decision-making (for example, giving indications to pursue the drainage of a wound, transfer from the intensive care unit, discharge from the hospital, vital function monitoring, etc.);
- Detailed information as to how the clinimetric system was validated;
- A clear knowledge of the index's characteristics in terms of internal and external validity;
- Detailed instructions on its use ('user's manual').

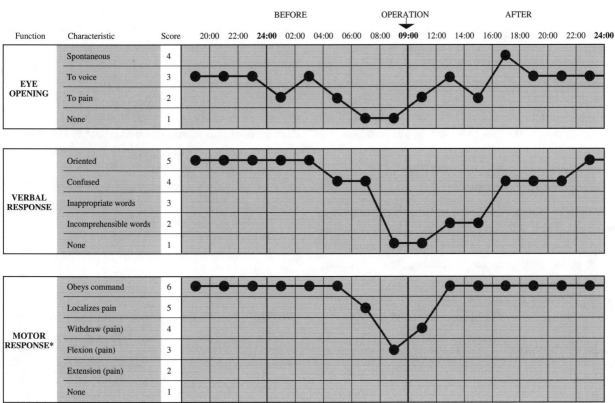

Figure 6.5 Follow-up of a surgical patient using the Glasgow coma scale. Source: Ref. 86, reproduced with permission from Elsevier Science (*The Lancet*)

The current challenge in the field of clinimetric indexes is two-fold. First, newly developed clinimetric tools must be more completely and thoroughly validated. Second, the old tools, often solidly entrenched in practice, require re-evaluation and re-assessment. This may mark the end of such indexes as the Apgar score[90,91] and others. Indeed, alternative algorithms for the care of the newborn (neonatal resuscitation) based on heartbeat frequency and other criteria[97] have already been proposed to replace that based on the Apgar score. Further validation may bring new challenges. For example, Rutledge et al[98–100] have found that diagnostic categories from the International Classification of Diseases (ICD) may have an even better prognostic value than trauma severity scoring as shown in evaluating the effectiveness of prehospital emergency services. In this case, simpler is not only better, but also more practical.

6.6 Comments on screening tests and screening programs

According to the current definition, **screening represents** '*the presumptive identification of unrecognized disease or defect by the application of tests, examinations, or other procedures which can be applied rapidly. Screening tests sort out apparently well persons who probably have a disease from those who probably do not. A screening test is not intended to be diagnostic. Persons with positive or suspicious findings must be referred to their physicians for diagnosis and necessary treatment*'[3,56]. It should be noted that, by definition, unrecognized symptomatic as well as pre-symptomatic disease is included; also, physical examination is considered part of the procedure so long as it can be classed as rapid. The term 'other procedures' may also embrace the use of questionnaires, which are assuming an increasingly important place in screening[56]. The relevance of screening programs, often representing large-scale activity, relies not only on how well the presumptive identification is performed and if the program reaches all people of interest, but also on what follows screening: other tests and, in particular, the treatment to be offered to subjects who need it. The last point was often forgotten in the past.

6.6.1 General rules for implantation of screening programs

A valid screening test still does not justify a screening program. Table 6.7 gives more details on the criteria justifying screening programs. The disease must first be a good candidate for screening, the screening test(s) must be valid, and the target population must receive suitable priority for any screening program. Tuberculosis[56] is an example of a disease suitable for

screening according to these criteria, and diabetes is not[101], breast cancer screening remains controversial. The situation has now evolved from global screening programs, focusing on multiple tests for multiple problems in large segments of the population, to selected and well-focused activities where every procedure is evaluated according to various criteria discussed in this chapter. The Canadian Task Force on the Periodic Health Examination reviews different aspects of screening activities. Results are periodically published. Recommendations are based on the quality of evidence for the cost and effectiveness of screening, diagnosis, and treatment[102].

6.6.2 Research implications of screening

Cases can be detected early (by screening) or later (by routine examinations). Such differences must be taken into account when evaluating the effectiveness

Table 6.7 Criteria for selection of screening program

Screening test	Disease to be detected	Community where screening program is considered
• Sensitive	• Disease well-defined according to precise operational criteria	• Community highly exposed to disease's etiologic factors
• Specific	• Gradient and spectrum of the disease is well-specified	• High prevalence of disease to be screened
• Good predictive value of results	• Prevalent	• Demographic data available (denominators for rates)
• Reproducible	• Serious (threat)	• Screening is perceived as necessary and a priority
• Inexpensive	• Easily distinguishable from normalcy	• Administrative facilities available
• Quick	• Natural and clinical courses of disease are known	• Human and material resources available
• Easy to apply	• Pre-symptomatic stage before clinical course is well defined	• Post-screening examinations for definitive diagnosis are available
• Acceptable for patients	• Can be treated	• Treatment facilities are available (screening without treatment is obviously not very useful)
• Operational criteria and definitions of disease and tests are given	• If treated, treatment at an earlier detected stage must give better results, than treatment given later to cases diagnosed later	• Good relations between the community, health teams, and civic leadership
• An appropriate phase of validation was carried out	• This disease is a priority among other diseases competing for similar programs	
• Satisfactory statistical requirements for validation (sample size)		

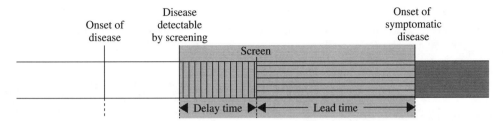

Figure 6.6 Delay time and lead time of screening. Source: Ref. 103, reproduced and adapted with permission from Blackwell Scientific Publishers

of treatment. Cases identified through screening, especially during an asymptomatic stage, will show a longer survival, or disease-free period after treatment, due to their earlier detection. Such a time span between the moment of screening and routine detection during the natural history of cases is called **lead time**[103]. It is the time gained in treating or controlling diseased cases when detection is made earlier than usual. When analyzing data, an 'equal chance should be given to all runners'. To do this, the lead time is deducted from the survival of cases detected by screening when compared to cases detected otherwise. For example, lead time of breast cancer in women is approximately one year[104], and five years in cervical cancer[105]. Figure 6.6 shows that knowing the **delay time** is also useful, i.e. the interval between the time when disease is detectable by screening and the actual moment of screening itself[103,104]. Delay time currently remains only a theoretical concept, while the natural history of chronic diseases is better known, described, and understood (see Chapter 7).

6.7 Studying the use of diagnostic tests in clinical practice

Once developed and validated, the use of a diagnostic test raises additional important questions:

- Why is it selected for practical use?
- How is it used and interpreted?
- What interventions and treatments are chosen based on its results?
- What is the performance of the whole clinical process, from selection of patients for a diagnostic procedure to treatment according to diagnostic evaluation and subsequent patient follow-up?

The field of clinical decision analysis deals with these questions and a subsequent chapter will be devoted to this topic.

6.8 Major criteria of a valid diagnostic study

Any study of any phase in a diagnostic process must be performed according to the general criteria of a research study in medicine, and according to the specific criteria for a diagnostic study itself. These criteria should be reviewed when preparing a clinimetric study; they should be followed and respected during the study itself; and they should be reflected in the reporting of results in a communication, research paper in a medical journal, poster, etc. Any research protocol must clarify several important points. Unclear or hidden information makes a study difficult and its results deceiving or unusable in practice if the reader, or purported future user, does not have enough information to make independent decisions about the test or any other clinimetric procedure (how to gather clinical data, how to use a test, what to do with a clinimetric index, etc.).

6.8.1 General criteria of an acceptable study in medical research

The most important 'commandments' of a study should be respected in a research proposal and protocol and reflected in the presentation of study results. A more detailed discussion of these criteria goes beyond the scope of this text. However, readers will also find useful information in Hulley and Cummings' monograph[106].

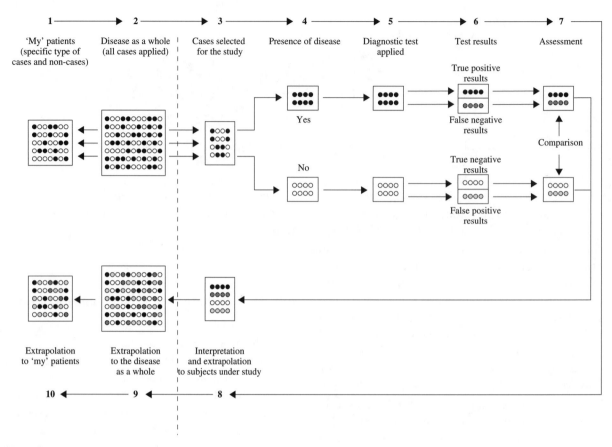

Figure 6.7 Flow chart of diagnostic test study

6.8.2 *Specific criteria and steps in a valid study on diagnosis*

As Figure 6.7 illustrates, clinimetric studies focus on some disease of interest. From this whole, only a part will apply to a group of patients in a particular institution (e.g. patients in the care of a given hospital, family clinics, etc.). Selection criteria for participation in the study apply; some patients are excluded. Non-diseased and diseased subjects are tested, giving true and false positive and negative results. Both groups are compared and interpreted **within** the study. Knowledge of the applicability of results beyond the study is valuable. Do the results apply to the disease as a whole (i.e. all cases in the community)? Do they apply to the kind of patients who are under the care of the reader, a potential user of the test?

1. Define the disease to be tested. Every disease has its evolutive stages (as seen in Chapter 2), its

spectrum, and gradient. They should be defined as follows:

Spectrum of disease: The term encompasses different systemic manifestations of the disease. (These manifestations are as different as colors in the spectrum.) Glandular, ulcero-glandular, oculo-glandular, oropharyngeal, pleuropulmonary and typhoid forms represent clinical spectrum of tularemia. Tuberculosis and syphilis have a wider clinical spectrum than the common cold. Qualitative clinimetric indexes (categorization, staging, classification) describe disease spectrum.

Gradient of disease: The term encompasses different grades of disease according to the severity of cases. The gradient of viral hepatitis is represented by subclinical infection, flu-like cases, benign acute hepatitis, chronic hepatitis and fatal necrosis. The clinical gradient of hepatitis is wider than the clinical gradient of chicken pox. Quantitative clinimetric indices are most often made to measure disease gradient.

NB In the past in infectious disease epidemiology, both terms were often used in a reverse sense. However, these new definitions reflect the basic meaning of spectrum and gradient common to other fields of science. It should be specified if the whole spectrum and gradient and/or all stages of disease are the subject of study, and if not, which parts will be selected.

2. *Define cases participating in the study*. As previously mentioned, the best possible **operational** as well as **conceptual** criteria should be defined. The example of toxic shock syndrome was already mentioned[39].

3. *Describe characteristics of patients participating in the study*. Demographic characteristics (age, sex, etc.) or social ones are not adequate. **Comorbidity** (other diseases which patients may have besides the disease tested) **and treatment for comorbidity** should be known and described. If patients in a diagnostic test study for a particular type of familial hyperlipidemia also have diabetes and are taking insulin, both their diabetes and their therapeutic regimens must be described.

4. *Identify what selected patients represent from the disease as a whole*. During the evaluation process, not all selected patients (even those well-defined) are accepted into the study. Philbrick et al[107] have shown the degree of attrition in the recruitment of patients in an evaluation study of a stress test in coronary

Table 6.8   Phases of validation of a diagnostic test

Phase	Disease cases	Non-diseased objects (controls)	Objectives
(1)	• Limited (narrow) disease gradient and spectrum, typical of disease	• No control group	• Performance of test procedure (technical feasibility, tolerance by patients, 'user and patient friendliness')
(2)	• Limited (narrow) disease gradient and spectrum, typical of disease	• Healthy individuals	• Separation of manifest cases from non-cases (healthy individuals) • Sensitivity, specificity within study predictive value determination
(3)	• Prevalent disease spectrum and gradient (expected clinical scope of disease)	• Healthy individuals	• Subtler distinctions on the basis of a more complete clinical scope of disease • Sensitivity, specificity, with study predictive value determination
(4)	• Expanded disease spectrum and gradients • Comorbidity included • Treatment of comorbidity included	• Non-diseased individuals • Comorbidity comparable to comorbidity of disease cases • Treatment for comorbidity comparable to comorbidity treatment of cases	• Test performance in a preponderant scope of relevant clinical situations • Sensitivity, specificity, predictive values in various conditions
(5)	• Full disease spectrum and gradient • Non-preselected group of patients	• Subjects with a full gradient and spectrum of conditions for which the test is ordered	• Equivalent of a clinical trial • Predictive values of test results as applied to expected clinical setting

Source: Reworked from Ref 108. Reproduced with permission of the American Medical Association (JAMA)

heart disease patients in comparison with coronary arteriography. From a group of entirely unknown patients, only a few are recognized and brought to attention in view of the study. Inadequate data have been collected in some patients, and other patients are not eligible for a reference examination, i.e. coronary angiography. Their example shows that a diagnostic test validation study may have an excellent internal validity but not necessarily a satisfactory external validity. Figure 6.8 shows that patients remaining in the study may represent only a fraction of the real spectrum and gradient of coronary disease cases in the community.

5. *Identify 'your' patients, or any group of patients to which results of the study would be applied.*

6. *Give a detailed technical description of the test* and how it will be administered. Explain possible pitfalls and errors which might be expected and ways to correct them.

7. *Specify the reference test* with which results of a new test will be compared. This is usually done when criteria for cases and non-cases are given.

8. *Decide if the study will be cross-sectional*, i.e. a 'single shot' comparison of diseased and non-diseased individuals at a given time, or if the study will be longitudinal, i.e. an ongoing study in time by testing and retesting diseased and non-diseased individuals over a time span (expected natural course) of disease.

9. *Define the evaluation phase of a diagnostic test under study.* It is impossible to evaluate a diagnostic test using a single study and it is impossible to evaluate the effectiveness of a new drug with a single clinical trial. Just as there are different phases of drug evaluation (see Chapter 9), diagnostic tests should also be evaluated step by step, as recently proposed by Nierenberg and Feinstein[108]. Table 6.8 represents a reworking of their concept. As a drug evaluation progresses from a basic study of its action (phase 1 trial) to post-marketing studies (phase 4 or 5), the basic performance of a diagnostic test is evaluated first (phase 1), and finally its performance 'in real practice' with 'real patients' (phase 5) is assessed.

10. *Determine how many subjects are needed to make a diagnostic test evaluation study.* Arkin and Wachtel's article[109] gives a statistical methodology to answer this important question.

Let us digress exceptionally into some biostatistical details to illustrate the importance of clinician input for computational methods. The most skilful biostatistician cannot work without knowing the clinical reality, relevance and importance of information needed for statistical problem solving like sample size determination. A clinician must estimate some proportion: sensitivity, specificity, or predictive values of the test result. He wishes to do these estimations with an acceptable type I error (error of falsely stating that two proportions are significantly different when they are actually equivalent), and type II error (error of falsely stating that two proportions are not significantly different when they actually are different), the latter in terms of statistical power or $1 - \beta$ (NB The probability of type I error is ζ, the probability of type II error is β). To determine the optimal sample size for comparing test A with test B, a clinician must assign the following values[109]: (1) an estimate of the expected value of the performance characteristic of interest for the reference test, (2) the smallest proportionate difference between the reference and the new test considered to be medically important, (3) the level of significance required to accept two proportions as different, which is γ (type I error), and (4) the level of certainty desired to detect the medically significant difference (statistical power). Authors of this methodology give computational formulas and tables to simplify the sample size determinations. However, it is the clinician's, not the statistician's, responsibility to define the above-mentioned values. No statistician is trained to determine what is 'medically or clinically important'. Articles on diagnostic tests should thus provide the information upon which clinicians and biostatisticians have agreed when defining the sample size for their study.

11. *At a chosen stage of evaluation, determine internal and external validity of the test.* The validity of any test depends on:
- The definition of disease itself;
- At what stage it is evaluated;

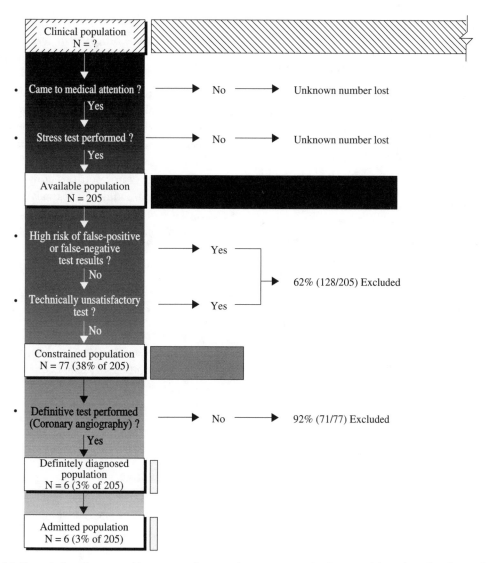

Figure 6.8 Attrition during the assembly process for exercise test research. Source: Adapted and redrawn from Ref. 107, reproduced with permission of the American Medical Association (*JAMA*)

- The reference diagnostic method (expert review, biopsy, autopsy, etc.);
- The type of patients; and
- The conditions under which the evaluation is made.

12. Mistakes (random errors) and biases (systematic errors) should be reviewed and results corrected accordingly.

13. A thorough review of the practical impact of false positive and false negative results should be

performed. What would happen to undetected cases left untreated? What would happen to healthy individuals needlessly exposed to more invasive diagnostic methods and/or aggressive treatments? Irreproducible tests should be discarded.

14. Readers should draw their own conclusions as to whether the test under scrutiny applies to their particular patients. Readers are potential users of the test, bearers of its good performance, and not perpetrators of its errors.

6.9   The question of differential diagnosis

Differential diagnosis, as a process of separating the right diagnosis from a set of competing diagnostic hypotheses, is traditionally one of the pinnacles of the mastery of medicine. Before the advent of rational and effective treatment, it was the only one, and the most cherished by physicians and patients alike. This field is relatively less methodologically developed than '*differential treatment*', i.e. a rational choice of the best treatment from many. Chapter 9 of this text provides more information on differential treatment.

Health problems subject to differential diagnosis abound in daily medical practice. The differential diagnostic process focuses on many items which may be found listed in the problem-oriented medical record as challenges to be solved: chronic headache, fever of unknown origin, joint pain, weight loss, syncope, fatigue, and occult bleeding, among others. Usually:

- The differential diagnosis begins by establishing a list of competing hypotheses, mostly deductively, triggered by few index manifestations.

- Physicians examine these alternatives using *intellectual processes outlined in section 6.3*. Knowledge of overlapping diagnostic manifestations and clues and their proportional distribution may be useful. Figure 6.9 shows such a situation in the differential diagnosis of joint pain and dysfunction in juveniles[110]. Venn diagrams (Euler diagrams for others, Hitchcock – personal communication) used here are pictorial presentations of the extent to which several manifestations common to competing diagnoses are mutually inclusive and exclusive.

- The best evidence is sought from various sources (literature, ongoing research, clinical experience) to obtain an idea about the validity of diagnostic methods and criteria constituting diagnostic entities.

- Pretest probabilities allow for the establishment of the first set of the most important diagnostic subsets (a 'working diagnosis'), which are subsequently analysed and reassembled if necessary[111]. These probabilities also help in choosing diagnostic tests and interpreting their results[112,113].

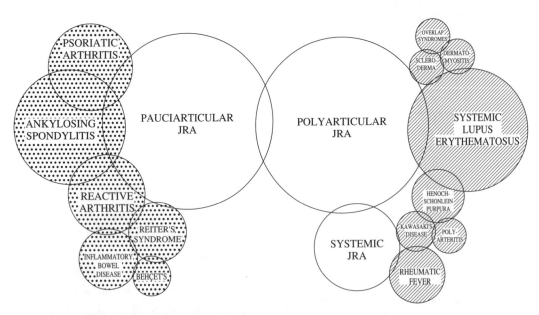

Figure 6.9   Differential diagnosis challenge of juvenile rheumatoid arthritis (JRA). Here, the Venn diagram represents three classes of childhood rheumatic diseases. *Unshaded circles:* JRA. *Dot-shaded circles:* Spondyloarthropathies. *Line-shaded circles:* Connective tissue and collagen–vascular disorders. Clinical and possible pathogenic similarities among certain diseases are presented by overlapping of circles. Sizes of circles roughly reflect relative frequencies with which diseases occur. Source: Ref. 110, reproduced with permission from Mosby Inc. (*J Pediatrics*)

- An attempt to structure the whole differential process may be useful if suitable for a more formal decision analysis, as discussed further in Chapter 13 of this text.

An effective differential diagnosis requires a larger array of evidence than, for example, the sensitivity or the specificity of a diagnostic test. Pre-test probabilities may be a good example of difficult choices of evidence of unequal quality and from various sources. Pre-test probabilities are derived not only from the prevalence of the disease (such as for the purpose of screening programs), but from other sources closer to clinical work: history and physical examination, 'impression' before or after the onset of signs/symptoms, subgroup of institution's patients, type of clinical practice, availability of clinical and paraclinical diagnostic tools, etc. Also, pre-test probabilities are one of many pieces of evidence needed for an effective diagnostic work-up. Further developments in differential diagnostic process methodology will also prove useful in refining valid clinical guidelines (see Chapter 13).

6.10 Diagnosis as seen in fuzzy theory

The fuzzy theory accepts the vagueness of our observations and expressions in daily life as a reality to deal with. It rejects 'crisp' demarcations[114] between diseased and non-diseased individuals and it emphasizes the ubiquitous vagueness of many terms like being ill, well, sick, healthy, fever, pain, chronicity, puffy face, chills, and innumerable others. In colloquial French, patients report of 'doing recently a bit of fever' or that their liver 'was more lazy these days'. Health, illness and disease are considered as fuzzy entities[115].

One way to deal with fuzzy terms is to 'defuzzify' them for practical decision-making. For example, we are already doing it by translating conceptual criteria of disease diagnosis into the operational ones. Another way is to keep clinical phenomena as fuzzy, analyze them as such, and use them in our decisions in a non-fuzzy way. Such dealing with diagnosis requires our understanding that fuzzy analyses require computerized computational techniques which cannot be so easily visualized in ones mind as

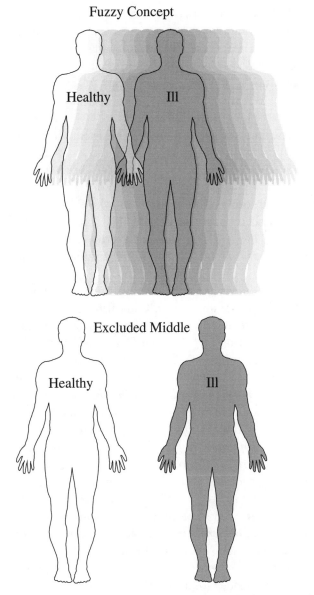

Figure 6.10 Fuzzy concept and 'excluded middle' concept of healthy and ill individuals

using 'crisp' demarcations (with an excluded middle) in Aristotelian reasoning. The latter can be used mentally without any technically sophisticated support. The former must still be brought to the level of mental operation by every layperson. Figure 6.10 illustrates the difference between crisp demarcation between healthy and sick individuals in Aristotelian logic and the fuzzy vision of health and disease which includes transitional measures and states between such entities.

For practical decisions in clinical medicine, however, one cannot accept that this patient 'is a bit pregnant', may have or not an incarcerated hernia, uterine prolapse, or pelvic fracture. Being healthy and unhealthy at the same time[116] may be at the first glance a repulsive idea for most practitioners. We may accept a theoretical plausibility of transitional states, but once again, our conclusions from an analysis of fuzzy situations and states must be 'defuzzified' in some way. However, fuzzy theory applies to diagnosis and nosology[117,118]. The fuzziness occurs throughout the whole clinimetric process, before the diagnosis is made. It is a reality of daily life and only through a proper analysis of fuzzy data we may reach some crispness of our decisions.

Fuzzy descriptions of disease in reputed textbooks of medicine are ubiquitous. Clinical features of viral hepatitis are described as follows[119] (fuzzy terms are in bold italics): '. . . *With the onset of* **clinical** *jaundice, the constitutional prodromal symptoms* **usually** *diminish, but in* **some** *patients* **mild** *weight loss is common and* **may** *continue during the entire* **icteric** *phase. The liver becomes* **enlarged** *and* **tender** *and* **may** *be associated with right upper quadrant* **discomfort.** **Infrequently** *patients present with a cholestatic* **picture** *. . .'*. As for appendicitis[120], '. . . *Patients with appendicitis* **generally** *present with a* **typical** *pattern of* **distress.** *. . . Patients who present* **late** *with appendicitis* **may** *have only* **general tenderness and rigidity** *. . . Hyperaesthesia or dysesthesia* **may** *occur in patients with . . .'*. Clinical medicine cannot avoid such soft and fuzzy information. However the most must be made from it. The challenge increases when such fuzzy elements are introduced into the process of arriving to the desired 'crisp' results. A similar view may be applied to the challenges of medical nosology (science of classification of diseases)[115,117,118]. Identifying and classifying people as diseased is an intellectual process superposed to the statement of an often fuzzy reality. For Sadegh-Zadegh[117], diagnosis may be:

- Categorical (Mr. Smith has epilepsy).
- Conjectural, by disjunction (Mr. Smith has either epilepsy or brain tumor) or by modal statement (possible epilepsy, or a probabilistic statement like being 80% sure that Mr. Smith has epilepsy).

- Nosological (International Classification of Diseases category of epilepsy).
- Abnormality statement based (history and clinical observation of seizures).
- Causal (related to some brain lesion confirmed by imaging).
- Fuzzy (a demarcation is made within some fuzzy states).

This author stresses that in most instances, cases are identified only after the disease was defined, but not before. Inclusion and exclusion criteria follow, not precede the definition of disease. Hence, the case is identified prescriptively, not descriptively[117]. The best way to define and identify disease remains still an open question, as partly outlined in Chapter 1.

More and more applications of dealing with diagnostic process and its results through fuzzy handling of data appear in the literature. In neurology, Helgason et al[121] applies fuzzy methodology to the problem of diagnosis and treatment of stroke. Surgeons rely on 'crisp' distinctions and decisions. They are nonetheless aware of the fuzziness of our observations and how they are verbalized[122]. Buchanan[123] expects that uses of fuzzy analysis will improve the prediction of outcomes in surgical patients. Amin and Kulkarni[124] developed a fuzzy Glasgow Coma Scale to improve the information content for prediction of the possibility of full cognitive recovery after head injury. More is yet to come. Together with the wider application of fuzzy theory, we will also need studies showing better results in favor of fuzzy or non-fuzzy methodologies.

6.11 Conclusions

Basic clinimetric process and diagnosis is part of a chain reaction. It is triggered by risk assessment and followed by treatment and prognosis, and must be evaluated in such a context. Chapters 9 and 10 of this text provide more details about this chain of events.

This chapter has outlined how clinical data are gathered, how they are converted into clinical information, how diagnoses are made, how diagnostic entities are constituted, and the validity of diagnostic methods. A distinction was made between a qualitative and a quantitative diagnosis in terms of clinimetric indexes measuring severity of disease.

In this field, most work evolves around the evaluation of diagnostic methods. However, the basic clinimetric process is also the subject of an increasing number of studies. Wiener and Nathanson's[113] study for the evaluation of physical examinations is a good example of the clinimetric assessment of physicians' work before diagnosis is made. Requirements of trauma surgery and intensive care greatly advanced the development of clinimetric indexes to better assess complex clinical situations of multiple life-threatening pathologies and trauma, especially in high-risk groups such as children and the elderly.

Some confusion still exists in practice and research about qualitative and quantitative clinimetric indexes. Qualitative clinimetric indexes often operate with numerical values, such as numbers of criteria needed for diagnosis. Such quantifications do not measure disease progress but rather, in quantitative or semi-quantitative terms, the predictive value of diagnosis. For example, the American Rheumatism Association propose criteria for the diagnosis of rheumatoid arthritis. Criteria include various manifestations such as morning stiffness, pain, swelling of joints, presence of subcutaneous nodules, and various paraclinical findings such as roentgenographic changes, rheumatoid factor in serum, synovial fluid, and histopathological anomalies. The presence of seven criteria leads to a classic diagnosis, five criteria a definite diagnosis, and three criteria a probable diagnosis of rheumatoid arthritis[125]. Another clinimetric index would be needed if such criteria were to measure disease progress.

Better practical application of clinimetric indexes is needed. Synthetic reviews of diagnostic problems in current practice applied to important health problems now help practising physicians translate theoretical principles of diagnostic methods assessment into practical decisions. Frank et al's[126,127] articles illustrate this issue well using AIDS as an example. However, several practical problems remain. For example:

- Unknown, poorly described and understood clinical work leading to diagnosis (inadequate clinimetric process);
- Reduced representivity for subjects and disease spectrum and gradient in studies of diagnosis due to recruitment attrition (assembly bias);

- Poor and incomplete evaluation of tests;
- Obscure use of diagnostic methods and tests in clinical decision-making;
- Poor evaluation of the impact of diagnostic procedures in conjunction with consecutive treatment(s).

These may now be priorities for future research and understanding of diagnostic work.

What diagnostic and screening tests or programs should be used in clinical practice? Which ones should be chosen? Two important sources guide practitioners today: the basic evaluation and its subsequent ongoing updates provided by the Canadian Task Force on Periodical Health Examination[102], and the United States Preventive Services Task Force's Guide to Clinical Preventive Services[128]. Both are highly recommended readings.

How should information about diagnostic tests be viewed within the framework of evidence-based medicine? Evaluating the quality of evidence in a diagnostic process is more difficult than evaluating evidence provided by analytical observational studies of risk or clinical trials. Diagnostic tests provide a wide array of evidence sought by more than one criterion: How does the test work in diseased individuals? How does it work in healthy subjects? How necessary is it to be confident in a positive diagnosis? Is the evidence solid enough to exclude this patient from care resulting from a negative diagnosis? Currently, there is no scale or hierarchy of evidence as outlined for a cause–effect relationship stemming from clinical trials and other types of studies that might be applied to the area of diagnosis. However, any diagnostician must be sure about the kind of evidence provided by a study of diagnosis or diagnostic test. The evidence must, in fact, be reviewed in terms of its internal or external validity and its screening power and it must be established to which kind of clinical setting and patients it applies.

The main question is not what kind of evidence it is, but rather what kind of evidence is provided about a particular patient, the nature of the disease, and the context in which a diagnostic process is made. It is impossible to qualify a diagnostic test as poor or as above reproach. As already mentioned in Chapter 2, evidence is not a term reserved exclusively for the degree or value given to the proof (clinical trial) of tested treatment effectiveness. It has a much broader sense and usefulness as illustrated here and in other chapters of this book. Current EBM recommendations also focus on various aspects of diagnosis: clinical manifestations of disease[129], mostly internal validity of a diagnostic method[130,131], differential diagnosis[111,112], or screening[132]. In general, authors of these recommendations focus on the quality and completeness of information provided by various approaches outlined in this chapter.

Will a diagnostic test aid in patient care? Is it appropriate for my patient(s)? Yes, if the patient or patients were eligible as participants in a study of validation of a given diagnostic test. Beyond this general rule, they should be compatible with criteria already outlined in Chapter 4, section 4.2.

Where can more information be found about clinimetrics and diagnosis? Both topics are extensively covered and discussed in several informative monographs[133–136].

Is there a recent publication that adequately illustrates the above-mentioned principles? The Ebell et al[137] evaluation of a clinical diagnosis of the streptococcal throat infection serves as a good example.

Does such a paper meet the requirements of medical journals for reporting studies on the validity of diagnostic tests? Readers may note that Bruns et al checklist[138] covers essential aspects outlined in this chapter.

Should we only pay attention to diagnostic tests based on new and advanced technologies? Certainly not. We still do not fully know the validity of the traditional, unpretentious, but ubiquitous clinical diagnostic methods that are often solely based on 'soft' findings or on tests that do not rely on advanced technologies. For example, what is the validity of the white blood cell count in the diagnosis of appendicitis[139]?

Is it important for us to better understand if and how our diagnosis is influenced by the context in which it is made? Definitely. The 'white coat hypertension', i.e. where blood pressure is persistently higher in the presence of a doctor or nurse, but normal outside the medical setting[140] illustrates how our findings depend on the setting in which they are made.

Do we better understand diagnostic work today? Yes, our understanding of the 'black box of reasoning' is enriched by a better and more complete methodology of reasoning and technical advances used to enhance it. However, diagnosis remains one of medicine's great intellectual challenges. It requires today more than one thought process: associative reasoning, parallel thinking, biological plausibility assessment, probabilistic considerations, awareness of strengths and weaknesses of new diagnostic technologies, all applied to a solid knowledge of human biology, physiology, and pathology. Such a process goes well beyond simple pattern recognition (Macartney's 'blunderbuss approach')[141]. In diagnostic logic, imaginative, but technically limited clinical reasoning will be combined more and more with unimaginative, but technically powerful computer facilities. Clinicians must possess a thorough knowledge of these processes and how to combine them to produce in a valid diagnosis. In any context, there is no good diagnosis without good clinimetrics. This is what our elders stressed as high quality clinical and paraclinical data and information. In reality, we have given a new catchy name to a more rigorous and better-structured diagnostic work-up and why not? After all, if it works, our patients will be its major beneficiaries.

REFERENCES

1. Feinstein AR. *Clinimetrics*. New Haven: Yale University Press, 1987
2. Feinstein AR. An additional basic science for clinical medicine: IV. The development of clinimetrics. *Ann Intern Med*, 1983;99:843–8
3. Last JM (ed.). *A Dictionary of Epidemiology*. 4th Edition. New York: Oxford University Press, 2000
4. Jenicek M, Cléroux R. *Epidémiologie clinique. Clinimétrie*. (Clinical Epidemiology. Clinimetrics). St. Hyacinthe and Paris: EDISEM and Maloine, 1985

5. Feinstein AR. Acquisition of clinical data. In: Huntington, Krieger RE eds. *Clinical Judgement*. Williams & Wilkins, 1967:289–349

6. Melzack R. The McGill Pain Questionnaire: Major properties and scoring methods. *Pain*, 1975;1:277–99

7. Finney DJ. *Probit Analysis*. Cambridge: Cambridge University Press, 1964

8. Bross IDJ. How to use ridit analysis. *Biometrics*, 1958;14:18–38

9. Jenicek M, Demirjian A. Age at menarche in French Canadian urban girls. *Ann Hum Biol*, 1974;1:339–46

10. Belloc NB, Breslow L, Hochstim JR. Measurement of physical health in a general population survey. *Am J Epidemiol*, 1971;93:328–36

11. Berkman PL. Measurement of mental health in a general population survey. *Am J Epidemiol*, 1971;94:105–111

12. American Cancer Society Workshop Conference: Methodology in Behavioral and Psychological Cancer Research. (Series of articles). *Cancer*, 1984;53:Supplement (May 15)

13. Feinstein AR. Clinical biostatistics. LVII. A glossary of neologisms in quantitative clinical science. *Clin Pharmacol Ther*, 1981;30:564–77

14. Charpak Y, Bléry C, Chastang C. Designing a study for evaluating a protocol for the selective performance of preoperative tests. *Stat Med*, 1987;6:813–22

15. Shelp EE, Perl M. Denial in clinical medicine. A re-examination of the concept and its significance. *Arch Intern Med*, 1985;145:697–9

16. Payer L. *Medicine & Culture. Varieties of Treatment in the United States, England, West Germany and France*. New York: Henry Holt & Co., 1988

17. Baron RJ. An introduction to medical phenomenology: I can't hear you while I'm listening. *Ann Intern Med*, 1985;103:606–11

18. Beckman HB, Frankel RM. The effect of physician behavior on the collection of data. *Ann Intern Med*, 1984;101:692–6

19. Gjerdingen DK, Simpson DE, Titus SL. Patients' and physician's attitudes regarding the physician's professional appearance. *Arch Intern Med*, 1987;147:1209–12

20. Burnum JF. Dialect is diagnostic. *Ann Intern Med*, 1984;100:899–901

21. Caster JH. Metaphor in medicine. *JAMA*, 1983;250:1841

22. Book HE. Empathy, misconceptions and misuses in psychotherapy. *Am J Psychiatry*, 1988;145:420–4

23. Brothers L. A biological perspective on empathy. *Am J Psychiatry*, 1989;146:10–19

24. Black DW. Laughter. *JAMA*, 1984;252:2995–8

25. Quill TE. Somatization disorder. One of medicine's blind spots. *JAMA*, 1985;254:3075–9

26. Epstein AM, McNeil BI. Relationship of beliefs and behavior in test ordering. *Am J Med*, 1986;80:865–70

27. Kassirer JP, Kopelman RI. Cognitive errors in diagnosis: Instantiation, classification, and consequences. *Am J Med*, 1989;38:433–41

28. Murphy EA. *The Logic of Medicine*. Baltimore and London: The Johns Hopkins University Press, 1976

29. Cebul RD, Beck JR. Biochemical profiles. Applications in ambulatory screening and preadmission testing of adults. *Ann Intern Med*, 1987;106:403–13

30. Hand DJ. *Discrimination and Classification*. New York: John Wiley and Sons, 1981

31. Jambu M, Lebeaux MO. *Cluster Analysis and Data Analysis*. Amsterdam: North-Holland, 1983

32. Wishart D. *CLUSTAN User Manual*. 3rd edition, Program Library Unit, Edinburgh University, 1978

33. Miyahara H. Cluster analysis of systemic lupus erythematosus. A case study of disease entities/ In: de Domball FT, Grémy F eds. *Decision Making and Medical Care*. Amsterdam: North Holland (Elsevier Biomedical Press BV), 1976:213–22

34. Manuila A, Manuila L, Nicole M, Lambert H. *Dictionnaire français de médecine et de biologie. (A French Dictionary of Medicine and Biology)*. Paris: Masson & Cie, 1972

35. Warkany J. Syndromes. *Am J Dis Child*, 1971;21:365–70

36. Feinstein AR. The Blame-X syndrome: problems and lessons in nosology, spectrum and etiology. *J Clin Epidemiol*, 2001;54:433–9

37. Cohen JR M. Syndromology: an updated conceptual overview. I. Syndrome concepts, designations, and population characteristics. *Int J Oral Maxillofac Surg*, 1989;18:216–22

38. Magalini S, Magalini SC. *Dictionary of Medical Syndromes*. 4th Edition. Philadelphia and New York: Lippincott-Raven, 1997

39. Wiesenthal AM, Ressman M, Caston SA, Todd JK. Toxic shock syndrome. I. Clinical exclusion of other syndromes by strict and screening definitions. *Am J Epidemiol*, 1985;122:847–56

40. Wulff HR. Rational Diagnosis and Treatment. An Introduction to Clinical Decision Making. Oxford: Blackwell Scientific Publications, 1981

41. Gale J, Marsden P. Diagnosis: Process not product. In: Sheldon M, Brooke J, Rector A eds. *Decision Making in General Practice*. New York: Stockton Press, 1985:59–90

42. Dowie J, Elstein A. *Professional Judgement A Reader in Clinical Decision Making*. New York: Cambridge University Press, 1988

43. Sackett DL. Clinical diagnosis and the clinical laboratory. *Clin Invest Med*, 1978;1:37–43

44. Price RB, Vlahcevic ZR. Logical principles in differential diagnosis. *Ann Intern Med*, 1971;**75**: 89–95

45. Kassirer JP. Diagnostic reasoning. *Ann Intern Med*, 1989;**110**:893–900

46. Emerson PA. Introduction to diagnosis by logical inference. *J Roy Coll Phys Lond*, 1979;**13**:193–4

47. Fu KS. Processing of chest X-ray images by computer, 271–86; Poppl SJ. Experience in computer classification of EEGs, 195–211; Nadler M. Effective and cost-effective real-time picture operators for medical imagery, 259–70 In: de Dombal FT, Grémy F eds. *Decision Making and Medical Care*. Amsterdam: North Holland (Elsevier Biomedical Press BV), 1976

48. Oreskovich MR, Carrico CJ. Stab wounds of the anterior abdomen. Analysis of a management plan using local wound exploration and quantitative peritoneal lavage. *Ann Surg*, 1983;**198**:411–9

49. Fox J. Formal and knowledge-based methods in decision technology. *Acta Psychol*, 1984;**56**:303–31

50. Miller RA, Popple HE Jr, Myers JD. Internist-I, an experimental computer based diagnostic consultant for general internal medicine. *N Engl J Med*, 1982;**307**:468–76

51. Lindberg G. *Studies on Diagnostic Decision Making in Jaundice*. Stockholm: Kongl. Karolinska Medico Chirurgiska Institutet, 1982

52. de Dombal FT. Computer-aided diagnosis of acute abdominal pain. The British experience. *Rev Epidémiol Santé Publique*, 1984;**32**:50–6

53. Fieschi M. *Artificial Intelligence in Medicine. Expert Systems*. London: Chapman and Hall, 1990

54. DeTore AW. Medical informatics: An introduction to computer technology in medicine. *Am J Med*, 1988;**85**:399–403

55. DeCosse JL. Early cancer detection. Colorectal cancer. *Cancer*, 1988;**62**:1787–90

56. Wilson JMG, Jungner G. *Principles and Practice of Screening for Disease*. Public Health Papers No 34. Geneva: World Health Organization, 1968

57. Goulston KJ, Cook I, Dent OF. How important is rectal bleeding in the diagnosis of bowel cancer and polyps? *Lancet*, 1986;**2**:261–5

58. Schulzer M, Anderson DR, Drance SM. Sensitivity and specificity of a diagnostic test determined by repeated observations in the absence of an external standard. *J Clin Epidemiol*, 1991;**44**:1167–79

59. Sackett DL, Straus SE, Richardson SW, et al. *Evidence-Based medicine. How to Practice and Teach EBM*. 2nd Edition. Edinburgh and London: Churchill Livingstone, 2000

60. Council on Scientific Affairs. Status report on the acquired immunodeficiency syndrome. Human T-cell Lymphotropic virus type III testing. *JAMA*, 1985;**254**:1342–5

61. Lembo NJ, Dell'Halia LJ, Crawford MH, O'Rourke RA. Bedside diagnosis of systolic murmurs. *New Engl J Med*, 1988;**318**:1572–8

62. Bayes T. An essay towards solving a problem in the doctrine of chances (Read 23 December 1763). *Biometrika*, 1958;**45**:296–315

63. Sox HC, Blatt MA, Higgins MC, Marton KI. *Medical Decision Making*. Boston: Butterworths, 1988

64. Black WC, Armstrong P. Communicating the significance of radiologic results. The likelihood ratio. *Am J Roentgenol*, 1986;**147**:1313–18

65. Halkin A, Reichman J, Schwaber M, et al. Likelihood ratios: getting diagnostic testing into perspective. *Q J Med*, 1998;**91**:247–58

66. Gallagher EJ. Clinical utility of likelihood ratios. *Ann Emerg Med*, 1998;**31**:391–7

67. Birthwhistle RV. Diagnostic testing in family practice. *Can Fam Phys*, 1988;**34**:327–31

68. Williams KL, Phillips BH, Jones PA, et al. Thermography in screening for breast cancer. *J Epidemiol Comm Health*, 1990;**44**:112–3

69. Fagan TJ. Nomogram for Bayes' formula. *N Engl J Med*, 1975;**293**:257

70. Cherian T, Simoes E, John TJ, et al. Evaluation of simple clinical signs for the diagnosis of acute lower respiratory tract infection. *Lancet*, 1988;**2**: 125–8

71. Hanley JA, McNeil BJ. The meaning and use of the area under a receiver operating characteristic (ROC) curve. *Radiology*, 1982;**143**:29–36

72. Hanley JA, McNeil BJ. A method of comparing the areas under receiver operating characteristics curves derived from the same cases. *Radiology*, 1983;**148**: 839–43

73. Galen RS, Gambino SR. Beyond Normality. *The Predictive Value and Efficiency of Medical Diagnoses*. New York: John Wiley and Sons, 1975

74. Fleiss JL. *Statistical Methods for Rates and Proportions*. 2nd Edition. New York: John Wiley, 1981

75. Chmura-Kraemer H. *Evaluating Medical Tests. Objective and Quantitative Guidelines*. Newburg Park: Sage Publications, 1992

76. Stollerman GH (chairman) and Committee to revise the Jones criteria. Jones criteria (revised) for guidance in the diagnosis of rheumatic fever. *Circulation*, 1965;**32**:664–8

77. Beahrs OH, Myers MH (eds), American Joint Committee on Cancer. *Manual for Staging of Cancer*. 2nd Edition. Philadelphia: JB Lippincott, 1983

78. Spiessl B, Scheibe O, Wagner G (eds), UICC (Union Internationale Contre le Cancer). *TNM-Atlas. Illustrated Guide to the Classification of Malignant Tumours*. Berlin, Heidelberg and New York: Springer-Verlag, 1982

79. Killip III T, Kimball JT. Treatment of myocardial infarction in a coronary care unit. A two-year

experience with 250 patients. *Am J Cardiol*, 1967; **20**: 457–64

80. Rovinsky JJ. Diseases complicating pregnancy. Diabetes mellitus. In: Romney SL, Gray MJ, Little AB, et al. eds. *Gynecology and Obstetrics*. 2nd Edition. New York: McGraw-Hill, 1981:747–53

81. Champion HR, Sacco WJ, Hunt TK. Trauma Severity Scoring to predict mortality. *World J Surg*, 1983;**7**:4–10

82. Gennarelli TA (Chairman) Committee on Injury Scaling. *Abbreviated Injury Scale. 1985 Revision*. Arlington Heights: American Association for Automotive Medicine, 1985

83. Greenspan L, McLean BA, Greig H. Abbreviated Injury Scale and Injury Severity Score: A scoring chart. *J Trauma*, 1985;**25**:60–4

84. Morris Jr JA, Auerbach PS, Marshall GA, et al. The Trauma Score as a triage tool in the prehospital setting. *JAMA*, 1986;**256**:1319–25

85. Champion HR, Copes WS, Sacco JW, et al. A new characterization of injury severity. *J Trauma*, 1990; **30**:539–46

86. Teasdale G, Jennett B. Assessment of coma and impaired consciousness. A practical scale. *Lancet*, 1974;**2**:81–4

87. Nelson KG. An index of severity for acute pediatric illness. *Am J Public Health*, 1980;**70**:804–7

88. Knaus WA, Zimmerman JE, Wagner DP, et al. APACHE – acute physiology and chronic health evaluation: a physiologically based classification system. *Crit Care Med*, 1981;**9**:591–7

89. Knaus WA, Draper EA, Wagner DP, Zimmerman JE. APACHE II. A severity of disease classification system. *Crit Care Med*, 1985;**13**:818–29

90. Apgar V. A proposal for a new method of evaluation of the newborn infant. *Curr Res Anaesth Analg*, 1953;**32**:260–7

91. Apgar V, Holaday DA, James S et al. Evaluation of the newborn infant – second report. *JAMA*, 1958; **168**:1985–8

92. Coté R, Hachinski VC, Shurvell BL, et al. The Canadian Neurological Scale; A preliminary study in acute stroke. *Stroke*, 1986;**17**:731–7

93. Coté R, Battista RN, Wolfson C, et al. The Canadian Neurological Scale: Validation and reliability assessment. *Neurology*, 1989;**39**:638–43

94. Wolfson CM, Coté R, Battista RN, Adam J. Quantitative scales for measuring neurological deficit in cerebrovascular disorders. *Ann RCPSC*, 1990; **23**:49–52

95. Shah S, Vanclay F, Cooper B. Improving the sensitivity of the Barthel index for stroke rehabilitation. *J Clin Epidemiol*, 1989;**42**:703–9

96. Rosenberg AA, Battaglia FC. The newborn infant. In: Hathaway WE, Groothuis JR, Hay WW Jr, Paisley JW eds. *Current Diagnosis & Treatment*. 10th Edition. Norwalk: Appleton & Lange, 1991:50–103

97. Koops BL, Battaglia FC. The newborn infant. In: Kempe CH, Silver HK, O'Brien D, Fulgitini VA eds. *Current Pedidatric Diagnosis & Treatment*. 9th Edition. Norwalk: Appleton & Lange, 1987:41–197

98. Rutledge R, Fakhry S, Baker C, Oller D. Injury severity grading in trauma patients: A simplified technique based upon ICD-9 coding. *J Trauma*, 1993;**35**:497–507

99. Rutledge R, Hyot DB, Eastman B, et al. Comparison of the Injury Severity Score and ICD-9 diagnosis codes as predictors of outcome in injury: Analysis of 44,032 patients. *J Trauma*, 1997;**42**:477–89

100. Rutledge R, Osler T, Emery S, Kromhout-Schiro S. The end of the Injury Severity Score (ISS) and the Trauma and Injury Severity Score (TRISS): ICISS, an International Classification of Diseases, Ninth Revision-based prediction tool, outperforms both ISS and TRISS as predictors of trauma patient survival, hospital charges, and hospital length of stay. *J Trauma*, 1998;**44**:41–9

101. Singer DE, Samet JH, Coley CM, Nathan DM. Screening for diabetes mellitus. *Ann Intern Med*, 1988;**109**:639–49

102. *Periodic Health Examination Monograph. Report of a Task Force to the Conference of Deputy Ministers of Health*. Cat No H39 -3/1980 E. Ottawa: Supply and Services Canada, 1980

103. Armitage P, Berry G. *Statistical Methods in Medical Resarch*. 2nd Edition. Oxford: Blackwell Scientific, 1987

104. Hutchison GB, Shapiro S. Lead time gained by diagnostic screening for breast cancer. *J Nat Cancer Inst*, 1968;**41**:665–81

105. Cole P, Morrison AS. Basic issues in population screening for cancer. *J Nat Cancer Inst*, 1980,**64**: 1263–72

106. Hulley SB, Cummings SR, Browner WS, et al (eds). *Designing Clinical Research. An Epidemiologic Approach*. Baltimore: Williams & Wilkins, 1988

107. Philbrick JT, Horwitz RI, Feinstein AR. The limited spectrum of patients studied in exercise test research. Analyzing the tip of the iceberg. *JAMA*, 1982; **248**:2467–70

108. Nierenberg AA, Feinstein AR. How to evaluate a diagnostic marker test. Lessons from the rise and fall of dexamethasone suppression test. *JAMA*, 1988; **259**:1699–1702

109. Arkin CF, Wachtel MS. How many patients are necessary to assess test performance? *JAMA*, 1990; **263**:275–8

110. Rosenberg AM. Advanced drug therapy for juvenile rheumatoid arthritis. *J Pediat*, 1989;**114**:171–8

111. Richardson WS, Glasziou P, Polashenski WA, Wilson MC. A new arrival: evidence about differential diagnosis. *ACP Journal Club*, 2000;**133**: A11–A12

112. Richardson WS, Wilson MC, Guyatt GH, et al. for the Evidence-Based Medicine Working Group. Users' guides to the medical literature. XV. How to use an article about disease probability for differential diagnosis. *JAMA*, 1999;**281**:1241–9

113. Wiener S, Nathanson M. Physical examination. Frequently observed errors. *JAMA*, 1976;**236**:852–5

114. Sadegh-Zadeh K. The fuzzy revolution: Goodbye to the Aristotelian Weltanschauung. *Artif Intell Med*, 2001;**21**:1–25

115. Sadegh-Zadeh K. Fuzzy health, illness, and disease. *J Med Phil*, 2000;**25**:606–38

116. Nordenfelt L. On the place of fuzzy health in medical theory. *J Med Phil*, 2000;**25**:639–49

117. Sadegh-Zadeh K. Fundamentals of clinical methodology. 4. Diagnosis. *Artif Intell Med*, 2000;**20**: 227–41

118. Sadegh-Zadeh K. Fundamentals of clinical methodology: 3. Nosology. *Artif Intell Med*, 1999;**19**:87–108

119. Dienstag JL, Isselbacher KJ. Acute viral hepatitis. In: Fauci S, Braunwald E, Isselbacher K, et al. eds. *Harrison's Principles of Internal Medicine*. 14th Edition. New York: McGraw-Hill, 1998:1677–92

120. Ferguson CM. Acute appendicitis. In: Morris PJ, Wood WC eds. *Oxford Textbook of Surgery*. 2nd Edition. Oxford: Oxford University Press, 2000: 1539–43

121. Halgason CM, Malik DS, Cheng S-C, Jobe TH, Mordeson JN. Statistical versus fuzzy measures of variable interaction in patients with stroke. *Neuroepidemiology*, 2001;**20**:77–84

122. Sawyer MD. Invited commentary: Fuzzy logic – an introduction. *Surgery*, 2000;**127**:254–6

123. Buchanan T. Invited commentary: Fuzzy logic, clear reasoning. *Surgery*, 2000;**127**:257

124. Amin AP, Kulkarni HR. Improvement in the information content of the Glasgow Coma Scale for the prediction of full cognitive recovery after head injury using fuzzy logic. *Surgery*, 2000;**127**:245–53

125. Harris ED Jr. Rheumatoid arthritis: The clinical spectrum. In: Kelley WN, Harris ED Jr, Ruddy S, Sledge CB eds. *Textbook of Rheumatology*. Philadelphia: WB Saunders, 1981:928–63

126. Frank JW, Goel V, Harvey BJ, et al. A critical look at HIV antibody tests: 1. How accurate are they? *Can Fam Phys*, 1987;**33**:2005–11

127. Frank JW, Coates RA, Harvey BJ, et al. A critical look at HIV-antibody tests: 2. Benefits, risks and clinical use. *Can Fam Phys*, 1987;**33**:2229–35

128. *Report of the US Preventive Services Task Force. Guide to Clinical Preventive Services. An Assessment of 169 Interventions*. Baltimore: Williams & Wilkins, 1989

129. Richardson WS, Wilson MC, Williams Jr JW, et al. for the Evidence-Based Medicine Working Group. Users' guides to the medical literature. XXIV. How to use an article on the clinical manifestations of disease. *JAMA*, 2000;**284**:869–75

130. Jaeschke R, Guyatt G, Sackett DL for the Evidence-Based Medicine Working Group. Users' guides to the medical literature. III. How to use an article about a diagnostic tests. A. Are the results valid? *JAMA*, 1994;**271**:389–91

131. Jaeschke R, Guyatt GH, Sackett DL for the Evidence-Based Medicine Working Group. Users' guides to the medical literature. III. How to use the article about a diagnostic test. B. What are the results and will they help me in caring for my patients? *JAMA*, 1994;**271**:703–7

132. Baratt A, Irwig L, Glasziou P, et al. for the Evidence-Based Medicine Working Group. Users' guides to the medical literature. XVII. How to use guidelines and recommendations about screening. *JAMA*, 1999;**281**:2029–34

133. King LS. *Medical Thinking. A Historical Preface*. Princeton, NJ: Princeton University Press, 1982

134. Cutler P. *Problem Solving in Clinical Medicine. From Data to Diagnosis*. 2nd Edition. Baltimore: Williams & Wilkins, 1985

135. Albert DA, Munson R, Resnik MD. *Reasoning in Medicine. An Introduction to Clinical Inference*. Baltimore and London: The Johns Hopkins University Press, 1988

136. Kassirer JP, Kopelman RJ. *Learning Clinical Reasoning*. Baltimore: Williams & Wilkins, 1991

137. Ebell MH, Smith MA, Barry HC, et al. Does this patient have strep throat? *JAMA*, 2000;**284**:2912–8

138. Bruns DE, Huth EJ, Magid E, Young DS. Toward a checklist for reporting of studies of diagnostic accuracy of medical tests. *Clin Chem*, 2000;**46**: 893–5

139. Bener A, Al-Suwaidi MHMO, El-Ghazawi I, et al. Remote general practice: diagnosis of appendicitis. *Can J Rural Med*, 2002;**7**:26–9

140. Manning G, Rushton I, Milklar-Craig MW. Clinical implications of white coat hypertension: ambulatory blood pressure monitoring study. *J Hum Hypertension*, 1999;**13**:817–22

141. Macartney FJ. Diagnostic logic. *BMJ*, 1987;**295**: 1325–31

Chapter 7

Describing what happens. Clinical case reports, case series, occurrence studies

*A clinical problem is more likely
to be an uncommon presentation
of a common disease than a common
presentation of an uncommon disease*
Anonymous

*I keep six honest servingmen,
(They taught me all I knew)
Their names are What and Why and When
and How and Where and Who*
Rudyard Kipling (1865–1933)

Principles of logic in medicine as outlined in Chapter 3 are not important solely for the theory of medicine. Often, we do not realize how much of our reasoning and decision-making depends on a solid logical discourse. Let us take an example: As a specialist in community medicine, you notice that cases of meningitis are suddenly unusually frequent in adolescents living in a given urban area. You also know that an effective immunizing agent is available. Hence, you conclude that a vaccination program in the area should be implemented to solve this public health problem. This kind of reasoning and decision can be seen as a syllogism or logical discourse:

Medical practice	Logical discourse	Evidence
You have received information about new cases of meningitis	There is an unusually high incidence of meningitis in this community **(Premise A)**	**Disease occurrence** from epidemiological surveillance
What should be done?	There is an effective vaccine available and it can be used in this community as the best alternative to other programs **(Premise B)**	Evidence on vaccine **efficacy, effectiveness** and **efficiency** and on other programs to control meningitis outbreak
An immunization program should be implemented and its effectiveness monitored	Immunization of high risk groups is mandatory and meningitis surveillance should follow **(Conclusion C)**	Estimating vaccine **effectiveness in this community**

Our conclusion will be only as good as the logical postulates that precede it. The best decisions will be based on **evidence-based postulates**. To know if our postulates are solid, we must know the appropriate criteria of good evidence and be familiar with the methods used to obtain it. In our example, valid evidence of a significant spread of meningitis, Postulate A, will be based on a well-designed occurrence (descriptive) study and surveillance of this disease in the community. We will read about these studies further in the present chapter. Valid evidence of the effectiveness of the vaccine Postulate B will depend on clinical and field trials of the vaccine, which will produce a quantifiable measure of vaccine effectiveness (see Chapter 9). Our choice of vaccination as a preventive measure (Conclusion C) will depend on the results of our decision analysis where competing strategies are taken into account and vaccination emerges as the best possible strategy to control this outbreak.

Reasoning and decisions in clinical and community care are most often based on a chain of logical discourses that must be evidence-based to produce expected results and to benefit the patient and the community. A clinician's primary goal is to know what a disease looks like as it spreads within a community. Once that information is known, the disease's origins can be studied and treatment options discussed. A priority for prevention or cure is knowing whether the disease is a numerically important and clinical problem.

Chapter 6 described the use of problem definition tools. This chapter outlines ways to answer the following questions about disease: How much? How many? How does it look? Epidemiologists call such endeavors **descriptive studies**. Because it is sometimes difficult to say if such studies describe prevalence or incidence of disease, the term **occurrence studies** is used when some events are counted and a prevalence/incidence problem may occur. The term **descriptive observational studies** is used when there are no control groups and events are recorded 'as they happen'. It is known that measuring the frequency of disease occurrence is not sufficient. Knowing what clinical cases or disease looks like is also important. Such portraits are becoming part of qualitative research, even if some observations are measured or otherwise quantified.

7.1 Three types of descriptive studies and their objectives

Three types of observational studies are discussed here:

1. Descriptions of single clinical cases as they are reported (**disease at an individual level**).
2. Portraits of case series or 'occurrence studies without denominators' (**disease in several individuals**).

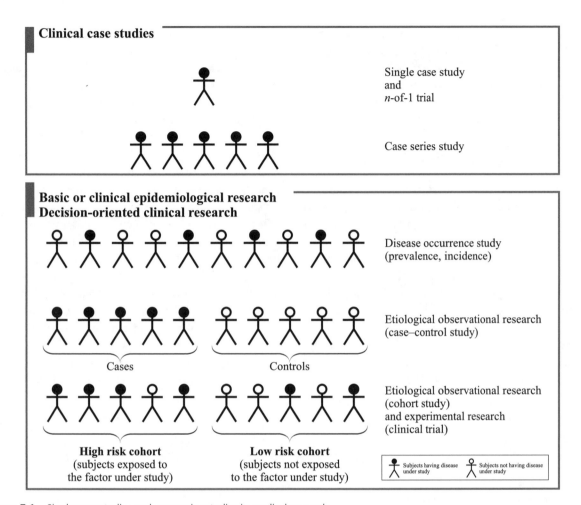

Figure 7.1 Single case studies and case series studies in medical research

3. **Disease occurrence and spread in the community** or 'epidemiological' descriptive studies, i.e. 'occurrence studies with denominators' where all rates, ratios and other expressions of quantification are related to a population database.

Figure 7.1 illustrates these types of studies. NB Case–control studies, cohort studies and clinical trials will be examined in Chapters 8 and 9.

Descriptive studies ask **'what happened' or 'what is happening'**. At this stage of dealing with clinical problems, questioning causes (hypothesizing) would be premature. Rather, an exact picture of events is obtained, leading to the questioning of causes (hypothesizing). The importance of descriptive studies must be emphasized at the outset. These studies are often frowned upon, even rejected, because 'they do not answer any questions'.

However, without a rigorous description and counting of events (disease cases, exposure to noxious factors, etc.), the analytical studies that follow are based on material that nobody understands. Thus, descriptive studies must be as thorough as analytical studies or clinical trials. Since each type of study answers different questions, they are all complementary in the eventual decision-making process.

7.2 Drawing clinical pictures or describing disease in an individual. Case reports

Physicians continually describe single cases in admission reports, progress reports, discharge summaries, on clinical wards, and in the medical press as **case reports**. If several single cases draw attention, **case series reports** are worthy of consideration. Given that these reports are the most frequent means of communication between health professionals, the argument for proper case reporting is strongly supported. This section first describes the clinimetric ingredients of case reports in terms of disease history and course, and introduces such pictures in case reports.

7.2.1 Disease history and disease course

Understanding disease requires not only the counting of cases from one circumstance to another, but also the follow-up of its evolution in time. The evolution of disease from onset to resolution is often called **the history of the disease**. The natural history or **natural course** of disease represents its spontaneous evolution, without any intervention to alter its severity, duration, or impact. The **clinical course** of disease represents a natural course altered by clinical interventions such as exploratory methods (diagnostic procedures), conservative (drugs) or radical (surgery) treatment, etc. The traditional term 'history

of disease' implicitly evokes the past. However, the picture of disease implies what happens or what will happen. Hence, the term '**course of disease**' is used in this text as synonymous for '**history of disease**'.

The natural history and course of many diseases is only poorly understood. This knowledge comes from the past, essentially from experience and careful observation. However, rules for uniform definitions of phenomena of interest, methods of counting, interpretation and classification (clinimetrics) were not established at the time the knowledge was acquired. Hence, narrative experience prevails in the body of knowledge of the natural course of many important health problems. Traditionally, the natural history of disease is defined as the course of a disease from its onset (inception) to its resolution. Figure 7.2 illustrates a hypothetical, contemporary understanding of disease history and course. The term 'course' appears more appropriate than 'history', indicating either '. . . a continuous progression or advance, progress, or . . . the continual or gradual advance or

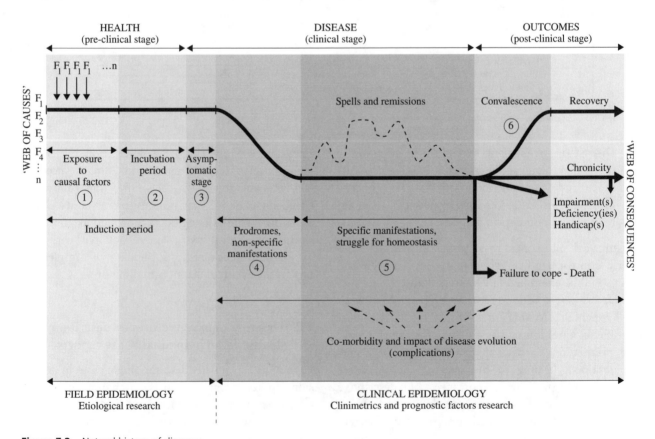

Figure 7.2   Natural history of disease

progress of anything'[1]. The natural course of disease may be altered by different clinical maneuvers, such as diagnosis and treatment, giving a picture of the **'clinical course of disease'**. Various comparisons of both these entities form the basis of evaluation of clinical practices and interventions, including prevention and treatment. Given the rapid development of specific treatment for many diseases (antibiotics for the treatment of bacterial infections, chemotherapy, radiation and surgery for many cancers, etc.), the clinical course of these diseases is better understood. For ethical reasons, however, it is necessary to rely on understanding of the natural course of disease from the imperfect experience of the past. Neither syphilis nor tuberculosis, diabetes or hypertension can be left untreated for the sole purpose of obtaining valid reference data for cooperative studies of prognosis in assessing the long-term effectiveness of clinical interventions.

A good clinimetric picture of disease cases gives important normative data that serves several purposes, the three most significant of which are quoted by O'Connor[2]:

1. Properly interpreted normative data are necessary for an accurate description of the natural history of clinical conditions.
2. Normative data are critical for developing appropriate standards of care for physicians.
3. Normative data enable the development and validation of illness nosology appropriate for primary care physician education and research.

Current descriptions of patients can be found under different denominations: case studies, natural history of disease, spectrum of disease, etc. One study may describe all clinical and paraclinical findings at a given time (usually when a clinician admits or discharges a patient). Less often, studies describe a chronological, ongoing picture of cases. A valid description of disease cases ideally requires several components. Such a composite picture, however, is the exception rather than the rule. Nonetheless, any attempt at drawing a good composite picture of a disease course in individuals is a useful exercise since it reveals how little (or how much) is actually known about the disease. Table 7.1 compares writing music to describing cases in medicine. The logic of both is very similar:

1. A musician clarifies the kind of composition desired (first ingredient): a simple song, a symphony, a mass. Just as a symphony evolves from one movement to another, or a mass from Kyrie to Gloria, Credo, Sanctus Dominus, and Agnus Dei, the natural or clinical course of disease evolves by **stages** from exposure to disease appearance and evolution, leading to several possible outcomes.
2. Just as melody (second ingredient) is the lifeline and bearer of a musical piece, with tones being important and necessary **components**, clinical **observations** of a pathological phenomenon under study should not be missed, and like notes in music, they should be put together.

Table 7.1 Understanding the logic of clinical course description through music

Writing music – necessary components	*Describing the clinical course of disease – necessary components*
(1) **Component structure (movements)**	All phases or **stages** of the natural and clinical course of disease should be well delineated, defined, and described in their proper, appropriate, natural sequence
(2) **Melody (notes)**	The essential **components** of the clinical picture must not be omitted. All ingredients should be included (good construct validity)
(3) **Harmony (chords)**	The entire **clinical spectrum** should be understood from one moment to the next
(4) **Dynamics (pp to ff)**	The evolution of the **disease gradient** should be known throughout the disease course ('ebb and flow' of disease)
(5) **Rhythm (3/4, 4/4)**	**Frequency, duration, and amplitude of disease spells** should be noted

3. Just as harmony (third ingredient) interrelates different tones (chords), the **clinical spectrum** of disease at a given time should be described.
4. Just as the dynamics of music (fourth ingredient) indicate all the required pianissimos and fortissimos and anything in between, **disease gradient** from one moment of the disease's course to another must be known.
5. Just as rhythm (fifth ingredient) must be given to music, **disease spells** should be described in time.

A more detailed examination of the aspects of disease course, methodological approaches, and the desired goal in describing disease cases from one disease stage to another is necessary at this point.

7.2.1.1 *Preclinical stages*

A proper description of cases of disease is based on a rigorous approach to all stages of disease including stages of exposure, incubation, the asymptomatic stage, the clinical stage, and the period of recovery (outcomes).

Period of exposure. in classical epidemiology covers exposure to noxious factors, such as breathing carcinogens, drinking contaminated water, or living in a stressful environment. In pharmacoepidemiology, the period(s) of treatment is submitted to similar attention. A proper description of this stage requires measurement of:

- Duration;
- Frequency of exposures (cigarettes smoked, occupational irradiation periods, drug doses taken, etc.), or the study of peaks of exposure (as in studies of air pollution in relation to exacerbations of respiratory problems);
- Quantity of exposure (e.g. total irradiation dose, quantity of lead or mercury ingested through contaminated food, etc.);
- Evolution of comorbidity (described in the same way as the clinical stage of the disease of interest; for more details see next section), in order to better understand its contribution to the evolution of the disease under study.

Incubation period is the time interval between the entry of an infectious agent into a macro-organism, or the critical (sufficient) exposure time to a noninfectious agent, and the appearance of the first clinical manifestation of the disease in question. Strictly speaking, the incubation period of an infectious disease includes such events as the infectious agent's multiplication in the macro-organism, its spread (bacteremia, viremia), and its fixation in target organs and systems. *NB The extrinsic incubation period is a term used in medical entomology to identify a time span between the initial vector infecting feeding (arthropods, or an animal host or reservoir) and the time at which vectors, hosts or reservoir species are capable of transmitting infections to man and others. For example, in arboviruses, this period varies from four days to 21 days, when the majority of infected insects transmit the virus*[3]. The concept of an incubation period is easy to understand in diseases based on a pinpoint exposure and the appearance of rather uniform cases, such as in measles. When exposure to a causal agent is long and disease counts many asymptomatic cases and/or a variable clinical picture of clinically manifest cases, the detection and understanding of incubation periods becomes difficult. This is the case with the epidemiological study of human cancer incubation periods[4,5]. In addition to the often insidious onset of diseases like cancer, stages of exposure, incubation, and the asymptomatic phase of disease may overlap.

Limits between exposure and incubation are often ill defined, such as in many cancers. In these cases, the term **'induction period'** as proposed by Rothman[6] appears more appropriate. This problem is very poorly understood at present. What represents a period of exposure versus an incubation period of cirrhosis in a chronic heavy drinker? With time variability in the moment of diagnosis, it must be acknowledged that a basic understanding of the natural history of cirrhosis according to contemporary rules and requirements of clinimetrics is inadequate. A proper study of this stage requires a rigorous clinimetric follow-up of cases, definition of exposure (episode, duration, etc.), and an operational definition of an inception moment (sometimes referred to as 'zero time') of disease and the diagnostic criteria of the latter at that time. For example, the incubation period of cervical cancer would be different if measured in relation to the moment of its detection at an asymptomatic stage (cancer *in situ*), or at a time when symptoms of an invasive cancer appear. To allow for practical decision-making in disease control, one must know the full interval of the incubation period of the disease in question. For example, if clinicians wish to know whether a particular case is the result of a nosocomial infection (infection acquired in hospital) or not, the terms must first be defined. A case of nosocomial infection may be regarded as any case in which the duration of hospitalization is longer than the lower limit (shortest interval) of an incubation period of disease. After a patient's discharge, any case of infection (while excluding other exposures after discharge) appearing during the period corresponding to the longest known incubation period (upper limit of incubation interval) should also be suspected as a possible nosocomial infection. For example, the incubation period of hepatitis B varies from 50 to 180 days. An elderly patient in poor health is hospitalized for one year. If the patient develops hepatitis B in the second half of the second month of the hospital stay, a nosocomial origin for the hepatitis should be evaluated (this case may have a very short incubation period). If the same patient were to develop hepatitis B at any time during the first six months after discharge from hospital, the hepatitis might also have been acquired during hospitalization. In this situation, the case might have involved an incubation period corresponding to the upper known limit for the disease.

Asymptomatic stage. In order for the time span of this stage to be known, morphological and physiological changes that might be detected using early diagnostic methods are of vital importance, both in theory and practice. This stage involves a variety of 'pre-clinical' changes, representing an already ongoing morbid process. Reactions at the primary site of infection, seroconversion, and other undetected morbid changes (if not anticipated) occur at this time. The asymptomatic stage further complicates any calculation of disease stage intervals in the course of disease. Studies of variability of these stages are practically nonexistent even if knowledge of this variability is of the utmost importance (ex. when deciding if screening programs should be implemented). Causal factors of the disease must appear before the disease starts. Only then are they identified as risk factors. If they continue to act after the beginning of the disease, they become prognostic factors (as detailed in Chapter 10) that might determine disease course and outcomes. From a theoretical point of view (and with considerable practical implications), the best possible measurement and knowledge of this stage by exacting clinimetric methods and criteria is essential if it is to be understood whether a given factor is responsible either for disease occurrence (**risk factor**), and/or for its course and outcome(s) as a **prognostic factor**. Only the knowledge of both problems leads to understanding, for example, if smoking is more serious before the appearance of lung cancer or whether continuing to smoke once the cancer is established can worsen the prognosis.

Obviously, the preclinical or asymptomatic stage of disease manifestation is often difficult to grasp. For practical reasons, a good knowledge of this stage is essential when considering the feasibility of screening for disease and when evaluating the impact of early treatment(s). The detectability of disease by specific methods and according to well-defined diagnostic criteria also allows for refinements of definition and calculation of the incubation period of the disease. Statistical problems related especially to the study of the first stages of the disease course were recently reviewed by Brookmeyer[7].

These first stages (exposure, incubation, asymptomatic, up to the appearance of prodromes) are of particular interest to classical or field epidemiology. For this reason, they are better known historically in infectious than in non-infectious disease epidemiology. The rest of disease course is mainly dealt with in clinical epidemiology.

7.2.1.2 *Clinically manifest period of disease; clinical stages*

The clinical stage of disease is the 'pièce de résistance' for clinimetrics. However, even today, cases reflecting clinicians' exceptional experiences are often expressed in an unorganised manner. A more thorough picture of cases should ideally include several elements, congruent with the logic of Figure 7.2.

Clinical stages. Disease becomes clinically patent through the appearance of various signs and symptoms. For many diseases, two consecutive periods exist: **The prodromal stage** is characterized by the appearance of various manifestations, signs or symptoms common to many diseases, and which are usually not sufficient for diagnosis. It represents a variable period during which patients exhibit non-specific signs and/or symptoms that are common to several disease entities. One or several days of fever, fatigue, pain, or coughing and sneezing are common to many infections. A longer period of dyspepsia may be common to many benign and malignant digestive disorders, such as gastritis, gallstones, hepatitis, or pancreatic cancer, among others. However, if such a period is recognized, practical implications can be important. For example, a few weeks after an AIDS primo-infection, an 'acute viral syndrome'[8] is diagnosed: fever, lymphadenopathy, pharyngitis, rash, sore throat, anorexia, headaches, etc. Such a period, as further investigations have shown[8–10], is associated with transient high levels of viremia and may precede seroconversion. This indicates that even in the early stages of this disease, patients may become a source of infection for their contacts, a fact that is significant for preventive and protective measures. Poliomyelitis, rabies, and measles are just a few examples of diseases having a prodromal stage. Sometimes, patients recover after the prodromal stage, representing so-called **abortive cases** of disease. There are in fact more cases of the abortive type of poliomyelitis than of the type that evolves into a paralytic stage.

The **stage of specific manifestations** ('classical' period, clinical stage, etc.) of disease represents a combination and sequence of signs and symptoms, as well as paraclinical findings (bacteriology, hematology, biochemistry, histology, etc.) that are diagnostic for the disease of interest and an indication for treatment and/or care. The clinical stage of disease encompassing specific manifestations of disease is often the best known. The greatest challenge remains the need for a structured description and understanding of disease evolution in time and space[16], which should extend beyond the counting of clinically manifest episodes (migraine, asthma, epilepsy, etc.) and remissions. All stages of disease should be defined, described, and delineated in operational terms. As for clinical stages of specific manifestations, staging of cancer is a classic example of such a procedure[11,12]. As often happens, the evolving

clinical spectrum of disease correlates with a worsening disease gradient.

The anatomical staging of disease may be further refined by clinical observation and recording of so-called **transition events** such as the appearance of new observations at clinical examination (new mass, retraction of skin over tumor site, etc.), allowing better timing of events and intervals between them. Such an improved follow-up of the time factor permits a more refined staging, relating to different prognostic characteristics. The procedure belongs to the description of disease course which has been termed '**auxometry of disease**' by Charlson and Feinstein[13]. Auxology in pediatrics represents the study of the growth and development of children (normal and abnormal) using, for example, measurements of pertinent somatometric variables (height, weight, etc.). The auxometry of disease thus performs the same function in the field of clinimetrics of disease.

The rate of disease progression from one stage to another often has different prognostic values. Rapidly evolving cases of cancer are lethal, and are sometimes missed in prevalence studies. If treatment is evaluated on the basis of the study of prevalent cases only, a '**prevalence – incidence bias**' (Neyman's bias) occurs, possibly leading to an overestimation of treatment effectiveness.

If taking treatment into consideration represents the mainstay of clinical course studies, much less is known about the **clinical course of diseases in relation to their co-morbidity** (in appearance and presence of other health problems), either before or during disease history. Most of the information in medical textbooks concerns disease in previously healthy subjects. Much less is known about the interaction between different pathologies (disease entities) and the impact of treatment of one disease on the evolution of co-morbidity, or, what impact the treatment of co-morbidity on the clinical course of the main disease of interest may have. Studies of prognosis would largely benefit from a more balanced understanding of disease outcome(s).

Comorbidity is now considered to be a powerful predictor of health outcome in terms of survival and disability. In fact, it contributes significantly to health services utilization and medical costs[14].

Coebergh et al[15] who focused their attention on co-morbidity in cancer patients, have even suggested the inclusion of frequent co-morbid conditions in prognostic research and guidelines for patient care.

Clinical components of a full disease portrait should be present in the description of cases. A description of the course of cancer given solely by the evolution of a patient's fatigue and weight loss would certainly have poor construct validity. Complemented by a chronology of precancerous tissue changes, appearance of primary site tumor, its growth, circumtumoral tissue changes, appearance of metastatic spread, etc. a more satisfactory clinical spectrum within a specific time frame is obtained. Any important abnormality should be noted, such as:

- Configuration or macroscopic **appearance** (region, organ);
- **Localization** (atopic organs, size, etc.);
- **Tissue abnormality** (histology, etc.);
- **Functional abnormality**, such as rhythm (cardiac arrhythmias), frequency (tachypnea, fibrillation), direction (gastro-esophageal reflux, arteriovenous shunt, blood circulation due to transposition of great vessels, etc.), volume (polycythemia, ascites, pus, etc.); or
- **Speed** (intestinal passage, growth rate of a tumor, etc.).

Impact levels should be described as well. In congenital problems, these levels may extend from dysmetabolism (e.g. Tay-Sachs disease) to dys-histogenesis (Marfan's syndrome), to organ or field malformation (trisomy-13), and to regional deformation (Potter sequence)[16].

Clinical and paraclinical spectrum of disease. Traditionally, pathological, histological, biochemical, or radiological spectra, etc. are produced. As for a clinical spectrum, it should involve a clear separation of:

- A spectrum of signs;
- A spectrum of symptoms;
- The picture of both at a given stage of disease; and
- Their evolution from one stage of disease to another.

Such a composite and well-organized clinical picture is the exception rather than the rule. Hattwick[17]

presents a good example of this in the evolution of the clinical spectrum of rabies (Figure 7.3).

Evans[18] describes an overall clinical spectrum of selected respiratory pathogens. His historical examples illustrate how narrow the clinical spectrum of streptococcal infections is (common cold-like, tonsillitis and pharyngitis, upper respiratory tract infection) compared to the overall spectrum of adenovirus infections (all of the above plus croup, bronchiolotis, pneumonitis, and pneumonia). For practical purposes, when clinicians want to know which type of disease case shows a particular period of communicability (infectivity), immunity, patency, latency, etc. indicative of preventive measures during and after disease, it is convenient to describe the course of the disease in terms of both its clinical and paraclinical spectra. Variation of laboratory findings, such as titers of a given antibody between individuals at one time, or in time from one individual to another, may serve as an example of a **paraclinical gradient of disease**. Conversely, variation of several antibody levels in infection sufferers, or the appearance of abnormal levels of several different serum enzymes in chronic alcohol drinkers represents a **paraclinical spectrum of disease**.

Disease spells (episodes, attacks). Chronic diseases often have an unstable course. Clinically manifest periods appear, followed by asymptomatic 'pauses', such as in migraine, gout, or asthma. *NB Chronic disease is defined for routine health statistics purposes as any phenomenon lasting three months and more*[2]. In clinical epidemiology, the time factor, always arbitrary, should be replaced by other criteria of chronicity, such as:

- Episodicity (running by spells);
- Pursuit of disease course if treatment is discontinued; or
- In cases of stagnation of disease course beyond a norm, i.e. if standard duration of treatment does not lead to cure.

Any disease occurring in spells requires the following descriptive data:

- Frequency of spells;
- Duration of spells;
- Clinical gradient (severity) of spells;

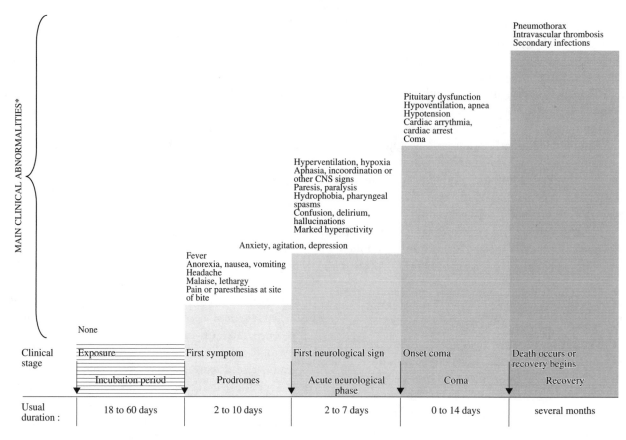

Figure 7.3 Evolution of clinical spectrum and gradient of rabies. Source: Ref. 17, reproduced with permission from Elsevier Science

- Duration of intervals between spells;
- Amplitude of spells; and
- Their clinical spectrum (uniformity).

Disease gradient. The most challenging clinimetric task is to properly describe disease dynamics in time. A good description of disease at the moment of examination progresses to the establishment of a longitudinal or evolving picture. A logical idea would be a multidimensional picture of the disease course, demonstrating relationships between time, space (body and/or mind), disease spectrum, and disease gradient. The latter is most often used for the description of disease dynamics. Simple clinical charts of body temperature or vital functions are elementary examples of a disease gradient study. Unfortunately, other clinical phenomena important for clinical decision-making, such as pain in other diseases, are not subject to similar follow-up, even if methodology for

these purposes is available[21]. Currently, there is no uniform system of tridimensional disease history and course description that would integrate the evolution of both gradient and spectrum in time. Most diseases of interest lack adequate structured information. Disease gradient is directional; disease spectrum is not.

7.2.1.3 Convalescence, recovery and other outcomes of disease

A considerable discrepancy in clinimetric rigor exists between the care taken to describe the initial clinical stage of disease and all ensuing events, including the eventual death certificate. Convalescence, or a period of waning signs and symptoms and the return to satisfactory morphology and function, is the least known. This is mostly due to poor clinimetric inception of the starting point and end point of convalescence. Frequently, periods such as the beginning of convalescence are defined by the end of the prescribed treatment or by the disappearance of specific manifestations of disease. The end of convalescence is measured in vague terms by a return to the asymptomatic state, daily habits, and working capacity. Studies and understanding of convalescence remain a weak point in the assessment of the impact of therapeutic interventions. Re-adaptation, physiotherapy, and any other measures of functional recovery and substitution rely on an equally rigorous clinimetric picture of what happens after the clinical stage of disease. Such an auxology of convalescence or, in other instances, of evolution 'ad pessimum' is equally important. Clinicians cannot abandon the patient by simply administering treatment. Clinimetrics stops only at the recovery of health or at death.

7.2.1.4 *Special comments on infectious diseases*

Clinimetric description of infectious diseases does not differ from the rest of human pathology, with the exception of a few specific additions related to the infection mechanism itself and its transmission, as outlined here. To complete aspects of the natural and clinical course of infectious diseases, two elements should be stressed: the **generation time** of infectious disease and the **period of communicability**. These are distinct from the generally applicable stages of disease course mentioned above.

In infectious disease epidemiology, knowledge needs to go beyond the incubation period. Transmission of an infectious disease to other persons does not always happen at the beginning of a clinically manifest stage of disease. **Generation time**[22] is the interval between the moment a subject is infected and the time when that subject becomes a source of infection for others. This does not completely coincide with the incubation period in many diseases. For example, chicken pox's generation time ends one or two days before eruptions appear. The period of communicability starts at this point, and it ends six days after their first appearance. If the spread of an infectious disease is to be controlled, its generation time should be known (some kind of patient isolation should be foreseen). An incubation period allows a

possible source of infection to be determined for this patient, but it will not give the same information as generation time. At present, only a minor fraction of infectious diseases have a well-known generation time useful for practical decision-making.

The **period of communicability** represents the time span during which an infected person can transmit disease to other individuals. This period does not often coincide with the clinical stage of disease. It may start at the moment of a pre-clinical stage (prodromes), or even towards the end of an incubation period. It may end before the clinical stage ends (e.g. as in pertussis, chicken pox, or measles), or it may extend well beyond the clinical stage, such as in convalescent and 'healthy' carriers in typhoid fever. Pertussis is highly communicable in the early catarrhal stage, but communicability becomes negligible after three weeks of disease despite a persistent spasmodic cough. The maximum infectivity of viral hepatitis A may occur during the later half of the incubation period (15 to 50 days) and continue for a few days after the onset of jaundice. In chicken pox, the period of communicability may start as early as five days before the onset of rash (usually one or two days before) and extend not more than five days after the appearance of the first crop of vesicles. In measles, communicability starts before the beginning of the prodromal period and becomes negligible after the first two days of rash. Communicability of typhoid fever extends into convalescence, with 10% of untreated patients becoming infectious three months after the onset of symptoms, and two to five per cent becoming permanent carriers.

The above-mentioned examples[23] illustrate the importance of solid knowledge of this period, so that isolation of patients and preventive measures focusing on all possible contacts (susceptible individuals) can be undertaken. Despite the demonstrable importance of knowing the generation time and the period of communicability of an infectious disease, a good body of literature specifies these periods wherever they are known, but it does not explicitly specify diseases for which these data are missing. An admission of uncertainty is as valuable a piece of information for readers as confirmation. The knowledge of uncertainties is also essential in making the best possible clinical decisions. **In summary, a good** description of a disease course requires the following fundamental components:

- Sufficient scope of **all possible stages** of the natural history and course of disease;
- Detection and appreciation of **all relevant clinical phenomena**, especially those which are important for diagnostic, therapeutic, and prognostic decisions;
- **Full clinical spectrum** at a given moment, and from one moment to another in disease course;
- Qualitative and quantitative portrait of **disease spells** if the disease is episodic;
- **Full clinical gradient** and its changes in time (disease dynamics);
- **Background characteristics of patients** (age, sex, occupation, medical and family history, etc.);
- Concurrent portrait of all relevant **clinical and paraclinical maneuvers** and their effects: diagnostic procedures and their undesirable effects, radical and conservative therapeutic regimens and their effect, secondary effects of treatments, clinical 'accidents' (machine failures, etc.) and errors, appearance of clinical emergencies and their control (shock, septic states, etc.);
- Precedence and/or concurrent appearance of **additional health problems**, i.e. **co-morbidity** (e.g. an asthmatic patient having a stroke), their courses, treatments and effects;
- **Exposure to additional important factors** (e.g. illicit drugs, drinking, or suicide attempts, etc.), and;
- **Explanation of the nature of biological responses** to various stimuli and events quoted above (reactions, adaptations, stress states, allergic reactions, shock, etc.).

It must be stressed that the **same picture must be obtained for comorbidity, including treatments for comorbidity and their effects.** A study of chronic obstructive lung disease in diabetic patients requires an equally solid description of diabetes and of respiratory problems. Since all of these requirements are needed for a good grasp of disease course, routine clinical charts are usually not suitable for a good clinimetric study of disease course. Such studies must be rigorously planned.

7.2.2 How to complete single case studies or clinical case reports.

A research protocol must be prepared in advance (not after data gathering is completed), and should cover the following elements:

- Review of the knowledge of the natural and clinical disease history and course;
- Theoretical and practical purposes (objectives) of description of cases;
- Components ('ingredients' as mentioned above) that will be followed according to specified operational criteria and definitions;
- Chronology and time frame of the study;
- The manner in which anticipated errors will be avoided and/or corrected; and
- Implications for clinical practice or for community medicine and public health.

This information should be present in all articles describing disease course. A well-informed reader will know what to expect from a good report on disease cases, course and history, what to read and retain for practice or research, and what to discard.

Case series studies, in comparison with studies of disease occurrence, are studies 'without denominators'. A simple occurrence of characteristics and events is established in patients. It is most often an in-depth study of 'numerators only', to which proper denominators remain to be assigned to establish rates in an epidemiological sense. It must be remembered that, for example, a characteristic present in 80% of patients does not mean that an individual bearing that characteristic has an 80% probability of having the disease; this might be concluded only on the basis of a prevalence rate. Neither does it mean that an individual in that community has an 80% probability of contracting the disease; only data on incidence would justify such a conclusion. Nor does it mean that there is a 80% probability that an individual bearing this characteristic will die of the disease under scrutiny; only mortality rates and case fatality studies would lead to such a conclusion. Such erroneous interpretations and conclusions of case studies still appear from time to time in the literature. These should be avoided. (See Chapter 3, section 3.1 on rates, proportional rates, and ratios.)

Are clinical case reports (CCRs) worthless, or are they valuable pieces of evidence? Even single clinical case reports are important pieces of evidence in medical practice and research. They are not proof of a disease's cause or effectiveness of treatment, but are an important source of hypotheses for such events. These hypotheses will validate themselves only in further, 'more serious' (i.e. having the power of proof) research. There are reasons for both the ebb and flow of interest in case reports in medicine. More than a century ago, the art of clinical case reporting was refined, particularly in French medicine, during Charcot's time at Paris' Pitié-Salpetrière Hospital. German medicine and the Prague and Vienna schools have all adopted **casuistics** as *the recording and study of the cases of any disease*[24] and synthesis of refined clinical observation. The subsequent attention in research to human biology, pathology and pharmacology, followed by epidemiology, clinical epidemiology and evidence-based medicine, has somehow neglected the fact that any practical and research activity starts at the bedside with a single patient, or with index cases in community medicine and public health.

CCRs are still presented for more than one reason:

- **To share a new or otherwise relevant observation** for the purpose of practice and research. There are several such good reasons justifying a CCR (*vide infra*).
- **To entertain.** Helping a patient who swallowed a toothbrush not only adds some flavor to the situation, but it also draws practical attention to a hidden problem of bulimia in this case[25].
- **To demonstrate the author's intelligence** in an overt or covert ego boost. In Sir Arthur Conan Doyle's or Agatha Christie's novels, the reader is immersed in the situation without obvious reason; only at the end is the mystery solved, underlying the author's brilliance.
- **To produce, as quickly as possible, a publication** enhancing the author's academic or professional standing and promotion chances.

CCRs are favored for the first two reasons. The last two discredit this important part of medicine. To remedy the situation, editors of several important periodicals have proposed better and more structured rules for good CCRs[26,27]. Pleas for relevant CCRs have also appeared in the literature[28,29], and the first textbook on how to write a CCR[30] is now widely available. A good clinical case report relies on **five basic qualities:**

- A relevant reason for choosing the topic of a CCR;
- A question to be answered by the CCR;
- A good presentation that follows the basic rules of clinimetrics and qualitative research;
- A structured form that is both reader-friendly and acceptable for the purposes of the medical press;
- Defined quality attributes including unexaggerated conclusions answering questions illustrated by the CCR.

What must be kept in mind when writing a CCR?

Choosing the topic. There are 20 reasons that justify the publication of a CCR:

1. Unusual presentation of unknown etiology;
2. Unusual natural history;
3. Unusual natural or clinical courses;
4. Challenging differential diagnosis;
5. Mistakes in diagnosis or treatment and their consequences;
6. Unusual and/or unexpected effect of treatment or diagnostic results;
7. Diagnostic and therapeutic 'accidents' (causes, consequences, remedies);
8. Unusual comorbidity (diagnosis, treatment, outcome);
9. Transfer of medical technology (from one disease, organ, or system to another);
10. Unusual setting of medical care (e.g. emergency or field conditions);
11. Management of an emergency case;
12. Patient compliance;
13. Patient/doctor interaction (as in psychiatry);
14. Single case clinical trial ('*n*-of-1' study);
15. Clinical situation as valuable experience, which cannot be reproduced for ethical reasons;
16. Limited access to cases (economy, ethics, social reasons, patient choices);
17. New medical technology (use, outcomes, consequences);
18. Confirmation of something already known (only if useful for a systematic case report review and synthesis);

19. Solving a challenging problem in medical ethics;
20. Evaluation of a potential burden of the case (family, health services, work environment, social services, economy).

Giving direction to a CCR. Any CCR may be developed either inductively or deductively. Most CCRs are inductive; an experience is described and conclusions are drawn from what was seen. A small number of CCRs are deductive; questions are asked first and the CCR speaks for or against a preconceived idea. Routine case reports, such as patient admission reports, are mostly of an inductive nature. Evidence-based clinical case reports as proposed by Reilly and Lemon[31] are based on deductive thinking.

Answering questions by researching and evaluating diagnostic, therapeutic or prognostic evidence, applied to the patient according to general or clinical characteristics[32], is the foundation of an **evidence-based clinical case report**. Simply reporting clinical and paraclinical results, information and experience means taking them at face value without questioning their validity and relevance to further decisions. In such cases, the ensuing patient management decisions are not always the most suitable. The evidence-based CCR is intended to remedy the situation.

In covering various components of a case report, such as diagnosis, treatment, or prognosis, a statement about them is accompanied by an explanation, on the basis of the best available evidence, of the reason for the clinician's preferred option. The reason for the conclusions drawn ('impression') should be clearly understandable and explained in the context of all available and relevant evidence. Also, as in Reilly and Lemon's experience[31], the case **generates more general questions** to which answers are sought across the available evidence. The best possible solution to the patient's problem is then **re-applied to** the question generating the **specific case.** An evidence-based clinical case report begins by identifying the patient and admitting physician, followed by a **search question** and subsequent **answer, with evaluation of the quality of evidence supporting such an answer.** On the basis of such an answer, a **patient care recommendation** is formulated. Evidence-based clinical case reports can also be found in surgery[33] and medicine[34].

Clinimetric considerations. Cases should be described according to the above-mentioned clinimetric rules covering patient risk characteristics, making a distinction between clinical data and clinical information, syndrome and disease, signs and symptoms, prognostic characteristics, comorbid states and their treatment. Criteria for all the above are available (on request), as is information about data recording and preservation covering all clinical and paraclinical actions in the patient.

Architecture (organization) of a CCR. A CCR for the medical press differs considerably from routine clinical case reports in focus, direction and structure. A routine CCR usually covers patient identification, chief complaint (reason for admission), patient history and views, concerns, expectations, values and ensuing preferences, physical and paraclinical examination, mental status assessment, 'impression' (working diagnosis), plan and orders for care, differential diagnosis work-up plan, prognosis and priority classification outlining alternative case management strategies.

An **ongoing clinical case report** summarizes either daily observations in a clinical setting or repeated observations of visiting patients in outpatient care. They are most often organized in a format known as 'SOAP':

- **Subjective** information covers the patient's version of the problem(s), its course and symptoms, how the patient is coping with the problem and subjective values given to the patient's state.
- **Objective** information represents a **focused** summary of physicians' observations like physical signs, results of paraclinical (laboratory) examinations, information provided by other health professionals (physical therapy results, dental or nursing care if relevant to the case), or social services and community medicine assistance.
- The **Assessment** section covers a revised and updated diagnosis and differential diagnosis, evaluation of the severity of the patient's state, and prognostic considerations.
- The **Plan** section includes additional clinical and paraclinical examinations and follow-up, conservative and radical treatment procedures like prescriptions and surgery, referrals to other specialists

Table 7.2 Architecture of a clinical case report

Summary*	• **Motives** and **reasons** for the report. 'Why are we reporting this?'
	• **Background** of the problem. 'In what context?'
	• **Highlights** of the report. 'What have we found?'
	• **Conclusions**. 'What does this mean?'
Introduction	• Definition of the **topic** (problem, disease, clinical activity).
	• General **context** of the topic (relevant knowledge, present clinical situation and challenges).
	• A **question** that this report should answer or a gap in knowledge that this report can fill.
	• **Objectives** and justification of this report.
Presentation of the case	• Situation, context and **triggering factor** of the report.
	• Clinical and paraclinical **initial state** of the patient.
	• **Evolution** of the clinical and paraclinical spectrum and gradient of the case.
	• Diagnostic and therapeutic **actions**, care and support.
	• **Expected** and actual **results** of actions carried out or omitted.
	• **Unexpected results** and events.
Discussion and conclusion	• Discussion of **observations** and **results**.
	• **Contribution** of the report to the fundamental knowledge of the problem represented by the reported case.
	• Proposals and **recommendations** for practice (clinical decisions) and research (new hypotheses generated by the case).
References	• Health problem and **disease** under study.
	• Clinical and paraclinical **actions**.
	• **Decisions** and actions under consideration.

*N.B. A summary of a clinical case report is not required by all medical journals

and care, advice given to the patient, and scheduling of further 'SOAP' encounters.

Considered too restrictive by some, a SOAP format is nonetheless useful as an organized source of information, necessary not only for the quality and completeness of clinical care but also for the administrative and legal aspects of a physician's practice. Ultimately, information from SOAP records is combined with admission and discharge records to constitute summary reports for other purposes, including clinical case reports in medical journals. Untidy and incomplete clinical charts are considered inadequate by governing medical bodies responsible for the quality of care. A **CCR for medical press** is more focused, less exhaustive, and oriented towards a specific problem. Table 7.2 illustrates the organization of a well-constructed CCR. A CCR written as an essay in the style of Michel Eyquem de Montaigne[35] is hard to follow. A structured CCR prevents that.

Desirable qualities of a CCR submitted for publication. An acceptable CCR should respond to criteria and expectations from medical journal editors[26,36]. Table 7.3 summarizes such requirements as formulated by the *Canadian Medical Association Journal*[27]. It provides the reader with a checklist of characteristics that make a CCR a good piece of evidence. Good CCRs are powerful evidence of what happened during a case. They are not representative of the disease or clinical actions beyond the case, and they do not bring any causal proof in etiology or treatment of the disease. They act as a stimulus for raising questions and for subsequent etiological and experimental research.

7.2.3 Evidence from multiple case observations. Case series and systematic reviews of cases

Even unusual and rare cases may reappear. For some, a case report is limited to one case only[37]. For others, two cases constitute a case report, and three[38] to

Table 7.3 *CMAJ* expectations with regards to case reports

Summary
- Does the summary give a succinct description of the case and its implications?

Introduction
- Is the case new or uncommon, with important public health implications?
- Is the rationale for reporting the case adequately explained?
- Has an adequate review of the literature been done?

Description of the case
- Is the case described briefly but comprehensively?
- Is the case described clearly?
- Are the results of investigations and treatments described adequately, including doses, schedule and duration of treatment?
- Are the results of less common laboratory investigations accompanied by normal values?

Comments
- Is the evidence to support the author's diagnosis presented?
- Are other plausible explanations considered and refuted?
- Are the implications and relevance of the case discussed?
- Is the evidence to support the author's recommendations presented adequately?
- Does the author indicate directions for further investigation or management of similar cases?

Source: Ref. 27. Reproduced with permission of the *Canadian Medical Association Journal*

ten[39] cases or more make up a **case series**. The study of more than one case has two main objectives:

- To determine prevailing characteristics of a given set of patients; and/or
- To determine the prevailing outcomes for these patients.

In occurrence (descriptive) studies in epidemiology as described in Section 7.3, numbers of cases are related as numerators to some larger numbers of individuals in the community of interest, yielding **rates** of disease. Case series studies are in some way 'studies of disease occurrence **without denominators**'. Such denominators in case series are most often unknown or extremely difficult to define. The presentation of a limited number of cases indicates that the first case is likely not unique, and that a more thorough descriptive study based on more complete numerators and denominators should be attempted. Such first cases brought to our attention can be considered as **index cases**, leading to more representative observations and their analysis. However, as in any other disease study, rules of clinimetrics apply fully to case series studies.

Case series studies may be classified from several points of view[30]:

According to the origin of cases

- Cases as observed by authors themselves;
- Cases assembled from several clinical sites;
- Cases assembled from the literature either in a somewhat random fashion, or systematically selected and uniformly described and analysed as a kind of 'meta-analysis of cases'.

According to the number of case examinations in time

- As a cross-sectional study yielding instant portraits of cases;
- As a longitudinal study of a single cohort (group of patients) only, yielding a better understanding of disease course and outcomes.

According to the number of case series involved

- As a single-set descriptive study;
- As a comparison of two or more sets in an analytical observational or quasi-experimental design focusing on treatment or other factors affecting these groups.

A combination of these three axes of classification may be found across the literature for each case series study. All such reports must conform to the general rules of any case-based paper[40,41]. The review of cases in the literature is an additional methodological challenge. It should be based on the **systematic review principles and methodology** as outlined later in this text. The review of the literature in a case series report can focus on pathology, management, or other topics, depending on the objectives, questions, and focus of the report.

7.2.3.1 *Cross-sectional or longitudinal portraits of cases*

When grouping several cases together, as in any other systematic review, information from the same categories (such as demographic characteristics, physical examination highlights, or laboratory test results) should be sought from one case to another and presented in the form of an **evidence table**, a technique well known in the field of meta-analysis and systematic reviews. This must be attempted when reviewing cases from one source, several sources, or from the literature in order to produce a **checklist of patient characteristics and findings**. In contrast to single case reports that are mainly inductive, case series reports are more often a form of deductive research. The enormous advantage offered by **case series from a single source** is the possibility of selecting and describing cases according to uniform clinimetric criteria of case detection, diagnosis, selection, measurement of selected variables, and final categorization and interpretation.

Longitudinal studies of case series as repeated examinations of case series in time focus most often on various disease outcomes. An outcome can be '. . . *all possible results that may stem from exposure to a causal factor, or from preventive and therapeutic interventions: all identified changes in health status arising as a consequence of the handling of a health problem . . .*'[42]: survival, longevity, cure, remission, pain resolution, normal organ function, return to normal values of biological variables, resumption of everyday activities, or social and professional re-integration of patients. Case series studies should not lack an *a priori* definition and justification of the choice of outcomes with regard to clinical decisions that have to be modified or made. Inherent characteristics of case series studies limit their conclusions. Nonetheless, since there are situations where case series can be carried out, they must be correctly prepared, executed and presented. Recommendations for case series reporting were formulated in the CMAJ[43]. Examples of good case series reports are primarily found in disciplines that depend more on this kind of reporting, such as psychiatry[44], occupational medicine[45], or clinical pharmacology[46].

7.2.3.2 *Systematic reviews and meta-analyses of cases*

Just as the results of original studies are heterogeneous, so are those of clinical case reports and case series reports. Can these results be integrated to obtain the most accurate picture of disease, especially when only isolated cases are available? The idea of systematic reviews of cases is relatively new, but it is a logical evolution of thinking in qualitative and quantitative research. Simultaneously but independently, conceptual proposals have appeared in the qualitative research[47–49] as well as in the first '*meta-analyses of case reports and case series reports*'[50–53]. Meta-analyses of cases are not explanatory. Only prevalent case characteristics and outcomes can be better assessed at this level of clinical research. Establishing prevalent characteristics, or average or typical values of observations in cases, is similar to other fields of meta-analysis and systematic reviews.

7.2.3.3 *Conclusions on case series reports*

Anyone who searches for evidence is not necessarily satisfied with conclusions drawn from single case and case series reports especially when treatment effectiveness is the topic of interest[54,55]. However, if no other, more adequate evidence is available, the best of this first line of evidence must be taken into account. Califf[56] states: '. . . *Case series without a control group will remain interesting because of the intrinsic importance of observation in medicine. . . . Although individual case reports should never be taken as definitive evidence that practice should be changed, the importance of astute, appropriate bedside observation cannot be underestimated.*' If an 'astute clinical observation' is at the root of clinical case reports, such astuteness should be a learned experience. Clinical case reporting is the clinician's most frequent exposure to medical research. The vast majority of clinicians will never carry out cohort or case control studies, or complex clinical trials. However, all of them should be proficient and astute clinical case reporters.

Case reports and case series reports may be the 'lowest' or the 'weakest' level of evidence of cause–effect relationship[54,57,58], but they often remain the '**first line of evidence**'. This is where everything else begins. Certainly, in case series without controls, '. . . *the reader is simply informed about the fate of a group of patients. Such series may contain extremely useful information about clinical course and prognosis but can only hint at efficacy.*'[54] Obviously, the 'information' and the 'hint' should be as accurate as possible as well. Many specialties such as psychiatry, clinical microbiology or surgery rely heavily on single case reporting or on case series follow-up. These reports remain prevalent in some of the literature of these specialties[59]. For example, case reports and case series reports were more prevalent in the core pediatric surgery literature in 1996–1997 than any other type of publication combined (reviews, laboratory studies, prospective studies, randomized controlled clinical trials). They are more than a part of medical culture: they are pieces of evidence to be used. Finally, clinical case reports may serve as a teaching tool to improve the quality of clinical data[60] or to illustrate desirable clinical knowledge, attitudes, skills and plans[61,62].

7.3 Picturing disease as an entity. Describing disease occurrence in the community. Descriptive or occurrence studies

Once a picture of disease cases has been obtained, it is necessary to know how such a disease appears in the community. Clinimetric studies show what coronary disease cases, measles cases or depression cases actually look like in patients. Community studies give a portrait or descriptive epidemiology of the disease. A portrait of disease must be addressed in terms of its spread. Community studies are important not only for field epidemiology and community medicine. Clinicians also need them, for two particular reasons:

- To improve diagnosis (looking back to Chapter 6 and the need to know the disease's prevalence to improve the predictive value of test results);
- To get ideas of new hypotheses about disease causes, possible success of treatment and other interventions, and prognosis.

A descriptive epidemiological study of disease is a study of disease occurrence as it appears in relation to different characteristics of time, place, and persons. Questions to be answered are: '**To whom, where and when did this happen?**' For example, one wishes to know where, in whom, and when obesity cases appear in the community. Or, it may be relevant to know the incidence of injury in the current year in agricultural workers, in relation to the region, the time of the year, age, sex, type of activity and other characteristics of farmers. The objective of descriptive studies is to obtain either an instant portrait of disease spread (cross sectional study, prevalence study), or an evolving portrait of disease in time (longitudinal study, incidence study).

Descriptive studies reveal disparities between disease occurrence according to time, place, and personal characteristics, thus producing hypotheses on possible causal relationships. However, the design (architecture) of these studies was not conceived to prove or disprove such *a posteriori*-obtained hypotheses. Indeed, one of the major objectives of descriptive studies is to generate hypotheses that should be better explored deductively by consecutive analytical studies, designed specifically to evaluate an *a priori*-proposed relationship between disease and its cause(s). For example, a descriptive study of the prevalence of depression shows that depression prevalence rates are higher in older subjects than in younger ones. A hypothesis may be formulated on the relationship between age and depression. It would be premature to state that age is a cause of depression. To make this statement, it would be necessary to have data on disease incidence and also on its relationships with other possible causal factors not included in the descriptive study, such as alcohol and drug abuse, stressful life events, various endogenous characteristics, etc. However, an intellectual basis is established from which to explore the relationships not only between age and depression, but also other possible risk factors that may be related to age.

7.3.1 Objectives of occurrence studies

Descriptive studies of disease have three major objectives:

1. To obtain a **portrait** of disease spread.

2. To formulate **hypotheses** on the cause of disparities of disease spread (*for a disease of unknown cause*).
3. To identify persons, time and places where the control of disease should be a **priority** (primary prevention in case of high incidence, secondary prevention in case of high prevalence and long duration of disease *for a disease of known etiology*).

7.3.2 Desirable attributes of occurrence studies

To attain such objectives, any descriptive study of disease must have several basic virtues. It must be:

- **Purposeful**, i.e. it should clearly indicate why it is done.
- **Useful**, i.e.
  - Relevant from the point of view of research and practice.
  - A priority in terms of explanation of disease causes and/or for disease intervention.
  - Beneficial for the patient and/or the community.
- **Comparable**, i.e.
  - Performed using reproducible methods,
  - In order to create possible links with other studies.
- **Representative**, i.e.
  - Of the disease under study (gradient, spectrum, course, etc.).
  - Of the framework of clinical activities implied by the disease (customary medical practices).
  - Of the population from which cases are derived (target population, population under study, population to which results of the descriptive study should apply).

Representativity should be enhanced:

- *From a qualitative point of view* by well-defined criteria and characteristics of disease, persons, time, and place; and
- *From a quantitative point of view* – enough subjects should be studied (sample size should be satisfactory from a statistical standpoint).

In practical terms, any descriptive study of disease should either generate a search for causes (etiological studies), or it should lead to well-oriented health interventions (programs) with a maximum relevance, priority of success in terms of prevention, control, or eradication of the disease under study in a population of interest.

7.3.3 How to understand an occurrence (descriptive) study, its structure and content

7.3.3.1 Structure

Any descriptive study in medicine, be it clinical or in community health, should follow a structured path and cover several elements, as summarized in Table 7.4. Some of these steps merit important observations.

How many subjects should be studied?

This is the most frequently asked question biostatisticians face regarding study design. Unless an exhaustive descriptive study is undertaken by examining all individuals concerned, in most situations for the sake of feasibility, a representative sample of subjects is selected. Any study based on reduced numbers of individuals remains an exercise in probability and a well-educated estimate. Such an estimate must be as accurate as possible. Studying too many individuals would be time-consuming and costly, but there must be sufficient numbers to obtain acceptable results. The statistical power of a study increases with the sample size (i.e. number of subjects examined), but between the two extremes an old statistical saying sums up the problem: '. . . with few subjects, you will demonstrate nothing, with very large numbers of individuals, you can demonstrate anything . . .'.

To determine the number of individuals to enrol in a study, physicians must provide biostatisticians with the best estimation of information (data) expected from the study, as well as their requirements, how rigorous the estimations of the reality (true values) should be on the basis of the study results. What is the most realistic estimation of disease incidence or prevalence rate? To what degree of certainty is it necessary to know that the study has estimated what it was supposed to (90%, 95%, or 99%?)? How close is it necessary to be to the disease occurrence (for example, a prevalence rate of obesity, incidence rate of influenza, etc.)? Specialized statistical

Table 7.4 General phases of a descriptive study of disease in the community

I   ***Acquisition of knowledge about the disease and the community to be described***

II   ***Definition of the study objectives (purpose)***
- Identification of high occurrence
- Generation of hypotheses
- Identification in whom, where, and when to set a priority for intervention (health program)

III   ***Definition of the health problem under study (disease – diagnostic criteria)***

IV   ***Identification of the study's design (cross-sectional? longitudinal?)***

V   ***Identification of the target population and of the population to be studied***

VI   ***Identification of the number of subjects to be studied (sample size)***

VII   ***Definition of the variables under study***
- Operational definitions
- Characteristics of variables (qualitative, quantitative)
- Scales and categories

VIII   ***Health indicators and clinical picture to be obtained (numerators and denominators)***
- Morbidity
- Mortality
- Case fatality
- Duration of cases
- Clinical gradient and spectrum of cases
- Comparative data, rates, and ratios
- Descriptive parameters of quantitative variables and outliers

IX   ***Identification of sources of data***
- Already available
- To be collected

X   ***Formulation of a picture of the disease***

XI   ***Verification that the study did not deviate from its previously fixed objectives (did we get what we wanted?) and that the target population was not missed (due to non-representative results)***

XII   ***Comparison of results with the characteristics of disease and disease indexes and indicators that are already known***

XIII   ***Conclusions: The problem under study is sporadic, epidemic, pandemic, or endemic***

XIV   ***Formulation of hypotheses for further studies***

XV   ***Recommendations for action (health programs) if necessary***

literature beyond the scope of this writing is devoted to basic statistical knowledge in medicine, to sampling and other fundamentals. However, any statistical sampling methodology, as elaborate as it may be, must be fueled by clinically relevant information, which health professionals provide to their partners in biostatistics.

Definition of variables under study

These definitions should not only be **conceptual** ('what') but also **operational**, ('how much, and how it will be obtained through measurement'). Looking back to Chapter 4, a good operational definition of a case states: 'That's what I will find and how I will find it (which method and technique will be used)'.

Inclusion criteria will say clearly 'who or what is in' and exclusion criteria will specify 'who or what is out'. The conceptual definition says only 'what is behind all this'. A **conceptual definition** of hypertension in pregnancy may be 'an unusually high blood pressure related to some poor prognosis and requiring proper control'. An **operational definition** would be 'a diastolic blood pressure equal to or more than 110 mmHg on any one occasion, or a diastolic pressure equal to or more than 90 mmHg on two or more consecutive occasions four hours or more apart'[63].

Equal attention must be paid to **dependent variables** (usually diseases under study) and **independent variables** (usually characteristics of persons, time, and place). Both groups must be equally well defined, studied, measured, described and classified. A multidisciplinary approach is often necessary. Physicians tend to pay excessive or even exclusive attention to disease, whereas environmentalists will describe pollutants very well, but describe ensuing morbidity or mortality less well in clinimetrically acceptable terms. Most releases from the US National Health Survey are good examples of careful and pragmatic definitions of all variables under study. For example, while studying injury, definitions of injuries are given with definitions of all relevant circumstances and possible causes, as well as risk characteristics under study[64]. All issues contain annexes giving operational criteria of variables under study. Wherever quantitative variables are described, their characteristics are routinely given in terms of different **descriptive parameters,** such as mean values, standard deviations, quantiles (percentiles, deciles, etc.), ranges, etc.

Outliers

Besides this vital information, attention should also be paid to the identification and interpretation of observations beyond the customary range of the current study. Such observations are called '**outliers**' in statistical–epidemiological language. They are defined as[65] '. . . *Observations differing so widely from the rest of the data as to lead one to suspect that a gross error may have been committed, or suggesting that these values come from a different population . . .*'.

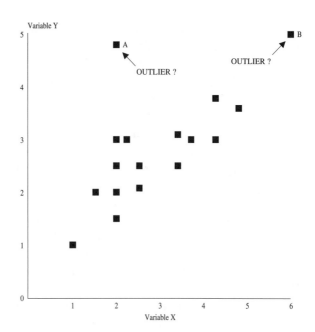

Figure 7.4 Outliers

Statistical methods to identify outliers are available[65]. Once outliers are identified (in the simplest situation, outside intervals plus or minus two or three standard deviations from the mean in the case of quantitative data, or cases located outside a given time or place), their position may signal errors in measurement, in recording of data (a schoolboy measuring 14.5 m is probably not acromegalic; rather, his height of 145 cm was not properly recorded), or individuals 'belonging to other populations' (highly abnormal or sick individuals). The question of an outlier is not only a statistical one. It depends primarily on the definition of the problem under study. Figure 7.4 illustrates a set of individual data; variables X and Y were measured in each individual. If the problem under study were a correlation between variables X and Y, individual A would obviously be an outlier. If the problem under study were the same correlation, where values of X between 1 and 5 only would be considered normal, individuals A and B would be outliers. If the objective of the study is to know how individual data of Y are distributed at the X level of 2, only the four individual values of X = 2 (including individual A) would not be outliers, but all others would.

Both the evaluation of typical values of descriptive parameters and their spread, and the assessment and interpretation of outliers, should be planned and carried out in every descriptive study. Moreover, a discovery of interesting outliers often leads to stimulating hypotheses for further study of abnormal findings, their occurrence, and causes. Also, it is desirable to look at 'outlying' studies in research synthesis, meta-analysis, systematic reviews (see Chapter 11) or while assessing participating centers in multi-center clinical trials (see Chapter 9). Such studies may signal not only possible errors, different methodology or target populations, but they may also signal innovative findings due to some factors which must be further elucidated by an in-depth study of local conditions (different patients, routines, care, conditions, etc.) that lead to 'outlying' or 'out of the crowd' results. As in daily life when eccentrics are often more interesting than 'ordinary' people. What is habitual may be essential but mundane. Unusual findings like 'outliers' are often stimulating, exciting, and thought-provoking.

7.3.3.2 Persons, time and place in occurrence studies. Establishing the portrait of disease spread

Identification of individual characteristics (persons)
If an unusual occurrence of disease is found in subjects having particular demographic or other characteristics, a hypothetical interpretation or hypothesis formulation remains the greatest challenge. For example, if a high incidence of trauma is found in adolescents, it may be due to several factors related to age: biological characteristics of adolescence (incoordination due to variable chronology and rate of body systems maturation), psychological characteristics (search for challenges, lack of experience, underestimation of risks, etc.), social characteristics (acquisition of new skills), etc. The same applies to differences between men and women. Biological factors, social roles, and preferential occupations play a part in the differential morbidity and mortality between genders. **Race** (hereditary, anthropometric characteristics) and **ethnicity** (acquired characteristics such as language, religion, or dietary habits), are often needlessly confounded. Epidemiological

analysis is more difficult wherever acquired characteristics are strongly bound to race or racial subgroups (such as Buddhism or Islam), adhering to particular faiths, with ensuing acquired habits and behaviors. Current epidemiological attention expands beyond individual demographical characteristics. Family endogenous characteristics, lifetime events, or daily life behaviors complete the epidemiological portrait of disease occurrence (Table 7.4).

Characteristics of time
As **chronobiology** has an important place in the study of biological functions, chrono-epidemiology studies the periodical variability of health phenomena in the community. Circadian, weekly, and seasonal periodicity of injury incidence, or seasonal variability of respiratory infections or incidence of affective disorders are just a few examples. Calendar time is most often used, such as in yearly studies of mortality (from January 1 to December 31 of a calendar year). **Chronological time** may be used, if disease occurrence between ages (e.g. from 10 to 19 years) is being studied, without consideration as to whether these ages were reached at a given calendar year. **Biological time** is given by time spans of biological events, which may vary. Health problems of women may be studied in relation to their menstrual cycles of variable duration, independently of calendar and chronological time. Similarly, **social time** may be given by the time span of various occupational, or social roles (climbing the career ladder), whose duration may vary from one individual to another. **Epidemiological time** (usually **epidemiological year**) is a period of more or less one year's duration during a periodical variation of disease occurrence, limited by moments of its lowest incidence in time. For example, the beginning of an epidemiological year of scarlet fever or diphtheria would not be January 1st, but a time in summer when the incidence rate is the lowest, and ending also at that time. Figure 7.5 illustrates an epidemiological year of varicella according to the same logic. In this example, calendar and epidemiological years do not coincide.

Arraiz et al[67] recently reported concurrent trends of incidence of corpus uteri cancer and purchases of sex hormone replacement therapy in Canada. Such a **study of concurrent time trends** may lead to

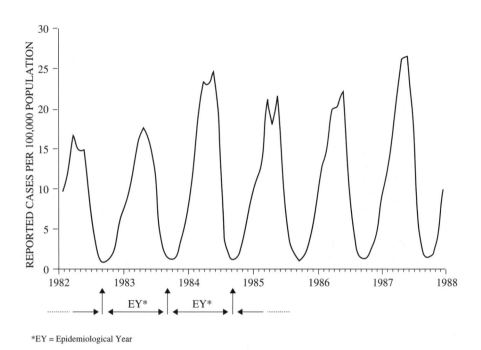

Figure 7.5 Epidemiological and calendar years of varicella, United States, 1982–1987. Source: Ref. 66 (Public domain), redrawn with modifications and reproduced after notification

hypothesizing on the causal relationship between estrogen and uterine cancer. It is not proof since it is not known which women took replacement therapy and which ones developed uterine cancer, and information is also lacking about non-users of hormonal therapy. In addition, one might speculate that a concurrent trend reflects a high carcinogenicity leading to a very short incubation or induction period of corpus uteri cancer. Studies of changes of disease occurrence over a long period of time, usually from one decade to another or from one generation to another, give a picture of a **secular or temporal trend of disease.** Secular trends are used for getting an estimate, usually from routine health statistics and data, about the possible impact of preventive or therapeutic measures (such as licensing and use of vaccines), or any other interaction between factors facilitating or blocking disease spread (Figure 7.6).

Place

Disease occurrence from one place to another may be studied by comparing city with country, different latitudes, altitudes, continents, and any other topographic characteristics. Geographical methods in the study of disease occurrence can lead to further studies of disease causes, related to particular place characteristics. For example, disease geography[69] may suggest an association between the population density in the eastern and western US states and the high mortality rates by cardiovascular disease in many of these areas. Further hypotheses should be generated, studied, and their validity demonstrated, to search for more direct causes of fatal cardiovascular problems (age of subjects, hypertension morbidity, dietary habits, other possible factors), possibly having a similar geographic distribution. This example also illustrates the limitation of this kind of association between places and disease occurrence. A simple geography of disease cannot itself explain disease causes.

When natural nidation of disease is understood and its natural foci defined, these foci (biotopes) can be studied wherever they are located, independent of continent or latitude. Such a topography of disease by ecosystems and biotopes is superior to a simple cartography of disease. In interpreting studies dealing with the geography of disease, errors known as ecological fallacy must be carefully avoided.

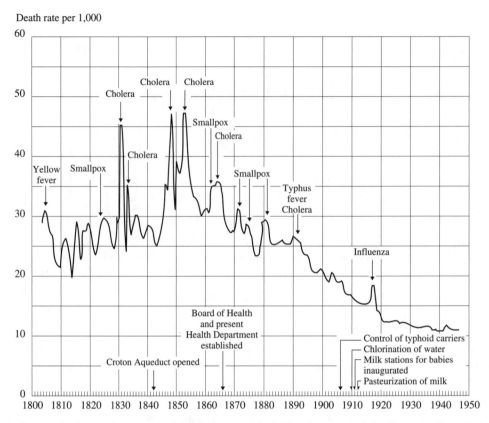

Figure 7.6 Secular trend of mortality rates. A historical example of 'The Conquest of Pestilence in New York City'. Source: Modified from Ref. 68

Ecological fallacy

Many observational studies combine data from different regions, groups, or instances where different conditions prevail. A comparison of such studies may lead to the conclusion that differences in disease occurrence are related to local exposure to a given factor. For example, indicators of perinatal and maternal health may be different in two areas. In one area, a special perinatal health care program exists; in the other, only routine primary care is offered to mother and child. In the first area, health indicators may be better than in the second. Is the special program more effective? If this question is re-evaluated by comparing **subjects rather than areas** (i.e. those who receive special attention vs. those under routine care), results might be different. Spurious interpretations can be produced if an individual experience is presumed on the basis of what was seen as a prevalent characteristic (experience) in

an area and its population as a whole. The process is called **ecological fallacy**[70,71]. Two definitions, one more statistical, the other more epidemiological, are currently given for this term[42]:

'1. *The bias that may occur because an association observed between variables on an aggregate level does not necessarily represent the association that exists at an individual level.*

2. *An error in inference due to failure to distinguish between different levels of organization. A correlation between variables based on group (ecological) characteristics is not necessarily reproduced between variables based on individual characteristics; an association at one level may disappear at another, or even be reversed.*'

For example, Martyn et al[72] recently found a geographical relation between Alzheimer's disease and aluminum in drinking water. It would be erroneous to infer from this finding alone that exposure to water with a given content of aluminum necessarily influences an individual's chances of getting Alzheimer's disease.

7.3.3.3   *Drawing conclusions*

Impressions derived from descriptive studies may yield hypotheses about possible causal relationships, but never firm proof. At present, the literature is flooded with assumptions based on simple observations of prevalent conditions in different groups of people and different health statistics in their areas of living. For example, an indirect correlation between alcohol consumption in different countries and mortality by atherosclerotic heart disease can be found: Higher consumption/lower mortality in Spain or Portugal, lower consumption/higher mortality in Canada or United States. Such assumptions (that alcohol protects against cardiovascular mortality) would certainly be revised if drinkers were to be compared to non-drinkers. Unfortunately, ecological fallacy-ridden assumptions are attractive for the popular press since they can impress the public and, at times, unwary health professionals as well. Better analytical studies as described in the next chapter usually clear up these problems.

Were study objectives reached? Representativity of results

A study may deviate from its objectives when selected individuals do not participate. **Non-participants** may in fact render the study non-representative from the point of view of individual characteristics, occurrence of disease, spectrum and gradient of disease, etc. At times, some individuals participate but do not give all the necessary information; these '**non-responses**' may further aggravate the non-representativity of the study. Because the main purpose of any descriptive study is to describe what it is supposed to describe, additional means should be taken to achieve this objective. Non-participants can be reached using a variety of methods, characteristics of non-participants can be compared to those of participants (if they are comparable, there may be fewer errors), and the study can be restricted (some individuals rejected) in such a way that it becomes a

representative study of a particular problem rather than a non-representative whole.

Identification of the magnitude of the problem

Besides establishing the mosaic of disease occurrence, the study 'describer' must determine if the problem under scrutiny is (according to considerations already given in Chapter 3) either:

- **Sporadic** (no relation between cases);
- **Epidemic**;
- **Pandemic**; or
- **Endemic**.

If the nature of the problem is undetermined, this should also be stated. Such information is necessary for the implementation of proper control measures for each of the four kinds of disease spread.

Formulation of hypotheses

If a described problem and its causes are unknown locally or in general, a simple description of facts is not enough. Hypotheses on this matter must be proposed. **In epidemiology, a hypothesis is a proposed explanation of epidemiological phenomena, provisionally accepted, until submitted for re-evaluation by an appropriate analytical study; such a proposition is then accepted or rejected by the study in question.** For example, an increase in the mortality rate of lung cancer with age is observed in men. It may be hypothesized that this mortality is related to some factor associated with age, such as duration of smoking, exposure to occupational factors in the workplace, biological susceptibility to neoplasia from one age to another, etc. Further analytical studies comparing smokers and non-smokers, exposure studies of cases in comparison to non-cases of lung cancer, or cessation studies (quitting smoking effect) will better clarify this original hypothesis (see Chapter 8).

Besides the picture of disease occurrence, reasonably formulated hypotheses are the most valuable acquisition of descriptive studies (providing that they are not exaggerated). Figure 7.7 gives two views on leukemia occurrence in Canada[74]. The left side of the figure shows percent of all cancer deaths represented by leukemia (proportional rates of leukemia mortality) and the right side shows true mortality and incidence rates of leukemia in Canadian men. First, when looking at proportional rates (leukemia is a major cause of death in children), it might be falsely hypothesized that leukemia is a disease of young individuals. However, when true mortality rates are studied, it can be observed that the risk of death increases with age, with a small peak during the first years of life. From the relationship between mortality and incidence rates (see section 3), it can be concluded that leukemia is actually more fatal in older individuals than in children. From this downward, convex, two-peak curve, even further hypotheses can be drawn:

1. The same disease may appear following two different exposures to the same etiological factor, one during childhood and the other at an advanced age;
2. Continuous exposure to one etiological factor may result in the same disease appearing during two periods of vulnerability (susceptibility), one at an early age and another at an advanced age (two identical biological responses);
3. The same situation as above (2) may prevail, but both biological responses facilitating the develop-

ment of disease are different (for example, some concurrent disease in childhood, aging of immunity mechanisms at an advanced age);
4. The same disease may be triggered by two different etiological factors, biological responses being identical;
5. The same as above (4), but with different biological responses;
6. Two different diseases (still to be differentiated from one another) as in situation 1 may be triggered by the same etiological factor;
7. There may be two different diseases in situation 2;
8. There may be two different diseases in situation 3;
9. There may be two different diseases in situation 4; and
10. There may be two different diseases in situation 5.

Obviously, such hypothesizing is highly speculative, but it shows limitations in the interpretation of descriptive studies as well as how innovative the generation of hypotheses must be, and how much more etiological research is needed by building specific analytical studies 'tailored to a given hypothesis' to confirm or disprove etiological proposals generated by descriptive studies at their origin. Other

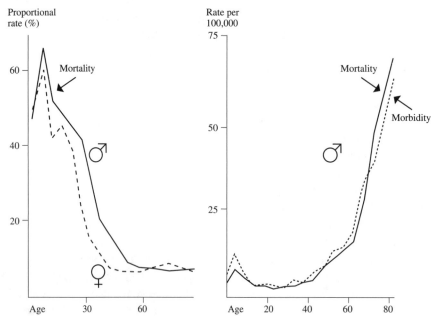

Figure 7.7 Leukemia rates in Canada, 1970–1972. Source: Ref. 74, reproduced with permission of Health Canada (Minister of Public Works and Government Services)

examples of hypotheses formulation in cancer epidemiology can be found in Higginson and Muir's chapter *ad hoc*[75].

Descriptive data cannot provide answers to these possible explanations. It might be clear that for each of the above-mentioned hypotheses, different analytical studies should be conceived (different designs, study of factors, different individuals, etc.). However, these descriptive data assist in the direction of further studies that would fully explain disease etiology.

7.3.4 Special kinds of occurrence (descriptive) studies

Four special types of occurrence studies are of interest, given their different specific objectives and ensuing methodologies: epidemiological surveillance; disease clustering; medical record linkage; and cohort analysis vs. analysis by cohort.

7.3.4.1 Epidemiological surveillance

Disease occurrence in time and space (people and places) is a product of the equilibrium between various factors facilitating or blocking its spread. Among others, such factors are:

- Evolving personal characteristics;
- Modifications of different components of the biotope (natural environment of disease);
- Interventions by people on the disease eco-system; or
- Infectious agents' properties.

Studies of these factors evolved from epidemics to what is now called **epidemiological surveillance**[76]. Langmuir[77] and Raska[78] coined the term in the sixties to identify a continuous study of disease in time, **independent of any immediate importance of disease occurrence**. This allowed for the forecasting of outbreaks, epidemics or pandemics and the establishment of appropriate and timely measures to prevent such events. From the surveillance of disease cases or deaths, the concept evolved into the surveillance of all relevant components of natural foci of disease, characteristics of agents (antigenic shifts, etc.), vehicles, vectors (arthropod or insect populations), reservoirs (multiplication of wild canine species in rabies), and preventive measures

(vaccine and immunization programs coverage and effectiveness), etc.

The concept applies to infectious and non-infectious diseases as well. For example, in the province of Québec (Canada), notifiable diseases (for declaration and surveillance) include not only certain infections but also acute intoxications or poisonings as well. In many countries, various national registries (e.g. cancer registries) serve a similar purpose of disease surveillance[79–81]. Injury surveillance illustrates the concept of surveillance as it applies to all major components of disease (sufficient causes or biotope). These were recently given by Foege[82]: Time, place, persons characteristics, type of injury, causes (vehicles, vectors), circumstances, medical care, outcomes of health. Local, national, and international levels of surveillance and their results are periodically reported in various World Health Organization periodicals (*World Health Statistics Quarterly*, etc.). At the national level, for example, the *Canada Communicable Disease Report* and the *Morbidity and Mortality Weekly Report (MWWR)* in the United States provide similar information together with outbreak investigations and other topics of interest.

Once again, the main purpose of disease surveillance is prediction or forecasting. Hypotheses on possible causes of disease occurrence represent only a byproduct (however important) of this activity. An example of such data is that of influenza surveillance in Canada[83]. On the basis of this activity, a 'habitual' occurrence and its seasonal periodicity may be established allowing for a better grasp of the situation if a given level of occurrence has or has not reached an epidemic level (see Figure 5.4). Other fields of application of surveillance methodology are as diverse as environmental factors[84], medical technologies[85], adverse drug reactions and other effects of treatment through pharmacoepidemiology[86,87], community follow-ups for genetic traits and congenital malformations, serological surveillance of prevailing strains of infectious agents such as the influenza virus, or others allowing for a timely and best possible (strain-specific) immunizing agents or other preventive measures.

Independent of the field of application of epidemiological surveillance, surveillance will remain in public health as an ongoing systematic collection, analysis, and interpretation of health data needed to plan, implement, and evaluate public health programs[88]. Surveillance of disease occurrence must serve some concrete purpose, if only a better orientation of further research. Epidemiological surveillance may be either passive or active: In **passive surveillance**, routine data such as hospital and other health service records or national demographic data are periodically explored. Observations and recommendations follow. In **active surveillance**, all information is gathered by a special *ad hoc* program, targeting data that are not available from current routine sources. Its objectives are set first and the surveillance program follows. For example, life expectancy is a subject of passive surveillance. Prevailing serotypes of influenza virus or herd immunity in school children against childhood infections are the subject of active surveillance. Several phenomena may currently be the subject of surveillance:

Cases of infectious disease;

- Vehicles, vectors, and reservoirs (natural foci of infection);
- Vaccine coverage (herd immunity by immunization);
- Immuno-biological state of individuals (serological surveillance);
- Marketing and use of physical and chemical agents (radiation sources in medicine and industry, pesticides in agriculture, polychlorinated biphenyls in communities);
- New technologies;
- Biological markers (cf. Chapter 8);
- Congenital malformations;
- Cancers;
- Injuries;
- Professional acts (state health systems and insurance companies);
- Any specific health problem of interest, such as modern threats (AIDS).

More information about contemporary concepts, techniques, and applications may be found in an *ad hoc* collection edited by Eylenbosch and Noah[89].

The major practical purposes of surveillance remain to:

1. Give estimates of disease occurrence;
2. Detect disease clusters (*vide infra*);
3. Direct better etiological research;
4. Direct better implementation of prevention programs at all levels; and
5. Allow the effectiveness of health interventions and programs to be evaluated.

Surveillance software[90] is now available to ease the handling of data. For the near future, Choi[91] recommends three classes of indicators: health outcomes; risk factors; intervention strategies. Surveillance data should also serve to evaluate measures taken on the basis of the surveillance information. The system must be systematic (evidence-based selection of indicators, not necessarily hypothesis-driven), ongoing, and population-based[91].

7.3.4.2 Disease clustering

Epidemiological surveillance or routine follow-up of health and disease may reveal an 'unusual aggregation, real or perceived, of health events, that are grouped together in time and space and that are reported to a health agency'[92]. Cases of disease may occur in close proximity either in time, in space, or both in time and space. Disease cases appearing close in time and space have been named '**clusters**'. If disease appears in such a way, its transmissibility and/or its relation to some etiological factors, appearing at a given place and at a given time, may be further studied. Knox' study of childhood leukemia[93] is one of the first historical examples. According to a given interval and distance between cases (all combinations are considered), contingency tables may be built giving frequencies of cases not associated, associated in time, associated in place, and associated both in time and place. If an aggregation in the time and space category is due to non-random events compared to other categories, a disease clustering may be considered. A statistical methodology[94] of aggregation in time, in place, and in both was reviewed recently by Armitage and Berry[95] and by other authors in several issues of specialized periodicals[96–98].

To state that a cholera epidemic exists does not usually require special quantitative techniques. If rare diseases such as tumors are involved, more sophisticated statistical techniques are required. If a 'new' disease appears, a study of its clusters may lead to etiological breakthroughs, such as the elucidation of angiosarcoma in workers exposed to vinyl chloride monomers, or of phocomelia after thalidomide exposure[92]. Once clusters are discovered, further etiological research follows based on methodology, as described in the next chapter. A study of disease clusters is subjected to rigorous methodology, as is any study of disease outbreaks. It relies on important clinical considerations such as the operational definition of cases (a cluster must be an aggregation of one disease and not of a mix of poorly defined, obscure cases of many different diseases). Statistical methodology, as diversified as it is today, goes beyond the scope of this reading and can be reviewed elsewhere (see Appendix to reference[92]).

In addition to the above-mentioned considerations, any descriptive study must yield either a representative sample of cases or as many cases as possible, if not all existing cases. It is often impossible to do this for economical and practical reasons. Providing that different sources of data (routine clinical records, various registries, national statistics, etc.) are of good quality from the point of view of comparability, representativeness, clinimetric acceptability, and subjects of interest, these data may be brought together for further in-depth study.

7.3.4.3 *Medical record linkage*
Medical record linkage does exactly what its name suggests. This term was coined by Dunn[99]: '. . . *Each person in the world creates a book of life. This book starts with birth and ends with death. Its pages are made of the records of the principal events in life. Record linkage is the name given to the process of assembling the pages of this book into a volume'.* The concept was further developed in terms of methodology and application by Acheson et al in Great Britain[100–102], Newcombe in Canada[103–105], and by others[101,106]. In contemporary terms, it is defined as: '. . . *A method for assembling the information contained in two or* more *records, e.g. in different sets of medical charts, and in vital records such as birth and death certificates, and a procedure to ensure that the same individual is counted only once. This procedure incorporates a unique identifying*

system such as a personal identification number and/or birth name(s) of the individual's mother. . . . Record linkage makes it possible to relate significant health events that are remote from one another in time and place or to bring together records of different individuals, e.g., members of a family. The resulting information is generally stored and retrieved by computer, which can be programmed to tabulate and analyze the data'[2].

Record linkage may serve to gather data from different sources about the same individual (e.g. family members' health data can be linked, occupational groups can be studied, etc). In etiological research, exposure of subjects to noxious factors cannot often be measured directly. It must be found in other sources, for example, company records in occupational epidemiology. The crucial problem of record linkage is not its technical feasibility from the point of view of informatics, but a comparable quality of different sources of data from which record linkage is meant to occur. Cases of cancer, coronary heart disease, injury, or depression may not always be defined according to comparable diagnostic criteria; they may be recorded, coded, and classified in different ways. If so, record linkage merits attention in disease study, provided that its often elevated cost is affordable.

Record linkage is therefore a technique for bringing together data from different data banks, files, or archives to answer a specific question. However, original sources of data have not been assembled to answer a specific question that a practitioner of record linkage might have in mind. For example, a particular relationship between mental disorders and drug abuse may be of interest. To study this relationship, related data may be found in hospital records, police records, occupational files, etc. These sources were not created to specifically study this problem. Interpretation of findings from studies based on record linkage must be done, keeping in mind the limitations of 'general purpose' data banks.

7.3.4.4 *Cohort analysis or analysis by cohort*
Cross-sectional studies often yield limited information about factors that might be related to disease occurrence. For example, a higher incidence or

mortality rate at age 60 compared to ages 40 or 50 may reflect the effect of age, of cohorts (groups of people aged 40, 50, and 60 are different individuals, exposed to different factors throughout their lives), or of both. Some instances occur when all individuals are exposed to particular events, such as the nuclear explosions in Hiroshima or Nagasaki, or disastrous failures of nuclear facilities, such as at Chernobyl in the Ukraine. The simplest, mostly visual method, the 'eye test' in epidemiological language, may be of interest for a reader to detect the effect of cohorts or of time.

But what is a cohort in epidemiology? In fact, it is a group of individuals with some defined characteristics, entering observation at the same moment and followed-up over time. By comparing several cohorts, the role of noxious or beneficial factors in disease occurrence or clinical course can be detected. Medical literature also uses two cohort-related terms. In etiological research (see Chapter 8), a 'real' **cohort study** refers to the comparison of two or more cohorts appearing most often at the same time. For example, one can consider the study of cancer or chronic obstructive lung disease in men born in 1930 by splitting the men into two cohorts, one represented by smokers and the other one by non-smokers. Some prior hypothesis about the etiology of disease can be verified using this kind of comparison.

In an **analysis by cohorts**, which is more like an extension of descriptive or occurrence studies as described in this chapter, changes over time from one cohort to a subsequent one are studied. For example, an analysis by cohort would focus on how disease occurrence changes between individuals (cohorts) born in 1930, and those born in 1940, 1950 and so on. One may only speculate or formulate hypotheses about what changes in which possible causal factors over time might be responsible for changes in health from one group of individuals to another. Using Table 7.5 as a fictitious example, from one decade to another, mortality rates for some disease increase in individuals of all ages. Is this due to biological, social, or occupational factors, or to some other unknown factors to which individuals are exposed from one age to another (throughout their occupational or social careers, residence mobility, etc.), or is it due to age-related factors such as biological changes coming

Table 7.5 Mortality rate per 100,000 for a fictitious disease according to different age groups in cross-sectional routine health statistics

Calendar year Age	1960	1970	1980	1990
0–10 years	**132**	128	122	115
20–39 years	145	**132**	128	122
40–59 years	182	145	**132**	128
60–70 years	195	182	145	**132**

with age, etc.? To better understand this example, data in different cohorts[107–109] may be compared, i.e. people reaching a given age in a given year (reading data diagonally from upper left to lower right). Data inside cohorts (diagonal readings) remain the same from one decade to another throughout the aging of the same cohort. All cohorts begin and progress at different levels. Thus, differences from one decade to another (horizontal reading of the table) are due to a cohort effect, i.e. different cohorts are exposed to different factors, but the effect of age does not appear (diagonal reading).

Figure 7.8 illustrates the evolution of cancer mortality rates in Canada during recent decades[110]. The left portion of the figure shows that at all ages illustrated, mortality by lung cancer increases from one decade to another. The right portion of the figure shows that mortality rates from one age to another in each cohort (subjects born in 1879, 1889, 1899, etc.) are higher at comparable ages from one cohort level to another. Such a notable cohort effect corroborates with increased tobacco smoking during the last century and a half. The left portion of the figure shows that these trends are higher from one age to another. The same data presented by cohorts, the right portion of the figure, shows very similar trends, as do data from one birth cohort to another. Breast cancer mortality rate differences from one age to another in women are due to biological and other possible factors related to age, while different life conditions of different birth cohorts have only a minor impact compared to age-related factors.

In summary, if disease occurrence varies from one cohort to another at comparable age (and other

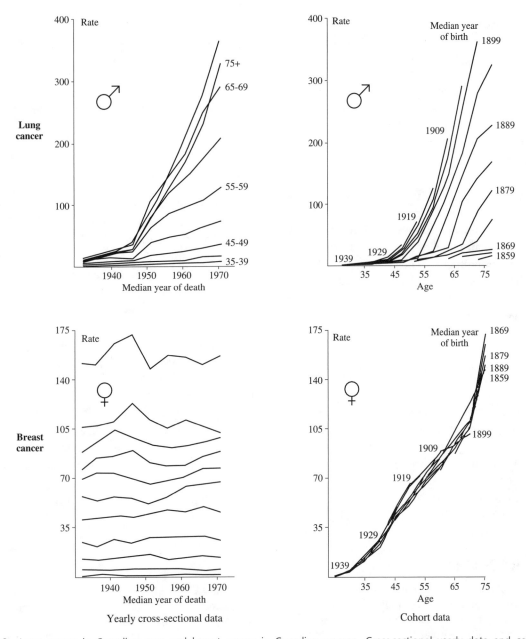

Figure 7.8 Lung cancer in Canadian men and breast cancer in Canadian women. Cross-sectional yearly data and cohort data, age-specific mortality rates per 100,000. Source: Ref. 74, reproduced with permission from the Minister of Public Works and Government Services (Health Canada)

characteristics) levels, it is due to a **cohort effect**, such as in lung cancer in men. If disease occurrence differs from one age to another, independent of instances identifying cohorts, age differences in disease occurrence are due mainly to the **age effect**, such as in breast cancer occurrence in women. If disease occurrence varies in relation to a calendar time, but independent of the age of subjects or any other criteria identifying cohorts, it is due to a **period effect**, such as in cancer occurrence after the Hiroshima bombing or after the Chernobyl nuclear disaster.

Cohort analysis may be used in the study of infectious diseases as well, such as in Fraser's tetanus analysis[111]. **Cohort analysis or analysis by cohorts** in this historical meaning must be differentiated from **cohort studies** in epidemiological research for causes. Cohort studies will be examined in more detail in Chapter 8. Statistical methodology[112] and additional comments on its applications (e.g. cancer[113]) may be found elsewhere.

7.4 Conclusions

Descriptive studies are fundamental to the understanding of what happens in an individual or in groups of individuals. Their representativeness, comparability, usefulness, and purposefulness are necessary attributes and criteria of their acceptability. Unfortunately, these criteria are not always respected. Five significant errors can still be found in many studies:

1. Cases are poorly described and defined from the clinimetric point of view;
2. The methodology of descriptive studies is poorly described, incomplete, or not explained at all;
3. Information on the quality control of data collection, measurement, recording and classification is incomplete or missing;
4. Descriptive studies are converted *a posteriori* into analytic ones, i.e. through inductive analyses, the authors try to explain causal relationships on the basis of the material (study) that was not designed to do this. Results and conclusions are exaggerated;
5. Descriptive studies are often 'dehumanized' by omitting clinically important soft data.

Many researchers and practitioners do not like descriptive studies[114] very much because 'they prove nothing'. While this is true, these studies were not conceived as a proof of some cause–effect relationship. Readers often erroneously search for them at any price! Descriptive studies are conceived to allow us to understand better the disease and its course, anticipate future disease trends and outcomes and, last but not least, generate hypotheses to be tested by other types of subsequent studies. No causal research is possible without the best possible description of observations. However, descriptive studies designed for reasons other than a causal search help only to identify characteristics of persons, time, and place, associated with a higher occurrence of disease (prevalence, incidence rates, etc.). Etiological studies (Chapter 6) and clinical trials (Chapter 7) are then necessary to elucidate which of these characteristics are risk or prognostic factors (which may be modified, consequently affecting the disease as well) and which are risk or prognostic markers (which cannot be modified). The next three chapters are devoted to these topics.

REFERENCES

1. *Webster's New Twentieth Century Dictionary of the English Language.* Unabridged. 2nd Edition. Cleveland: William Collins Publishers, 1979
2. O'Connor PJ. Normative data: Their definition, interpretation, and importance for primary care physicians. *Fam Med*, 1990;22:307–11
3. Monath TP (ed.). The Arboviruses: *Epidemiology and Ecology*. Boca Raton: CRC Press, 1988
4. Armenian KH, Lilienfeld AB. The distribution of incubation periods of neoplastic diseases. *Am J Epidemiol*, 1974;99:92–100
5. Armenian KH, Incubation periods of cancer: Old an new. *J Chron Dis*, 1987;40:(Suppl. 2 – Time Related Factors in Cancer Epidemiology):9S–15S
6. Rothman KJ. *Modern Epidemiology*. Boston: Little, Brown and Co., 1986
7. Brookmeyer R. Statistical problems in epidemiologic studies of the natural history of disease. *Environ Health Persp*, 1990;87:43–9
8. Cooper DA, Gold J, Maclean P. Acute AIDS retrovirus infection. Definition of a clinical illness associated with seroconversion. *Lancet*, 1985;1:537–40
9. Clark SJ, Saag MS, Decker WD, et al. High titers of cytopathic virus in plasma of patients with symptomatic primary HIV-1 infection. *N Engl J Med*, 1991;324:954–60
10. Daar ES, Moudgil T, Meyer RD, Ho DD. Transient high levels of viremia in patients with primary human immunodeficiency virus type 1 infection. *N Engl J Med*, 1991;324:961–4
11. Speissl B, Scheibe O, Wagner G (eds). TNM Atlas. Illustrated Guide to the Classification of Malignant Tumours. Berlin: Springer-Verlag, 1982

12. Beahrs OH, Myers MH, American Joint Committee on Cancer. *Manual for Staging of Cancer.* 2nd Edition. Philadelphia: JB Lippincott Co., 1983

13. Charlson ME, Feinstein AR. The auxometric dimension. A new method for using rate of growth in prognostic staging of breast cancer. *JAMA,* 1974;**228**: 180–5

14. Gabriel SE, Crowson CS, O'Fallon WM. A comparison of two comorbidity instruments in arthritis. *J Clin Epidemiol,* 2001;**52**:1137–42

15. Coebergh JWW, Janssen-Heijnen MLG, Post PN, Razenberg PPA. Serious co-morbidity among unselected cancer patients newly diagnosed in the southeastern part of Netherlands in 1993–1996. *J Clin Epidemiol,* 2001;**52**:131–6

16. Cohen Jr MM. Syndromology: an updated conceptual overview. II. Syndrome classifications. *Int J Oral Maxillofac Surg,* 1989;**18**:223–8

17. Hattwick MAW. Rabies virus. In: Mandell GL, Douglas RG Jr, Bennett JE eds. *Principles and Practice of Infectious Diseases.* New York: John Wiley & Sons, 1979:1217–28

18. Evans AS. Acute respiratory infections. In: Top FH ed. *Communicable and Infectious Diseases. Diagnosis, prevention, treatment.* 5th Edition. St. Louis: CV Mosby Co., 1964:476–501

19. Paul JR. Poliomyelitis. In: Debré R, et al. *Poliomyelitis.* WHO Monograph Series No 26. Geneva: World Health Organization, 1955:9–29

20. Kitchen SF. Falciparum Malaria. In: MF Boyd MF ed. Malariology. *A Comprehensive Survey of All Aspects of This Group of Diseases from a Global Standpoint.* Philadelphia: WB Saunders Co., 1949: 995–1016

21. Melzack R. The McGill pain questionnaire: Major properties and scoring methods. *Pain,* 1975;**1**: 277–99

22. Sartwell PE (in collaboration with WH Price). General Epidemiology of Infections. In: PE Sartwell PE ed. *Maxcy-Rosenau: Preventive Medicine and Public Health.* 10th edition. New York: Appleton-Century-Crofts, 1973

23. Chin J (ed.). *Control of Communicable Diseases Manual.* 17th Edition, Washington: American Public Health Association, 2000

24. *Mosby's Medical Dictionary.* 5th Edition. St. Louis: Mosby, 1998

25. Faust J, Schreiner O. A swallowed toothbrush. *Lancet,* 2001;**357**:1012

26. Huth EJ. *Writing and Publishing in Medicine.* 3rd Edition. Baltimore: Williams & Wilkins, 1999: 103–110

27. Huston P, Squires BP. Case reports: Information for authors and peer reviewers. *CMAJ,* 1996;**154**:43–4

28. Vandenbroucke JP. Case reports in evidence-based world. *J Roy Soc Med,* 1999;**92**:159–63

29. Vandenbroucke JP. In defense of case reports and case series. *Ann Intern Med,* **2001**:330–4

30. Jenicek M. *Clinical Case Reporting in Evidence-based Medicine.* 2nd Edition. London: Arnold, 2001

31. Reilly B, Lemon M. Evidence-based morning report: A popular new format in a large teaching hospital. *Am J Med,* 1997;**103**:419–26

32. Tandan VR, Harmantas A, Gallinger S. Long-term survival after hepatic cryosurgery versus surgical resection for metastatic colorectal carcinoma: a critical review of literature. *Can J Surg,* 1997;**40**:175–81

33. Parker MJ. Managing an elderly a patient with a fractured femur. *Br Med J,* 2000;**320**:102–3

34. Del Mar C. Asymptomatic haematuria in the doctor. *Br Med J,* 2000;**320**;165–6

35. de Montaigne M-E (AD 1533–1592). Essays. London: Penguin Books, 1993

36. Squires BP. Case reports: What editors want from authors and peer reviewers. *CMAJ,* 1989;**141**: 379–80

37. Coates M-M. Writing for publication: Case reports. *J Hum Lact,* 1992;**8**:23–6

38. Instructions for authors. *Obstet Gynecol,* 1994;**83**: six title pages (unnumbered)

39. Simpson RJ Jr, Griggs TR. Case reports and medical progress. *Persp Biol Med,* 1985;**28**:42–6

40. Huth EJ. The Review and the Case-Series Analysis. In: *How to Write and Publish Papers in Medical Sciences.* Philadelphia: iSi Press, 1982:64–8

41. Milne R, Chambers L. Assessing the scientific quality of review articles. *J Epidemiol Comm Med,* 1993; **47**:169–70

42. Last JM (ed.). *A Dictionary of Epidemiology.* 4th edition. New York: Oxford University Press, 2001

43. Squires BP, Elmslie TJ. Reports of case series: What editors expect from authors and peer reviewers. *CMAJ,* 1990;**142**:1205–6

44. Cohen D, Flament M, Dubos P-F, Basquin M. Case series: Catatonic syndrome in young people. *J Am Acad Child Adolesc Psychiatry,* 1999;**38**:1040–6

45. Delzell E, Beall C, Rodu B, et al. Case-series investigation of intracranial neoplasms at a petrochemical research facility. *Am J Ind Med,* 1999;**36**:450–8

46. Merren MD. Gabapentin for treatment of pain and tremor: A large case series. *South Med J,* 1998; **91**:739–44

47. Jensen LA, Allen MN. A synthesis of qualitative research on wellness-illness. *Qualit Health Res,* 1994;**4**:349–69

48. Eastbrooks CA, Filed PA, Morse JM. Aggregating qualitative findings: An approach to theory development. *Qualit Health Res,* 1994;**4**:503–11

49. Jensen LA, Allen MN. Meta-synthesis of qualitative findings. *Qualit Health Res,* 1996;**6**:553–60

50. Fraser EJ, Grimes DA, Schultz KF. Immunization as therapy for recurrent spontaneous abortion: A

review of meta-analysis. *Obstet Gynecol*, 1993;**82**:854–9

51. Nordin AJ. Primary carcinoma of the fallopian tube: a 20-year review. *Obstet Gynecol Survey*, 1994;**49**:349–61

52. Drenth JPH, Michiles JJ, Ozsoglu S. Erythermalgia Multidisciplinary Study Group. Acute secondary erythermalgia and hypertension in children. *Eur J Pediatr*, 1995;**154**:882–5

53. Cook MW, Levin LA, Joseph MP, Pinczover EF. Traumatic optic neuropathy: A meta-analysis. *Arch Otoralyng Head Neck Surg*, 1996;**122**:389–92

54. Sackett DL. Rules of evidence and clinical recommendations. *Can J Cardiol*, 1993;**9**:487–9

55. Peipert JF, Gifford DS, Boardman LA. Research design and methods of quantitative synthesis of medical evidence. *Obstet Gynecol*, 1997;**90**:473–8

56. Califf RM. How should clinicians interpret clinical trials? *Cardiol Clinics*, 1995;**13**:459–68

57. Canadian Task Force on the Periodic Health Examination. *Canadian Guide to Clinical Preventive Health Care*. Ottawa: Health Canada, 1994

58. Preventive Services Task Force. *Guide to Clinical Preventive Services*. 2nd Edition. Baltimore: Williams & Wilkins, 1996

59. Hardin WD Jr, Stylianos S, Laly KP. Evidence-based practice in pediatric surgery. *J Pediatr Surg*, 1999;**34**:908–12, discussion: 912–3

60. Soler M, Porta M, Malats N, et al. Learning from case reports: Diagnostic issues in an epidemiologic study of pancreatic cancer. *J Clin Epidemiol*, 1998;**51**:1215–21

61. Rourke JTB, Goertzen JH, Goldsand G, et al. Rural patient stories / physician management narratives. 2. Mental care. *Can J Rural Med*, 2000;**5**:80–2

62. Rourke JTB, Goertzen JH, Hatcher SN, et al. Rural patient stories / physician management narratives. 3. Trauma care. *Can J Rural Med*, 2000;**5**:141–3

63. Davey DA, MacGillivray I. The classification and definition of hypertensive disorders of pregnancy. *Am J Obstet Gynecol*, 1988;**158**:892–8

64. *Vital and Health Statistics. Types of Injuries by Selected Characteristics: United States, 1985–1987.* Series 10. Data from the National Health Survey No 175. DHHS Publ. No (PHS) 91–1503, Hyattsville: US Department of Health and Human Services, December 1990:54–8

65. Bolton S. *Pharmaceutical Statistics. Practical Applications*. New York and Basel: Marcel Decker Inc., 1984:294–300, 485

66. Centres for Disease Control. Summary of Notifiable Diseases. *MMWR*, 1987;**36**(54)

67. Arraiz GA, Wigle DT, Mao Y, Sylvain M. Recent trends of cancer of a corpus uteri and estrogen replacement therapy in Canada. *Chron Dis Canada*, 1991;**12**:4–5

68. Dublin LI, Lotka AJ, Spiegelman M. Length of Life. *A Study of the Life Table*. New York: The Ronald Press Co., 1949

69. Marcus S, Leaverton P (eds). *Proceedings of the 1976 Workshop on Automated Cartography and Epidemiology*. DHEW Publ. No (PHS) 79–1254. Hyattsville: US Dept. Health, Educ. Welfare, 1979

70. Morgenstern H. Uses of ecology analysis in epidemiologic research. *Am J Public Health*, 1982;**72**:1336–44

71. Piantadosi S, Byar DP, Green SB. The ecological fallacy. *Am J Epidemiol*, 1988;**127**:893–904

72. Martyn CN, Osmond C, Edwardson JA, et al. Geographical relation between Alzheimer's disease and aluminium in drinking waters. *Lancet*, 1989;**1**:59–62

73. LaPorte RE, Cresanta JL, Kuller LH. The relationship of alcohol consumption to atherosclerotic heart disease. *Prev Med*, 1980;**9**:22–40

74. Bureau of Epidemiology Laboratory, Center for Disease Control. *Cancer Patterns in Canada 1931–1974*. Ottawa: Health and Welfare Canada, 1977

75. Higginson J, Muir CS. Epidemiology. In: Holland JE Frei, E eds. *Cancer Medicine*. Philadelphia: Lea and Febiger, 1973:214–306

76. International Journal of Epidemiology. Symposium on Methods of Surveillance in Planning for Health. *Int J Epidemiol*, 1976;**5**:13–91

77. Langmuir AD. The surveillance of communicable diseases of national importance. *N Engl J Med*, 1983;**268**:182–92

78. Raska K. National and international surveillance of communicable diseases. *WHO Chron*, 1966;**20**:315–21

79. Muir CS, Nectoux J. Role of the cancer registry. *Natl Canc Inst Monogr*, 1977;**37**:3–6

80. Goldberg J, Gelfand HM, Levy PS. Registry evaluation methods: a review and case study. *Epidemiol Rev*, 1980;**2**:210–20

81. Kurtzke JF. Data registries on selected segments of the population: veterans. *Adv Neurol*, 1978;**19**:55–67

82. Foege WH (Chairman) Committee on Trauma Research. *Injury in America. A Continuing Public Health Problem*. Washington: National Academy Press, 1985

83. Peacocke JE. The epidemiology of influenza in Canada, 1977–78. *Can J Public Health*, 1979;**79**:321–8

84. Leaverton PE, Massé L, Simches SO (eds). *Environmental Epidemiology*. New York, Praeger, 1982

85. Thacker SB, Berkelman RL. Surveillance of medical technologies. *J Public Health Policy*, 1986;**7**:363–77

86. Strom BL (ed.). *Pharmacoepidemiology*. New York: Churchill Livingstone, 1989

87. Lasagna L. Are drug benefits also part of pharmaco-epidemiology? *J Clin Epidemiol*, 1990;**43**:849–50

88. Graitcer PL. The development of state and local injury surveillance systems. *J Safety Res*, 1987;**18**:191–8

89. Eylenbosch WJ, Noah ND (eds). *Surveillance in Health and Disease*. Oxford: Oxford University Press, 1988

90. On L, Semenciw RM, Mao Y. Orius software: Calculation of rates and epidemiologic indicators, and preparation of graphical output. *Chron Dis Canada*, 2000;**21**:134–6

91. Choi BCK. Perspectives on epidemiologic surveillance in the 21st century. *Chron Dis Canada*, 1998;**19**:145–51

92. Centers for Disease Control. Guidelines for Investigating Clusters of Health Events. *MMWR*, 1990;**39**(RR–11):23

93. Knox G. Epidemiology of childhood leukemia in Northumberland and Durham. *Br J Prev Soc Med*, 1964;**18**:17–24

94. Mantel N. The detection of disease clustering and a generalized regression approach. *Cancer Res*, 1967;**27**:209–20

95. Armitage P, Berry G. *Statistical Methods in Medical Research*. 2nd Edition. Oxford: Blackwell Science, 1987

96. National Conference on Clustering of Health Events. *Am J Epidemiol*, 1990;**132**(Suppl 1):S1–S202

97. Olsen SF, Martuzzi M, Elliott P.Cluster analysis and disease mapping – why, when, and how? A step-by-step guide. *BMJ*, 1996;**313**:863–6

98. Alexander FE, Boyle P (eds). *Methods for Investigating Localized Clustering of Disease*. IARC Sci Publ. 135. Lyon: Int Agency Res Cancer, 1996

99. Dunn HL. Record linkage. *Am J Public Health*, 1946;**36**:1412

100. Acheson ED. *Medical Record Linkage*. London: The Oxford University Press, 1967

101. Acheson ED. Techniques and problems in record linkage. In: *Proceedings of the 5th International Scientific Meeting of the International Epidemio-logical Association, Primosten, Yougoslavia, 25–30 August 1968*. Belgrade: Savremena administracija, 1970: 203–15

102. Baldwin JA, Acheson ED, Graham WJ (eds). *Textbook of Medical Record Linkage*. Oxford: Oxford University Press, 1987

103. Newcombe HB. Record linking. The design of efficient systems for linking records into individual and family histories. *Am J Hum Genet*, 1967;**19**:335–59

104. Newcombe HB. Value of Canadian hospital insurance records in detecting increases in congenital anomalies. *Can Med Assoc J*, 1969;**101**:121–8

105. Newcombe HB. The use of medical record linkage for population and genetic studies. *Methods Inf Med*, 1969;**8**:7–11

106. Acheson JE (ed.). *Record Linkage in Medicine. Proceedings of the International Symposium, Oxford, July 1967*. Edinburgh and London: Livingstone, 1968

107. Sartwell PE. Cohorts. The debasement of a word. *Am J Epidemiol*, 1976;**103**:536–8

108. Springett VH. What is a cohort? *Br Med J*, 1979;**1**(6156):126

109. Jacobs AL. What is a cohort? *Br Med J*, 1979;**1**(6158):266

110. Bureau of Epidemiology Laboratory, Center for Disease Control. *Cancer Patterns in Canada, 1931–1974*. Ottawa: Health and Welfare Canada, 1977

111. Fraser DW. Tetanus in the United States, 1900–1969. Analysis by cohorts. *Am J Epidemiol*, 1972;**96**:306–12

112. Glenn ND. *Cohort Analysis*. Beverly Hills: Sage Publications, 1977

113. Newell GR, Boutwell WB, Morris DL. Epidemiology of cancer. In: DeVita VT Jr, Helman S, Rosenberg SA eds. *Cancer. Principles and Practice of Oncology*. Philadelphia: JB Lippincott, 1982:3–32

114. Grimes DA, Schultz KF. Descriptive studies: what they can and cannot do. *Lancet*, 2002;**359**:145–9

Chapter 8

Search for causes of disease occurrence. Why does disease occur?

Every what hath a wherefore
William Shakespeare (1564–1616)

Some circumstantial evidence is very strong,
as when you find a trout in the milk
Henry David Thoreau (1817–1862)

The world is full of bright researchers
and highly competent methodologists.
However, what are needed, in equal numbers, are not only
discoverers, but also astute and discerning
users of new evidence who are able to put to
good use relevant evidence and to discard the irrelevant

Patients want to know why they contracted a disease. Politicians and health planners want to know why there are so many cases of cancer, injury, heart disease or infection in the community and which preventive measures should be put in place. The answers to these questions should be logical and supported by the best evidence available:

Clinical practice:	Logical discourse:	Evidence:
'You are suffering from of a rather serious liver disease'	This is a case of liver cirrhosis **(Premise A)**	**Valid diagnosis** liver cirrhosis and exclusion of other competing diagnoses
'Your disease is due to excessive drinking!'	Liver cirrhosis is due to alcohol abuse **(Premise B)**	Alcohol abuse causes liver cirrhosis (**causal proof** from etiological research)
'You should stop drinking right away before things become worse!'	Liver cirrhosis course might improve if patient stops drinking **(Conclusion C)**	**Clinical trials** or **other effectiveness studies** like **prognostic studies**

For this kind of logical argumentation, a clinician needs evidence:

- That the patient really has liver cirrhosis (from the field of diagnosis; see Chapter 6);
- That liver cirrhosis is caused by alcohol abuse (from the field of etiological research as outlined in this chapter); and
- That stopping alcohol consumption will improve the patient's health and survival (from studies of health intervention and prognosis as outlined in Chapters 9 and 10 of this text).

This chapter is devoted to the evidence of causes of disease (i.e. how to justify Premise B in the above example).

Descriptive studies do not explain the causes of disease. They give information about disease spread. To explain whether some characteristics of persons, time, or place cause health problems, analytical studies based on single or multiple comparisons are required. Analytical studies are the basis of what is

called etiological, or causal, research. This chapter focuses on:

- The concept of causes in medicine;
- Judgmental and computational criteria of the cause–effect relationship;
- The two main types of etiological studies and the contribution of their computational products to causal inference;
- The most important clinical precautions required to avoid errors and bias in analytical research;
- Etiological research of unplanned events, such as the investigation of disease outbreaks;
- The challenges of multiple causes and multiple consequences; and
- The implications of the results of etiological studies for practical decision-making in preventive medicine and clinical care.

As mentioned in Chapter 4, one classification of medical research distinguishes between observational and experimental research. This chapter deals with observational analytical studies, whereas Chapter 9 will be devoted to experimental research (the search for causes) through clinical trials.

8.1 Concept of cause(s) in medicine

The concept of cause in medicine is no different from the concept of cause in general, which classical philosophers like David Hume, John Stuart Mill, Bertrand Russell and Karl Popper thoroughly examined. The only difference, perhaps, is the fact that the primarily speculative thinking of classical philosophers is enriched by experience from the experimental domain and that it is better adjusted to our desire and means of controlling disease by controlling its causes. The *Encyclopaedia Britannica* identifies a cause as '. . . *that factor which is possible or convenient for us to alter in order to produce or prevent an effect . . . This concept contains two components, production of an effect and an understanding of its mechanisms.*'[1] In medicine, three groups of factors can be considered **causes**:

- All endogenous and exogenous phenomena, events, characteristics of individuals, as well as of groups of individuals, which determine and modify health status and the occurrence of health phenomena (disease) in the community (domain of **risk**);

- All decisions (medical or otherwise), and other factors modifying disease occurrence and influencing disease course (field of **prognosis**); and also
- All phenomena determining clinical decisions and public health measures.

Any disease **outcome** (cure, death, incapacitation, chronicity, costs) can be considered a **consequence** in cause–effect relationships in our field of interest. Primary prevention is not possible without knowledge of the first group of factors, and there is no effective secondary or tertiary prevention without knowledge of the exact role of prognostic markers and factors and/or the impact of clinical intervention on disease outcome (how this modifies the natural course of disease in terms of its clinical gradient and spectrum). Hence, causal relationships are considered from one stage of disease course to another: causes of occurrence of new cases of disease (risk); causes of disease outcomes (prognosis); clinical and community health interventions as causes of improvement of community health. Valid causal proof is of vital importance for all levels of prevention, as defined in Table 8.1.

According to the general definition, a 'cause' (etiological factor) must be modifiable, and its modification must lead to the change of its effect (patients' status, disease spread). Causes of disease are sometimes mistakenly called risk factors since this term represents only a part of what are known as risk characteristics (i.e. any variable which is associated

with a high probability of disease). As mentioned in Chapter 2, Grundy[2] sees **two components of risk characteristics: risk markers** (age, sex, etc.), which cannot be modified, but nevertheless give a high probability of disease in the future; and **risk factors**, which are modifiable (smoking, diet, etc.). In this chapter, the term 'cause' is taken to mean Grundy's risk factors. (NB Based on this logic, the same can be said about prognostic factors and markers as described in Chapter 10.) However, current literature uses the term **risk factors** to signify 'factors' and 'markers' as well. In statistical terms, according to the cause–effect sequence, studies explore relationships between **independent variables** (risk factors or markers, causes such as smoking or air pollution) and **dependent variables** (consequences, diseases such as respiratory problems resulting from tobacco or air pollution exposure). Depending on the hypothesis of the causal relationship under study, **indirect causes** (such as smoking) or **direct causes** (i.e. exposure of bronchi and lung tissue to polycyclic hydrocarbonates contained in smoke) can be studied.

The identification of direct causes remains one of the greatest challenges of etiological research in medicine. Webs of causes (see Chapter 2) can occur at a given moment or in a particular sequence. If more than one 'cause' is needed to produce an effect, 'minimum sufficient causes' should be known[3]. For example, a cholera outbreak is due not only to the presence of *Vibrio cholerae* in the environment, but also to the availability of untreated water to the population, to close contact between sick and healthy individuals, to poor hygiene in both, to malnutrition, to comorbidity and other factors enhancing the expressivity of cholera and its consequences.

8.2 Basic concept and design of causal studies

The way cause(s) whether single, multiple, isolated, or interacting are viewed will largely determine study design. Several possible cause–effect relationships exist in medicine including those connecting 'bad' causes (e.g. smoking) and 'good' causes (treatment and the cure it produces) and their effects. For ethical reasons, evaluation of 'bad' causes must be done by **observational studies** (the subjects themselves choose their own exposure to cause), or **experimental**

Table 8.1 Causes in relation to different levels of prevention

Level	Causes of interest	Characteristics under study
Primary:	Causes of disease incidence	Risk factors (not becoming ill)
Secondary:	Causes of disease prevalence (by controlling causes of disease duration)	Prognostic factors (healing)
Tertiary:	Causes of endogenous spread, disease extent, and severity	Prognostic factors (staying alive)

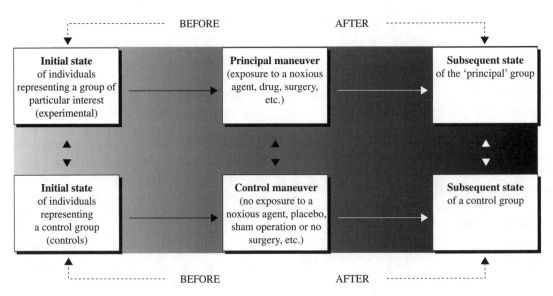

Figure 8.1 Basic model of an analytical study. Source: Ref.5 and personal communication. Redrawn with modifications

studies, such as a clinical trial in which a health professional decides who will receive a drug, an expected 'good' cause of cure. **Both types of studies are, however, in synonymous terms, analytical or etiological studies of cause–effect relationships, or causal studies. They are both subject to the same causal reasoning.**

The basic concept of causal proof stems from experimental research in the health sciences (physiology, pathology, pharmacology, etc.) as well as from clinical trials. In epidemiological terms, an analytical study is based on the comparison of two or more groups of subjects. Descriptive studies describe **in whom, when and where disease occurs.** Analytical studies answer a fourth question: **why does disease occur?** Claude Bernard's basic experimental approach[4] was translated by Feinstein[5] into a pragmatic structure, illustrated by Figure 8.1. For example, the effects of vitamin-deficient diets are studied in laboratory animals. The experimental group is given an inadequate diet, and the control group receives an optimal diet. After a given period of different dietary regimens, the occurrence of vitamin-deficient states is compared in the two groups. Obviously, the initial state of both groups (before diet programs), maneuvers (feeding programs), and the final evaluation of all animals (subsequent state) should be comparable in order for the study to be as objective as possible. These simplified

basic rules apply to all etiological research and although such logic might appear simplistic on paper, it is frequently difficult to respect.

In an observational study, overeaters (by their own choosing, for whatever reason) are compared to normal eaters in order to establish differences in the occurrence of cardiovascular or metabolic problems between the groups. This simple example demonstrates that following the rules of an analytical (comparative) approach is often much more difficult for observational studies than for experimental ones. How do the researchers obtain comparable initial states of individuals becoming overeaters and normal eaters? Is it necessary for their dietary regimens (frequency of meals, activity, other factors) to be comparable in all aspects except the number of calories ingested? Do some 'hidden' maneuvers appear (such as comorbidity, etc.), and what should be done with them? What should the evaluation of the subsequent state include? These are challenging questions for which appropriate answers, research methods, and techniques are difficult to find.

8.3 Fundamental philosophy and criteria of the cause–effect relationship

In etiological research, the vocabulary of medical literature is extensive:

Disease '. . . *is associated with* . . .'
          '. . . *correlates with* . . .'
          '. . . *is linked to* . . .'
          '. . . *is closely associated with* . . .'
          '. . . *is strongly related to* . . .' a habit,
            exposure, etc.

Do these expressions mean different things, or are they all synonymous? Perhaps different terms are used to describe something that is not clear. If a tabloid mentions that two pop stars are 'romantically linked', it can mean that they are friends, lovers, spouses or have just had twins. Such convenient ambiguity is, needless to say, unacceptable when looking for causes in health sciences. **Events of interest must be related by more than just 'links' or 'associations'.**

8.3.1 *Basic considerations*

An association is a term used in statistical language to imply a dependency between two or more events, characteristics, or other variables. An association is present if the probability of occurrence of an event or characteristic (for example, disease), or the quantity of a variable (high blood pressure) depends on the occurrence of one or more other events, the presence of one or more other characteristics, or the quantity

of one or more other variables (high salt intake, stress, abnormal renal or endocrine functions, etc.)[6].

Statistical correlations (i.e. the degree to which variables change together) do not necessarily imply causal relationships. Caricatured examples abound. In a direct correlation throughout time, the numbers of nesting storks in cities correlates with human birth rates in the same cities, yet we remain unconvinced that more storks bring more babies. In an indirect correlation, an increasing trend in time for the number of dishwashers sold in North America is associated with a decreasing trend in mortality from stomach cancer. Does automatic dishwashing prevent and/or cure stomach cancer (mortality = incidence × case fatality)?

Relationships between variables such as causal factors and disease may be put in hierarchical order, as illustrated by Figure 8.2. It must be clearly demonstrated that such observations and conclusions are not purely coincidental. In reality, they have a logical basis. Moreover, such **associations may be symmetrical**, as in the equation linking mortality, incidence and case fatality (any change in the left or right side of the equation brings a change to the other side); **or asymmetrical** (i.e. smoking leads to cancer, but cancer does not lead to smoking). Asymmetrical associations in a proper time sequence are of particular interest in a causal proof although they represent a considerable challenge.

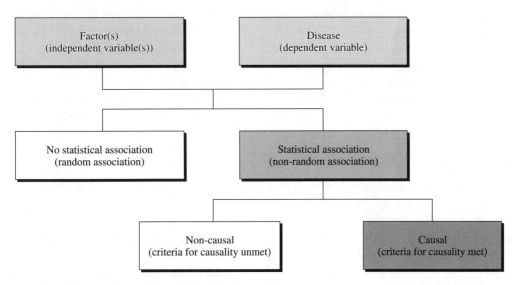

Figure 8.2   Associations between factors (suspected causes) and disease

In observational studies, epidemiological proof is just **circumstantial evidence. Conclusions are drawn, if possible, without error and bias** from events themselves and the way in which they occurred. In experimental studies (trials used as a standard of causal proof), we must proceed deductively when trying to reproduce at the bedside or in the community and without sacrificing, if possible, the reality of subjects' normal daily life conditions, the rigor of experimental studies in a laboratory setting. Before discussing the design of analytical studies, let us review the logic and reasoning surrounding a causal proof in medicine and other health sciences. Such a proof is much more difficult to obtain than in exact sciences, given the biological nature of events and characteristics of both dependent and independent variables.

Any relation between a cause (independent variable) and its effect (dependent variable) is a **question of both measurement and judgment.** Both of these components have become increasingly solid during the last 50 years[7-10]. A. Bradford Hill's bridging observation and experiment in search for causes[11], J. Yerushalmy's and C.E. Palmer's[12], A.M. Lilienfeld's[13], A.B. Hill's[14], A.S. Evans'[15] and others[16] contribution to establishing criteria of causation represent the basis of causal thinking today. Several authors also tried to better understand relationships in time and space between etiological factors and their causes: K.J. Rothman's concept of minimal sufficient causes[16] brought different factors together. Their relationship is seen as a sequence through path analysis or other models[19-21] and their joint effect (synergy – additive and potentialization, or antagonism) is under study as well[22]. Throughout these contributions, it is stated that a good causal proof relies on the following prerequisites and criteria (see also Table 8.2).

8.3.2 *Prerequisites of a causal proof*

1. **The association under study is not due to chance alone.** Tests of significance as the cornerstone of statistical analysis represent only an introduction to causal analysis; they are not a substitute for it. Unfortunately, incomplete etiological research sometimes stops at a simple demonstration of statistical significance.

2. **The researched association should be 'anticipated' or predictable.** The result should be consistent with prediction. Generally, possible causal associations are studied by **induction** (material gathered without a particular hypothesis in mind is analyzed and hypotheses are proposed from observed associations) or by **deduction** (hypotheses are formulated first, studies built accordingly and their results used to confirm or disprove the pre-established hypotheses in question). Hence, if a causal relationship is first demonstrated through inductive research, the deductive research must bring the same results. The deductive approach has the advantages of 'predictability' and 'testability'[23].

3. Selected variables are introduced in an observational design, which is built **ideally in such a way that it respects at a maximum the criteria and virtues of an experimental study** (clinical trial, if the latter might be done in such circumstances)[24,25].

4. Both dependent and independent **variables under study** must be clearly **observable, measurable, defined and classified.** In other terms, they must be satisfactory from the clinimetric point of view. For example, in psychiatry, this prerequisite is particularly arduous because not only is mental illness (dependent variable) seen through such soft data as symptoms (sorrow, grief, etc.) and clinical signs (e.g. flat affect, antisocial behavior, hyperactivity in a child, etc.), but the independent variables (presumed causes) represent soft data as well (rejection, verbal assault, abusive behavior, etc.). Hence, hardening of such soft data is often a double challenge.

5. The study should represent **unbiased observation, comparison and interpretation.** Observations must be as complete as possible and not based on 'confounding' factors, which are hard to interpret.

6. **Uncontrollable and uninterpretable factors should ideally be absent from analytical studies.** In observational studies, uncontrollable factors may be other causal factors which are impossible to measure or which are not followed by the study. If a study of respiratory problems were limited only to smoking, other factors might be missed such as exposure to occupational factors

causing the same or similar problems, possibly drugs, etc.

Other types of factors belonging to this category are variables bearing social stigma or shame, whose reporting is often distorted: drinking, drug abuse, income, sexual orientation and behaviors, criminal activities, interpersonal relationships, etc.

A special challenge in etiological research is the control of **confounding factors** or '**confounders**'. A **confounding factor** is, by the most commonly understood definition[3,26] any variable that distorts the observed effect of exposure on a health condition under study. These factors are variables **that are associated with both the dependent and independent variables under study**[3,27]. For example, in a study of the etiology of lung cancer, both cigarette smoking and age are related to the disease. In relation to the 'cigarette–cancer' hypothesis, age is a confounder, being related both to the duration (and quantity of carcinogen inhaled) of smoking and to the risk of cancer as well. For Feinstein[28], a confounder is a phenomenon external to the two main variables of maneuver and outcome that can distort their relationship as calculated from a fourfold table or other statistical expression[26,29,30]. For others[31] a confounding variable is a variable related to the dependent variable only, but not to the cause (it may be another causal factor independent from the one under study). Confounding factors do not have the role of **intermediate factors**[31], i.e. factors in the middle of a causal chain between the direct cause and its consequence (for example, malnutrition aggravating the risk of measles or cholera infections and the severity of cases). The overabundance of definitions for confounding factors aptly illustrates the saying: 'the more definitions there are, the greater the uncertainty'. For now, the initial definition given[3,27] may be the best, the most concrete and practical. For many methodologists, confounding factors represent the specter of analytical studies. They may be eliminated or controlled by two means:

1. By carefully designing analytical studies, i.e. by avoiding them in advance[3,26,27]. Matching individuals, restricting and/or stratifying data and individuals for the purpose of comparison are often used to control confounding. Any researcher in a search for causes must be armed with correct information. The most complete knowledge of up-to-date (even imperfect) possible etiological factors must be acquired. The most relevant information may then be chosen and fit into the best architecture of research design.

2. The second requirement is a perfect knowledge (if possible) of all clinimetric data on the disease under study, its natural history and course. Mechanical studies of whatever factor is available (such as demographic or social characteristics, etc.) inevitably lead to a plethora of confounders, in turn leading to a more complex analysis of data. On one hand, increasingly complex quantitative methods are being developed to 'control' (i.e. understand and improve the interpretation of results) 'confounders' and 'effect modifiers'. On the other hand, a careful design is always better than *a posteriori* problems in analysis and interpretation. It is often preferable to anticipate and prevent the existence of confounding, effect-modifying or interacting factors rather than attempt to 'cure' or control them *a posteriori*.

Only after the appropriate prerequisites of acceptable studies are fulfilled can observations and comparisons be submitted to the proper criteria of causation. In other words, studies:

- In which the effect of chance was not evaluated;
- Giving unpredictable results (conditional);
- Inconsistent with rigorous design;
- With undefined or poorly defined variables under study;
- In which observations are biased and full of errors; and
- In which many obscure and uninterpretable factors appear;

do not merit assessment of causality using the criteria presented in the following section. Surprisingly enough, the authors of criteria of causation in epidemiology did not always have the above-mentioned prerequisites in mind, thereby enumerating their criteria as if all studies under consideration were inherently good.

8.3.3 Criteria of a causal relationship

Hill's often quoted criteria of causality[11], which are also common to Yerushalmy and Palmer[12], Sartwell[21], Susser[7], or Lilienfeld[13] among others[32,33], may be logically organized, as summarized in Table 8.2.

Table 8.2 Fundamental prerequisites and assessment criteria of the cause–effect relationship

Prerequisites of causal assessments (before causal criteria apply)

- Exclusion that observed differences are due to **chance** alone
- Results are consistent with **prediction**
- Observational studies are based and built on the same logic and with similar precautions, **according to the fundamental rules of experimental research**
- Studies are based on **clinimetrically valid data**
- **Unbiased observations, comparisons and analysis** of the former
- **Uncontrollable and uninterpretable factors** are ideally absent from the study

Criteria of causation

Major

- **Temporality** ('cart behind the horse')
- **Strength** (relative risk)
- **Specificity:**
  o **Manifestational** ('pattern' of clinical spectrum and gradient) i.e. one result among others
  o **Causal** (etiological fraction, attributable risk percent) i.e. one factor among others
- **Biological gradient** (more exposure = stronger association)
- **Consistency** (assessment of homogeneity, e.g. by meta-analysis or evaluation of the spectrum of minimal sufficient causes)
- **Biological plausibility** (explanation of the nature of association)

Conditional

- **Coherence with prevalent knowledge**
- **Analogy**

Reference

- **Experimental proof** (preventability, curability): of Golden standard or 'cessation study'

Confirmation

- **Systematic review** and **meta-analysis** of evidence

Temporality

The precedence of presumed cause to the effect is not obvious in all fields of medicine. In a smoking → cancer relationship, 'the cart is clearly behind the horse'. While studying an association between alcohol abuse and depression, each may be considered as the dependent or independent variable according to different hypotheses under study and according to the temporal precedence of one to another. Alcohol abuse can be studied as a risk factor of depression, but it can also be studied as an outcome of depression. Hence, temporality determines if this is a study of risk or a study of prognosis. In other cases, examples of which are frequent in psychiatry, the clinical inception point of disease does not represent its beginning, such as in psychosis or endogenous depression. It is often difficult to say whether we are studying a real risk factor of disease or a causal role of a prognostic factor of subsequent episodes or spells of an already existing health problem (e.g. a bipolar affective disorder, antisocial behavior, or ischemic heart disease). Proper temporality should be the first and absolute criterion of causality of disease occurrence.

Strength of association

This criterion is based on measurement. For example, the higher the disease occurrence (incidence rate) in exposed subjects compared to unexposed ones, the stronger the association. Thus, the distance or contrast between the groups compared gives the appropriate information. In cohort studies, relative risk (syn. rate ratio) is an appropriate quantitative expression of the causal link's strength. In case–control studies, the odds ratio (exposure ratio, exposure odds ratio) serves a similar purpose. These ideas are detailed in Sections 8.4 and 8.5.

Biological gradient (dose–response relationship)

This is an extension of the previous criterion (strength), indicating directionality between the amount of exposure (duration, intensity, or quantity) and the size of impact. It is also based on measurement. The strength of association should correlate with the degree of exposure. As the relative risk of lung cancer increases with duration and frequency (number of cigarettes) of smoking, the frequency of anxiety reactions or suicide attempts increases in relation to the frequency of stressful life events or with the degree of social support (or lack of it). A **reverse gradient** indicates a diminishing risk with diminishing exposure, such as progressively fewer respiratory problems if smokers quit smoking for one, five, ten years etc. as seen in cessation studies.

Specificity of association

Two aspects of specificity[34] should be studied. The **manifestational specificity** reveals that a factor (cause under study) leads to a consistent pattern of consequences. In other terms, clinical spectrum and gradient of morbid manifestations (one or more diseases) should be exclusive to a given exposure. Cluster analysis and analysis of categorical data may be helpful in the study of manifestational specificity. For example, the 'four D's' of pellagra (dermatitis, diarrhea, dementia, death) are specific to this kind of malnutrition. The **causal specificity** is based on a measure of how important one factor is relative to others. This criterion may be evaluated by assessing differences between rates of occurrence in exposed and unexposed subjects, in absolute terms of attributable risk (syn. risk difference), or in relative terms as etiological fraction (syn. attributable risk percent, attributable fraction). Absolute specificity means that all cases are due to one factor (100% of cases are attributable to the factor under study). The less specific the factor (and the causal association linked to it), the lesser the proportion of disease cases are due to exposure. This is discussed in detail in Section 8.4. *NB Readers of specific literature should not be surprised that the summation of all known etiological fractions of various factors, as provided by different studies, can yield more than 100% of the total etiology. In each original study, the combination of the factors under study and all other etiological factors (minimal causes) can be different. The information on etiological fraction of a causal factor is primarily valid within the study. A proper integration of information on etiological fractions coming from various studies is still being developed.*

Consistency of association

The consistency of an etiological link should be demonstrated across different independent studies of the same problem. The same association should be confined in different populations, different regions, times, and in various combinations with different factors and characteristics. For example, smokers develop lung cancer whether they are Caucasians or not, residents of North America or not, or whether they smoked before, during, or after the industrial revolution in their country. Again, meta-analysis (see Chapter 12) may help to assess studies across this criterion.

Biological plausibility

The explanation of morphological and functional mechanisms linking a supposed cause and its effect must be attempted and found. For example, anemia in women and its etiology is understood on the basis of our knowledge of folic acid and iron turnover and metabolism during pregnancy, reproductive cycles, and aging. Sometimes, some new and interesting mechanisms are noted before the etiology of disease is known, allowing for a better search for still unknown causes, such as the discovery of the importance of endorphins or dopamine in relation to mental disorders, dependency, etc. If biological plausibility cannot be explained, its proof may be attempted by exclusion, i.e. by eliminating the plausibility of all other known biological mechanisms and factors (the 'Sherlock Holmes method', i.e. 'whatever is left, is it!').

Readers of medical literature may be familiar with three types of etiological studies: The first relies mainly on impeccable quantitative analysis and explanations of biological plausibility are more or less neglected. The second type is based on biological plausibility, but neglects quantitative analysis and assessment of strength, specificity, or biological gradient (poor statistical analysis). The third covers both quantitative and qualitative considerations of cause–effect relationships.

The next criteria[7,8] are enforcing and complementary in causal proof (in the epidemiological sense), but not necessary.

Coherence with prevalent knowledge

In most cases, associations found are not in conflict with contemporary, generally known and/or admitted facts around disease history and course. On the other hand, many innovative findings may be lost if contradictory results are not explored sufficiently.

Analogy

A finding of analogous associations between similar factors (i.e. other cancer-producing) and similar diseases (other and different cancers) may strengthen a conviction of causality, but it is not a condition '*sine qua non*' of a causal link.

Experimental proof as a reference criterion

An experimental study of exposure and its consequences (a well controlled clinical or community trial) is an obvious standard for observational studies. A **cessation** (syn. withdrawal) **study**, as the mirror image of the former, remains an alternative wherever experimentation is impossible for ethical and/or other reasons. For example, instead of forcing people to smoke for defined periods, the risk of respiratory problems may be studied in ex-smokers in relation to the duration of nicotine cessation (the longer the cessation period, the lower the risk).

Before drawing conclusions about causality on the basis of a maximum of criteria met (Section 8.5.2), two basic designs of analytical studies, their challenges, and the meaning of their product (risks) must be understood.

8.3.4 Measures (indices) of strength and specificity of associations

There are two measures of **strength**: relative risk and odds ratio.

> Relative risk is a ratio of two individual risks, the one in subjects exposed to a presumed causal factor compared two that in unexposed ones. Incidence rate, attack rate, incidence density, or mortality rate are used as individual risks for comparison purposes. This measure comes from cohort studies as described after the following basic definitions.
>
> **Odds ratio** (odds exposure ratio) is the ratio of the odds in favor of exposure among cases to the odds in favor of exposure among non-cases of disease[6]. This measure comes from case–control studies, a description of which follows.

Specificity of a causal relationship may also be evaluated by two measures: by attributable risk and etiological fraction assessments.

> **Attributable risk** or risk difference is the rate of disease in exposed subjects, which is due to a given factor and not to other factors, representing a web of causes of the disease under study. This rate is obtained from cohort studies by subtracting the rate in unexposed subjects from that of the exposed ones.
>
> **Etiological fraction** (attributable risk percent, attributable fraction) is a proportion represented by the attributable risk to the whole risk, either in exposed subjects only (exposed group etiological fraction) or in the whole population under study, i.e. exposed and unexposed individuals together (population attributable fraction). The etiological fraction may be calculated from cohort studies and estimated also from case–control studies.

Number needed to harm (NNH)[35,36] is the most recent addition to our evaluation of the impact of a health problem-causing factor. It comes from the field of trials and observational studies of the adverse effects of medical interventions such as drugs. In more general terms, NNH is the number of individuals who, if exposed to a harmful factor, would lead to one additional person contracting the health problem under study compared with unexposed individuals. It is calculated as a reciprocal value of attributable risk. However, at the time of writing, the use of NNH has not yet been sufficiently expanded and refined beyond the field of adverse drug reaction studies.

It is important to know, on the basis of practical examples from cohort and case–control studies, how these measures are obtained and how they should be interpreted. To this end, the strengths and weaknesses of these studies will also be presented. Symbols and notation in the text follow those of the International Epidemiological Association's *Dictionary of Epidemiology*[6]. Figure 8.3A illustrates two basic approaches to analyzing causes in epidemiology. Assuming multifactorial etiology of many health problems, variability of observations and of diagnosis, errors in classification, difficulties in measurements of exposure to causal factors, etc., all exposed subjects do not inevitably 'fall ill', and also all non-exposed individuals (who are exposed to the same etiological factors as the group exposed to the studied factor) will not remain healthy. A cohort study is based on 'hunting for cases' in both the exposed and unexposed groups, waiting for cases to occur. As demonstrated in Figure 8.3A, the cohort study is read from left to right. The study proceeds in terms of a time sequence from cause to consequence. A case–control study proceeds in the reverse order, from consequence to cause. Cases and non-cases are identified at a given moment in time. Then, individuals in each group who were or were not exposed to the factor under study are identified. Once again, a similar two-by-two table is obtained, but, as demonstrated in Figure 8.3A, the study is read from top to bottom. Both approaches, which have practical and scientific advantages and disadvantages, allow for the estimation of different risks and ratios, with varying degrees of precision.

8.4 Cohort study

A cohort study (syn. prospective, prolective, 'looking forward', concurrent, follow-up) is a longitudinal study of the occurrence of disease in a group of exposed subjects compared to that of individuals not exposed to a presumed causal factor of interest. At a given point in time, the study begins with individuals in both groups; the individuals **are all healthy, i.e. they do not have the disease under study, but all are susceptible to the disease in the future.** This susceptibility is not always equal (reason for the study).

In military terms, a **cohort** (from the Latin *cohors*, the tenth part of a legion) represented a square of soldiers marching in closed ranks to probable death. In epidemiology[6], in a similar sense, the term describes 'any designated group of persons who are followed or tracked over a period of time' (i.e. 'who advance from exposure to disease'). Depending on the question asked, an entry moment, i.e. 'recruitment' of the individual to a cohort, is defined preferably by the **beginning of exposure,** such as starting to smoke, take drugs or drink contaminated water. **The follow-up ideally spans a complete period of time, allowing for the full potential of development of disease cases or other health phenomena of interest.** Duration of exposure, incubation period, sufficient

time for a healing effect, becoming immune, etc. are taken into consideration. More often, but less adequately, a **calendar period** of follow-up of selected individuals represents a 'cohort study' (for example, from January 1, 1991 to December 31, 2000). There are two variants of cohort studies:

- A **'true' cohort study** (syn. prolective study) would begin on the current date by following groups of exposed and unexposed individuals. The identification of incident cases would take place during a defined period of time in the future. The current date (i.e. the date of exposure to the event, such as starting to smoke) marks the beginning of the follow-up period.
- A **historical cohort study** (syn. retrolective study, prospective study in the past, etc.) began at a given moment in the past by identifying exposed and unexposed groups and finding incident cases occurring up until the current date, which marks the end of the follow-up period.

For example, instead of today beginning a 30-year study of individuals who start smoking and later develop cancer, it would be faster and less expensive (providing that good quality records exist) to identify a population of healthy individuals 30 years ago, part of whom became smokers. The impact of 30 years of smoking could then be evaluated to this day.

Historical cohort or prospective studies in the past, rely heavily on the availability of high-quality data and documentation in routine archives, which have not been created for these studies. The quality of such historical studies is therefore variable, but their cost is much lower than that of a true cohort study.

8.4.1 Information provided

The following fictitious example is both simple and explicit. A community study might demonstrate that out of one million individuals, 400,000 were exposed to environmental air pollution since adolescence and 600,000 were not exposed to such pollution. After 20 years of living in different conditions as described above, 320 individuals in the first group developed chronic respiratory problems, and 120 similar cases

A. Directionality of cohort and case–control studies

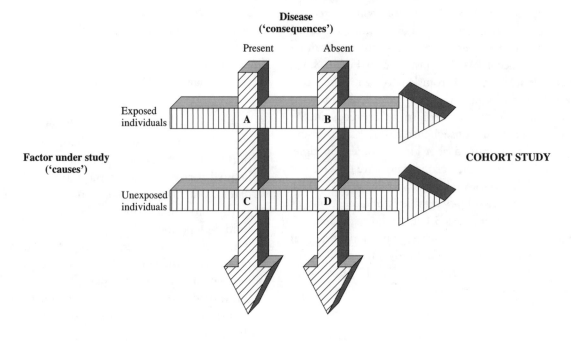

At the moment of evaluation:
A: Number of subjects exposed and who have developed the disease
B: Number of subjects exposed and who did not develop the disease
C: Number of subjects unexposed and who have developed the disease
D: Number of subjects unexposed and who did not develop the disease

B. Size of cohort and case control studies

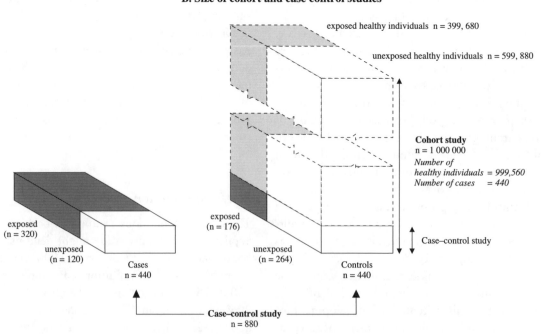

Figure 8.3 Directionality and size of cohort and case–control studies. For comments see Sections 8.3.4 (A) and 8.5.1 (B)

Table 8.3 An example of basic epidemiological information provided by cohort studies

	cases	non-cases	
exposed	320	399,680	400,000
	A	B	e
unexposed	C	D	u
	120	599,880	600,000
	440	999,560	p
			1,000,000 (population under study)

Key:
A, B, C, D: as in Figure 8.3
e: number of subjects exposed to the factor under study (**A** + **B**)
u: number of unexposed subjects (**C** + **D**)
p: number of all subjects under study (**A** + **B** + **C** + **D**)

appeared in the non-exposed group. Is there a strong and specific association between air pollution and respiratory problems? Table 8.3 illustrates the basic steps of analysis and computation of risks. Comments on interpretation follow.

Steps of analysis and basic information:

1. Is a different **distribution of cases** and non-cases in relation to exposure due to **chance only**? Statistical analysis (x^2 test for homogeneity) precedes epidemiological evaluation.

2. **Incidence rate in the population** under study. (Note for beginners: Before proceeding to comparisons of rates, note that the sizes of the groups in the example are not equal, i.e. 400,000 and 600,000 respectively. The group sizes must be made equal by establishing rates per 100,000. Rates of interest can then be compared, having denominators of equal size.)

$$I_p = \frac{A+C}{p} \times 10^n = \frac{320+120}{1,000,000} \times 100,000$$
$$= 44/100,000$$

3. **Proportion** of the population that is **exposed**. (prevalence of exposure in the population under study).

$$P_e = \frac{e}{p} = 0.4 \quad \text{(or 40\%)}$$

4. **Incidence rate**, i.e. cumulative incidence in this example (individual risk) **among the exposed.**

$$IR_e = \frac{A}{A+B} \times 10^n = \frac{320}{320+399,680} \times 100,000$$
$$= 80/100,000$$

5. **Incidence rate** (individual risk) **among the unexposed. 'Baseline risk' in EBM.**

$$IR_u = I_u = \frac{C}{C+D} \times 10^n$$
$$= \frac{120}{120+599,880} \times 100,000$$
$$= 20/100,000$$

6. **Relative risk** (risk ratio).

$$RR = \frac{I_e}{I_u} = \frac{80/100,000}{20/100,000} = 0.4$$

7. **Risk difference** (attributable risk).

$$RD \text{ (or AR)} = I_e - I_u$$
$$= 80/100,000 - 20/100,000$$
$$= 60/100,000$$

8. **Attributable fraction** (etiological fraction, attributable risk percent).

$$AF_e \text{ (EF or AR\%)} = \frac{RD}{I_e}$$
$$= \frac{I_e - I_u}{I_e} \times \ldots$$
$$\frac{80/100,000 - 20/100,000}{20/100,000}$$
$$= 75\%$$

9. **Attributable fraction** in the whole population under study.

$$AF_p = \frac{I_p - I_u}{I_p} \times 100 =$$
$$= \frac{44/100,000 - 20/100,000}{44/100,000} \times 100$$
$$= 54.5\% \quad \text{also: } \frac{e(I_e - I_u)}{p.I_p} \times 100$$

NB *An alternative (see case–control studies for comments) would be:*

$$AF_p = \frac{P_e(RR-1)}{1+P_e(RR-1)} \times 100 =$$

$$= \frac{0.4(4.0-1)}{1+0.4(4.0-1)} = \frac{1.2}{2.2} = 54.5\%$$

10. **Re-adjustment of individual risk estimates according to the internal validity of a diagnostic method (test) which identifies cases**[31,39].

S_p = test specificity (in decimal fraction). (For example, specificity, S_p, of the test used is 90% or 0.9.)

$$I_e = \frac{A - e(1-S_p)}{e}$$

$$I_u = \frac{B - u(1-S_p)}{u}$$

RR, RD, and AF are re-calculated on the basis of these two formulas, wherever relevant.

11. **Number needed to harm (NNH)**[35]:

NNH = 1 / [a/(a + b)] – [c/(c + d)]

NNH was proposed and is being used in the study of undesirable effects of treatment, such as adverse drug reactions. At present, its uses in other fields of etiological research require further development and evaluation.

Bender and Blettner[36] propose the following calculation of the 'number needed to be exposed for one additional person to be harmed (NNEH):

$$NNEH = \frac{1}{(OR-1) \times UER} + \frac{OR}{(OR-1) \times (1-UER)}$$

where
OR > 1 (harmful exposure) is the adjusted OR and UER is the unexposed event rate
(for derivations see Ref. 36).

The smaller the number of individuals exposed to a harmful factor needed to produce one additional case of disease, the more dangerous the factor. This might be used as an additional argument in defending health programs or other interventions against health problem-producing factors.

8.4.2 Comments on findings and their interpretation and meaning

In the comments that follow, a line is drawn between statistical analysis (tests of significance) and epidemiological analysis (comparisons of risks). In reality, both steps are based and their results interpreted on both statistical and epidemiological considerations. However, assessment of causality and of its criteria is primarily an epidemiological matter. Steps 2 to 10 give point estimates (^) of various measures for the purpose of basic understanding only. For all these measures, confidence intervals of the former are computed and are routinely given in the literature. This methodology is explained elsewhere[26,37]. In principle, the interpretation of confidence interval estimations is similar to the principles and philosophy of estimations of rates, as given in Section 5.6.3.

Step 1 – Statistical evaluation of the basic contingency table

A simple look at the table suggests unequal numbers of subjects in cells A, B, C, D. Is this the result of some random effect only, or is there more to be considered? Are differences in such a distribution according to health status and exposure due to factors beyond the sole effect of chance? In practical terms, are the differences between risk in exposed and unexposed individuals due to chance alone, or do these differences reflect more than random variation (i.e. a possible causal action of exposure)? Readers wishing to learn more about these concepts should consult Kleinbaum, Kupper and Morgenstern[26], Fleiss[38] or Breslow and Day's[39] monographs.

If this basic statistical evaluation of data from a cohort study yields **statistically significant results** (distribution of individuals according to their health status and exposure is not due to chance alone), the data merit further epidemiological analysis and interpretation. Insignificant results do not warrant further examination of data. Such a statistical evaluation is nothing more than a screening corridor (albeit a fundamental one) if further epidemiological analysis is warranted. It indicates the presence of differences, but does not indicate how important they are for assessing the causality, nor how important they are from the clinical or public health point of view. **Epidemiologically significant findings** are defined by the magnitude of the strength and specificity of the association under study and by fulfilling other criteria of causality. **Clinically significant findings** will depend on various values given to cure, care or failures.

Step 2 – Incidence rate in the population under study

This information gives an idea of the overall impact of disease on the whole community under study. (NB It is necessary to make a distinction between the population sample under study, if this is the case, or the target population, or the population to which the study results should apply or be extrapolated.) This information is also necessary to estimate attributable fraction (Step 9) for the whole population (exposed and unexposed together).

Step 3 – Proportion of the population exposed

Since a higher occurrence of disease is expected in exposed subjects, this measure is associated with the greater impact of disease in the community, once its association is established. The proportion of population exposed is required for computations of attributable fraction in the whole population under study (Step 9, alternative formula) and for adjustment of individual risk estimations according to the internal validity of diagnostic tests (Step 10).

Steps 4 and 5 – Incidence rates in exposed and unexposed groups

These are measures of individual risk in each of the groups, which can then be compared. If duration of exposure does not vary from one individual to another, simple incidence rates are used. If exposure does vary, incidence density rates are more appropriate to estimate individual risks. If the entire possible period of exposure is involved, attack rates are often used. For diseases with a high fatality rate, mortality rates reflect individual risk (NB Mortality =

incidence × case fatality). Prevalence rates are not a proper measure of risk, especially if disease duration varies. Fast-evolving cases (either benign or highly lethal) 'disappear' from prevalent cases, and may distort considerably the degree of individual risk (Neyman's or 'prevalence–incidence' bias).

Step 6 – Relative risk

This ratio of individual risks is a measure of the strength of an association. The greater the distance (contrast) between the rates in exposed and unexposed subjects, the stronger the association under study. If the relative risk is 1.0, there is no association, i.e. individual risks in exposed and unexposed subjects are the same. The greater the value of the relative risk of a disease-producing factor, the stronger the association between the presumed cause and the disease it produces. A relative risk of less than 1.0 is due to the fact that the individual risk in exposed individuals is lower than in unexposed individuals. Thus, the factor under study has a protective effect and not a harmful one.

How strong are the associations reflected by relative risk values? *Very arbitrarily, values under 2.0 (without any additional information) are not considered particularly strong with regard to practical decision-making. Given the prevalent size of studies, especially those of the case–control type (number of participants), low relative risks often have confidence intervals straddling values of 1.0. For example, a relative risk of 1.5 indicates a 50% excess of risk in the exposed group. If its confidence interval were 0.8–2.2, for example, the factor under study may play a putative role (the relative risk may be as high as 2.2), a protective role (the 'real' relative risk may be as low as 0.8), or no role at all (1.0 relative risk is also possible). In this range of relative risk (below 2.0), the lower limits of the confidence interval are often very close to a value of 1.0. Such study results, important for research, usually lead to more solid (and greater) studies, yielding better estimates of the strength of association. In practice, decision-makers look for 'overwhelming evidence', preferably without any doubt.*

Step 7 – Attributable risk

This measure gives a true rate in exposed subjects, due exclusively to the factor under study. The underlying logic is that both exposed and unexposed subjects are equally exposed to other factors that may cause the same health problem. For example, if smokers are compared to non-smokers in terms of the occurrence of respiratory problems, it is assumed that both groups breathe the same polluted air, or that an equal proportion of them are exposed to occupational hazards (toxic agents) provoking similar problems. Hence, their effect in unexposed individuals is subtracted from the effect in exposed individuals, because the same proportion of cases are due in probability to the other factors, in both unexposed and exposed groups. Understandably, from this 'residual rate', i.e. rate attributable to the factor under study only, it is possible to calculate the number of cases due to the factor. In the earlier example, it would be 4×60, i.e. 240 cases. Eighty (80) cases would be due to factors common to the unexposed group. Attributable risk is the measure of the specificity of association in terms of true rates. The closer the risk difference (attributable risk) to the whole individual risk in the exposed, the more exclusive (prevalent) is the causal role of this factor among others, representing the web of causes of the disease under study.

Step 8 and Step 9 – Attributable or etiological fraction

The concept of multiple causes means that cases can be due to any factor from this web. Besides attributable risk (risk difference), the proportion of the total risk (total of cases) represented by risk difference can be of interest. Such an etiological fraction (attributable risk percent) may be evaluated for the exposed group only (Step 8) or for the whole population (unexposed included – Step 9). In the latter case, the etiological fraction will depend on the proportion of the total population that is exposed to the factor. The smaller it is, the smaller the population attributable fraction compared to that of the exposed group.

The etiological fraction is another measure of the specificity of an association. The closer the value to 100%, the more specific the association is, i.e. the

factor under study occupies a preponderant place among all factors which are involved in disease etiology, known or unknown. This concept can be interpreted in two ways:

1. It indicates the part the factor plays in the overall impact of the whole web of causes; or
2. It allows for an estimate of the proportion of cases that might be prevented by the control of the factor under study. Such a possibility must, however, be verified by a clinical or community health trial (see Chapter 9). Results from an observational study may differ from those of an experimental study.

Step 10 – Estimation of the number needed to harm (NNH)[35,36]

There is no concrete number indicating what is 'acceptable' and what is not. While comparing the effect of two noxious factors, it can only be estimated which one is worse (i.e. requiring fewer exposed individuals to produce additional cases).

Step 11 – Correction of risk estimation according to the internal validity of tests

The considerations described above were made based on 'perfect' diagnostic methods identifying cases and non-cases in exposed and unexposed subjects. Sensitivity and specificity of tests, however, may vary, and consequently risk estimations may also vary. Formulas were proposed[31,40] for correction of rates and ratios computations according to the internal validity of the diagnostic method used. (NB Specificity, entered in the work-up of these formulas, disappeared during multiple transformations leading to the final formulas recommended by the authors.) If the internal validity of the tests is known, this procedure allows for a more realistic estimation of risks. Otherwise, false positive and false negative results can lead to misclassification of the subjects under study.

8.4.3 Advantages and disadvantages of cohort studies

Cohort studies within the limitations of the observational method produce reliable results, providing a good follow-up in time of both individuals and their exposure. Researchers wait for cases to appear and so cases rarely escape detection. The study can be planned. The risk of systematic errors (bias) is lower than in case–control studies. The assessment of exposure is not biased by the presence of disease. However, cohort studies:

- Are difficult to reproduce;
- Require a great deal of uniformity of study throughout time;
- Suffer from a considerable migration of participants (moving away, change of occupation, etc.);
- Have considerable sample sizes;
- Are costly.

Liddell's review[41], Breslow and Day's monograph[42] and others[28,43] will complete the reader's grasp and understanding of cohort studies.

8.5 Case–control study

The case–control approach also has its advantages and drawbacks. Before discussing these, however, the fundamental structure of case–control studies and their underlying logic should be understood. Case–control studies (syn. retrospective studies, 'trohoc' – as anagram of 'cohort', looking backward studies, case–compeer studies, case history studies, case referent studies, case comparison studies) are cross-sectional studies by definition. Instead of multiple measurements of health status and exposure as in cohort studies (at least two, at the beginning and at the end of a defined period), case–control studies are based on a single identification of health status and past or present exposure of each individual under study. In terms of direction, a case–control study 'starts by the endpoint of the natural history of disease' and 'looks backward' on exposure, which might lead to the consequence (disease) under study. Often, information on risk (incidence rates) is not available and the case–control approach must use other quantification tools, as partly outlined in Section 3.3.1.1:

> **Proportions** are any numbers of individuals (observations) with a given characteristic divided by the total number of individuals (observations) in the group of interest. Percentages or other decimal fractions are used to quantify a proportion.

Odds are ratios of the probability of an event occurring (like becoming ill) to the probability of the event not occurring (like staying healthy). Their values range from zero to infinity. *NB Probabilities range from 0 to 1.*

Odds ratios are ratios of two odds.

The following describes how the situation from Table 8.3 would be studied using a case–control approach. Usually, fewer subjects are studied than in cohort studies. Often, a limited number of cases are identified, and a control group of non-cases is chosen (one or more controls per case). It is only once this is done that exposure or non-exposure is identified in all participants. Another 2 × 2 basic table is obtained, with a great economy of time and means, allowing for several estimations of strength and specificity of causal relation.

8.5.1 Information provided

Consider the same situation as in the previously discussed cohort study of one million subjects, some of whom are exposed to air pollution (see Figure 8.3B). This might be studied based on a case–control approach: At a given moment, chronic respiratory problem sufferers would be detected, i.e. 440 individuals. A control group of non-cases, say 1:1, would be selected (unmatched). The following starting picture would be obtained.

	Cases	*Non-cases*
Exposed	A	B
Unexposed	C	D
	440	440

Once this information is available, cases and non-cases would reveal if they live in a polluted or unpolluted environment. A completed picture would follow:

	320	176
	A	B
	C	D
	120	264
	440	440

From this situation, estimations of strength and specificity can be obtained in a slightly different way. Individual risks in exposed and unexposed subjects cannot be computed in a case–control study. These studies are most often based on prevalent (not incident) cases, and denominators are unclear or unknown. Given the small size of the control group (in this example, 440 instead of 999,560), in 880 subjects (instead of one million), incidence rates would be quite different from a cohort approach. In addition, every second subject in this study suffers from respiratory problems, a situation once again different from that of a cohort. If rates of disease are low (approximately less than 5%) this reasoning can be used: In a cohort study of rare events, the relative risk formula can be simplified by excluding cases from the denominators of risk (320 and 120 respectively), these being even rarer in unexposed subjects:

$$RR = \frac{\dfrac{A}{A+B}}{\dfrac{C}{C+D}} = \frac{\dfrac{320}{320+399,680}}{\dfrac{120}{120+599,880}} = \frac{\dfrac{A}{B}}{\dfrac{C}{D}}$$

$$= \frac{AD}{BC} = \text{again appr. } 4.0$$

Risk ratio $\longrightarrow$ Odds ratio (cross ratio)

Hence, the risk ratio is approximated by a ratio of exposure or odds ratio.

If a case–control study adequately reflects a situation that might otherwise be evaluated by a cohort study, the odds ratio produced by the case–control approach may be used (as relative risk is elsewhere) to evaluate the strength of a causal association. The exposure–odds ratio for a set of case–control data is the ratio of odds[6] in favor of exposure among the cases (a/b) to the odds in favor of exposure in non-cases (c/d); this reduces to ad/bc. In the above example, the odds ratio is then 320 × 264 / 176 × 120, i.e. 4.0.

It may be said that the risk ratio is a risk ratio and the odds ratio is an odds ratio. The interpretation of the odds ratio, however, tends to approach that of the former. How was the same result produced, i.e. 4.0? In this case–control study, all incident cases were obtained (an ideal condition to facilitate understanding). In addition, the proportion of exposure in

controls as it exists in a real (cohort) situation was artificially estimated. Both estimations of the strength of causal association, cohort and case–control, lead to the same result.

Unfortunately, case–control studies often take place under much less favorable conditions; based on few prevalent cases (not incident ones) with denominators unknown or poorly known. For the sake of internal validity, controls are often matched by age or selected in some other way to resemble cases as closely as possible (by age, sex, etc.). The proportion of exposure in controls may differ considerably from what can be seen in a target population as a whole or in its non-diseased individuals. However, if a case–control study succeeds in evaluating odds as they exist in a cohort study, i.e. getting incident cases (all or their representative sample) **and** if the proportion of exposure in the control group found in the case–control study adequately reflects a proportion of exposure in the undiseased part of the target population, the odds ratio may well estimate the relative risk which would be obtained if the same situation were studied using a cohort approach.

8.5.2 *Matched pairs case–control studies*

In many studies, control groups are selected by choosing one more control for each case having one or more similar characteristics, such as age, sex, or any other risk marker or factor. These matched pairs require a different analysis. Theoretically, a basic 2×2 table (different from the previous tables) is created based on the concordance or discordance of exposure and disease in individuals representing each matched pair one by one. An estimation of odds ratio in such a table is made according to the ratio of the numbers of pairs, classified as discordant:

		Controls		
		Exposed	Unexposed	
	Exposed	r	s	
Cases				
	Unexposed	t	u	
				½ N

The estimation is then: OR = s / t

Relating pairs in cell s (case individual was exposed and control is found unexposed, i.e. the greatest distance between disease and exposure) and in cell t (cases are unexposed and their matched controls are found exposed, i.e. the shortest distance between exposure and disease). This ratio of within cell discordant pairs estimates the strength of association. Cases may be matched to more than one control. Detailed quantitative methodology of analysis is available elsewhere[38,39,43].

8.5.3 Estimation of specificity of a causal relationship in a case–control study

In a case–control study, there is no way to directly estimate individual risks. The above example contained 880 study subjects instead of one million, in which the ratio of respiratory problems was 1:1 (every second individual in the target population did not have respiratory problems). In case–control studies, the cohort situation is unknown. However, the odds ratio is known as an approximation of relative risk. Several substitutions can be made. Instead of an unknown **individual risk in exposed individuals**, it can be said that their (unknown) risk is four times higher (odds ratio = 4) than that of unexposed individuals. Instead of the **individual risk in unexposed individuals**, an odds ratio (as if they were compared to another unexposed group) of 1.0 characterizes them. Using these two approximations, Step 8 can be reproduced from cohort analysis (see above) to estimate the attributable fraction in the exposed group by:

$$AF_e\ (AR\%) = \frac{I_e - I_u}{I_e} \times 100 = \frac{OR - 1.0}{OR} \times 100$$

$$= \frac{4.0 - 1.0}{4.0} \times 100 = 75\%$$

An attributable fraction for the whole population can be estimated in a similar way, replacing the relative risk by an odds ratio in the formula:

$$AF_p = \frac{P_e (RR - 1.0)}{1.0 + P_e (RR - 1.0)} \times 100 = \frac{P_e (OR - 1.0)}{1.0 + P_e (OR - 1.0)}$$

$$= \frac{0.4 (4.0 - 1.0)}{1.0 + 0.4 (4.0 - 1.0)} \times 100 = 54.5\%$$

NB The proportion of exposure in a target population P_e, 40% in this example, must be obtained from other sources: routine data, other studies, small sample or pilot study estimations, etc.

In this example, both approaches give the same result, as ideally comparable (identical) data have been examined. Once again, the more prevalent the exposure in the target population (to which this case–control study applies), the closer the attributable fraction is to the attributable fraction in the exposed group.

8.5.4 Occurrence of disease and validity of odds ratio

The higher the prevalence of disease, the further the odds ratios are from relative risk estimations. Table 8.4 illustrates a fictitious situation in which the relative risk is always the same, but prevalence rates of disease are not. Roughly speaking, beyond 5%

Table 8.4 Relationship between disease occurrence and estimation of relative risk and odds ratio

	CA	NC			
Disease occurrence : 50%					
E	800	200	1,000	$RR = \dfrac{80\%}{20\%}$	**= 4.0**
NE	200	800	1,000	$OR = \dfrac{800 \times 800}{200 \times 200}$	**= 16.0**
Disease occurrence : 19%					
E	300	700	1,000	$RR = \dfrac{30\%}{7.5\%}$	**= 4.0**
NE	75	925	1,000	$OR = \dfrac{300 \times 925}{75 \times 700}$	**= 5.29**
Disease occurrence : 2.5%					
E	40	960	1,000	$RR = \dfrac{4\%}{1\%}$	**= 4.0**
NE	10	990	1,000	$OR = \dfrac{40 \times 990}{10 \times 960}$	**= 4.1**
Disease occurrence : 1.25%					
E	20	980	1,000	$RR = \dfrac{2\%}{0.5\%}$	**= 4.0**
NE	5	995	1,000	$OR = \dfrac{20 \times 995}{5 \times 980}$	**= 4.06**

E = exposed individuals; NE = non-exposed individuals; CA = cases; NC = non-cases

prevalence (as it is usually reported in textbooks), relative risks and odds ratios differ considerably.

Nevertheless, if the case–control approach is applied to a well-known cohort situation (where all individuals cannot be evaluated, such as in the investigation of large outbreaks of disease and their causes), and assuming both previously mentioned conditions exist (incident cases and a good knowledge of exposure), reliable estimations may be obtained. As a matter of fact, a case–control approach may be applied to the study of causes of disease outbreaks (see the following section *ad hoc*) or, for that matter, to any situation where a cohort would be too large to make a cohort study economical and feasible.

8.5.5   Numbers needed to harm derived from case–control studies

Once odds ratios (OR) are known, and knowing the adverse event rate in groups of individuals who are not exposed to the putative factor (PEER, i.e. patient expected event rate), NNHs can be estimated from case–control studies using the formula proposed by Sackett et al[35]:

$$NNH = 1 - [PEER \times (1 - OR)] / (1 - PEER) \times \ldots$$
$$PEER \times (1 - OR)$$

8.5.6   Advantages and disadvantages of case–control studies

Like cohort studies, case–control studies have their own advantages and disadvantages. They are **advantageous** because they:

- Are of short duration;
- Are relatively easy to do (but often much more difficult to conceive and build intellectually);
- Are repeatable (to some extent);
- Are less costly than cohort studies;
- Allow the study of rare diseases;
- Allow the use of more sophisticated methods of evaluation of subjects;
- Allow a considerable array of independent variables to be studied.

Disadvantages are also numerous:

- Often unclear identity of cases (prevalent, incident, some, all, from which denominators, etc.);
- Biases are difficult to identify and control;
- Subjects' recall of exposure in the past is limited, similar data do not often exist in clinical charts or other sources of data;
- Diagnostic criteria for cases and criteria for exposure are not always met if information is obtained only from existing data, like routine hospital or primary care records.

8.6   'Hybrid' designs of analytical studies

Because of the inherent disadvantages of cohort and case–control studies, several 'hybrid designs' were developed to make analytical studies as feasible as possible from the point of view of time and subjects involved. These designs are used and studies based on them are reported more often in the literature: case–control within control design[44,45], case–cohort design[46], nested studies[44], case–control studies 'with no controls'[47]. The principle of hybrid designs is a mix of cohort data introduced in case–control comparisons. Groups of interest (communities, industry, employees, etc.) are followed prospectively, their exposure or lack of it being identified at the beginning of the cohort follow-up.

8.7   Conclusions on causality

In any analytical study, conclusions regarding the presence or absence of a cause–effect relationship are a question of careful overall judgment and review of all important causal criteria. Unfortunately, this crucial rule is omitted in most studies. Authors are often happy with statistically significant results perpetrating a 'myth of small *p*'s'. Analysis and conclusions should go beyond this[48]. It should be remembered that a *P* value calculated from data only says that *'the probability that a set of observations as extreme as, or more extreme than, those actually observed would happen by chance alone'*[49,50]. It explains absolutely nothing about the magnitude of differences observed and their clinical and practical significance and meaning. In some cases,

Table 8.5 Demonstration of causality in epidemiology for certain cases

Criteria of causality	Smoking and lung cancer (Surgeon General, 1973)[51]	Adrenocorticosteroids and osteoporosis (Guyatt et al 1984)[52]	Social support and mental health (Broadhead et al 1983)[53]
Temporality	Yes	?	Yes
Strength	Yes	Contradictory results	Yes
Specificity			
Manifestational	Poorly known	Poorly known	Possible
Causal	Yes	?	?
Biological gradient	Yes	Possible	Yes
Consistency	Yes	No	Yes
Biological plausibility	Yes	Not well established yet	Yes
Coherence with prevalent knowledge	Yes	To be established	Yes
Analogy	Hard to assess	Hard to assess	Unknown
Experimental proof	Yes	Hard to make	Yes

relative risks or odds ratios are given, suggesting an unspecified 'association'. Any causal study should, however, clearly state which criteria are met. Table 8.5 illustrates that this may be done not only for the classical example of smoking and lung cancer[51], but also in studying clinical problems in internal medicine, such as the role of adrenocortico-steroids in osteoporosis[52] or the role of social support in mental health in psychiatric evaluative research[53]. Often, a lack of information, intellectual laziness, epidemiological ignorance, competition for research grants, or all of the above lead to unsatisfactory conclusions concerning the presence or absence of a causal relationship.

Very often, the weakest point of causal interpretation is the review of **'neglected' criteria**, such as a demonstration of biological and other, i.e. theoretical, factual, and statistical plausibility[54]. Table 8.6 illustrates the useful proposals of biological and social plausibility to better understand the possible role of toothpaste use in Crohn's disease (regional ileitis)[55]. Such explanations are often hypotheses to be pursued in future studies, but they also reinforce results of other studies. There is no scoring system for the demonstration of causality, especially when the demonstration is available only on the basis of observational studies. The final conclusion is a product of judgment.

Table 8.6 Consideration of plausibility of the etiological role of toothpaste in Crohn's disease

Observations about Crohn's disease	Possible explanation
19–20th century disease	Toothpaste is a modern development
Western disease	More toothpaste in the West
Recent epidemic	Dental hygiene improved
May occur in families	Families use same toothpaste
More common in Ashkenazi Jews	More Westernized
More common in smokers	Smokers brush more
More common in urban women	Less likely to spit after brushing
More common in white-collar workers	Brush more than blue-collar workers
Crohn's patients eat more sugar	Have to brush more
Very rare in infants	Teeth develop at about one year
Chronic disease	From chronic exposure to toothpaste
Most common in ileocecal area	Area of stasis
Panenteric disease	Whole gut exposed to toothpaste
Granulomas	Common histological response to foreign material
Transmural/local nodes	Material in migratory phagocytes
Postresection recurrence	Continued exposure to toothpaste

Source: Ref 55. Reproduced with permission from Elsevier Science (*The Lancet*)

8.8 Major prerequisites for valid etiological studies

Needless to say, any consideration of causality must be based on results of studies with satisfactory validity. Good **internal validity** relates to the design (architecture) of the study (how it is built), and **external validity** relates to the property of the study in order to accurately reflect the situation in the community (group of patients) to which study results apply. Table 8.7 outlines several of the most important prerequisites of good etiological studies. They require more comments as reviewed here.

8.8.1 *Exclusion of the effect of chance*

Chance and random variation are taken into account at two levels of epidemiological work: when making basic comparisons between study groups; and when presenting results. For example, in the cohort study in Table 8.4, a chi-square test[38] should be performed first. A result indicating a higher value than that in tables of critical values of χ^2, shows that the unequal distribution of observations in the exposed and unexposed groups is not due to chance alone. The

epidemiological analysis is justified and should follow. Later, when results are presented and interpreted, point estimates of risks must be associated with the presentation of interval estimates of resulting rates, ratios, and odds. The reason is the same as that presented in Chapter 1. For example, a 95% interval estimate of the relative risk in the above-mentioned example would be[56]:

$$RR_{IC95} = \underline{RR}.\overline{RR} = \hat{RR}^{1 \pm (1.96/\chi)}$$

A 'true' relative risk may be situated anywhere between the upper and lower limits of its confidence interval. For example, MacMahon et al[57], in their highly criticized study of the association between coffee drinking and pancreatic cancer, obtained point and interval estimates of odds ratios, reflecting a possible dose–effect relationship as illustrated by Table 8.8. A less experienced reader might notice that point estimates of odds ratios show some overall increasing trend with the number of cups of coffee per day. However, overlapping confidence intervals for these odds ratios without any detectable trend does not support such a conclusion (NB A statistical test for trend might be considered here.) Once again, the most conservative estimations are often taken into account (lower limits) in interpreting results for practical decision-making. Statistical formulas for interval estimations of relative risk, attributable risk, etiological fraction, or odds ratio are available in several original articles[58–60] and in specialized monographs[61,62] as well.

Table 8.7 Pre-requisites for consideration of causality

Pre-requisites for consideration of causality

- Exclusion of the effect of **chance** (tests of significance, statistical analysis), i.e. the association under study is not due to chance alone.
- Results consistent with **prediction**, i.e. if demonstrated through inductive research, the deductive approach should bring the same results.
- Observational study is designed in such a way that it closely follows the **golden rules** of the experimental approach.
- Studies are based on clinimetrically **valid data** (isolation, observation, classification, inference, definition).
- Sufficient **data** (sample size).
- **Unbiased** observation, comparison, analysis, interpretation.
- **Absence (or, more realistically, a strict minimum)** of uninterpretable and/or uncontrollable factors ('**confounders**').
- **Criteria of causality** satisfied.

Table 8.8 Is there any dose–effect relationship between coffee drinking and cancer of the pancreas in women?

Category	Coffee drinking (cups per day)				
	0	*1–2*	*3–4*	*> 5*	*Total*
Cases (no.)	11	59	53	28	151
Controls (no.)	56	152	80	48	336
Adjusted relative risk	1.0	1.6	3.3	3.1	2.3
95% confidence interval	–	0.8–3.4	1.6–7.0	1.4–7.0	1.2–4.6

Source: Ref 57. Abstracted and reproduced with permission from the Massachusetts Medical Society (*N Engl J Med*)

8.8.2 Predictable results

Predictable results require *a priori* formulation of hypotheses and studies constructed to refute or accept them. The deductive approach in causal analysis gives the opportunity to construct a study with less bias and uncontrollable factors than inductive research, which is based on currently available data.

8.8.3 Bringing observational analytical studies closer to the standards of experimental research

In experimental research (laboratory, clinical drug trials, etc.), studies are organized to obtain, if possible, irrefutable findings. Individuals in compared groups are similar in their characteristics: they are eligible for any maneuver under study; their prognosis and/or risk (excluding the principal maneuver) is comparable either by selection or by random assignment of subjects in groups, giving an equal representation of 'unequal' subjects (if *n* is large enough) in all groups to be compared. To do this, Horwitz et al[24,25] advocate the careful selection of subjects for observational studies, i.e. ideally those with no ethical or other obstacles, who would also be enrolled in an experimental study. Clinimetric assessment of cases (gradient and spectrum of disease), prognostic characteristics, equal susceptibility to exposure to the factor under study, to clinical maneuvers, and the clinical or paraclinical evaluation of their state (diagnostic procedures) among others should be considered. A similar approach is useful *a posteriori*, whenever the information is available, to assess the quality and validity of a cohort or case–control study already finished and presented to the public.

8.8.4 Good (clinimetrically valid) data

It is not enough to thoroughly define exposure in operational terms. As already stated in Chapters 5 and 6, operational criteria of qualitative and quantitative diagnosis for any relevant stage or end point of the natural or clinical course of disease are the absolute prerequisites of analytical studies. Without these criteria, the studies are uninterpretable. Health professionals, not statisticians, are responsible for the production of high-quality clinical and paraclinical data. This burden should never be shifted to statisticians, sociologists, demographers, or any other person who, many clinicians feel might 'better know how to perform studies involving many subjects'.

8.8.5 Sufficient number of study subjects (sample size)

The number of subjects in analytical studies, like elsewhere, should be 'just right'; not too few (the study would demonstrate nothing), or too many (even small relative risks would become significant; the study would demonstrate 'almost anything'). Basic computational formulas are currently available in the literature[60–63]. They may be used to calculate *a priori* sample sizes of a cohort or case–control study, or they may be used to evaluate what strength and specificity might be evaluated satisfactorily given the number of subjects involved in the *a posteriori* evaluated study[63,64]. (NB Smith and Bates[65] suggest that confidence limit analyses should replace *a posteriori* reassessment of epidemiological study power.) Most clinicians and other investigators will collaborate with biostatisticians to ensure that the right **study sample size** is determined. To perform these computations, basic elements are required[60,61].

For both cohort and case–control studies:
1. Alpha, or type I error (level of significance, or the rigor to confirm the null hypothesis, i.e. failure to confirm no difference between groups compared),
2. Beta, or type II error (probability of not detecting a significant risk that must be considered clinically and/or epidemiologically important),

and,

For a cohort study:	*For a case–control study:*
3. Relative risk value, which is considered important, and	Odds ratio value, which is considered important, and
4. Incidence of the disease in unexposed individuals.	Prevalence of exposure in the target population.

These computations go beyond the scope of this introductory text, but readers must realize the importance of these elements in designing and interpreting analytical studies. Statistical sampling and analysis will depend highly on these elements, given by clinicians and other health professionals to biostatisticians. Personal and professional experience must be shared here to achieve optimal results. Only health professionals can and must say what they want and what is important. Otherwise, they risk being forced by quantitative methodology specialists into some unexpected territories, sometimes salvaging a study, sometimes not. It is the primary responsibility and obligation of any health professional to provide specialists in quantitative methodology with scientifically and practically relevant requirements for objective expected results. Quite understandably, studies involving few subjects will detect only considerable risks, while large studies will allow the evaluation of more subtle associations.

8.8.6 Absence of bias

Assessing bias in analytical studies is paramount not only for providers of evidence (researchers), but also for consumers in their critical reading of the medical literature. As already mentioned, observational analytical studies should respect the rigors of experimental proof in all possible ways. For example, to obtain valid information on disease and exposure, multiple blinding is used in clinical trials: participants and clinicians are unaware of the identity of the maneuver (drug), outcome measures, and who belongs to which group under comparison. Similarly, it is desirable, **even in observational research,** to blind subjects, interventions, and outcomes. Thus, in a case–control study, interviewers or reviewers of records should not know who is a case and who is a control. Similarly, when several exposures are assessed, these interviewers should not be aware which one is of real interest and which outcome measure (from several under study) is 'real'.

Many controversial topics remain in the literature (Mayes et al[66] reviewed 56 of them) mainly due to faulty reasoning, design, and lack of ability to translate clinical knowledge such as disease history and course, diagnostic practices, treatment ordering, outcome assessment and follow-up into the study. Either **random errors** are made which are often

unavoidable, or **systematic errors (bias)** appear in study design, clinimetrics, interventions, evaluations, or interpretations. The latter represent a definition of bias. Hence, random errors, bias, or confounding factors may lead to erroneous conclusions and must be avoided. It is best to prevent these before the study begins and thus avoid later errors. The worst-case scenario is *a posteriori* recourse to various sophisticated quantitative techniques, aimed at salvaging the often unsalvageable. From the extensive array of bias[67–73], clinicians and other health professionals are primarily responsible for bias related to various omissions of clinical realities at various stages of analytical studies: initial state, maneuver, subsequent state. Table 8.9 gives some of their most important examples.

Correcting bias due to differences in demographic or other non-medical characteristics is not enough. Other systematic errors are due to a lack of attention to various clinical characteristics related to patients themselves, clinical practices and health professionals involved. Some are worthy of quoting as examples.

Susceptibility bias[72,73] can be produced by inequality of risk or prognosis in individuals, which cannot be randomized in observational studies. It may be caused by some confounding factor or by any other factor related to the way and moment of detection of disease, to different diagnostic practices, etc. These factors are often related to health problems other than the disease under study. For example, in the past, diethylstilbestrol may have been given to women who had problems with bleeding and/or pregnancy loss. These manifestations may be considered indicative of a future risk of clear cell carcinoma of the vagina, thus possibly unrelated risk markers and not risk factors (causes), common to some other health problems having these manifestations in their history of course. Susceptibility bias can arise if individuals in the groups to be compared are matched or subjected to stratification according to demographic characteristics only, and not according to their prognostic characteristics.

Remedies to susceptibility bias include:

- Clinically comparable initial states;
- Indications for treatment (maneuver) are comparable (hemorrhage, threatened abortion, etc.);

Table 8.9 Clinically important bias in etiological studies

Bias	Definition	Example	Precautionary measures
Initial state-related			
Susceptibility bias[74,75]	• Unequal risk or prognostic characteristics leading to unequal probability of outcome event	• Diethylstilbestrol and clear-cell vaginal carcinoma • Sex steroids and birth defects • Menopausal syndrome and endometrial cancer	• Randomization (if possible) • Adequate and stringent selection criteria • Narrow spectrum and gradient of cases • Knowledge of comorbidity and etiological co-factors (webs of causes and consequences) • Application of criteria of eligibility to randomization even if the study is observational
Protopathic bias[76,77]	• Reversal of cause–effect temporal sequence; presumed causal exposure is enhanced, modified, stopped, or avoided because disease (consequence) is already present	• Estrogens and endometrial cancer • Oral contraceptives and benign breast disease • Bronchodilators and death from asthma	• Understanding and respect of disease history and course
Lead time bias[78]	• Different methods of diagnosis lead to assembly of cases at unequal moments in disease history and/or course	• If cases detected by screening at an earlier stage are treated earlier, their survival is longer (difference between the screening and routine moments of detection): treatment is more efficient in screened cases	• Proper timing of diagnostic procedures and follow-up with respect to disease course and history
Maneuver-related			
Proficiency bias[5]	• Inadequate dosage, route, site, frequency of interventions within and between compared groups (maneuvers)	• Better compliance with principal maneuver (treatment, etc.) leading to principal maneuver having more impact than a control maneuver.	• Comparable quality and quantity of principal and control maneuvers • Blinding
Attrition bias[28]	• Losses of participants and/or information during the period of application of maneuvers or movement of individuals from one group to another	• Cases that are too light or too serious are withdrawn from one of the groups, making maneuvers more or less outcome-related	• Larger samples • Analysis of comparability of dropouts, migrants between groups and complying of participants
Subsequent state-related			
Detection bias[5]	• Outcome noted in two compared groups has been detected in an unequal manner	• Unequal diagnostic methods, criteria, frequency and timing, or interpretation lead to different frequencies of outcomes in groups compared	• Identical diagnostic maneuvers, frequencies, and moments of outcome assessments • Multiple blinding

- Prognosis is comparable (age, sex, comorbidity, cotreatments, diagnostic and therapeutic maneuvers in the past).

More generally, comparability at the moment of initial state must include the following:

- State of health;
- Equal probability of having the problem diagnosed;
- Equal probability of treatment (access, etc.);
- Equal probability of follow-up;
- Comparable clinical spectrum and gradient;
- Equal probability and access to exposure to the factor under scrutiny;
- Equal prognosis;
- Guarantee of equal access to information;
- Quality of information is comparable concerning reading and interpretation of patients' information, clinical and paraclinical data; and ideally
- Eligibility of subjects to randomized controlled clinical trials.

Protopathic bias[76,77] can best be defined as the use of any clinical procedure (diagnostic, treatment), influenced by an already present early manifestation of disease, which has not yet been detected. The clinical procedure can be started, modified, or withdrawn in response to the clinical features of the disease under study. Hence, the consequence replaces the cause. For example, if estrogens are prescribed as treatment for bleeding as an early manifestation of an already present endometrial cancer, they may erroneously be considered as its cause. **Whereas susceptibility bias concerns several pathologies, protopathic bias is a problem within a single pathology** ('within disease' bias). The cause of this bias is that clinical intervention follows (and is indicated for) the first, often non-specific, manifestations of the disease, or that the treatment is initiated before the diagnosis is made, whatever the reason may be. Protopathic bias can be avoided by knowing and respecting the natural and clinical history and course of disease, current clinical practices and decisions, and by choosing individuals in the study not only according to their manifestations (prodromes), which are often non-specific, but also according to a comparable moment in their disease history and course.

In the case of **detection bias,** the unequal performance of maneuvers or observations in all groups compared is responsible for the problem. Any loss of study subjects, information, or any other kind of non-uniform assessment of outcome as the subsequent state may produce detection bias[5,79]: unequal general medical surveillance of subjects; frequency and types of diagnostic procedures; and criteria of their interpretation. When the problem of interpretation arises, serious challenges stem from the application of the law of initial value[70], where distinctions must be made between reaction, adaptation or faulty adaptation (e.g. when interpreting changes of levels of circulating hormones, etc.). Detection bias is essentially due to the inequality of clinical process, be it the frequency of examinations or treatment plans. It concerns diagnosis, assessment of exposure (risk), but mainly evaluation of results (outcome). One or all may occur. Wells and Feinstein[80] performed a case–control study to determine whether the autopsy suggestions of detection bias in the diagnostic pursuit of lung cancer were confirmed by the way that sputum and Pap smears were ordered in an outpatient setting. Results suggested that female non-smokers may be deprived of appropriate diagnosis and therapy unless a diagnostic work-up for this neoplasia is guided by radiographic findings and presenting manifestations. In etiological considerations, detection bias has probably led to an overestimation of the strength of association for male smokers and to a falsely low estimate of incidence rates in women.

Remedies to detection bias are: uniform observation of individuals and groups ('no peeking into data by curiosity'), identical study protocols for groups to be compared, and verification that other maneuvers do not lead to unequal follow-up.

One of the most important components of advanced training in epidemiology is the acquisition of skills for the avoidance and control of a maximum number of random errors and bias. Elsewhere, many **spurious correlations** (cause–effect considerations) stem from a lack of biological plausibility in the associations made between presumed causes and their effects. Sometimes, early consequences are incorrectly taken to be causes: The rapid fall of a barometric reading in summer is not the cause of a storm[90], erratic mitoses and multiplication of cells are not the cause of cancer. Readers of medical articles should know these potentially undesirable characteristics of studies and be able to assess the real quality of scientific information and its relevance for practical use and adoption.

8.8.7 Satisfactory presentation of resulting data

Any study must provide enough data to enable the reader to understand the method of description and the analysis used. All observations cannot be presented, but all basic frequencies and descriptive parameters should be. It may be interesting to note the relative risk or etiological fraction but such a finding is less interesting if basic contingency table(s) are not provided. Essential raw data are needed to judge the strong and weak points of the study.

8.8.8 Realistic and critical interpretation and conclusions

It is not a sign of weakness or incompetence to reveal and review points where a study may have failed or did not stand up to expectations. On the contrary, this information is extremely valuable in assessing the importance of findings, and it also gives direction to further research. Conclusions must include what the study brings to scientific research and what it means for medical practice: how should results be used in medical decision-making? Specifically, in the case of analytical observational studies, demonstrations of causality are not final in terms of the identification of risk factors. Also, associations must be shown as biologically plausible and any independent variable remains a risk characteristic as long as it is not confirmed as a risk factor by an experimental study, i.e. in a clinical trial or community health program trial. Until then, conclusions on the role of risk factors remain only provisional, no matter how closely they correspond to most criteria of causality.

8.9 Advanced quantitative methods in etiological research. Multivariate and multivariable analysis

Any reader of current medical literature will quickly find that studying one cause and one consequence is the exception rather than the rule. Nowadays, such analyses are based most often on more complex models than 2×2 tables, and they are more difficult to visualize.

8.9.1 Studying more than one cause at a time

Until recently, examples of studies given here concerned simplified 'one cause → one consequence' models. Now, several causal factors are very often implicated (web of causes) in disease occurrence, and exposures lead to several health problems (web of consequences). The development of remarkable biostatistical techniques in **multivariate** (several independent variables, 'causal factors') and **multivariable** (several dependent variables, consequences, ensuing health problems) research and their execution through electronic computing led to their widespread use in clinical and epidemiological research. They must be used and interpreted critically[81–84].

Linear regression, logistic regression, discriminant function analysis and proportional hazards regression (Cox regression) seem to be the most prevailing multivariate methods in the current medical literature[85,86]. If these methods (less familiar to readers of medical literature) are becoming standard, at least their basic characteristics and principles[3,78,81–83] should be outlined here for future basic understanding. References are also given for more advanced readings[26]. Several factors (smoking, drinking, dietary habits, etc.) can be studied in relation to one disease without paying attention to the temporal–spatial relationship between those factors. **Logistic regression analysis**[86], which the reader will find most often in research papers on etiology or treatment, can serve as an example. This methodology is introduced more in depth to health professionals in several reader-friendly papers[87–92] and chapters[93].

In other situations, it may be interesting to study how various causes (factors) interact in which sequence, and which is the strongest trajectory in such a web of simultaneously and successively appearing causes. For example, path analysis and more recently, structural equation models (G. Norman – personal communication) belong to this second category. In a good body of medical research, it is valuable to know how one variable depends on (predicts) another one. For example, how does pulse rate increase with workload? A similar evaluation of a web of causes requires the study of more than one independent variable. An internist may be interested, for example, to see if blood pressure is related to salt intake (X_1), lifestyle (X_2), various endocrine gland activity (X_3), age (X_4), renal function (X_5), etc. Such a relationship becomes a **multiple linear regression** equation. When studying such relationships, not only are basic relationships established, but a subset of independent variables that still satisfactorily predict the dependent variable under study can be selected.

A **multiple logistic regression model** is used when the dependent variable is binary, like dying from or surviving some exposure (noxious factor, beneficial treatment), developing or not some health problem of interest. This model allows the estimation of individual or relative risks (or odds ratios) when taking into account not only a particular exposure (factor) under study, but also other possible causal factors representing webs of causes. This model, like multiple linear regression, also has the additional advantage of allowing quantitative and qualitative (categorical) independent variables to be studied as well. Regression coefficients for each independent variable under study (beta coefficients), obtained from logistic regression analysis, can be used to estimate individual risks of disease on the basis of all contributing causal factors found in a patient and covered by the study. Also, beta coefficients from the logistic regression analysis can be transformed into odds ratios for the purposes of etiological research. Contributing variables are tested for their statistical significance (their *p*-values). Confidence intervals are also established and published together with point estimations of associations of interest. Those worthy of further attention are evaluated for their contribution as one of several potential causes. Further analyses, as well as their advantages and disadvantages, extend beyond these introductory comments and may be found elsewhere[92].

Logistic regression is appropriate if response (dependent) variables are qualitative or binary, i.e. yes or no (like becoming ill or staying healthy, dying or staying alive, etc.). If more than two categories of outcomes are of interest, like stages of disease or prognostic subgroups, **ordinal logistic regression** is recommended[88]. Logistic regression can be used for risk predictions on the basis of cross-sectional and longitudinal data as well. Estimations of individual and relative risks (odds ratios) through logistic regression and further analyses are included nowadays in most major statistical packages (programs) like SPSS[94], making them available to a large number of users.

Readers of medical journals will often find 2×2 tables presented in articles, relating a particular causal factor to its consequence. However, various risks are not computed solely from this table, but from all relevant information available (i.e. several independent variables through logistic regression). Hence, discrepancies between estimations from simplified tables of categorical data and numerical information from multivariate analysis are understandable.

Besides logistic regression, other etiological research focuses, for example, on various moments in disease history and course, during which various causal factors appear. They often have a different impact from one moment in disease history to another. Etiological factors can also be studied in relation to morphological stages of disease, such as in the molecular epidemiology of cancer.

In psychiatry, Brown, Harris and Peto[33] and Paykel[95] introduced the notion of '**brought-forward time**', i.e. average time by which the spontaneous onset of mental disorders can be considered to be advanced by life events like the death of a close one, illness, financial ruin, etc. Some life events provoke several weeks of brought-forward time in schizophrenia or depression, suggesting a **triggering effect**. The **formative effect** is considered if brought-forward time represents more than 12 months[33], such as bereavement in mixed psychiatric illness[24].

8.9.2 Studying relationships in space and time between various possible causal factors

Multivariate analysis as described above allows obtaining some kind of hierarchy between causal factors accordingly to their strength (odds ratios) and specificity (attributable risk percent, syn. etiological fractions). In addition to that, we may be also interested in 'what leads to what', i.e. if there is any chaining or sequence between various possible causal factors and their consequences in time and space. What is the right path through the maze of interlinked factors and their consequences? In such an additional approach, sequence and interactions between various factors can be studied through **path analysis**[21]. The method of path coefficients is a form of structured linear regression analysis with respect to standardized variables in a closed system (formally complete)[21]. This technique invokes hypothetical linear relationships among variables and assesses the nature of these and consequential relationships by estimating correlation coefficients and their functions[96]. Path analysis was used to study interactions between risk factors of mortality in very low birth weight children[97] or interrelationships between health determinants of infant mortality[98], predicting fatigue in systemic lupus erythematosus[99], possible causal factors of respiratory problems in children and adults[100], utilization of medical services due to the post-traumatic stress disorder and other factors[101]. In nursing sciences, factors influencing the academic performance of students were also studied this way[102]. In operational research, various factors determining the use of physician services can be studied, such as age, sick days, or chronic health problems.

Path analysis evaluates, through various path coefficients, the one most likely 'path' or sequence of factors leading to the consequence of interest. Introduction to this methodology can be found in Li's monograph[21]. Path analysis and its results will depend largely on a prior knowledge and concept of webs of causes and their temporal spatial relationships. Relevant variables must be introduced in the model, and the model must reflect as much as possible the reality of the phenomena under study. Figure 8.4 shows such a model on the utilization of physician services[21]. By looking at the size of path coefficients, the most plausible 'causal path' may be 'age – chronic problem – sick days – use of physician services' (i.e. bold-faced path). Sewall Wright's path analysis[103], conceived in the 1920s was criticized for its qualities and shortcomings as well[96,104].

Biostatisticians prefer nowadays **structural equation modeling**[105] to path analysis[106]. Structural equation modeling studies also 'paths' or relationships between multiple causes and their consequences. The main difference between path analysis and structural equation modeling is that path analysis looks at relationships among measured variables only, whereas structural equation modeling examines both measured variables and the latent ones[106]. Latent variables are those which are not measured directly, like for example patient cultural and religious values (non measured) defining his or

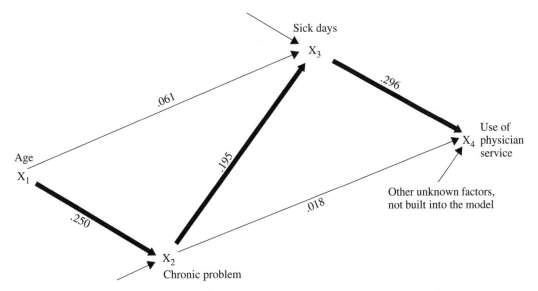

Figure 8.4 A model for path analysis. Utilization of physician services in relation to age, chronic conditions and sick days. Source: Adapted from Ref. 21

her compliance (measured) with some treatment regimen. This kind of modeling, however, allows for testing hypotheses, which cannot be studied by other multivariable methods like multiple regression only and others. This model takes into account also measurement error and brings together the measurement model and the structural model (relationships between variables). All paths in both models are estimated and evaluated simultaneously. It incorporates the strengths of several multivariable analytical methods in a single model that can be evaluated statistically and it permits directional predictions among variables and modeling of indirect effects as well[105]. As an example of its practical applications, we may quote studies describing such diverse topics as how objective and perceived neighborhood and environment predict mental health and behavior in adolescents[107], factors influencing adherence to cancer control regimens[108], factors important in self-reporting symptoms, awareness, and fear of hypoglycemia in insulin-treated diabetes patients[109], or the role of various factors acting upon nurses' role performance and ultimately patient outcomes[110].

8.9.3 Study of genetic factors as causes of disease

The study of genetic factors as causes of disease represents another challenge. Classical epidemiology focused essentially on environmental factors. Once all etiological fractions attributed to exogenous factors were accounted for, reasoning short-circuited the problem of web of causes, often stating that the rest (often unknown) were or had to be due to hereditary factors. Most health problems are not exclusively of environmental or genetic origin. The contribution of both factors varies from one disease to another. Primary liver cancer, acute respiratory problems, peptic ulcers are mostly due to environmental factors; hypertension, diabetes or breast cancer may carry more weight from endogenous factors; galactosemia or phenylketonuria are mostly due to genetic factors.

From the wider methodological array of **genetic epidemiology**[111–121], it must be stressed that the basic reasoning in genetic epidemiology is not alien to analytical reasoning as mentioned above. It is, however, applied to studies and populations which are more specific in the study of genetic factors, such as studies of families, subsequent generations, siblings, homozygotic and heterozygotic twins sharing or not sharing similar living conditions, and exposure to competing environmental factors, which complete the expected webs of causes. In etiologic research focusing on genetic factors, studies are also based on comparisons of disease occurrence. Groups of individuals having a more or less close genetic link are compared to assess the weight of genetic and environmental factors. For example, in studies of twins, disease occurrence in both monozygotic and heterozygotic twins can be compared. These concepts were applied to various problems. In psychiatry, Gregory and Smeltzer[116] attributed an etiological fraction between 38 and 100% to genetic factors in the etiology of manic-depressive psychosis, and between 19 and 84% in schizophrenia. Other approaches are based on judgment. Both approaches are summarized in Table 8.10 (see also Childs[121]), reviewing several situations and allowing the possibility of a genetic rather than an environmental etiology. Genetic epidemiology is a young but very promising field with many interfacing domains. Exploration of the human genome is one of its challenges[122]. Results of studies indicating an endogenous or exogenous etiology are crucial for prevention programs. In the former, problem solving is based in the laboratory; in the latter, it depends on the community.

More recently, **biological markers** have become an additional focus of etiological research. Biological markers, which may be found in body liquids or tissues, fall into two categories. In medicine, biological markers include measures of **exposure**[123,124], categories such as levels of solvents or lead in the blood, chemical metabolites in body tissues (e.g. trichloroacetic acid in urine from trichloroethylene exposure) as measures of **reaction to exposure**[125]. Elsewhere, some target or surrogate tissues are studied, such as acetylcholinesterase activity in pesticide poisoning, tumor markers or chromosome aberrations in lymphocytes. These are rather **diagnostic tools**[125–128]. The former imply a study of risk (etiological research), the latter should be

Table 8.10 Some considerations on prevalent causes of diseases

Mostly hereditary (genetic) factors	*Mostly environmental factors*
1. Clustering of cases in chronological time (e.g. 20-year-olds are mainly affected, independent of the calendar year)	1. Clustering in calendar time
2. Higher occurrence in monozygotic than dizygotic twins	2. The occurrence is independent of multiple births
3. Random occurrence in birth order	3. Occurrence according to a particular birth order (kwashiorkor – 'third child disease')
4. Occurrence independent of mother's age	4. Occurrence associated with the age of the mother
5. Occurrence higher in natural than adopted children	5. Equal occurrence in natural and adopted children
6. Excess occurrence in some racial or ethnic group (Tay-Sachs disease)	6. Occurrence unrelated to race or ethnic characteristics
7. Occurrence parallel with some already-known hereditary problems or characteristics (blood group A and diabetes, O and peptic ulcer)	7. No link between hereditary phenomena and occurrence under study
8. A hereditary trait demonstrated in animals for disease(s) common to man and animal	8. No hereditary trait in animals, no known model of occurrence
9. Occurrence higher in relatives than in non-relatives	9. Occurrence unrelated to family relation
10. Occurrence of problems elevated at specific anatomic and/or physiological sites in related subject, more so than in general population	10. Occurrence unrelated to a particular site in relatives
11. Excessive consanguinity in cases of recessive traits	11. No excess consanguinity in recessive traits
12. Higher occurrence in natural children of parents having the disease than in adopted ones (toxemia)	12. Occurrence similar in natural and adopted children of parents having the problem under study
13. The problem appears at a typical age, independent of any known or foreseeable provoking or precipitating event	13. The problem appears at a given age but it is preceded by a known provoking or precipitating event or factor

the subject of assessment of the markers' internal and external validity among others. In psychiatry, '*biological markers*', also called '*trait markers*'[124], are (for example) twins, relatives or living in adoption. On the other hand, the tyramine challenge test in depressed patients, the dexamethasone suppression test in affective and psychotic disorders, or enzymatic abnormalities in alcoholics represent 'biological markers' which are helpful for diagnosis. Before biological markers are further described, they must be better specified. It should always be specified in which sense the term 'biological markers' is being used: biological markers of exposure or risk on one hand; or biological markers of susceptibility[129], early biological response[130], and early or surrogate diagnosis on the other.

8.10 Investigation of disease outbreaks and their causes

The term 'outbreaks', often substituted for epidemics, is most often used when speaking of common source epidemics, like any diarrheal disease after a common meal or from a particular water source. The term 'outbreak' is less often used in studies of person-to-person spread. An **outbreak** is currently defined as an epidemic limited to a localized increase in the incidence of disease, e.g. in a village, town, or closed institution[6]. It is a disease occurrence beyond its usual expectations at a given place and at a given time. Any physician may witness and be involved to a variable degree in an investigation and control of a disease outbreak. He or she must know how an investigation is performed and why. Consider this detailed explanation: In essence, epidemiological investigations of epidemics regroup all steps of epidemiological work:

- Description of event;
- Identification of cause(s);
- Intervention (i.e. control of an outbreak); and
- Evaluation of the success.

From the point of view of causal research, an investigation of an outbreak represents a simultaneous evaluation of many possible causes (hypotheses). Wedding banquet attendees or community members sharing meals at a county fair may become ill by eating one or more meals contaminated by a diarrhea-provoking microbial agent. Elsewhere, noxious gases (carbon monoxide), heavy metals (lead, mercury), or simple irritants (heat, sulfur dioxide) may provoke signs and/or symptoms, and non-specific manifestations common to microbial (bacterial and viral) infections, chemical poisoning, or to a mass psychogenic illness[131] (a more socially acceptable euphemism for mass hysteria reactions).

What is the cause, what is the diagnostic entity, where should intervention take place? The general approach is multidisciplinary. Clinical medicine evaluates cases, paraclinical methods are used (bacteriological analysis of food samples), epidemiological studies focus on the establishment of causal links by multiple comparisons of exposure and cases and on the evaluation of the impact of control measures. The latter is often 'left alone' if biological material is not available, and environmental factors and individuals under study become out of reach. Table 8.11 gives an overview of the steps of an epidemiological investigation in an outbreak, along with the elements of a report on the investigation and control of an outbreak. Many elements of the investigation are found in the report. Many of the steps mentioned should be commented on. Any health professional should know how these investigations work. Even when not directly involved, the kind of information, which might be requested, what to look for, what to pay attention to, and what reported results mean should be understood.

To perform an epidemiological analysis, multiple comparisons are made to verify multiple hypotheses. Table 8.12 represents such a result based on an outbreak of gastrointestinal disease in Ottawa in 1975[132]. From 126 persons eating different meals at a social gathering, eaters and non-eaters of various meals were identified, and attack rates of disease were identified in each of them. A cohort approach was chosen in this example, but if the situation were suitable for a case–control study for any reason (e.g. a large outbreak for which it is not possible to follow all cases of exposure and disease), this approach might be advisable[133]. Essentially, several cohort comparisons are performed here, and the strongest and most specific association is sought between exposure to a given meal and disease. Differences in attack rates, i.e. attributable risks, lead to the implication of sauce, carrots, potatoes and peas as possible vehicles of infection. As a matter of fact, more than one vehicle is often found; meals may be contaminated by the same person (carrier), may be mixed together, stocked in poor conditions, etc. Comparable attributable risks may be re-evaluated by the additional computation of etiological fractions of each exposure yielding comparable high attributable risk.

In addition to this, cross-tabulations may be performed linking the distribution of a case according to either or both exposures (meals) under study in this example:

		Sauce	
		Eaters	*Non-eaters*
	Eaters	cases (n)	cases (n)
Carrots		x	w
	Non-eaters	y	z
		cases (n)	cases (n)

A comparison of discrepant cases **w** and **y** may yield additional useful information. Once again, all causal criteria must be reviewed and final conclusions drawn in connection with the clinical assessment of cases and laboratory results (cultures, serology), veterinary inquiry into cases of anthropozoonoses, biology (assessment of vectors), toxicology, etc. For a more practical example, readers may be interested in Goldsmith's monograph on the investigation of various infectious and non-infectious problems in communities[134].

In **mass psychogenic illness outbreaks**[135–137] (see other cases in these references), subjects report

Table 8.11 Phases of an investigation: components of a report dealing with the investigation of an outbreak

Investigation of an outbreak	*Report of an outbreak investigation and control*
1. Verification of the diagnosis of index and subsequent cases	1. Introduction – description of the sanitary situation before the occurrence of the outbreak
2. Confirmation that disease occurrence reached epidemic proportions	2. Description of the situation leading to the investigation (what happened and who brought it to the attention of the investigators)
3. Notification of cases	3. Definition of cases (with inclusion and exclusion criteria)
4. Active search for additional (hidden and forgotten) cases	4. Description of data collection and of laboratory and other techniques of analysis of clinical and paraclinical data
5. Identification of common exposure and formulation of first hypotheses	5. Description of the epidemic: • Chronology; • Morbidity, mortality, case fatality; • Assessment of a possible 'iceberg' of the event
6. Epidemiological description of common experiences (attack rates)	6. Epidemiological analysis: • Tabulation of individual experiences and cases; • Comparison of attack rates and exposures; • Statistical analysis; • Epidemiological interpretation; • Rectifications taking into account late-occurring cases
7. Comparison of common experiences by cohort approach (if small epidemic)	7. Laboratory results (isolations, typing, concentration of toxic chemicals, etc.)
8. Laboratory analysis of all suspect sources, vehicles or vectors	8. Explanation of possible causes and modes and ways of spread
9. Formulation of the hypothesis of outbreak cause(s), usually by induction	9. Description of individual and collective measures to control disease spread (treatment, immunization, testing, sanitary measures in the environment, etc.)
10. Elaboration of the outbreak's control program, aimed at: • Sources of agent; • Modes of spread; • Agent carriers; • Diseased individuals; • Still-healthy individuals	10. Evaluation of the effectiveness of outbreak control measures
11. Verification of the effectiveness of control measures	11. Long-term recommendations dealing with the problem causing the outbreak and disease under investigation
12. Sanitary protection of the territory	
13. Writing the report on the epidemic	
14. Epidemiological surveillance, sequel to the investigation and event reported	

Table 8.12 Food-specific attack rates – what is the cause (vehicle of agent)?

Food	Number of persons who ate specific food				Number of persons who did not eat specific food				Difference in percent*
	ill	well	total	percent ill	ill	well	total	percent ill	in percent*
	❶	❷	❸	❹	❺	❻	❼	❽	❾ = ❹ – ❽
Steak	58	11	69	84	1	2	3	33	51
Sauce	59	8	67	88	–	5	5	0	88*
Mushrooms	54	7	61	89	5	6	11	46	43
Carrots	59	8	67	88	–	5	5	0	88*
Potatoes	59	11	70	84	–	2	2	0	84*
Peas	59	9	68	86	–	4	4	0	86*
Tomato juice	52	10	62	84	7	3	10	70	14
Parfait	52	9	61	85	8	3	11	73	12
Coffee	48	10	58	83	12	2	14	86	–3
Drinks	57	9	66	86	2	4	6	33	53
Ice	55	13	68	81	4	–	4	100	–19

*Possible vehicles as suggested by highest attributable risks.
Source: Based on data from Ref. 132, reproduced with permission of Health Canada (Minister of Public Works and Government Services)

manifestations similar to index cases of other organic problems (intoxications, etc.), or show signs or report symptoms which may otherwise be confounded with other health problems. In the presence of such non-specific manifestations, investigators proceed by exclusion. Often, food poisoning, pesticide intoxication, heavy metal or solvent exposure must be excluded by clinical, paraclinical, and laboratory toxicological methods before a mass psychogenic illness outbreak is declared. These cases are often socially and politically delicate and evidence must be strong. Enquiries by exclusion may also be very expensive.

Participants in an outbreak investigation will find an increasing number of statistical packages for personal computers on the market. Such software facilitates user recording of individual data and experiences, their comparisons, computations of risks and the production of descriptive information. It also gives proposals for possible causal agents on the basis of computed incubation periods and other descriptive data provided.

8.11 Epidemiologic proof of causality in court. Contributions of physicians to decision-making in tort litigation

Individual patients and whole communities sometimes complain and sue when they doubt medical decisions, effects of industrial and other environmental factors, or their possible role in perceived poor health. Did a physician's care and decisions during a difficult labor lead to a newborn's brain damage? Did exposure of a population to air pollutants in an urban area lead to a high occurrence of respiratory problems? Does toxic waste disposal lead to leukemia outbreaks and clusters? Is cancer in military veterans due to exposure to chemical warfare agents? The notion of 'evidence' is important not only to physicians in times of 'evidence-based medicine', but equally, if not more broadly, in the field of law. A common language is currently being constructed[138,139]. Common understanding is vital wherever and whenever medical findings are used outside, 'in the real world', such as in tort litigations in courts of law. Physicians and other providers of health information who may be potential expert witnesses must all know the fundamentals of doctor–lawyer interplay. Physicians and epidemiologists are increasingly called upon as expert witnesses to express their opinions about such kinds of cause–effect relationships. They are requested to answer two kinds of questions:

1. Is there in general a cause–effect relationship between a presumed medical or non-medical factor (treatment, pollution, etc.) and a particular disease (cancer, etc.)?
2. Did this particular factor cause a health problem in this particular individual?

Levin defined a general approach to these proofs as follows[140]: '. . . *The standard of proof in the courtroom is similar to that in clinical medicine. To be indicted as a causative factor in an illness, an agent must be shown to a reasonable degree of medical certainty to cause or substantially contribute to that illness. This standard of proof is true for infectious and toxin associated diseases in clinical medicine . . .*' More specifically, two levels of decision must be made. In **civil law**, it must be demonstrated that a particular agent or act is a ***more probable than improbable cause*** of a given health problem (in other words, 'this one rather than the other one'). In **criminal law**, proof beyond a reasonable doubt is not enough, and it must be demonstrated that a health problem in litigation (paralysis, coma, death) is ***due to and* only to** a given factor (cause). In other terms, 'it cannot be the other one'. Hoffman[141] summarizes this point as follows: '. . . *Whereas scientific proof and statistical significance rest by convention on demonstration of a 95 per cent or greater probability that the results of an experiment or investigation were not due to chance, in civil tort cases the most widely used standards of proof require a 'preponderance of evidence', 'more likely than not' a '50.1 per cent or more probability', 'but for', or 'reasonable medical certainty'. Probable is defined as 'having more evidence for than against'. 'Preponderance of evidence' is defined as 'evidence of greater weight or more convincing than the evidence which is offered in opposition to it . . . 'preponderance' denotes a superiority of weight'. In criminal cases, the usual standard of proof is 'beyond a reasonable doubt'.*

Therefore, quantitative epidemiologic data must be expressed more qualitatively in the courtroom . . .' In general, it must be drawn from up-to-date knowledge of specific evidence and research. The question of whether the criteria of causality (as reviewed in this chapter) were met[142,143] is also important. (NB The latter are not fixed, but they evolve with technology[143].)

First and foremost, were all variables (cause, effect, etc.) well defined qualitatively and quantitatively? Was exposure well defined and quantified? Are health problems defined satisfactorily from the point of view of clinimetrics? What is fatigue? What is malaise? What is a lack of concentration? Frequently, very soft and non-specific clinical data are presented as evidence, and only physicians can help the court make a 'right' decision. Did cause really precede effect? Did the plaintiff begin to lose weight before or after using a suspect household cleanser? Many cases are motivated by greed and come from poorly defined areas; others are much more serious.

Is the causal link under review strong and specific enough?

In civil law, if one cause is known, its etiological fraction should be superior to 50%; if more etiological factors are known, should the etiological fraction of the factor under scrutiny be superior to any other known? In criminal law, an absolutely specific relationship is sought in terms of attributable fraction approaching 100%. For example, based on Cole and Goldman's review[144], while studying occupational exposure to vinyl chloride monomers as a cause of liver cancer, a 200.0 odds ratio (giving approx. 99.5% attributable fraction) was found. A 2.0 odds ratio relating benzene occupational exposure to bone marrow neoplasia[144] (giving a 50% attributable risk percent) is less convincing than the former.

Similar attention must be paid to **all other criteria of causality**. Rose[145] rightly distinguishes causes of disease incidence, i.e. causes of disease as a mass phenomenon in the community and cause(s) of a particular case. High national salt intake may be responsible for an important occurrence of hypertension in such a community in general, but what is the reason for developing hypertension in a particular patient? This demonstration is more difficult, causes of cases are less known than causes of incidence, and

Table 8.13 Rules of evidence: Criminality and causality

Mayhem or murder and criminal law	*Morbidity, mortality and causality*
1. Criminal present at the scene of the crime	Agent present in lesion of the disease
2. Premeditation	Causal events precede onset of disease
3. Accessories involved in the crime	Co-factors and/or multiple causality involved
4. Severity or death related to state of victim	Susceptibility and host response determine severity
5. Motivation – the crime must make sense in terms of gain to the criminal	The role of the agent in the disease must make biologic and common sense
6. No other suspect could have committed the crime in the circumstances given	No other agent could have caused the disease under the circumstances given
7. The proof of guilt must be established beyond a reasonable doubt	The proof of causation must be established beyond reasonable doubt or role of chance

Source: Ref. 15, reproduced with permission of Oxford University Press (*Am J Epidemiology*)

presently conclusions must be based on rigorous judgment and inference from a knowledge of causality at the community level.

Remember that **the burden of proof rests with the plaintiff**[146]. If this were generally known, there would be fewer court cases concerning health problems of individuals or communities. Judges and lawyers are now aware of epidemiology, and the issue of causal proof in health and disease is the subject of attention in law and medicine[146–153], as well as in a growing body of literature. Surprisingly for many, the reasoning processes of people of law and medicine are very similar. Table 8.13 represents Evans' postulated logical similarities between reasoning processes in the worlds of health and law[15].

All health professionals, not just epidemiologists, must be cognizant of the rigor of causal proof in the face of the law. Considerable amounts of money and the health and well-being of subjects are at stake. Conclusions are made on solid evidence and not on hearsay or demagogic statements from positions of authority, function or qualification. Meta-analysis[154,155] will play an increasingly important role in such endeavors. Causal demonstrations in courts are challenging and difficult. Credibility, competence, and experience of all experts involved must be rebuilt from scratch before the judge. Everything is recorded, and records become public domain. Inevitably, expert witnesses are brought to the court both by the plaintiff and the defendant. They are recruited to one side or another no matter their objectivity. Work ethic must be scrupulously respected, as

in all fields of epidemiology; its rules are now available in literature[156]. **Ultimately, physicians giving their advice to courts must realize that courts are certainly interested in a general truth, e.g. that a particular chemical causes cancer. However, decisions are made for the specific and precise case of the plaintiff.** So the issue goes from general to specific. Do studies giving a general proof apply to a specific individual? This is similar to the question 'does this research result apply to my patient?' General rules of admissibility have been partly listed in Chapter 4, mostly concerning the theoretical eligibility of a particular individual to studies of evidence brought to the attention of the courts.

Most recently, epidemiological experience from the investigation of causes of outbreaks can be applied to such unusual 'outbreaks' as a series of clinical course complications or patient deaths in hospitals, which might be related to such a cause as a mentally disturbed or criminal employee, or any other responsible 'cause' of such a situation. Multiple cause–effect hypotheses (which employee might be related to the occurrence of cases) must be and have been successfully analyzed in courts as contributing evidence to strengthen final conclusions about the guilt of suspected individuals[157–160].

8.12 Conclusions

A causal proof through analytical observational studies in medicine is a challenging task: intellectually, professionally, and ethically. It is the primary responsibility of physicians and other health professionals to formulate questions, lead and interpret studies. It is unjust to place this burden on methodologists and specialists in quantitative analytical methods, simply because they are key partners in etiological research.

This chapter has outlined some important principles in the search for causes in medicine:

- Assessment of risks;
- Study of contrasts;
- Assessment of impact;
- Assessment of imputability of effect to a cause.

How can it be concluded that an analytical study is of good quality and therefore an acceptable contribution to a causal proof? Deductive thinking is primordial[32]. Innovative parallel thinking, associative reasoning, and biological plausibility considerations are essential to move ahead with new ideas. Careful assessment of initial states, maneuvers and subsequent states of subjects of etiological research require a perfect knowledge of disease history and course, medical practices and decisions, and human biology and pathology. Figure 4.3 in Chapter 4 illustrates the sequence of stages of analytical studies, either observational or interventional. The above-mentioned assessment of stages 4 to 7 concerns the **internal validity** of the study; the evaluation of stages 1, 2, 3, 8, and 9 concerns the **external validity** of the study. Internal validity is primordial. An internally valid study, representing only a fraction of the problem defined at the beginning, is far more acceptable than an all-encompassing study poorly built and based on poor measurement, analysis, and interpretation. For example, in a cohort study, occupational radiation exposure and cancer association is evaluated. Only cancers of some sites (not all) are detected, the rest of the sufferers being unavailable for some reason. The remainder of the study is well done. Conclusions of the study apply to cancer at the observed sites, but not to the whole cancer problem. The study has a limited external validity, but a good internal one. Four ensembles of criteria must, however, be considered for each evidence (study):

1. Conceptual criteria, i.e. the respect of criteria of causality as outlined in this chapter;

2. Necessary components of etiological studies as proposed by Lichtenstein et al[161];
3. Proper architecture and precautions of studies, as proposed for case–control studies by Feinstein[28]; and
4. Confirmation of findings based on the available body of knowledge as provided through meta-analysis in medicine[154,155].

At the time of writing, there are currently no available or generally structured and accepted criteria for observational cohort analytical studies, or for analytical studies as a whole. However, the following **rules** must apply in order **for any analytical study** to be acceptable:

- Reason for doing the study is known through well-defined objectives;
- Hypothesis is clearly formulated;
- Variables are appropriate in view of the hypotheses stated;
- Variables are well defined according to precise inclusion and exclusion criteria and those of measurement;
- Clearly presented design, allowing reproducibility of the study;
- Good evaluation of the initial state;
- Good evaluation of maneuvers;
- Good evaluation of subsequent state;
- Appropriate review of statistical associations and of cause–effect relationships leading to the distinction between scientific and practical importance of results; consideration and explanation of biological plausibility is not omitted;
- Conclusions follow a careful review of errors and bias, clearly stating whether the hypothesis was confirmed or rejected, and if the objectives of the study were attained.

Observational research and its results are like diagnostic tests[162]: a positive test result does not mean that the patient has the disease; and a significant p value does not necessarily confirm a causal link. Large studies (involving many subjects) are very sensitive; small studies yielding low p values are specific. While assessing study results, significant results must not be considered alone, but with the study's power and p value and the characteristics of the hypotheses under evaluation. Browner and Newman's assessment of this problem is worth quoting: '. . . *All significant p values are not equal. Just as accuracy of a diagnosis depends on how well the clinician has estimated the prior probability and considered alternative diagnoses and laboratory errors, the interpretation of a research study depends on how well the reader has estimated the prior probability and considered confounders and biases . . .*'[162].

Analytical observational studies represent only one link, one of the most important in the path of causal proof. Figure 8.5 represents an algorithm of such a path. These studies identify risk characteristics, but only experimental research (i.e. through interventions) such as clinical trials or health program trials and evaluations will clarify what is a risk marker and what is a risk factor. Evaluative and operational research eventually help to evaluate the priority of a cause–effect relationship under study as a priority for research, for clinic intervention, or for programs in the community. The next chapter is devoted to analytical studies based on intervention.

Results of many studies conclude that no significant statistical and/or epidemiological associations were found ('big *p* – small risk findings'); authors succumb to scientific depression and nihilism; and many journals refuse to publish 'negative results', rejecting the hypothesis under scrutiny. However, if statistically acceptable and epidemiologically valid, these results are of equal importance, and more reliable journals publish them. Refuting a possible causal association and avoiding future misdirection, perpetrating errors and ultimately threatening patient health (e.g. treating a patient with an ineffective treatment) or restricting healthy individuals by prohibiting their daily living pleasures is equally important from the point of view of practical decisions based on the results of causal research. The relevance of analytical observational research starts when research questions are formulated and ends with the production of convincing results.

Until now, etiological research in medicine has often been disproportionate between risk markers (which cannot be practically controlled, such as age, sex, social class) and risk factors (which can be controlled, such as drug abuse, heavy drinking, pharmaco-dependency, etc.). Very often, surrogate risk factors are studied. For example, Davidson et al[163] published a well-executed case–control study of risk factors in two teenage suicide clusters. Previous attempts, previous knowledge of violent deaths in a teenager's environment, emotional break-ups, school mobility and living with parents were identified as important risk characteristics. However, control of such factors is not feasible in efficiently preventing suicide in these subjects. It identifies subjects at high risk, but not factors which might be realistically modified. The challenge of psychiatry and medicine is dealing with such a problem. While smoking is implicated in lung cancer, its control is straightforward. Only a more refined study of realistically modifiable factors is beneficial in such an instance. As an example of this type of study, an endpoint production of results must be as convincing as possible. Several authors[164,165] stress the explicitness of presented facts and conclusions. *P*'s, relative risks or attributable fractions speak, but in terms of increased risk or loss of life expectancy, the impact is more tangible. Knowing that the risk of lung cancer increases in smokers by 700–1500% and coronary artery disease by 30–300% may convince some smokers to stop. Smokers will also better comprehend the hierarchy of risks to avoid if they know that smoking will lead to the loss of 2,250 days of life expectancy in men. Being 30% overweight will lead to a loss of 1,300 days for an average person, medical roentgenograms 6 days, and all radiation from the nuclear industry will represent a loss of only 0.02 days or 30 min of life expectancy in the population[145]. Such a pragmatic translation of the results of etiological research is reassessed further by interventional studies as an ultimate test of their relevance.

Identification of modifiable risk factors leading to the modification of disease occurrence and course is the ultimate and foremost objective of all causal research in medicine. One of the greatest challenges remains the need for equal knowledge of risk factors responsible for disease occurrence at the population level (causes of incidence), and of 'personal' risks of disease (causes of cases)[145]. At present, more is known about causes of incidence, given their importance in prevention, and less about causes of cases, so important in clinical medicine. More is known about causes of disease occurrence (risk factors) than about

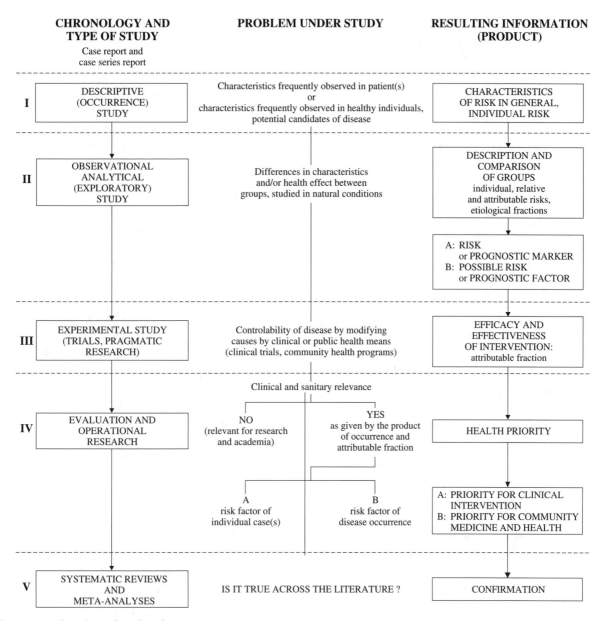

Figure 8.5   Flow chart of studies of causes

causes of disease course (prognostic factors; more about this in Chapter 10). A more balanced knowledge of the above will greatly improve medicine.

A final problem in medical etiological research is the frequent inability to propose and study etiological models beyond our specialties. For example, comprehensive studies are done on the hereditary aspects of psychiatric disorders[116]; elsewhere, the same field is analyzed as a problem of immunity and infection[166]. It would be interesting to study more integrated models, such as the role of immunity and infection in subjects carrying different hereditary traits or factors. The same applies to studies of such disorders as Alzheimer's disease[167–172] or anxiety[173]. Most often, in better reviewed causes, such as Eaton's recent overview of the epidemiology of schizophrenia[174], different factors and markers are reviewed one by one rather than side by side in their respective interaction according to some plausible causal model.

In the methodological field, the case–control approach is increasingly more refined conceptually and methodologically. Given its economical and temporal advantages, this approach remains a focus of attention and innovation. For example, Rodrigues and Kirkwood recently debunked the 'rare disease' assumption and propose possible ways of obtaining estimates of relative risk instead of relying on the odds ratio as an indirect estimate[175]. Computerized data banks and sophisticated analytical software are putting research involving dozens of dependent and independent variables within the reach of many computer literate health professionals. From computerized check-ups performed in California, Friedman and Van Den Eeden[176] analyzed 779 characteristics in individuals in relation to pancreatic cancer. However, the meaning of any association found in such research is limited by its inductive nature. Etiological research still remains an uncharted path. It is to be hoped that this will be a 'deductive' path rather than an uninformed pursuit of all possible associations through inductive research[177], since the statistical methodology for the latter may be more refined. The epidemiological search for causes is currently reaching new crossroads. Two major questions arise:

1. Is the hypothesizing and hypothesis-testing pathway as described in this chapter the best and only way to search for causes[179,180]? To answer this question, there is no alternative clear and operational intellectual pathway proposed, published and tested to successfully replace the deductive–inductive iterative process. Ultimately, it is people and not studies that generate hypotheses.
2. How is the 'black-box' problem to be overcome, i.e. what happens between the action of a presumed 'cause' and disease occurrence?

Vandenbroucke[179] compares the present state of epidemiological research to the miasma theory reign in the history of infectious disease. Similarly, the current understanding of pathogenic mechanisms underlying a 'cause–disease' link is often missing. Two streams of research may develop in the future: on the one hand, epidemiological research may try to open the 'black box' by studying its 'parts' through molecular epidemiology. On the other hand, Loomis and Wing[180] propose to study not only the partitioning of causal problems by 'webs of causes', but also as systems having their own properties. These collective properties may ultimately be seen as 'causes'. The recent development of molecular epidemiology is based on Potter's question in cancerology[181]: '*Who gets cancer – the genes, the cell, the organ, the organism, or perhaps even the population?*' Classical epidemiology focused mainly on organ–organism–population levels, whereas molecular epidemiology targets the problem at the cellular and subcellular level.

After Higginson's pioneering approach[182], Perera and Weinstein[183] originally defined molecular epidemiology as '. . . *an approach in which advanced laboratory methods are used in combination with analytical epidemiology to identify at the biochemical or molecular level, specific exogenous agents and/or host factors that play a role in human cancer causation . . .*' Dorman[184] sees it rather in broader terms as '. . . *a science that focuses on the contribution of potential genetic and environmental risk factors, identified at the molecular and biochemical level, to the etiology, distribution and prevention of disease within families and across populations. It differs from traditional genetic epidemiology in that it equally focuses on environmental and inherited cases of disease . . .*' The study of biological markers at the cellular and subcellular level, of genetic damage, or mutations are just a few examples of this more refined approach, which tries to elucidate mechanisms 'inside the cause–effect black-box'. First used in the field of cancer[185,186], concepts, methods, and techniques of molecular epidemiology expanded into other fields such as atherosclerosis[187], diabetes[188], or infectious diseases[189–191], to name just a few.

A multidisciplinary approach, well beyond the most sophisticated computation and comparison of risks, is necessary as a modern alternative to a 'renaissance man' in causal research. The best evidence about disease causes is required. Health planners need the best evidence about disease occurrence and etiological fractions to calculate their priorities for health programs and their target groups in the community (more information on this topic in Chapters 9 and 10). Clinicians need the best evidence about causes to guide the patient in primary and secondary prevention. Moreover, if a patient asks 'why do I have this problem?' 'Why do you suggest that I do or not do this or that?' or 'what are my chances?' professionals owe this patient evidence-based answers instead of spontaneous emotional outbursts of their beliefs and societal clichés. Giving unjustified advice if evidence is available is not only malpractice, but against the Hippocratic oath. This advice may not benefit the patient as much as possible and may even be harmful. A patient asking for a reason is owed an explanation, not only evidence-based in general, but specifically applicable to the patient (some rules are listed in Chapter 4, and in Section 8.11 of this chapter).

The epidemiological and experimental search for disease causes will never end, due to constantly emerging new problems. Innovative ideas are needed more than sophisticated refinements of methodology, especially in the case of 'robust' (i.e. strong) evidence when conclusions are the same. Kuller[192] and Davey Smith[193] warn against 'circular epidemiology' and poorly focused research where many good studies of the same problem are carried out repeatedly without any justification or need to evaluate consistency of findings, or if such endeavors have a poor biological rationale. A great deal of innovative thinking and imaginative interpretation of biological mechanisms and plausibility is needed when studying cause–effect relationships. For example, it takes a biologically reasoning physician to propose mechanisms behind the effect of music on health[194]. In such a case, hard quantitative evidence may follow sooner or later. Readers of this book may master critical reading of etiological observational studies, but they risk wasting precious time by consuming *art for the sake of art* within an abundance of identical information, however well written. It is solely up to the readers to read accurately and make rational choices for practice and research.

REFERENCES

1. *Encyclopaedia Britannica*. Chicago: Encyclopaedia Britannica Inc., W. Benton, 1968
2. Grundy PF. A rational approach to the 'At risk' concept. *Lancet*, 1973;2:1489
3. Rothman KJ. *Modern Epidemiology*. Boston: Little, Brown, 1986 (2nd Edition: 1998)
4. Bernard C. *An Introduction to the Study of Experimental Medicine*. New York: Macmillan, 1927 (Introduction à l'étude de la médecine expérimentale). Paris: JB Baillière et fils, 1865
5. Feinstein AR. *Clinical Biostatistics*. St. Louis: CV Mosby, 1977
6. Last JM (ed.). *A Dictionary of Epidemiology*. 4th Edition. New York: Oxford University Press, 2001
7. Susser M. *Causal Thinking in the Health Sciences. Concepts and Strategies of Epidemiology*. New York: Oxford University Press, 1973
8. Greenland S (ed.). *Evolution of Epidemiologic Ideas. Annotated Readings on Concepts and Methods*. Chestnut Hill, MA: Epidemiology Resources Inc., 1987
9. Buck C, Llopis A, Najera E, Terris M(eds). *The Challenge of Epidemiology. Issues and Selected Readings*. Part III. Etiologic Investigations. Washington: Pan American Health Organization, 1988:147–806
10. Rothman KJ (ed.). *Causal Inference*. Chestnut Hill, MA: Epidemiology Resources Inc., 1988
11. Hill AB. Observation and experiment. *N Engl J Med*, 1953;248:995–1001
12. Yerushalmy J, Palmer CE. On the methodology of investigations of etiologic factors in chronic disease. *J Chron Dis*, 1959;10:27–40
13. Lilienfield AM. On the methodology of investigations of chronic diseases – Some comments. *J Chron Dis*, 1959;10:41–6
14. Hill AB. The environment and disease: Association or causation? *Proc Roy Soc Med*, 1965;58:295–300
15. Evans AS. Causation and disease. A chronological journey. *Am J Epidemiol*, 1978;108:249–57
16. Rothman KJ (ed.). *Causal Inference*. Chestnut Hill: Epidemiology Resources Inc., 1988
17. Rothman KJ. Causes. *Am J Epidemiol*, 1976;104:587–92
18. Rothman KJ, Greenland S (eds). *Modern Epidemiology*. 2nd Edition. Philadelphia: Lippincott & Raven, 1998
19. Blalock HM (ed.). *Causal Models in Social Sciences*. Chicago: Aldine-Atherton, 1971
20. Hirschi T, Selvin H. *Principles of Survey Analysis* (formerly Deliquency Research). New York: Free Press, 1973
21. Li CC. *Path Analysis – a primer*. Pacific Grove, CA: The Boxwood Press, 1975
22. Rothman KJ. Synergy and antagonism in cause–effect relationships. *Am J Epidemiol*, 1974;99:385–8. (See also 103:506–11 and 108:9–11)

23. Weed DL. Causal criteria and Popperian refutation. In: Rothman KJ ed. *Causal Inference*. Chestnut Hill: Epidemiology Resources Inc, 1988:15–32

24. Horwitz RI, Feinstein AR. The application of therapeutic clinical trials principles to improve the design of etiological research. *J Chronic Dis*, 1981;**34**: 757–83

25. Horwitz RI. The experimental paradigm and observational studies of cause–effect relationships in clinical medicine. *J Chron Dis*, 1987;**40**:91–9

26. Kleinbaum DG, Kupper LL, Morgenstern H. *Epidemiologic Research. Principles and Quantitative Methods*. London: Lifetime Learning Publications, 1982

27. Jenicek M, Cléroux R. *Épidémiologie clinique. Clinimétrie.* (Clinical Epidemiology. Clinimetrics.) St. Hyacinthe and Paris: EDISEM and Maloine, 1985

28. Feinstein AR. *Clinical Epidemiology. The Architecture of Clinical Research*. Philadelphia: WB Saunders, 1985

29. Miettinen OS, Cook EF. Confounding: Essence and detection. *Am J Epidemiol*, 1981;**114**:593–603

30. Ely JW. Confounding bias and effect modification in epidemiologic research. *Fam Med*, 1992;**24**:222–5

31. Copeland KT, Checkoway H, McMichael AJ, Holbrook RH. Bias due to misclassification of relative risk. *Am J Epidemiol*, 1977;**105**:488–95

32. Buck C. Popper's philosophy for epidemiologists. *Int J Epidemiol*, 1975;**4**:159–68

33. Brown GW, Harris TO, Peto J. Life events and psychiatric disorders. Part 2. Nature of causal link. *Psychol Med*, 1973;**3**:159–76

34. MacMahon B, Pugh TF. Causes of entities of disease. In: Clark DW, MacMahon B eds. *Preventive Medicine*. Boston: Little, Brown, 1967:11–18

35. Sackett DL, Straus SE, Richardson WS, et al. *Evidence-Based Medicine. How to Practice and Teach EBM*. 2nd edition. Edinburgh: Churchill Livingstone, 2000

36. Bender R, Blettner M. Calculating the 'number needed to be exposed' with adjustment for confounding variables in epidemiological studies. *J Clin Epidemiol*, 2002;**55**:525–30

37. Altman DG, Machin D, Bryant TN, Gardner MJ (eds). *Statistics With Confidence. Confidence Intervals and Statistical Guidelines*. 2nd Edition. London: BMJ Books, 2000

38. Fleiss JL. *Statistical Methods for Rates and Proportions*. 2nd Edition. New York: John Wiley & Sons, 1981

39. Breslow NE, Day NE. *Statistical Methods in Cancer Research. Volume II – The Design and Analysis of Cohort Studies*. IARC Sci. Publ. No 82. Lyon: International Agency for Cancer Research, 1987

40. Rogan WJ and Gladen B. Estimating prevalence from the results of a screening test. *Am J Epidemiol*, 1978; **107**:71–6

41. Liddell FDK. The development of cohort studies in epidemiology: A review. *J Clin Epidemiol*, 1988;**41**: 1217–37

42. Breslow NE, Day NE. *Statistical Methods in Cancer Research*. Volume I – The Analysis of Case–Control Studies. IARC Sci. Publ No 32. Lyon: International Agency for Cancer Research, 1980

43. Schlesselman JJ. *Case–Control Studies. Design, Conduct, Analysis*. New York: Oxford University Press, 1982

44. Wacholder S, Boivin J-F. External comparisons with the case–control design. *Am J Epidemiol*, 1987;**126**: 1198–1209

45. Liddell FDK, McDonald JC, Thomas DC. Methods of cohort analysis appraisal by application to asbestos mining. *J Roy Stat Soc (A)*, 1977;**140**:469–91

46. Prentice RL. A case–cohort design for epidemiologic cohort studies and disease prevention trials. *Biometrika*, 1986;**73**:1–11

47. Khoury MJ, Flanders WD. Non-traditional epidemiologic approaches in the analysis of gene-environment interaction: Case–control studies with no controls *Am J Epidemiol*, 1996;**144**:207–13

48. Goodman SN, Royall R. Evidence and scientific research. *Am J Public Health*, 1988;**78**:1568–74

49. Ware JH, Mosteller F, Ingelfinger JA. P values. In: Bailar JC III, Mosteller F eds. *Medical Uses of Statistics*. Waltham, MA: NEJM Books, 1986:149–69

50. Holland BK. *Probability Without Equations. Concepts for Clinicians*. Baltimore and London: The Johns Hopkins University Press, 1998

51. 51. Surgeon General's Advisory Committee on Smoking and Health. *Smoking and Health*. Washington: Public Health Service Publ., No 1103, 1973

52. Guyatt GH, Weber CE, Mewa AA, Sackett DL. Determining causation – a case study: adrenocorticosteroids and osteoporosis. Should the fear of inducing clinically important osteoporosis influence the decision to prescribe adrenocorticosteroids? *J Chron Dis*, 1984;**37**:343–52

53. Broadhead WE, Kaplan BH, James SA, et al. The epidemiologic evidence for a relationship between social support and health. *Am J Epidemiol*, 1983; **117**:521–37

54. Susser M. What is a cause and how do we know one? A grammar for pragmatic epidemiology. *Am J Epidemiol*, 1991;**133**:635–48

55. Sullivan SN. Hypothesis revisited: Toothpaste and the cause of Crohn's disease. *Lancet*, 1990;**2**:1096–7

56. Miettinen O. Simple interval-estimation of risk ratio. *Am J Epidemiol*, 1974;**100**:515–6

57. MacMahon B, Yen S, Trichopoulos D, et al. Coffee and cancer of the pancreas. *N Engl J Med*, 1981; **304**:630–3

58. Miettinen OS. Estimability and estimation in case–reference studies. *Am J Epidemiol*, 1976;**103**: 225–35

59. Fleiss JL. Confidence intervals for the odds ratio in case–control studies. The state of the art. *J Chron Dis*, 1979;**32**:69–77

60. Schlesselman JJ. Sample size requirements in cohort and case–control studies. *Am J Epidemiol*, 1974;**99**: 381–4

61. Schlesselman JJ. *Tables of the sample size requirements for cohort and case–control studies of disease.* Bethesda: Nat Inst Child Health Hum Develop Biometry Branch: Jan. 1974

62. Lemeshow S, Hosmer Jr DW, Klar J. Sample size requirements for studies estimating odds ratios or relative risks. *Stat Med*, 1988;**7**:759–64

63. Hsieh FY. Sample size tables for logistic regression. *Stat Med*, 1989;**8**:795–802

64. Walter SD. Determination of significant relative risks and optimal sampling procedures in prospective and retrospective comparative studies of various size. *Am J Epidemiol*, 1977;**105**:387–97

65. Smith AH, Bates MN. Confidence limit analyses should replace power calculations in the interpretation of epidemiologic studies. *Epidemiology*, 1992;**3**: 449–52

66. Mayes LC, Horwitz RI, Feinstein AR. A collection of 56 topics with contradictory results in case–control research. *Int J Epidemiol*, 1988;**17**:680–5

67. Sackett DL. Bias in analytic research. *J Chron Dis*, 1979;**32**:51–63

68. Murphy EA. *The Logic of Medicine*. Baltimore: The Johns Hopkins University Press, 1976:239–62

69. Cole P, Morrison AS. Basic issues in cancer screening. In: Miller AB ed. *Screening in Cancer*. A Report of a UICCC International Workshop, Toronto, Canada, April 24–27, 1978.UICC Technical Report Series – Vol. 40. Geneva: International Union Against Cancer, 1978:7–39

70. Wilder J. Modern psychophysiology and the law of initial value. *Am J Psychother*, 1958;**12**:199–221

71. Zelen M. Theory of early detection of breast cancer in the general population. In: Henson JC, Mattheim WH, Rosencweig M eds. *Breast Cancer: Trends in Research and Treatment*. New York: Raven Press, 1976:287–300

72. Jenicek M, Cléroux R. *Epidémiologie. Principes, techniques, applications. (Epidemiology. Principles, techniques, applications.)* St. Hyacinthe and Paris: EDISEM et Maloine, 1982, Chapter 10

73. Grimes DA, Schulz KF. Bias and causal associations in observational research. *Lancet*, 2002;**359**:248–52

74. Horwitz RI, Feinstein AR. Analysis of clinical susceptibility bias in case –control studies. Analysis as illustrated by the menopausal syndrome and the risk of endometrial cancer. *Arch Intern Med*, 1979;**139**: 1111–13

75. Horwitz RI, McFarlane MJ, Brennan TA, Feinstein AR. The role of susceptibility bias in epidemiologic research. *Arch Intern Med*, 1985;**145**:909–12

76. Horwitz RI, Feinstein AR. The problem of 'protopathic bias' in case–control studies. *Am J Med*, 1980;**68**:255–8

77. Horwitz RI, Feinstein AR, Harvey MR. Case–control research. Temporal precedence and other problems of the exposure-disease relationship. *Arch Intern Med*, 1984;**144**:1257–9

78. Armitage P, Berry G. *Statistical Methods in Medical Research*. 2nd edition. Oxford: Blackwell Science, 1987

79. Feinstein AR. Clinical biostatistics. LVII. A glossary of neologisms in quantitative clinical science. *Clin Pharmacol Ther*, 1981;**30**:564–77

80. Wells CK, Feinstein AR. Detection bias in the diagnostic pursuit of lung cancer. *Am J Epidemiol*, 1988;**128**:1016–26

81. Sadegh-Zadeh K. Fundamentals of clinical methodology: 2. Etiology. *Artif Intell Med*, 1998;**12**:227–70

82. Cupples IA, Heeren T, Schatzkin A, Colton T. Multiple testing of hypotheses in comparing two groups. *Ann Intern Med*, 1984;**100**:122–9

83. Hanley JA. Appropriate uses of multivariate analysis. *Ann Rev Public Health*, 1982;**4**:155–80

84. Evans SJW. Uses and abuses of multivariate methods in epidemiology. *J Epidemiol Community Health*, 1988;**42**:311–5

85. Khan KS, Chien PFW, Dwarakanath LS. Logistic regression models in obsterics and gynecology literature. *Obstet Gynecol*, 1999;**93**:1014–20

86. Kleinbaum DG, Kupper LL and Chambles LE. Logistic regression analysis of epidemiologic data. Theory and practice. *Commun Statist Ther Math*, 1982;**11**:485–547

87. Vollmer RT. Multivariate statistical analysis for pathologists Part I. The logistic model. *Am J Clin Pathol*, 1996;**105**:115–26

88. Bender R, Grouven U. Ordinal logistic regression in medical research. *J Roy Coll Phys London*, 1997;**31**: 546–51

89. Preisser JS, Koch GG. Categorical data analysis in public health. *Ann Rev Public Health*, 1997;**18**: 51–82

90. Duleba AJ, Olive DL. Regression analysis and multivariate analysis. *Sem Reprod Endocrinol*, 1996; **14**:139–53

91. Ananth CV, Kleinbaum DG. Regression models for ordinal responses: A review of methods and applications. *Int J Epidemiol*, 1997;**26**:1323–33

92. Ostir GV, Uchida T. Logistic regression: A non–technical view. *Am J Phys Med Rehabil*, 2000;**79**:565–72

93. Logistic regression. In: Norman G, Streiner D eds. *Biostatistics. The Bare Essentials*. Hamilton and London: BC Decker Inc., 2000;139–44

94. SPSS Inc. *SPSS for Windows. (Statistical Package for Social Sciences)*. Version 11.0.1. Chicago: SPSS Inc., 2002

95. Paykel ES. Contribution of life events to causation of psychiatric illness. *Psychol Med*, 1978;**8**:245–53

96. Karlin S, Cameron EC, Chakraborty R. Path analysis in genetic epidemiology: a critique. *Am J Hum Genet*, 1983;**35**:695–732

97. Sulkes J, Fields S, Gabbay U, et al. Path analysis on the risk of mortality in very low birth weight infants. *Eur J Epidemiol*, 2001;**11**:377–84

98. Vaconcelos AGG, Rodrigues Almeida RMV, Nobre FF. Path analysis and multicriteria decision making: An approach for multivariate model selection and analysis in health. *Ann Epidemiol*, 2001;**11**:377–84

99. Tayer WG, Nicassio PM, Weisman MH, et al. Disease status predicts fatigue in systemic lupus erythematosus. *J Rheumatol*, 2001;**28**:1999–2007

100. Goldsmith JR, Berglund K. Epidemiological approach to multiple factor interaction in pulmonary disease: the potential usefulness of path analysis. *Ann NY Acad Sci*, 1974;**221**:361–75

101. Deykin EI, Keane TM, Kaloupek D, et al. Post-traumatic stress disorder and the use of health services. *Psychosom Med*, 2001;**63**:835–41

102. Ofori R, Charlton JP. A path model of factors influencing the academic performance of students. *J Adv Nurs*, 2002;**38**:507–15

103. Wright S. On 'path analysis in genetic epidemiology: A critique'. *Am J Hum Genet*, 1983;**35**:757–68

104. Cloninger CR, Rao DC, Rice J, et al. A defense of path analysis in genetic epidemiology. *J Hum Genet*, 1983;**35**:733–56

105. Hoyle RH, Smith GT. Formulating clinical research hypotheses as structural equation models: A conceptual overview. *J Consult Clin Psychol*, 1994;**62**:429–40

106. Path analysis and structural equation modeling. In: Norman G, Streiner D eds. *Biostatistics. The Bare Essentials*. Hamilton and London: BC Decker Inc., 2000:178–96

107. Stiffman AR, Hadley-Ives E, Elze D, et al. Impact of environment on adolescent mental health and behavior: Structural equation modeling. *Am J Orthopsychiatry*, 1999;**69**:73–86

108. Gritz ER, DiMatteo MR, Hays RD. Methodological issues in adherence to cancer control regimens. *Prev Med*, 1989;**18**:711–20

109. Hepburn DA, Deary IJ, MacLeod KM, Frier BM. Structural equation modeling of symptoms, aware-ness and fear of hypoglycemia, and personality in patients with insulin-treated diabetes. *Diabetes Care*, 1994;**17**:1273–80

110. Doran DI, Sidani S, Keatings M, Doidge D. An empirical test of the Nursing Role Effectiveness Model. *J Adv Nurs*, 2002;**38**:29–39

111. Newman HH, Freeman SN and Holzinger K. Twins: *A Study of Heredity and Environment*. Oxford: Pergamon Press, 1937

112. Hanna BL. Genetic studies of family units. In: Neel JV, MW Shaw, Schull WJ eds. *Genetics and the Epidemiology of Chronic Diseases*. Washington: US Dept Health, Educ Welf, Publ No 1163, 1965:7–21

113. McKusick VA. Genetic aspects of epidemiology and preventive medicine. In: *Maxcy-Rosenau Preventive Medicine and Public Health*. 9th edition. New York: Appleton–Century–Crofts.1965:629–38

114. MacMahon B and Pugh TF. Genetics and Epidemiology. In: *Epidemiology, Principles and methods*. Boston: Little, Brown, 1970:301–32

115. Morton NE. Some aspects of the genetic epidemiology of common diseases. In: Inouye E, Nishimura H eds. *Gene–Environment Interaction in Common Diseases*. Baltimore: University Park Press, 1977:21–40

116. Gregory I and Smeltzer DJ. Biological determinants of personality and psychopathology. In: Psychiatry. *Essentials of Clinical Practice*. Boston: Little, Brown, 1977:77–87

117. Murphy EA. Epidemiologic strategies and genetic factors. *Int J Epidemiol*, 1978;**7**:7–14

118. Schull WJ, Weiss KM. Genetic epidemiology: four strategies. *Epidemiol Rev*, 1980;**2**:1–18

119. Pardes H, Kaufmann CA, Pincus HA, West A. Genetics and psychiatry: Past discoveries, current dilemmas, and future directions. *Am J Psychiatry*, 1989;**146**:435–43

120. Lynch HT, Hirayama T (eds). *Genetic Epidemiology of Cancer*. Boca Raton: CRC Press, 1989

121. Childs B. *Genetic Medicine. A Logic of Disease*. Baltimore and London: The Johns Hopkins University Press, 1999

122. Clayton D, McKeigue PM. Epidemiological methods for studying genes and environmental factors in complex diseases. *Lancet*, 2001;**358**:1356–60

123. Hulka BS, Wilcosky TC, Griffith JD (eds). *Biological Markers in Epidemiology*. New York: Oxford University Press, 1990

124. El-Guebaly N. Risk research in affective disorders and alcoholism: Epidemiological surveys and trait markers. *Can J Psychiatry*, 1986;**31**:352–61

125. Monster AC. Biological markers of solvent exposure. *Arch Environ Health*, 1988;**43**:90–3

126. Woodside B, Zilli C, Fisman S. Biologic markers and bipolar disease in children. *Can J Psychitary*, 1989;**34**:128–31

127. Virji MA, Mercer DW, Herberman RB. Tumor markers in cancer diagnosis and prognosis. *CA – A Cancer J for Clinicians*, 1988;**38**:104–27

128. Collins PM. Tumor Markers and Screening Tools in Cancer Detection. *Nurs Clin of North Amer*, 1990; **25**:283–90

129. Murray Jr RF. Tests of so–called genetic susceptibility. *J Occup Med*, 1986;**28**:1103–7

130. Schober SE, Constock GW, Helsing KJ, et al. Serologic precursors of cancer. I. Prediagnostic serum nutrients and colon cancer risk. *Am J Epidemiol*, 1987;**126**:1033–41

131. Colligan MJ, Pennenbaker JW, Murphy LR (eds). Mass Psychogenic Illness. *A Social Psychological Analysis*. Hillsdale, NJ: Lawrence Erlbaum Associates, 1982

132. Mobley J, Machin J, Kennedy ME, et al. *Clostridium perfringens food poisoning* – Ontario. *Canada Diseases Weekly Report*, 1976;**2–23**:90–1

133. Pereira Fonseca MG, Armenian HK. Use of the case–control method in outbreak investigations. *Am J Epidemiol*, 1991;**133**:748–52

134. Goldsmith JR (ed.). *Environmental Epidemiology: Epidemiological Investigation of Community Environmental Health Problems*. Boca Raton: CRC Press, 1986

135. Levine RJ. Epidemic faintness and syncope in a school marching band. *JAMA*, 1977;**238**:2373–6

136. Goh KT. Epidemiological enquiries into a school outbreak of an unusual illness. *Int J Epidemiol*, 1987;**16**:265–70

137. Arcidiacono S, Brand JI, Coppenger W, et al. (and Editorial Note). Mass sociogenic illness in a day-care center, Florida. *MMWR*, 1990;**39**:301–4

138. Special Issue. Evidence: Its Meanings in Health Care and in Law. *J Health Politics Policy Law*, 2001;**26** (Number 2)

139. Waller BN. *Critical Thinking. Consider the Verdict.* Englewood Cliffs: Prentice Hall, 1988

140. Levin AS. Science in court. *Lancet*, 1987;**2**:1526

141. Hoffman RE. The use of epidemiologic data in the courts. *Am J Epidemiol*, 1984;**120**:190–202

142. Norman GR, Newhouse MT. Health effects of urea formaldehyde foam insulation: evidence of causation. *Can Med Ass J*, 1986;**134**:733–8

143. Evans EA. Causation and disease: Effect of technology on postulates of causation. *Yale J Biol Med*, 1991;**64**:513–28

144. Cole P, Goldman MB. Occupation. In: Fraumeni JF Jr. ed. *Persons at High Risk of Cancer*. New York: Academic Press, 1975:167–84

145. Rose G. Sick individuals and sick populations. *Int J Epidemiol*, 1985;**14**:32–8

146. Brennan TA, Carter RF. Legal and scientific probability of causation of cancer and other environmental disease in individuals. *J Health Politics and Law*, 1985;**10**:33–80

147. Black B, Lilienfeld DE. Epidemiologic proof in toxic tort litigation. *Fordham Law Review*, 1984;**52**:732–85

148. Lilienfeld DE, Black B. The epidemiologist in court: some comments. *Am J Epidemiol*, 1986;**123**:961–4

149. Teret SP. Litigating for the public's health. *AJPH*, 1986;**76**:1027–9

150. Norman GR. Science, public policy, and media disease. *CMAJ*, 1986;**134**:719–20

151. Cole P. Epidemiologist as an expert withnes. *J Clin Epidemiol*, 1991;**44**(Suppl 1):35S–39S

152. Editorial. Greater use of expert panels proposed as additional means of presenting epidemiologic evidence to the courts. *Epidemiol Monitor*, 1989; **10**:1–3

153. Holden C. Science in court. *Science*, 1989;**243**:1658–9

154. Jenicek M. Meta-analysis in medicine. Where are we and where we want to go. *J Clin Epidemiol*, 1989; **42**;35–44

155. Jenicek M. Méta-analyse en médecine. Evaluation et synthèse de l'information clinique et épidémiologique. (Meta–analysis in medicine. Evaluation and synthesis of clinical and epidemiological information). St. Hyacinthe and Paris: EDISEM et Maloine, 1987

156. Fayerweather WE, Higginson H, Beauchamp TL (eds). Industrial Epidemiology Forum's Conference on Ethics in Epidemiology. *J Clin Epidemiol*, 1991;**44** (Suppl I)

157. Rothman KJ. Sleuthing in hospitals. *N Engl J Med*, 1985;**313**:258–9

158. Istre GR, Gustafson TL, Baron RC, et al. A mysterious cluster of deaths and cardiopulmonary arrests in a pediatric intensive care unit. *N Engl J Med*, 1985;**133**:205–11

159. Buehler JW, Smith LF, Wallace EM, et al. Unexplained deaths in a children's hospital. An epidemiologic assessment. *N Engl J Med*, 1985;**313**:211–6

160. Sacks JJ, Stroup DF, Will ML, Harris EL, Israel E. A nurse-associated epidemic of cardiac arrests in an intensive care unit. *JAMA*, 1988;**259**:689–95

161. Lichtenstein MJ, Mulrow CD, Elwood PC. Guidelines for reading case–control studies. *J Chron Dis*, 1987;**40**:893–903

162. Browner WS, Newman TB. Are all significant p values created equal? *JAMA*, 1987;**257**:2459–63

163. Davidson LE, Rosenberg ML, Mercy JA, et al. An epidemiologic study of risk factors in two teenage suicide clusters. *JAMA*, 1989;**262**:2687–92

164. Cohen BL, Lee I–S. A catalog of risks. *Health Physics*, 1979;**36**:702–22

165. Berger ES, Hendee WR. The expression of health risk information. *Arch Intern Med*, 1989;**149**:1507–8

166. King DJ, Cooper SJ. Viruses, immunity and mental disorder. *Br J Psychiatry*, 1989;**154**:1–7

167. Henderson AS. The epidemiology of Alzheimer's disease. *Br Med Bull*, 1986;**42**:3–10

168. Henderson AS. The risk factors for Alzheimer's disease: A review and a hypothesis. *Acta Psychiatr Scand*, 1988;**78**:257–75

169. Kay DW. The genetics of Alzheimer's disease. *Br Med Bull*, 1986;**42**:3–10

170. Corsellis JAN. The transmissibility of dementia. *Br Med Bull*, 1986;**42**:111–4

171. Heyman A, Wilkinson WE, Stafford JA, et al. Alzheimer's disease: A study of epidemiological aspects. *Ann Neurol*, 1984;**15**:335–41

172. Ball MJ. Alzheimer's disease – Some contemporary etiological hypotheses. *Annals RCPSC*, 1984;**17**: 569–71

173. Reich J. The epidemiology of anxiety. *J Nerv Ment Dis*, 1986;**174**:129–36

174. Eaton WW. Epidemiology of schizophrenia. *Epidemiol Rev*, 1985;**7**:105–26

175. Rodrigues L, Kirkwood BR. Case–control designs in the study of common diseases: Updates on the demise of the rare disease assumption and the choice of sampling scheme for controls. *Int J Epidemiol*, 1990;**19**:205–13

176. Friedman GD, Van Den Eeden SK. Risk factors for pancreatic cancer: An exploratory study. *Int J Epidemiol*, 1993;**22**:30–7

177. Skrabanek P. The poverty of epidemiology. *Persp Biol Med*, 1992;**35**:182–5

178. Cole P. The hypothesis-generating machine. *Epidemiology*, 1993;**4**:271–3

179. Vanderbroucke JP. Is 'The Causes of Cancer' a miasma theory for the end of the twentieth century? *Int J Epidemiol*, 1988;**17**:708–9

180. Loomis D, Wing S. Is molecular epidemiology a germ theory for the end of twentieth century? *Int J Epidemiol*, 1990;**19**:1–3

181. Potter JD. Reconciling the epidemiology, physiology, and molecular biology of colon cancer. *JAMA*, 1992;**268**:1573–7

182. Higginson J. The role of the pathologist in environmental medicine and public health. *Am J Pathol*, 1977;**86**:459–84

183. Perera FP, Weinstein BI. Molecular epidemiology and carcinogen-DNA adduct detection: New approaches to studies of human cancer causation. *J Chron Dis*, 1982;**35**:581–600

184. Dorman JS. Genetic epidemiology of insulin-dependent diabetes mellitus. International comparisons using molecular genetics. *Ann Med*, 1992;**24**:393–9

185. Wogan GN. Molecular epidemiology in cancer risk assessment and prevention: Recent progress and avenues for future research. *Environ Health Persp*, 1992;**98**:167–78

186. Perera FP. Molecular cancer epidemiology: A new tool in cancer prevention. *JNCI*, 1987;**78**:887–98

187. Davignon J, Gregg RE, Sing CF. Apolipoprotein E polymorphism and atherosclerosis. *Atherosclerosis*, 1986;**6**:357–77

188. Drash AL, Lipton RB, Dorman JS, et al. The interface between epidemiology and molecular biology in the search for the causes of insulin–dependent diabetes mellitus. *Ann Med*, 1991;**23**:463–71

189. Hide G, Tait A. The molecular epidemiology of parasites. *Experientia*, 1991;**47**:128–42

190. Tompkins LS, Falkow S. Molecular biology of virulence and epidemiology. In: Gorbach SL, Bartlett JG, Blacklow NR eds. *Infectious Diseases.* Philadelphia: WB Saunders, 1992:30–7

191. Busch MP. The need for rigorous molecular epidemiology. *AIDS*, 1991;**5**:**1379**–80

192. Kuller LH. Invited commentary: Circular epidemiology. *Am J Epidemiol*, 1999;**150**:897–903

193. Davey Smith G. Reflections on the limitations of epidemiology. *J Clin Epidemiol*, 2001;**54**:325–31

194. Storr A. The enigma of music. *J Roy Soc Med*, 1999;**92**:28–34

Chapter 9

The impact of treatment and other clinical and community health interventions.
A 'does it work?' evaluation

*The experiment is the most powerful and most reliable
lever enabling us to extract secrets from nature . . .
The experiment must constitute the final judgment
as to whether a hypothesis should be retained or be discarded.*
Wilhelm Conrad Röntgen, Würzburg, 1894

*As I see it, however, the medical profession
has the responsibility not only for the cure of the sick
and for the prevention of disease but for the advancement
of knowledge upon which both depend. This third responsibility
can only be met by investigation and experiment . . ..*[1]
R. A. McCance, Cambridge, 1950

To do nothing is also a good remedy
Hippocrates, Greece, *c*.460–*c*.400 BC

Hippocrates is particularly right if there are
solid pieces of evidence that 'to do nothing' is the
best and the most effective option of them all

9.1 Basic paradigm and general consideration

Without treatment, medicine would be limited to contemplation. Identifying a patient's health problem must lead to prevention, to cure, or if the causes of disease are unknown, to the alleviation of suffering. Ultimately, further research may elucidate causes and conditions, and allow for the control of disease and the maintenance of health. Some of Rudyard Kipling's 'six honest serving men' have been discussed in Chapters 5 and 6 ('**What**'), 7 ('**Who**', '**When**', '**Where**'), and 8 ('**Why**'). The next step is understanding the validity of these questions by transforming conclusions derived from observations into a deliberate and controlled action (the essence of experimental research), be it in laboratories, drug trials, surgical procedures in clinical settings or field trials of health programs in community medicine. '**Really?**', as in 'Does it really work?', is an important 'seventh honest man' in the understanding of human biology and pathology.

Clinical practitioners are mostly interested in papers on diagnosis or treatment. Is there a new way to treat increasingly drug resistant tuberculosis? Is a new antineoplastic drug more effective than current treatment? Moreover, any practicing physician can choose to be involved in clinical and field trials of new preventive or curative procedures. Challenges in this area must be understood as this chapter points out. Historically, treatment has not always been based on what actually works or on what is the best, taking all considerations into account. Several reasons motivate the decision to treat or not to treat:

- Standard procedures (customary practice);
- Orders from senior colleagues;
- Gut decisions and flair;
- Conditioning by industries and market (drugs, etc.);
- Patient's insistence;
- Pleasing practices ('rewards');
- Fear of doing nothing;
- Fear of doing something;
- Unsubstantiated pseudo-logic of spiraling empiricism (term coined by Kim and Gallis[2] for such fallacies as 'more severe disease = more, bigger, and newer drugs', or 'failure to respond = failure to cover', or fear of not doing enough, etc.);
- Defensive practice of medicine (fear of being sued if not treating aggressively enough);
- Ultimately, right decisions.

Treatment considerations and decisions are another exercise in logic. As in any logical discourse, premises must be made sustainable by the best available evidence. Consider this example of a patient being diagnosed with rheumatoid arthritis, followed by treatment considerations:

Practice	Logical discourse	Evidence needed
'You have rheumatoid arthritis.'	The patient has a well-defined clinical problem. **(Premise A)**	**Valid diagnosis**.
'Your problem is not easy to treat, but some drugs may offer you relief.'	There are drugs which relieve arthritis symptoms **(Premise B)**	**Effectiveness** of non-steroidal anti-inflammatory drugs **proved in clinical trials**.
'You will benefit from the medication for which I am writing a prescription right now. Here is what you will do . . .'	The treatment of this patient is mandatory **(Conclusion)**	**Prognosis worse if not treated.** *This* treatment applies to *this* particular patient.

As the challenges of evidence in the field of diagnosis have been shown (Chapter 6) to support Premise A, the challenges of treatment effectiveness evidence (Premise B), its prognostic value and its applicability to a specific patient lead to the decision to treat (conclusion of the argument). Making clinical decisions or decision analysis will be the subject of the final chapter. The present chapter explores how to make decisions about the validity of evidence on the success of the treatment and about whether it is worth consideration in specific clinical situations involving specific patients. Medicine in this century has become increasingly interventionist. North Americans especially want to act, to do something regardless of the cost (and with little concern for the old saying 'if it ain't broke, don't fix it'). However any treatment, preventive or curative, must:

- Bring about a desired **effect**;

- Represent an improvement in the **quality of care;**
- Have a reasonable **cost** (economical);
- Do **more good than harm** ('primum non nocere').

9.1.1 Treatment and cure as a cause–effect relationship

If disease is understood as an undesirable (for some reason) product of interaction between man and various endogenous and exogenous factors, corrective measures must be undertaken. Five types of intervention can be considered:

- **Modification of the factor** or cause of disease. For example, sodium chloride intake in relation to hypertension may be partly replaced by the consumption of other salts.
- **Modification of exposure,** in terms of avoidance, lesser doses, or its spread in time: abstention from some foods or alcohol, gluten-free diet in phenylketonuria, etc.
- **Modification of the response,** such as augmenting subject resistance through vaccines, better nutrition, drugs, operations, etc.
- **Avoidance of response,** such as in personal hygiene.
- **Suppression of the target organ (modification of the morphology),** such as performing an appendectomy or hernia repair. For example, a woman whose mother and sister died of breast cancer may ask her surgeon to perform a bilateral mastectomy, eliminating the biological terrain for a high-probability cancer, given that various endogenous and exogenous factors or causes remain unknown.

In any of the above-mentioned situations, an active intervention is proposed and a positive sequence or beneficial effect is expected, such as healing, cure, alleviation of symptoms, non-appearance of disease, etc. **This theoretical concept of cause–effect relationship from the previous chapter also applies to any kind of intervention in medicine at any level of prevention as already defined (Chapter 8): control of exposure to noxious factors; immunization in primary prevention; treatment in secondary prevention; avoiding metastases; or ensuring the comfort of a terminal patient in tertiary prevention. The same criteria of cause–effect relationships apply as well as various risk measurements (absolute, relative,** attributable). **Any evaluation of treatment impact, such as effectiveness or adverse effects and their evaluation by additional methods, are derived from this basic consideration and approach.**

Intervention in health sciences encompasses drug or surgical treatment, nursing care, mental health support, vaccination, health education, cessation of smoking or drinking, rehabilitation, or social re-integration of a patient in the family or social and professional environment. Any diagnostic process in medicine ends with the decision to treat or not to treat a patient. To make such a decision, the value of treatment must be known. Many treatments, which by tradition and history are incorporated in the practice of medicine, still need to be evaluated, as all new treatments must be.

9.1.2 Evaluation of treatment

Treatment represents the second cause of the rising cost of health care, diagnosis being the first. **Its evaluation consists of various procedures, methods, and techniques needed to determine as objectively as possible the relevance, effect and impact of various therapeutic activities relative to their pre-established objectives**[3]. Does a new analgesic control arthritis pain? Does a coronary bypass improve cardiac function? Does psychotherapy relieve anxiety in a patient under stress? As mentioned earlier, all these interactions as cause–effect relationships must be examined with the same logic as that used for the assessment of criteria of causality, as explained in the previous chapter. In interventional or experimental studies, however, it is not the subject who chooses to be exposed (or not) to the factor under study, but rather the health professional, be it the researcher or practicing clinician, who decides who will be exposed to the active treatment or its inactive alternative (placebo). Since the factor under study (treatment, nursing care, rehabilitation, etc.) is expected to bring about a cure, healing, functional improvement, alleviation of pain, or comfort to the patient, there are fewer ethical obstacles to 'voluntarily and deliberately' exposing the patient to such factors. With the well-being of patients or a community in mind, it is hoped that interventions will have the best possible impact on disease or health. Three areas and levels of intervention have their own specificities, requirements, and resulting methodologies requiring special comments:

- Disease treatment and cure;
- Disease prevention; and
- Health maintenance or health promotion.

This chapter is devoted to these three topics. In terms of health programming, any treatment is an intervention, and it represents a cause in relation to the expected impact (result effect). In health evaluation, four questions are usually explored:

- Is the proposed action **sound** ('*does it make sense*')?
- Is the **structure** of the intervention adequate ('*how is it organized*')?
- Is its **process** acceptable ('*does it happens as desired*')?
- What is the **result** or impact of the treatment ('*what does it do*')?

For example, antibiotic treatment for various bacterial infections may be very effective, but it may be decided, prescribed or available in a non-uniform way. The result of therapy may be acceptable, but not its structure (e.g. patients may not comply with orders to take pills for a fixed period of time; thus the process of antibiotic therapy is rendered unsatisfactory). The following question is obvious: If the treatment works, does it have some result? Any result may be evaluated on four different levels:

- Does the treatment work in *ideal conditions* (uniform, laboratory or hospital)? This represents the **efficacy** of the treatment ('Can the treatment work'? In other terms, 'are treatment or prevention specious and consistent'?);
- Does the treatment work in *habitual conditions* ('everyday life')? The **effectiveness** of the treatment is then understood ('does the treatment work'?);
- Does the treatment work *adequately* in relation to the amount of money, time, and resources spent[2]? The **efficiency** of the treatment is examined this way. ('What is the price of such gains'?);
- Does the treatment *continue to work* once put into action? The **constancy** of the performance is highly desirable.

Health economics, operational research and health care organizations focus on the efficiency of interventions. Experimental research, clinical trials and community trials focus primarily on the understanding of treatment efficacy and effectiveness. The latter two topics are discussed in greater detail further in this chapter. The epidemiological approach[4–6] is essential to the assessment of the impact of treatment (assessing 'doing good') and its collateral effects (secondary or adverse effects, harm). This chapter is devoted to the evaluation of therapeutic procedures and of their impact. Chapter 13 is devoted to clinical decisions (such as to treat or not to treat, which procedures to choose, and when to act). The following is a review of fundamental concepts, methods of analysis, and the interpretation of results of therapeutic interventions. Many specialized, high-quality monographs focus on the subject of clinical trials, some being more comprehensive[7–9] and others more technical[10–11]. These and other excellent references[12–14] may be considered as ancillary reading to this chapter.

9.2 Evaluation of treatment in disease cure

Any evaluation of treatment must be based on sound knowledge of the target pathology, its physiology, pharmacology or technology of intervention (drug, surgery, etc.), as well as the clinico-epidemiological methodology of a valid clinical trial. A clinical trial is a research activity that involves the administration of a test regimen to humans in order to evaluate its efficacy and safety[3]. For Lawrence[15], a clinical trial is a carefully controlled and highly ethical human experiment that is designed to test a hypothesis relating to possible improvements in patient management.

Historical note: The first clinical trials come from the field of nutrition[16,17]. First, Daniel[16] under the rule of Nebuchadnezzar (The Bible, Book of Daniel, Chapter 1) compared the effects of a vegetarian diet (pulse and water) with the Babylonian court diet (meat and wine):

'. . . 11. *Then said Daniel to Melzar, whom the prince of eunuchs had set over Daniel, Hananiah, Mishael, and Azariah,*

12. *Prove thy servants, I beseech thee, ten days; and let them give us pulse to eat and water to drink.*

13. *Then let our countenances be looked upon before thee, and the countenance of the children that eat the portion of the king's meat; and as thou seest, deal with thy servants.*

14. *So he consented to them in this matter, and proved them ten days.*

15. *And at the end of ten days their countenance appeared fairer and fatter in flesh than all the children which did eat the portion of the king's meat.*

16. *Thus Melzar took away the portion of their meat and the wine that they should drink; and gave them pulse. . . .'*

(Certainly, the n-of-4 experimental group was compared to a control group of unknown size in this non-randomized and unblinded trial, but the methodology has come great distances since then.) Later, in the eighteenth century, a British navy physician, James Lind[17], performed a better documented trial of the beneficial effects of citrus juice in scorbutic sailors.

9.2.1 The basic design of treatment study in disease cure and prevention

Since then, any evaluation of treatment in medicine implies a study of the cause–effect relationship. Hence, by definition, two or more groups are compared with regard to the effect of exposure and non-exposure to treatment or its equivalent (standard). **A classical clinical trial is an excellent experimental study** and should be considered as such. Figure 4.2 may then be translated in terms of a clinical trial as is illustrated in Figure 9.1. *(NB Steps 3 and 4 from Figure 4.2 are inverted to reflect differences between an observational and an experimental study.)*

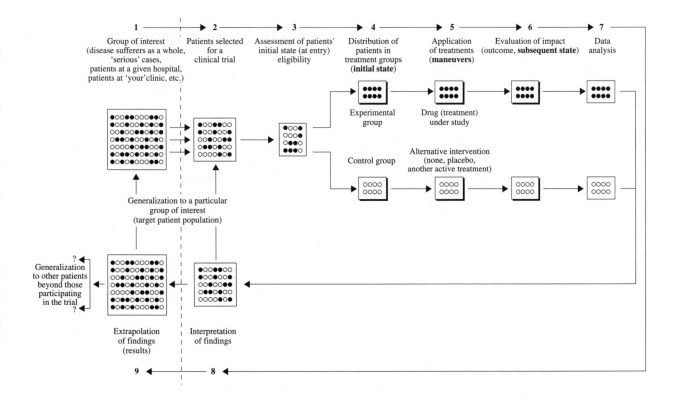

Figure 9.1 Basic architecture of clinical trials

Szmuness et al[18] evaluated the effectiveness of a new hepatitis B vaccine. First, all subjects at risk of hepatitis B were considered for possible enrolment in the study (Step 1). For several theoretical and practical reasons (high risk, collaboration, accessibility, cost, etc.), the male homosexual community was selected for the trial (Step 2). Subjects contacted were evaluated by serological and other means as to their 'initial state' (not infected, susceptible to develop hepatitis B – Step 3). Subjects were then randomized (Step 4) and received either the experimental vaccine or a placebo as 'maneuvers' (Step 5). After a period of possible exposure, participating subjects were re-evaluated by clinical (diagnosis of incident cases) and paraclinical (seroconversion, etc.) methods to confirm hepatitis B as a 'subsequent state' (Steps 6 and 7). Data from both groups were compared for risk of hepatitis. Relative and attributable risk findings, as well as etiological fractions, confirmed the high protective efficacy of the vaccine (Step 8). Results were critically evaluated as a possible extrapolation of findings beyond the findings of the high-risk group involved in the study (Step 9).

9.2.2 Assessment of the impact of treatment. Treatment efficacy and effectiveness

Once comparisons of outcomes in treatment groups are made, investigators bring their experiences to the attention of readers. Results are interpreted as being 'significant', 'highly significant' or 'statistically significant'. *P* values from the statistical analysis of data are used to show the strength of evidence in analytical studies, be they observational or experimental. *P* values are also used to evaluate the degree of dissimilarity between two or more series of observations. Once again, remember that as a measure of the impact of treatment in clinical or epidemiological terms, *p* values can only 'clear the way' (if they are small) for the epidemiological and clinical assessment of results of clinical trials. **The *p* value is** *'usually the probability of obtaining a result as extreme as, or more extreme than, the one observed if the dissimilarity is entirely due to variation in measurement or in subject response – that is, if it is the result of chance alone'*[19]. Some funding agencies or

institutions may still be happy with 'small p_s', indicating that a drug leading to different outcomes shows a very low probability of not working (null hypothesis would be true). This, however, does not indicate the magnitude of the effect. Hence, *p* values and significance of findings in terms of inferential statistics should be carefully interpreted and given their proper meaning[19,20].

Any clinical trial must confirm or reject a cause–effect relationship between a treatment modality and the modification of the history or course of the disease under study. It is thus a special kind of etiological study. Its conclusions must confirm or reject a causal relationship according to the criteria explained in Chapter 8: does the treatment really precede an expected disease outcome? Is the relationship strong? Is it specific? Is there a dose–effect gradient? Does it conform to the rest of the cause–effect criteria? If authors are happy stating that differences in disease outcomes between groups are statistically significant, they must keep the following in mind: **What is statistically significant is not necessarily significant from an epidemiological point of view. Statistically significant studies may still show low relative risks (a poor strength of association) or etiological fractions (specificity of improvements due to the treatment under study).**

All epidemiologically important results are not necessarily of equal clinical importance. For rare phenomena and outcomes that are not severe or life-threatening, strong associations may exist but they are of lesser clinical importance in comparison to more frequent and serious health problems, where even less epidemiologically important findings might be of more clinical interest. In other terms, if one needs to know some *p* value beyond its customary clearing power in the chain of quantitative analysis of clinical trial results, findings are probably not relevant ('significant') from the point of view of clinical reasoning and decision-making. For example, smoking is epidemiologically more important in relation to lung cancer than in relation to cardiovascular problems. However, given the frequency of cardiovascular problems, control of smoking may be more clinically important for this area than for lung cancer. The fundamental epidemiological measures of treatment (or prevention modality) efficacy and effectiveness are the relative risk (strength of association) and the etiological fraction (specificity of association)[21]. These risks are calculated traditionally based on the occurrence of undesirable events (complications of disease, disease cases, deaths), using tradition and experience from field studies in community medicine. The same can be done for expected improvements, provided they are well defined in clinimetrically acceptable terms.

The following example is from the field of primary prevention of an infectious disease. Its logic and essentials of interpretation apply equally to the evaluation of effectiveness of drugs, surgery and other components of care in disease cure or improvement (secondary and tertiary prevention): Before an influenza epidemic, one community is immunized and another is not. The fictitious influenza attack rates for the evolved period of the epidemic were 10% for the former and 65% for the latter. Based on knowledge of the etiological fraction (see Chapter 8), it is interesting to note what proportion of cases in the non-immunized community is due to the community's non-immunization. In addition, by taking the attack rate in the community at higher risk for an event in the 'exposed' (language of the previous chapter) and the other for 'unexposed' (i.e. at lower risk), **vaccine effectiveness** or **efficacy** or **protective efficacy rate** may be calculated. (NB At times, these terms are used erroneously in the literature, and readers must often read 'between the lines'.) VE, on the basis of disease attack rates in unvaccinated subjects (ARU) and in vaccinated ones (ARV)[21–23] is calculated as follows:

$$VE = (ARU - ARV)/ARU = 1 - ARV/ARU$$

Where:

VE = vaccine efficacy or effectiveness
ARU = attack rate in the unvaccinated group
ARV = attack rate in the vaccinated (immunized) group

In this example, immunization efficacy or effectiveness (etiological fraction due to non immunization; vaccine efficacy or effectiveness; protective efficacy rate)

$$= \frac{65\% - 10\%}{65\%} \times 100 = 84.6\%$$

A frequent novice error is to attribute treatment effectiveness simply to the proportion of subjects in one group of interest who do not develop the disease, or to the number of individuals who do not develop an undesirable outcome when treated. Probabilities of a beneficial effect (staying healthy, being cured, alleviated) may also be counted. Uses of etiological fractions in the evaluation of treatment impact and their interpretation will depend on the choice of an outcome, which is supposed to measure the impact of treatment. If it is an undesirable outcome, such as death or complications, an etiological fraction quantifies the proportion of the whole of the undesirable event prevented or avoided by intervention. If a positive outcome, such as a cure, is considered, the etiological fraction quantifies the proportion of the whole of the success, which may be attributed to the intervention (treatment) of interest. However, there are now more ways to evaluate the impact of treatment than by just applying attributable fractions[24], as in the above-mentioned example. Table 9.1 summarizes various measurements of treatment impact based on the occurrence of good or bad events while comparing treated and untreated groups of patients. Information from each measurement is complementary, each index giving a different piece of evidence. For example, a bad event in the table may indicate an adverse reaction to the drug, lack of improvement, worsening, development of complications and death. Good events indicate cure, alleviation of pain and other manifestations of disease, regaining of autonomy, having a better quality of life, leaving the hospital and staying alive. In this table, it may be noted that all quantifications of treatment impact are based (with few exceptions) on classical notions of attributable risk or etiologic fraction (attributable risk percent) as explained in Chapter 8. The use of bad or good events in these computations measures two sides of the same issue. Overall, however, these quantifications give clinical and family medicine practitioners more meaningful expressions than those used currently in epidemiological research.

Relative risk of events, absolute risk reduction (or benefit increase) (ARR or ABI), and relative risk increase (RRI) or relative benefit increase (RBI) are increasingly used in evidence-based medicine and beyond. The original EBM contribution to the

Table 9.1 Qualification of bad and good events in clinical trials and prevention

Counting bad (undesirable) events	*Counting good (desirable) events*
Individual risk (probability) in the higher-risk group: Incidence (attack) rate of bad events in the non-vaccinated (non-treated) group (controls). In EBM, usually **CER**	**Individual risk (probability) of good events in the higher risk group**: Incidence (attack rate) of good events in a higher probability of such events group; usually EER
Individual risk (probability) in the lower-risk group (or baseline risk): Incidence (attack) rate of bad events in the vaccinated (treated, experimental) group. In EBM, usually **EER**	**Individual risk (probability) of good events in the lower-risk group**: Incidence (attack rate) of good events in a lower probability of such events group; usually CER
Relative risk of bad events: Incidence rate in the higher-risk group/incidence rate in the lower-risk group	**Relative risk of good events**: Incidence rate of good events in the expected higher-risk group (EER)/incidence rate in the expected lower-risk group (CER)
Attributable risk of bad events: Incidence rate in the higher-risk group – Incidence rate in the lower-risk group. It is an equivalent of **ARR (absolute risk reduction)**, the absolute arithmetic difference in event rates, ER, in the experimental (EER) and control (CER) group: IEER – CERI. It is also known in EBM as **absolute risk increase (ARI)**, if the experimental treatment harms more patients than the control treatment (e.g. adverse effects)	**Absolute benefit increase (ABI)** in EBM is the absolute arithmetical difference in good event rates, i.e. IEER – CERI
Etiological (attributable) fraction of bad events (not to be treated): Incidence rate (control group) – Incidence rate (experimental group)/incidence rate (control group): CER – EER/CER. **Relative risk reduction (RRR)** in EBM is calculated as ARR/CER	**Attributable fraction of good events (attributable benefit fraction, ABF)** is an increase in the rate of good events based on the comparison of those rates in the experimental and control patient groups in a trial, calculated as IEER – CERI / EER
Relative risk increase (RRI) as proposed in EBM is based again on an absolute arithmetical difference of IEER – CERI, i.e IEER – CERI/CER	**Relative benefit increase (RBI)** in EBM is an increase in the rates of good events based on the comparison of such events in the experimental and control groups IEER-CERI/CER
Number needed to treat (NNT) is the number of patients who need to be treated to achieve one additional favorable outcome. NNT = 1/ARR. It is a reciprocal of ARR	**Number needed to treat (NNT)** in EBM denotes the number of patients who must receive the experimental treatment to create one additional improved outcome in comparison with the control treatment: 1/ABI. It is a reciprocal of an absolute benefit increase (ABI)
Number needed to prevent (NNP) is the number of individuals not to be exposed to a putative factor to prevent one additional case: NNP = 1/ARR. It is a reciprocal of ARR in primary prevention. (N.B. Yet to be tested in practice. **Number needed to harm (NNH)** is the number of patients who, if they received the experimental treatment, would lead to 1 additional person being harmed, compared with patients who receive the control treatment: 1/ARI , hence a reciprocal of ARI	

For all of the above:

All the above quoted computations are **point estimates of various risks or proportions.** The uncertainty of these measurements is quantified by computing **confidence intervals (CI)**, usually reported as ranges within which those true values for the whole population (of patients) lie, 95% CI or 99% CI

evaluation of treatment impact is the development and use of the 'number needed to treat' or **NNT**[25–32]. As defined in Table 9.1, NNT allows the clinician an additional meaningful expression of clinical or preventive intervention impact. *The lesser the NNT, the more effective the drug.* A **'number needed to harm'** or **NNH**, developed and used originally in the study of undesirable (adverse) effects of treatment, may also be used (perhaps after other methodological refinements) in studies of different harmful factors in the etiology of disease. For now, clinicians seem to prefer NNTs, while biostatisticians prefer more traditional measures of impact such as attributable risk and etiologic fraction[32]. Journals devoted to EBM[33–36] regularly update the repertory of the most important treatment impact indexes. Both intervention efficacy or effectiveness (as discussed later) are measured the same way; only the nature of the clinical trial will decide what is measured (ideal or field conditions).

Returning to the example, vaccine effectiveness (attributable fraction of cases due to the prevention, or relative risk reduction (RRR) in EBM) was 84.6%. This does not mean that 85% of immunized subjects will not develop the disease. Rather, it means that in the non-immunized group of subjects, 85% of cases occurring in this group are due to the fact that they have not been immunized. Only this meaning applies to treatment effectiveness and efficacy. Vaccine efficacy (VE (%)) can also be estimated from case–control analysis, using formulas[18] from an unmatched analysis, as:

$$VE(\%) = (1 - OR) \times 100 = (1 - ad/bc) \times 100$$

or from a matched pair analysis, where odds ratio (OR) is s/t, in the notation used in Section 8.5.2. of Chapter 8, as

$$VE(\%) = (1 - OR) \times 100 = (1 - s/t) \times 100$$

In field epidemiology and community medicine, information from cohort or case–control approaches is not always available. In these circumstances, 'screening' formulas for vaccine effectiveness were proposed. An introduction of the proportion of the population vaccinated (PPV) in computations of vaccination impact allows the possibility of evaluating vaccine effectiveness rather than its efficacy (the proportion of individuals exposed to a favorable factor may vary from one community to another; in a cohort evaluation of efficacy one entire cohort is vaccinated, the other is not). In addition, the information most often available is the proportion of cases that were vaccinated (PCV). For such situations where vaccine coverage varies and limited observations are available, the appropriate screening formula is either[19,18]

$$VE(\%) = \frac{PPV - PCV}{PPV(1 - PCV)} \times 100$$

derived from the formula[18,19]

$$PCV = \frac{PPV - (PPV \times VE)}{1 - (PPV \times VE)}$$

or[20]

$$VE(\%) = 1 - \frac{PCV}{1 - PCV} \times \frac{1 - PPV}{PPV} \times 100$$

Obviously, the above-mentioned approach may be extended and applied to other situations where an impact (efficacy and effectiveness) of a beneficial factor, either preventive or therapeutic, is of interest. For example, such an approach might prove useful in phase IV clinical trials or post-marketing studies of drug effectiveness (see Section 9.2.3 of this chapter). This kind of 'borrowing methodology' from one field to another (with proper adjustments) should only be encouraged. From the infectious disease vaccination concept and model, cases of disease are replaced in a broader framework by cases that fail to improve or to respond to treatment in an expected way, and vaccination is replaced by treatment of interest.

In clinical evaluations, distinctions must be made between findings in ideal (experimental) and field (real-life) conditions. In absolute terms, the effectiveness of an immunization program is measured as it happens, and not the vaccine effectiveness at an individual level when leaving the manufacturer's laboratory. Vaccine storage, transportation, way of inoculation, and other factors such as health status and co-morbidity in immunized subjects may affect the overall impression obtained through epidemiology. Such an 'etiological' experimental study, however, is only part of the more complex process of treatment evaluation. It does not take place right away, but is preceded by several important phases of assessment.

9.2.3 Phases of evaluation of treatment

Any evaluation of medical intervention is a sequential procedure, beginning with trials on animals. Surgeons first try procedures on pigs, dogs or apes (monkeys). Pharmacologists test drugs on mice, rats or guinea pigs. Short-term trials in animals last one to four weeks or more, and studies of toxicity last from three to 12 months. About one-third of substances toxic to animals are also toxic to humans. Finally, the 'vertical impact' of drugs must be assessed. This involves the potential cancerogenicity in descendants of parents treated by the drug under study. Such an assessment aims to prevent occurrence, such as the risk of primary clear cell carcinoma of the vagina in daughters of mothers who have taken diethylstilbestrol. Once the risks of a 'horizontal impact' (between experimental animals) and a 'vertical' one (impact on descendants) are eliminated, four phases of evaluation in humans[37–39] take place. Table 9.2 summarizes these procedures.

A **phase one study** evaluates the basic biological responses of healthy individuals to the drug. The procedure may start with approximately 2% of the effective dose in animals, and is progressively doubled to reach a biologically effective dose in humans. Both expected responses and undesirable effects are noted. Once life-threatening or other disease-forming (cancerogenicity) risks are eliminated, and other side effects ('trade-offs' for the efficiency of a drug, such as nausea or blood dyscrasia in cancer chemotherapy) are detected, palliative co-treatment may be planned. For example, Jones et al[40] tested the response of female volunteers in good health to a new birth control vaccine. There were no important adverse reactions over six months, and potentially contraceptive levels of antibodies to human chorionic gonadotropin developed in all 30 subjects. Gustavson and Carrigan[41] evaluated the pharmacokinetics of a new hypnotic (estazolam). Absorption, plasma concentration and elimination were shown to be independent of the dose and dosage strength administered. These characteristics were found compatible with the drug's effect on sleep latency and duration.

A **phase two study** evaluates the treatment under study in subjects suffering from the target disease[42,43]. Most of these studies do not include control groups. Foon et al[44] evaluated the efficacy of interferon in 19 chronic lymphocytic leukemia sufferers. Toxicity was found to be dose-dependent. Given the different responses of patients to the treatment, it was established to be ineffective.

A **phase three study** is, by definition, an experimental etiological study of a drug (cause) and its healing effect (consequence). The efficacy of treatment is evaluated at this stage. Szmuness et al[18] conducted an excellent field trial of a new type of hepatitis B vaccine. In their placebo-controlled, randomized, double-blind trial (as detailed later), the reduction of the incidence rates of disease was found to be as high as 92.3% when comparing two high-risk groups, i.e. vaccinated and unvaccinated (placebo recipients) for a total of 1083 homosexual men. This is a phase three study. In another, still disputed controlled clinical trial, the Anturane Reinfarction Trial Research Group found that sulfinpyrazone (Anturan) modified the prognosis of sudden death (reinfarction) during the high-risk period between two and seven months after the first heart attack[45].

A **phase four study** (i.e. a post-marketing study after the licensure of the drug) assesses drug effectiveness 'in field conditions', i.e. in daily hospital practice or in primary care, either with non-selected individuals who have the disease under study, or in sufferers of multiple health problems for which the medication may have multiple positive or negative impacts or unexpected effects by interacting with other drugs given to these patients for other health problems. For example, anticancer drugs are often given to elderly patients who have coronary problems, liver and/or kidney insufficiency or arthritis, and who are hypertensive, hyperlipidemic, depressed, etc. The subjects of post-marketing studies[48,49] may be numerous. Drug effectiveness, side effects with prolonged use, drug incompatibilities, effects on comorbidity or compliance (respecting treatment plans such as dosage, frequency and duration) may be the objects of study. Pierce, Shu, and Groves[47]

Table 9.2	Phases of clinical evaluation of drugs				
Phase of trial	*Fundamental question to be answered*	*Individuals involved*	*Clinical problem to be solved*	*Design*	*Example in literature (ref.)*
I.	How will healthy individuals respond to the drug?	Healthy subjects (volunteers)	– Pharmacokinetics – Drug safety	Descriptive observational study	40,41
			Early phase:		
II.	How will patients respond to the drug?	Pre-selected sufferers of the target disease (usually hospital patients)	– Establishment of dose range – Potential benefits – Side effects	Observational case study (descriptive)	42–44
			Late phase:		
			– Estimation of the efficacy relative to competing drugs	– Small samples – Observational case studies, or studies with historical controls, or with groups from 'outside the trial' – Comparative studies of immediate impact – Comparative studies of the modification of disease course (comparative studies of prognosis); impact in time	
III.	Can and does the treatment really work?	Pre-selected target disease sufferers in hospital setting <u>or</u> in the community	Efficacy of the drug (impact in ideal conditions)	– Randomized double-blind controlled clinical trial, or its alternatives (sequential design, 'n-of-one' study, etc.) – Large enough samples	18, 45,46
			Early phase:		
			Efficacy in a limited spectrum and gradient of disease	'Model' or 'typical' cases	
			Late phase:		
			Full spectrum and gradient of disease	All kinds of cases	
			Early phase:		
IV.	How will the treatment work once it is put to general use?	Non-selected patients in the population at large (hospital or community – 'whoever comes through the door')	Effectiveness of the drug (impact in habitual conditions)	'Clean', 'neat' cases	47
			Late phase		
V. (proposal)		Post-marketing studies	– Rare, late, and chronic toxicity and secondary effects – Drug interactions – New, unknown effects – Better dosage	Cases with comorbidity and co-treatment(s)	

evaluated the safety of Estazolam (triazolobenzo-diazepine), already marketed in over 40 countries and used as a hypnotic. Their study on 1,320 insomniac volunteers showed no effects on vital signs, some side effects, and no effects on psychomotor performance, including memory. The drug was found to be safe and effective in this post-marketing study. Hence, a phase III experiment assesses basic causal associations under 'clean' conditions, while a phase IV trial evaluates the impact in the context of the 'messy' realities of clinical practice[50]. For some[50,51], the former represents a fastidious or explanatory trial, while the latter is more pragmatic.

A **phase five study** might be a phase four trial in which are enrolled patients suffering also from other diseases that the disease of main interest (comorbidities) and who are treated also for these additional problems (cotreatment for comorbidities). Such an additional classification is still open to discussion.

Such a step-by-step (phase after phase) assessment of treatment is similar to the classification of validation studies of diagnostic techniques and methods as proposed by Freedman[38], Nierenberg and Feinstein[52,53]. Table 9.3 illustrates the corresponding phases of trials of treatments and diagnostic methods (see also Table 6.16 in Chapter 6).

At all phases of drug evaluation, the essential rigor of clinimetric follow-up of the disease must be respected. In the analytical phases (phases three and four), all precautions to avoid bias must be taken (see Chapter 8). Cause–effect relationships must be demonstrated according to the generally applicable criteria of causality (also explained in Chapter 8). Unfortunately, the latter is seldom done, and the

authors (and often pharmaceutical or other companies) remain satisfied with 'statistically significant' results. The epidemiological assessment of the treatment's impact must be established.

9.2.4 Designs of clinical trials

The basic architecture of a clinical trial as illustrated in Figure 9.1 can be determined in several ways, some more appropriate than others. A strict experimental approach cannot in fact be used to study all health problems and interventions.

9.2.4.1 The golden standard. Randomized trials with parallel groups

The clinical trial closest to the experiment is the 'randomized, double-blind, placebo-controlled' trial. Its title reflects three fundamental precautions (added to observational design) to ensure maximum objectivity of findings and their interpretation. **Randomization** is the procedure of assigning subjects to treatment groups using the effect of chance. **Blinding** is the procedure that makes the nature of the observations and actions unknown to the participants (patients) and the investigators. Unbiased reading and interpretation of findings is sought this way. **Placebo** represents an inactive, 'sham' treatment (drug, surgical procedure, etc.) to which the active procedure under study is compared. Starch pills, saline solution injections or skin-deep incisions instead of full operations may serve as placebos. It is, however, sometimes desirable that the placebo imitate the side effects of the active procedure (for example, extrapyramidal effects of psychoactive

Table 9.3 Phases of studies evaluating clinical procedures

Phase	Diagnostic procedure	Therapeutic procedure
I	Feasibility, promise	Toxicity, feasibility
II	Studies of diagnostic accuracy	Screening for activity against disease
III	Studies of clinical value (or randomized comparisons where feasible)	Randomized, controlled comparison in a clinical setting
	End-points: diagnosis; treatment; patient outcome	
IV	Before-and-after studies for monitoring routine use	Monitoring routine use and outcome

Source: Adapted from Ref. 52.

drugs, etc.), thus being called an 'active placebo'. The placebo procedure is selected at the moment of trial planning as soon as control groups are considered. Randomization is performed at stage 4. Blinding applies to the whole trial except for its planning and interpretation after the statistical analysis of findings.

Randomization

Randomization as defined above allows for the distribution of patients into comparable treatment groups according to characteristics that are either **unknown** or hard to identify. Subjects are assigned (by the will and decision of the experimenter) **at random** into one of the groups to be compared. One method of randomization would be to flip a coin; other methods considered in the past were based on some nominal (names) or numerical identification (hospital or telephone numbers) of patients. Especially in the latter case, the effect of chance may be dubious. The method most often used today involves the use of **tables of random numbers**. Tables of random numbers are easily generated by computer or found in most biostatistics books. They give horizontal and vertical sequences of numbers suitable for randomization and are constructed so that there is no possible distinguishable periodicity or predictable sequence of numbers. The main purpose of this procedure is to eliminate susceptibility bias. However, not all inequalities (be they in state of health, prognosis, chance for diagnostic procedures, follow-up or other uncontrolled factors) are eliminated. They are merely equally distributed between the comparison groups. Table 9.4 illustrates a portion of such a table, generated for a previous reading[23]. If even numbers were chosen for an experimental drug and odd numbers for placebo treatment, patients numbered 1, 2, 4, 7, 8, 10, etc. in presenting order should receive

the drug; others would receive the control treatment (placebo).

For example, a trial is constructed for a new analgesic used to control simple tension headaches in patients visiting a clinic. The attending physician may choose even numbers for treatment A and odd numbers for treatment B (placebo). Active pills or placebo pills would be put in unidentified envelopes. If the second line of numbers in the table were to be used (starting at any line, column or place), the first two patients would get the first two envelopes containing the active pill (unknown to the physician), the third one would get the placebo envelope, the fourth the active pill, the fifth and sixth patients would get the placebo, etc. Other, more detailed procedures of randomization are available in the statistical literature[54–57].

Randomization does not:

- Replace other methods that make groups comparable, such as restricting cases to those who have only certain characteristics (representativity is compromised);
- Replace more structured designs, such as prognostic stratification (see Chapter 10), whose aim is to increase the comparability of the stratification variables in treatment groups[58,59];
- Exclude confounding factors[4,60].

Randomization does:

- Eliminate bias from the assignment of treatment;
- Balance treatment groups in covariates (susceptibility bias control, prognostic factors, other intangible characteristics)[58,61] if the sample size is large enough;
- Guarantee the validity of the statistical tests of significance that are used to compare treatment[60].

Randomization is used essentially to neutralize inequalities due either to **unknown factors** (e.g. hereditary predisposition, unrecognized drug abuse, sexual orientation, etc.) or to those that are **hard to recognize**, or, in case of **inequalities, those which cannot be compensated by other means**, usually reserved for the control of **known factors**: stratification (i.e. making subgroups according to differences in disease spectrum, gradient, prognosis, etc.); matching; restriction (dropping some marginal

Table 9.4	Table of random numbers (excerpt)

	30702	52673	36233	46610	25127
Start→	**2 8** 5 **2** 5	9 **2 2 9 2**	41238	84734	34654
	44188	36785	10133	85052	46077
	70306	87207	04549	16669	36734
	76025	09747	22705	12843	54251

Source: Drawn from Ref. 23 and reproduced with permission.

subjects from the study); multivariate analysis, etc. However, if patients' characteristics are known (for example, if the prognosis is known), stratification according to these known characteristics may be considered first before any other method of 'balancing the trial'. For example, cancer patients may be enrolled in groups according to their cancer stage, and treatment effectiveness may be compared from one stage to another. Findings from studies may differ from similar, 'unstratified' ones[62]. More information about this can be found in the chapter on prognosis.

Blinding

The second characteristic of a clinical trial is the necessity of **blinding**. Blinding's main purpose is to avoid bias by a preconceived impression of initial state or maneuver, or a subsequent state, or of various measures, readings, etc., either by the experimenters or the participating subjects. For example, if trial subjects were to know who received an experimental drug and who received a placebo, they may declare the 'new' drug to be more effective, thus corresponding to their preconceptions. In the same spirit, buyers of art purchase the latest dated paintings of an artist (the more recent the painting, the better it must be), which is why some artists 'blind' their paintings by not indicating the year of creation of their work. Blinding (or masking) is any procedure designed to make observations in clinical trials as objective as possible:

1. **Physicians** are blinded, i.e. they do not know what therapeutic regimen the patient is undergoing. If this were not so, they might consciously or subconsciously assess a patient's status differently by knowing, for example, who receives the inactive placebo or the active drug.
2. **Patients** are blinded; they do not know what therapeutic regimen they are undergoing. Otherwise, they might report effects differently: for many, the 'new' drug (or second in a sequence) 'must be better', etc.
3. The way **randomization** occurs is blinded. Patients may be randomly assigned in different ways (random numbers, choice of days, etc.). Experimenters should not know how randomization is carried out. Otherwise, pre-treatment risk factors

may be distributed unequally[58], or patients and/or physicians might recognize some 'pattern' of responses, etc.

4. Investigators must be blinded as to **trends**[63]. In long-term studies to which patients are continuously being admitted and in which withdrawals occur, the knowledge of trends (expected results) may bias the final make-up of the treatment groups.
5. **Outcome variables** must be hidden. For example, investigators do not know if blood pressure, body temperature or heart rate are supposed to measure the effect of a therapeutic procedure. Biased attention and reading may be improved in this way.
6. **Biostatisticians** must be blinded when they are analyzing trial results (which group receives what).
7. In studies where blinding of therapies is absent or imperfect, **patients removed during or after data collection** (observation period) should be unknown to the investigators: (i.e. from which compared group are they coming, and how well the patient was responding when the decision to remove him or her from the study was made).

It is important that all possible kinds of blinding be implemented wherever relevant and possible. In all cases, a 'double blind (patient and physician), randomized placebo controlled clinical trial' represents the standard, even in the need of further improvements[64]. The degree of blinding (simple, double, or more) is dictated by the nature of the problem, and no general rule can be proposed as to how advanced it must be. For example, if only one measure of outcome is available (i.e. survival), there is no need to blind the outcome variable.

As already mentioned, randomization is used essentially to control (to spread evenly among groups under comparison) subjects according to **unknown** characteristics (e.g. possible competing causal factors) or those which are hard to obtain because of cost, falsifiability (characteristics bearing social stigma such as drug abuse, sexual orientation, income), etc. For beginners, randomization may appear as a way of blinding. This is not so. One procedure does not replace another; each is done for different purposes. Randomization evenly distributes characteristics of patients in various groups under comparison. Blinding makes the reading of these characteristics and treatment impact(s) more objective and unbiased.

Even a best possible randomized double-blind controlled clinical trial (RCT), in its classical form, may still carry several imperfections. For Kaptchuk[64], the knowledge of possibly receiving a placebo may decrease the response to either drug or placebo. The participation in RCT itself may affect the detection of beneficial or adverse responses. What about individuals who, for any reason, have not been enrolled in an RCT – their characteristics, diagnosis, treatment and fate? A better understanding of the placebo and nocebo effect and the whole patient pool (refusals, dropouts, ineligibility and all other factors) may lead to a greater understanding of treatment and its effects.

Placebo and other reference procedures

The choice of a reference procedure depends on the question the clinical trial is meant to answer. A reference procedure may be a placebo such as an inactive substance, the best available treatment or procedure, the most often used treatment or anything else depending on the question: Does the new treatment work, does it work better than the best available drug, does it work better than the most popular treatment? In a fastidious or fundamental approach of efficacy studies (establishing a basic causal relationship), a placebo may be preferred. In a pragmatic trial or effectiveness study, the best available treatment or any other active treatment (e.g. the one which is most often prescribed in practice, etc.) may be chosen. The best available treatment as a reference procedure is dictated by medical ethics wherever the disease has a serious prognosis (with or without treatment) and wherever such a treatment is available. Sometimes, a placebo ('just getting the pill') may seem to work. The placebo response has been a subject of laic and professional interest for centuries[65].

The **placebo effect** (or halo effect) is attributable to the expectation that the regimen will have an effect, i.e. the effect is due to the power of suggestion[3]. Hence, a placebo may appear to have an effect. If the placebo has some effect, this may have two meanings[66]: effect of placebo intervention itself and/or effect of patient–provider interaction, a 'white coat effect'. The **'placebo effect'** is also defined as '*any effect attributable to a pill, potion, or procedure but not to its pharmacodynamic or specific properties*'[67]. In practice, the placebo effect is not necessarily bad. If a placebo works to the benefit of the patient, why not prescribe it? In designing clinical trials, this effect must be taken into account[68]. Brody[69] estimates that the placebo effect may be responsible for as much as 30% of many treatment effects. It should still be better understood[70,71].

Nocebo effect

Good news offered to patients may act as a placebo by contributing to improvement in the patient's health. Bad news may cause the opposite effect. Reminders of real or perceived deleterious effects of a particular habit, or of threatening environmental or psychologic factors, act as a **nocebo** by having a negative effect on health[72]. Hahn[73] defines the nocebo effect as '. . . *the causation of sickness (or death) by expectations of sickness (or death) and by associated emotional states.*' The patient may expect a specific problem or have vague expectations resulting in imprecisely anticipated problems. A surgical patient may anticipate death from surgery and die because of such an expectation and not because of the surgery itself. Unexpected complications may occur because of vague, non-specific negative expectations, such as those stemming from depression. Such phenomena must be distinguished from **placebo side effects**, which occur when expectations of healing produce sickness (positive expectations leading to negative outcomes), like a rash after receiving a placebo[73]. In the nocebo situation, negative outcomes are expected. Inversely, nocebos may exert side effects when negative expectations produce positive outcomes.

The nocebo effect may play an important social and cultural role. Such is the case, for example, in voodoo death[74], 'tapu' or 'taboo' death among New Zealand Maoris[75], sociogenic (psychogenic, mass-produced) illness (hysteria), or unexplained responses to exposures to unpleasant sensations such as odors or mild irritants in environmental health and occupational medicine. The nocebo effect is confirmed in these cases by an often complex and extended exclusion of known specific harms. Victims of wars, refugees or dispossessed, or otherwise socially alienated persons may become subjects of specific or non-specific expectations and ensuing nocebo consequences. The nocebo effect may be a clinical problem at the bedside and a public health problem in a community setting.

9.2.4.2 *Other types of randomized clinical trials*

As discussed earlier, parallel trials[76] are (most) often performed. A parallel follow-up of experimental and control groups may be performed in a reasonable time, but larger samples (numbers of patients participating) are often necessary. One must also attempt to control the feeling that 'the next, the second or the following treatment must be better'. **Crossover design**[76,77] have been put into practice for these reasons.

Another problem stems from the limited availability of patients who would satisfy the statistical requirements of a valid trial (see further). Although most trials involve a pre-calculated number of patients (fixed designs), an 'open design' has also been developed. **Sequential design**[78] is a good example of this second category, which may prove useful in situations where results must also be

obtained as soon as possible (life threatening disease if untreated).

Crossover design

In chronic diseases with episodic manifestations and a protracted course, several therapeutic options (i.e. two drugs) may be evaluated by comparing two groups of patients who, at a given time, receive two therapeutic or preventive regimens in reverse order. Figure 9.2 illustrates such a crossover design. More information from a limited number of patients is provided, intra-patient variation is smaller, and groups serve as their own controls in time. Therapeutic sequences must, however, be preceded by a proper **'run in'**[79] **or qualification period**[80] and interspaced thereafter by a proper **'washout' interval**. The qualification period also serves to become better acquainted with patients (characteristics, course of cases, clinimetric data, as well as introducing the trial after a proper washout period). Washout periods are intervals before or between treatment regimens during which therapeutic and secondary effects (or any other factors which might bias patients' evaluations) should disappear. Proper clinimetric information on disease course and treatment itself (pharmacodynamics etc.) must be available to estimate

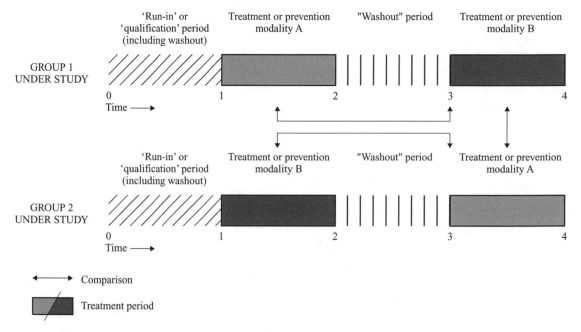

Figure 9.2 Schematic representation of a crossover design: Evaluation and comparison points in time of groups under study

sufficiently long washout periods. Studies of migraine[79–81] or chronic angina[82,83] can serve as examples of problems assessed through crossover trials.

Both parallel and crossover designs have their own advantages and disadvantages, as summarized by Kunkel[81]. Parallel studies do not need a washout period, a longer follow-up detects better some side effects, blinding is easier. However, larger samples of patients are needed. Crossover studies permit intra-patient comparisons as patients serve as their own control, fewer patients are needed, fewer patients drop out, and the randomization is easier. 'Blindness' is more difficult to maintain and a washout period is often necessary.

N-of-1 clinical trials

Randomized trials in individual patients, or the **'n-of-1 study'**, are clinical trials whose purpose is 'to tailor the treatment modality to a specific patient', not to seek some universal truth about treatment superiority. A single patient (i.e. sample size, N, being 'one', hence the name of the design) may serve as the subject of a randomized trial[83–89].

Many chronic diseases have episodic courses, like angina, migraine, tension headache, herpes, asthma, vasovagal syncope, atopic dermatitis, bulimia binges, irritable bowel syndrome, gout or arthritis, among many others. The sufferer is a subject of a pair of treatment periods (two drugs to choose from). The order of drugs within each pair is randomized. Pairs of treatment periods are repeated. Three pair periods are usually enough to recognize which drug is more effective, but they may be repeated as often as necessary or be stopped any time for ethical reasons, or in the case of overwhelming evidence in favor of one treatment modality. This type of crossover design (*n*-of-one trial) may prove useful in the following situations[84]:

- Where no randomized trial was conducted;
- When the health problem is rare;
- When the patient does not meet the criteria of eligibility for a trial;
- When the decision must be specific to an individual patient;

- When some patients would not benefit from treatment in a randomized controlled clinical trial in its classical form; and
- When a randomized clinical trial came to negative conclusions, but some participants benefited from treatment.

Short, clearly delineated episodes with rapidly appearing and disappearing manifestations (clinical or paraclinical) and short washout periods are desirable for this kind of trial[85].

Treatment modalities are allocated at random in a sequence within the pair, and multiple blinding is feasible as in a classical design. Conventional trials mainly evaluate the overall effect on a group, whereas a single case experiment will determine whether treatment is beneficial for a specific individual[86]. Given the latter benefit and feasibility, the *n*-of-1 study may be increasingly attractive for many practicing clinicians[87]. It will provide individualized information complementary to classical randomized clinical trials[85]. Prolonged treatments associated with recurrent symptoms or infections are also suitable for a single patient trial. For example, Metronidazole efficacy in controlling infection in ileostomized patients was evaluated in this way[88]. Rochon described a more detailed statistical approach to this design[90].

Sequential design

Another form of clinical trials was developed taking into account the minimum number of patients to enroll in a clinical trial. **Sequential design**, described by Wald[91] and subsequently developed in medicine by Bross[92] and Armitage[93], is an example of an open design, where the number of patients is not fixed *a priori*. Rather, it is determined by the experiment itself, i.e. by the nature of the results appearing from patients entering the study in stages.

In this kind of trial, patients enter the study in pairs. The first pair receives a random treatment modality. The treatment that works best is noted. These preferences are drawn into an *ad hoc* sequential plan, representing a 'checkerboard configuration[92]' (Figure 9.3 and 9.4), whose boundaries of 'significant results' are obtained from the binomial distribution[92,93]. The upper section of the plan above the significance boundary for a treatment under study indicates a preference for this kind of intervention. The lower boundary (and its crossing) represents a preference (or significant result) in favor of the reference treatment (placebo or another drug). The first pair of patients entering the study is

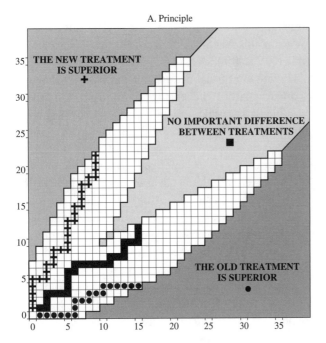

A. Principle

Figure 9.3 Principle of a sequential trial plan. Source: Ref. 92, reproduced and adapted with permission from the International Biometric Society

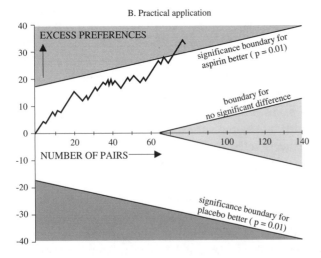

B. Practical application

Figure 9.4 Sequential design of a clinical trial. Practical application. Source: Ref. 94, reproduced with permission of the Massachusetts Medical Society (*N Engl J Med*)

evaluated and the results marked in the upper direction of the vertical axis if the experimental drug is more effective, in the down direction if the reference treatment is more effective (the result is not registered if the effect is the same in both patients, i.e. if both recover or die). For the next pair, the preference is marked relative to (from) the position reached by the previous pair of patients, and so on as shown on Figure 9.3.

Figure 9.4 illustrates the results of the evaluation of the protective effects of aspirin against acute myocardial infarction and death in men with unstable angina[94]. The significance boundaries were crossed on the 75th patient pair, hence 75 pairs were enough to demonstrate the preferential effects of aspirin in this study.

Sequential design has its own limitations[95]. Pairs must be suitably matched (disease, characteristics, etc.), and they should preferably enter the trial in a reasonably rapid sequence (succession). The time required to record results should be less than the time required to collect the cases. Inequality of the duration of responses within and between pairs is also not desirable. Hence, every method has its own trade-offs. Sequential trials demonstrate, by a succession of results, the direction of treatment preference. They do not allow the assessment of treatment effectiveness in terms of relative and attributable risks.

Other, non-randomized studies of treatment effects to consider are uncontrolled trials, field studies[96], series of consecutive cases, natural experiments (as they happen), studies with historical control groups[97] or assessments of effectiveness of preventive and curative interventions by observational studies[98] such as case–control analytical methods[99]. Each of these methods has its advantages, such as economy, availability of data or ethical ease. Their main disadvantage is a more limited power of proof of treatment effectiveness or efficacy.

9.2.5 Assessment of a clinical trial's quality

The quality of any clinical trial depends on three main components:

- How a clinical trial is prepared. Research protocols are vital for this purpose ('what will happen?');

- How a clinical trial was realized ('what happened?');
- How the findings are analyzed, interpreted and presented ('what was done with the results?').

9.2.5.1 Research protocols. A priori prerequisites
Research protocols of clinical trials are written records of stated problems indicating how they will be studied and how they will be solved. The following fairly standard elements of a research proposal and protocol usually reflect and give details on the nine steps of a clinical trial as represented by Figure 9.1.

- **Title;**
- Research **question** that the clinical trial should answer (hypothesis);
- **Background**, i.e. justification of the trial given past experience, missing information, relevance of expected findings, gains in health, resources, and care;
- **Design** of the trial (RCT or its alternatives);
- **Sample** size considerations, data **collection** and strategies of **analysis;**
- **Methodological challenges** of measurement, analysis, interpretation, and implementation;
- Blank forms, data **sheets,** dummy **tables** (how results will be presented);
- **Ethical considerations** and consents;
- Other administrative and technical **authorizations** wherever needed, resources, budget.

This kind of thorough preparation defines the final success of the trial. The quality of a research protocol depends on how clearly the problem is stated, to whom it applies (step 1), on whom will it be studied (step 2), how patients will be recruited into the study (step 2), how their initial state will be evaluated (step 3), how they will be spread into comparison groups (step 4), how maneuvers will be applied (step 5), how outcomes will be evaluated in patients (step 6), how data will be analyzed (step 7), interpreted and explained within the study (step 8), and how they may and will be generalized beyond the study (step 9). As will be seen later, similar criteria apply to the evaluation of quality of a clinical trial once it is complete. In detail, research protocols of clinical

trials include (in varying complexity) several components[9,100–102] as represented in Table 9.5.

All of these components appear in variable combinations and details as required by the funding agencies of clinical trials[9,100,101]. In general, subsequent results of clinical trials are only as good as their initial protocols. Given this crucial fact, protocols of important studies are worthy of publication on their own, before the trial is begun. More and more study designs are being published[103–105] including the characteristics of the subjects enrolled[106] before the presentation of intermediate[107] or final results[108]. Prepublication of trial design, methods and techniques is a valid, but unsparing exposure of the investigators' competence, as well as a warranty of the trial's success and a source of valuable information for other investigators wishing to produce data and findings comparable to the ongoing study. Several important additional aspects of good clinical trials are worth mentioning.

Deductive building of trial design
Any decision to match, stratify, or randomize must be made beforehand. This applies particularly to prognostic stratification[109,110], or to the potency and timing of the therapeutic maneuver. It is easy to do this after data is collected, rearranging the findings to the investigator's liking to make them 'significant', but this is inappropriate.

Particular attention to the handling of soft data
As one of the objectives of a clinical trial is not only to find a cure, but also to ease a patient's suffering, soft data often represent outcome variables. Pain, anxiety, itching, anger, etc., are often targeted by treatment. Clear operational criteria (both for inclusion <u>and</u> exclusion[111]) must be given to these variables (hard data presents less of a problem). Exclusion criteria should not only be observations outside a certain range, but they should be complementary to the inclusion criteria. For example, pain beyond a certain duration and frequency is excluded by definition, but a 'real' exclusion criterion would be the presence of a brain tumor in a study of simple tension headache. Hence, attention is paid not only

Table 9.5 Desirable components of a research protocol

Formulation of the problem:
1. Background and rationale for the trial ('why is it done').
2. Hypothesis to be tested.
3. General objective of the study (point to reach in qualitative terms).
4. Specific objective (point to reach in quantitative terms).

Clinimetrically valid definition of dependent (health problem, disease) and independent (treatment modality, control modality) variables under study with clear inclusion and exclusion criteria:
5. Definition of the disease in terms of its spectrum, gradient and course.
6. Operational definition of the experimental treatment (or prevention) modality.
7. Operational definition of control (reference) treatment (placebo, other active intervention, etc.).
8. Clinimetrically valid definition of outcomes or expected results of impact (endpoints of the trial).
9. Equally valid definitions of comorbidities and cotreatments, if these are relevant to the problem under study.

How subjects will be recruited into the trial:
10. Target disease, population of patients, community from which they come.
11. Sampling plan, size, and accession rate.
12. Clinimetrically precise and unequivocal inclusion **and** exclusion criteria of subjects for the trial.
13. Subjects' informed consent (including information provided to patients).

Architecture or design of the trial:
14. Type of trial.
15. How it will be controlled: randomization; blinding; matching; stratification; other techniques, all well described.
16. Possible biases of the trial or possible accidental errors and how they will be controlled before, during, and after the trial.
17. Baseline data needed and how data will be obtained.
18. Other relevant information such as comorbidity and/or cotreatment(s), whenever relative to the hypothesis under study.

Information on preventive or therapeutic maneuvers:
19. Clinimetrically valid (qualitative and quantitative) description of experimental and control treatment modalities.
20. How they will be applied (schedule of treatments).

Information on evaluation of subsequent state:
21. Schedule of evaluations.
22. Way of dealing with unexpected outcomes (undesirable, secondary effects, etc.).

How the trial will be conducted:
23. Methods of data collection and recording (including sample forms of questionnaires, data sheets, etc.).
24. Responsibilities for data management.
25. Methods and responsibilities for data analysis: statistical; epidemiological; clinical.
26. Procedures and rules for discontinuing treatment.
27. Handling dropouts (nonresponders, nonresponses).

How results will be presented:
28. Descriptive and analytic parameters to be obtained.
29. Which clinical, statistical, and epidemiological information will be presented.
30. Form of presentation of findings ('dummy tables', blank graphics, or other relevant forms).
31. Plans for publication of results.

Administrative aspects of the trial:
32. Material resources required (hardware, software).
33. Human resources required (research, clinical, technical staff, archives, etc.).
34. Chronology of the trial.
35. Cost of the trial (budget).

Ethical evaluation of the trial:
36. Approval by the ethics committee where the study will be done (hospital, university, research institution).
37. Informed consent given or a copy of the consent form made available.

to the control of diagnostic entities but also to specific manifestations, signs or symptoms[112]. Both inclusion and exclusion criteria must be defined not only in conceptual but also in operational terms. Even if this is more challenging, it must also be done for soft data, such as in migraine[111] and elsewhere.

Attention to human biology (chronopharmacological consideration)

As mentioned in Chapter 1, **chronobiology** has resulted in new advances in the understanding of circadian rhythms, these being of particular importance in sick individuals. The new domain of **chronotherapy** enhances effectiveness of treatment modalities by adjusting the timing and potency of treatments to physiological and pathological biorhythmicity. These considerations should be respected in preparing clinical trials and in making therapeutic decisions in practice, wherever this knowledge is available and relevant. Recent findings show how useful these refinements are, for example, in the use of asthma and non-steroidal anti-inflammatory drugs for arthritis control[113,114].

Sample size considerations

Wherever possible, the number of subjects enrolled in clinical trials must be calculated beforehand. A clinician usually does this with the help of an expert biostatistician. However, it is the clinician's primary responsibility to provide valid and realistic clinical estimations on which sample sizes are calculated.

If a *qualitative variable* is studied, such as the frequency of improvements of disease spells, complications, etc., the following are needed[8,114]:

1. Expected rate of success in the control group, i.e. what the reference treatment does;
2. Rate of success in the experimental work, i.e. a difference between both groups, expected (realistically) from what is known of the tested treatment;
3. Alpha error (Z_α). Only the physician may decide how important this is (in making an error by choosing a false promising treatment, which in reality is completely ineffective or not as effective as another treatment already available);

4. Beta error (Z_β, or a power in terms of $1 - beta$). Again, the physician should determine the degree of certitude required so as not to miss a more effective treatment. Alpha error of 0.05 and beta error of 0.2 (a 1 : 4 ratio) is not a rule.

Wherever sensitivity and specificity are important in diagnosis (on the basis of a Bayesian approach, see Chapter 6), sample sizes may be defined by taking into account sensitivity, specificity, and the prevalence of the disease under study in the design of a randomized trial[116].

In trials where *quantitative variables* such as blood pressure or glycemia are measures of effect, similar premises need to be clarified:

1. The variance of the variable of interest;
2. The desired difference to be reached by the treatment under study. For example, the investigator wants to lower the average diastolic blood pressure by 5 mmHg;
3. Alpha and beta errors;
4. The proportion of patients in each group to be compared (from the whole sample);
5. The expected number of non-responders.

These parameters, corresponding as much as possible to the clinical reality, must be defined by a health professional. Otherwise, statisticians may use caution by adopting excessively severe criteria that yield either unrealistic numbers of patients for the trial, or trials that are more costly than necessary. Small sample sizes of clinical trials lead to a low statistical power. Trials of preventive measures, in particular, often require large sample sizes[117]. Sample sizes for cross-over designs are given by Tfelt-Hansen and Nielsen[118].

Ethical considerations

Any clinical trial must be submitted to an appropriate ethics committee (institutional or inter-institutional), which approves its acceptability, provided that:

1. The patient is well informed about the trial, its course and its outcomes;
2. No unacceptable harm will be done to the patient by using a new treatment, or by not treating the patient with the modality of interest.

3. No harm will be done to the patient's children (remember diethylstilbestrol and clear cell vaginal cancer in daughters of mothers who took it, or the thalidomide tragedy);

4. No breach of confidentiality will be made, especially in this era of informatics, record linkage, and collaborative studies.

These basic criteria are well detailed in the literature[119–122]. In addition to the basic requirements of medical ethics, physicians must approach a clinical trial with **equipoise**, i.e. with a genuine uncertainty regarding the comparative therapeutic merits of each arm of the trial, existing within the expert medical community[123]. If such an uncertainty disappears during the trial (new information obtained on treatment efficacy), the best available treatment is then given to the patient.

The physician must also respect the finding of **medical futility**[124,125]. A futile action is one that cannot achieve the goals of the action, no matter how often it is repeated[120]. Any treatment, which overwhelmingly provides evidence of its inability to improve a patient's prognosis, comfort, well-being, or general state of health, should be discontinued right away, whether in the context of a trial or elsewhere. Schneiderman et al[124] propose that when clinicians conclude (either through personal experience, experiences shared with colleagues, or consideration of published empiric data) that in the last 100 cases a medical treatment has been useless, they should regard the treatment as futile. Outside clinical trials, consideration of futility is important when discontinuing therapy in medical practice[125].

The **ethical guidelines** for clinical trials and experimental research also extend to **epidemiological research**[126], which is often observational. Beauchamp et al's[127] recommendations reflect this point well:

'**Obligations to the subjects of research**: *to protect their welfare; to obtain their informed consent; to protect their privacy; to maintain confidential information.*

Obligations to society: *to avoid conflicts of interest; to avoid partiality; to widen the scope of epidemiology; to pursue responsibilities with due diligence; to maintain public confidence.*

Obligations to founders and employers: *to specify obligations; to protect privileged information.*

Obligations to colleagues: *to report methods and results; to confront unacceptable behavior and conditions; to communicate ethical requirements*'.

Treatment modalities or 'maneuvers' in clinical trials

In the beginner's mind, a clinical trial is run to evaluate drugs. However, treatment modalities are extremely diversified, and many of them are worth evaluation in controlled clinical trials. The following examples reflect this diversity:

- Alteration of type A behavior to reduce cardiac recurrences[128];
- Using oscillating beds to reduce apnea in premature babies[129];
- Social work in children suffering from chronic illness to reduce psychosocial maladjustment[130];
- Bed-rest in acute low back pain[131];
- Health care delivery[132];
- Home care after surgical procedures[133], etc.

Even less traditional is the increasing attention given to **maneuvers or co-maneuvers representing soft data.** Two categories of these maneuvers should be mentioned. The first, less serious, is an ensemble of maneuvers stemming from **alternative medicines**, such as homeopathy, magnetotherapy, herbal medicines, etc.[134–138]. These maneuvers are seldom, if ever, the subject of controlled clinical trials and as long as this continues to be the case, their roles will be considered as that of a placebo. Far more serious is the increasing attention needed to evaluate the human side of treatment[138]. Non-verbal messages from the physician such as the 'bedside manner' (interest, empathy, attention, availability, motivation, etc.) represent an as yet poorly defined maneuver. The effect of this maneuver, called **iatrotherapy**[139], is still unknown but may be important. Before it is recognized, it must be better defined in clinimetric terms, as shown in the first findings of a qualitative meta-analysis[140] (see

Chapter 11). Reiser and Rosen[141] propose four components for what may be considered iatrotherapy:

1. **Acceptance** of the patient's state by the physician ('doctor's big heart');
2. **Empathy** as the ability to fully understand and share in another's feelings, coupled with the ability to know that those feelings are not identical to one's own;
3. **Competence**, which is not knowledge or intelligence, but rather the ability to use these attributes in real-life clinical practice and to apply them to individual patients;
4. **Conceptualization**, i.e. 'patient-oriented' care, in contrast to problem solving and treatment at the tissue or organ level. Conceptualization goes well beyond the patient by acknowledging the impact of the situation on the family, community, workplace, etc.

Hence, the iatrogenic effect as formulated above must be differentiated from its traditional meaning, i.e. illness resulting from the physician's or other health professional's activities or from simply going to the hospital. The former is desirable, the latter should be preventable[142]. Studying bedside manners or iatrotherapy and its effectiveness as a principal maneuver or co-maneuver remains a considerable methodological challenge.

Despite this challenge, it is worthy of increasing attention not only for the domain of psychiatry, where these concepts are already more solidly anchored, but also for medicine in general.

Process assessment in trials and practice (audit)

The quality of a clinical trial also depends on the evaluation of its run (process of treatment). The impact of treatment does not depend solely on its exact timing or potency[109], but also on patients' compliance (how they respect the treatment plan and orders). For Meador[143], compliance is a human experience which has a web of causes – lack of money, lack of trust in doctor, dementia, hidden side effects of treatment, malingering, cultural differences, family sabotage, alcohol abuse, inconvenience of drug administration (frequency, site, pain) or

misunderstanding of instructions. These causes should all be anticipated and controlled, and their role explained. Among others, blinding of phenomena of interest[144] and early side effects in quantitative and qualitative terms (their occurrence and severity)[145] must be monitored, evaluated and corrected. Dropouts should not be completely discarded. Their characteristics should be known and compared to participants so as to exclude biased findings if the latter differ substantially. Replacements should also be considered.

The process of any therapeutic intervention, either in a clinical trial or in general practice (treatments already at work), must be evaluated given the fact that the patient's outcome depends not only on the stage, spectrum, and gradient of the disease or on the potency of treatment, but also on the quality of diagnostic tests, clinical performance (competence, motivation, barriers), and patient compliance[146]. The **medical audit** is a way of evaluating the process of treatment representing already accepted methods, techniques, and therapeutic procedures. Its main objective is to reach and maintain the best possible quality of care. A medical audit is currently defined as '*an examination or review that establishes the extent to which a condition, process or performance conforms to predetermined standards or criteria*'[3]. Hence, in industrial terms, process surveillance in clinical trials focuses on the quality of scientific findings (research and development quality). The medical audit is a sort of '*quality of production assessment*', once the product is developed. The focus of a medical audit is the quality of care as a '*level of performance or accomplishment that characterizes the health care provided*'[3]. It depends on changing value judgments as well as on more easily measurable determinants such as structure, process, and outcome. The assessment of the quality of care was largely developed and may be found in more detail in Donabedian's writing[147]. In other terms[148], the medical audit is '*the systematic critical analysis of the quality of medical care, including the procedures used for treatment, the resulting outcome and quality of life of the patient*'. Batstone attributes the following to a medical audit[149]:

- It is a system of peer review;

- It involves the setting of standards, which, although often implicit, are best made explicit;
- It reviews current practice against these standards;
- It determines the actions to be taken to remedy any shortfall in performance;
- It requires that the actions taken achieve the desired effect.

Therapeutic interventions are not the only focus of the medical audit. Early detection of disease, diagnostic procedures and plans, patient guidance, education, follow-up, health professionals' performance, etc., may be evaluated. An audit as a form of **continuous** peer review may be internal (done by an institution's insiders) or external (done by an institution's outsiders). The medical audit focuses on clinicians, the clinical audit focuses on the ensemble of providers of clinical care. In these terms, Stone[150] classifies short-term (ad hoc) activities and types of evaluation. Rutstein et al[151] stress the difference between quality and efficiency of medical care. Quality is concerned with outcome and efficiency is related to the process of care. The medical audit should encompass both. For Dixon[152], the medical audit as an evaluation methodology must respect the scientific approach to measurement: explicit objectives; valid measures; clear and precise operational definitions of the concepts to be measured; valid analysis of data; and fair and unbiased interpretation of the audit's findings are required. However, contrary to clinical trials and other experimental and observational analytical studies, the medical audit does not analyze effectiveness, but rather examines conformity to accepted standards and norms. The audit uses outcomes only as indirect evidence that the structure and process of care were appropriate.

Clinical trials or other research methodologies determine a cause–effect relationship between a maneuver (its nature, structure, and process) and its result. Medical and clinical audits use outcomes as indirect evidence that the structure and process of a maneuver (once put into practice) were appropriate[152]. The antibacterial properties of an antibiotic and its proper use are demonstrated by a clinical trial; appropriateness of its use in clinical practice is evaluated by a medical audit.

Assessment of outcome

Consider **statistical considerations** first. By comparing subsequent states, in a clinical trial, investigators first conclude if the findings between the groups are 'statistically significant' on statistical grounds. Their

---

Table 9.6 Conceptual comparison of results of diagnostic tests and clinical trials

Diagnostic test

		If breast mass is actually:	
		Malignant	*Benign*
The result of a fine-needle aspirate is:	**Positive**	This is a true-positive test: result is correct.	This is a false-positive test: result is incorrect.
	Negative	This is a false-negative test: result is incorrect.	This is a true-negative test: result is correct.

Clinical trial

		True state of affairs:	
		Treatment makes a difference	*Treatment does not make a difference*
Conclusion drawn from a clinical trial:	**Treatment makes a difference**	Correct conclusion (true positive)	Type 1 error and *P* value (false positive)
	Treatment does not make a difference	Type II error (false negative)	Correct conclusion (true negative)

Source: Combined from Ref. 154 (test) and 153 (trial). Reproduced with permission of the American Medical Association (*JAMA* and *Arch Int Med*)

conclusions are subject to Type I or alpha and Type II or beta errors. By drawing a parallel between results of diagnostic tests and results of clinical trials, Detsky and Sackett[153] and Browner and Newman[154] linked p values to 1– specificity (i.e. false positive rate) and the power (1 – beta error) to sensitivity (i.e. true positive rate). Table 9.6 illustrates this concept. Hence, results of clinical trials must be reviewed once the trials are finished to determine whether they were large enough to truly demonstrate that the treatment does not work ('negative' results) or that, on the contrary, it does work ('positive' results). The problem concerns 'negative' results in particular. Was the sample size sufficient to detect a clinically important effect if, in fact, it existed? This may be evaluated using an estimation of the size of the difference treatment makes, the rate of events among the control group, and the alpha level in use (see section 9.2.5.1). Tables[153], formulas[155] or nomograms[156] to do this are already available. Clinicians may retrospectively assess how 'powerful' their trial was or what they have been able to detect as differences in treatments given the number of patients in the trial.

Clinical reality dictates the numbers of patients available, thus it is not always possible to produce a sufficient number of patients to conform to the biostatistician's requirements. Hence, retrospective assessment of a clinical trial may be necessary to underline the relevance of findings. These considerations are important in deciding whether or not it is worthwhile or necessary to repeat a trial. There is a tendency in some clinical research to repeat studies that bring positive results (studies that 'pay off' academically and in grants) while negative results are often abandoned for the opposite reason. Finally, as previously noted, the epidemiological relevance of findings (causal criteria and their quantification) and their clinical importance must be elucidated.

Efficiency of treatment or cost-effectiveness is also important

Outcomes of trials first indicate treatment impact. Relative risks, attributable fractions, or other frequencies or proportions of outcomes from Table 9.1 are obtained. Such quantified effectiveness must also be related to material and other resources (cost) invested in intervention to assess the efficiency of treatment or prevention. The basic formula for cost-effectiveness assessment of health and medical practices was proposed by Weinstein and Stason[157]. It clearly illustrates the ingredients necessary for such an evaluation. Their cost-effectiveness ratio requires comparison of the following:

$$\text{Cost-effectiveness ratio} = \frac{\text{Net health care costs}}{\text{Net health program effectiveness}} =$$

$$\frac{\Delta C}{\Delta E} = \frac{\Delta C_{RX} + \Delta C_{SE} - \Delta C_{Morb} + \Delta C_{RX}\, \Delta_{LE}}{\Delta Y + \Delta Y_{Morb} - \Delta Y_{SE}}$$

where:

ΔC_{RX} = All direct medical and health care costs (hospitalization, physician time medications, laboratory services, counseling, and other ancillary services)

ΔC_{SE} = All health care costs associated with adverse side effects of treatment

ΔC_{Morb} = Savings in health care, rehabilitation and custodial cost due to the prevention, cure, or alleviation of disease

$\Delta C_{RX}\, \Delta_{LE}$ = Cost of treatment of diseases that would not have occurred if the patient had not lived longer as a result of the original treatment

ΔY = Expected number of unadjusted life years (net increase in life years)

ΔY_{Morb} = Improvements in the quality of life years due to the alleviation, cure, or prevention of morbidity

ΔY_{SE} = Side effects of treatment

As the formula shows, this approach balances the impact of treatment and its outcomes, while taking into account the impact of substituting other health problems. Several examples of such an evaluation may be quoted: immunization programs[158], hypertension management[159], cancer prevention[160]; various aspects of control of coronary heart disease[161–163]; large-scale use of new drugs[164] or their pricing[165]; surgical versus medical treatment options[166]. Cost-effectiveness analysis allows for the comparison of cost-effectiveness ratios of competing preventive or therapeutic modalities, thereby allowing the best choice to be made. This strategy was well reviewed by Detsky and Naglie[167] and Eisenberg[168]. The full methodology of the assessment of treatment from the point of view of health economics must be found in an *ad hoc* literature, well beyond the scope of this reading. The assessment of treatment outcomes in terms of impact (efficacy and effectiveness) was previously described in section 9.2.2.

Assessment of a clinical trial

In general, the quality of a proof that treatment works will depend on:

- How its trial (evaluation study) is designed;
- How it was realized;
- Its result; and
- How it is reported.

These four criteria should be reviewed in more detail. Only the results of valid clinical trials are worth integrating into routine practice and clinical decision-making. Each trial is only as valid as its components. These may be evaluated by searching for unacceptable characteristics, or the 'fatal stab'. For example, if disease care or the therapeutic maneuver is not well defined, it is not worth pursuing. This is one of the main arguments for detractors from checklists and scoring methods for the quality of clinical trials. An acceptable study (trial) may be the subject of different systems of evaluation, giving various scores of quality. Padgett et al[169], DerSimonian et al[170] and Chalmers et al[171] (in increasing order of complexity) proposed *ad hoc* scoring systems. For example, in Chalmers et al's system[171], a perfect clinical trial earns a maximum of 60 points for the way the trial is built and run (design, components), 30 points for the analysis and interpretation of findings, and 10 points for the way the study is presented (total of 100 points maximum). Nicolucci et al[172] used a similar system in their evaluation of clinical trials for the treatment of lung cancer, grouping original criteria into internal validity and external validity considerations.

Internal (scientific) validity items:

- Methods of randomization;
- Analysis of efficacy of randomization;
- Blinding the evaluation of response to treatment;
- Blinding the evaluation of interim results;
- Compliance;

- Follow-up schedules;
- *A priori* estimate of sample size;
- Withdrawals;
- Analysis of withdrawals;
- Response evaluation; and
- *A posteriori* estimate of study power (1 – beta error).

External (generalizability) validity items:

- Patients' characteristics;
- List of eligible but non-enrolled patients;
- Description of principal and reference therapeutic maneuvers;
- Timing of events; and
- Discussion of side effects.

These scoring systems and other proposals on how clinical trials should be reported (structure)[173] or on what should be included[174], do not give 'pass' or 'fail' scores to a trial. Rather, they help the clinician assess more objectively the strengths and weaknesses of the reported trials and their findings, the organization of the information and its content. All trials without 'fatal stabs' are acceptable, some more than others. However, qualitative assessment of acceptable studies is important for the analysis and synthesis of findings from different trials focusing on the same problem. This procedure is fundamental to meta-analysis and systematic reviews, to which Chapter 11 is devoted. In evidence-based medicine, clinical trials are often abstracted and subject to systematic review (see Chapter 11). For such purposes, additional criteria of quality and acceptability were established[175–177] providing that the study topic is relevant for clinical practice:

- Patients are randomly allocated to comparison groups;
- Outcome measures under study have known or probable clinical importance;
- These outcome measures were obtained for at least 80% of participants who entered the investigation;
- The data analysis is consistent with the study design;
- Study design and analysis are consistent with pre-established research question(s), hypotheses, and objectives.

Other pragmatic requirements originate in evidence-based medicine:

- The results of the study must fulfill the above-mentioned requirements for the overall quality of a trial[178].
- They should help the clinician in patient care[179]. Findings should be clinically meaningful, outcomes relevant and the treatment produce more benefit than harm.
- Study results should be applicable to an individual patient[180]. In short, the patient should be potentially eligible to complete the study given his or her characteristics, health problem, health care and compliance. The patient should also respond to the criteria listed in Section 4.6.3 (Chapter 4).
- Often, surrogate end points are used in the study, i.e. findings which are substitutes for clinically meaningful end points, like blood pressure instead of stroke or cholesterol levels for myocardial infarction. In those cases, a detailed relationship between surrogate and real end points should be known[181] in terms of risk, prognosis and modification.
- If possible, it should be known if the drug under study exerts more than a class effect[182]. Beta-blockers, minor tranquillizers or anti-inflammatory drugs belong to groups of drugs having some common basis and a particular effect (class effect). Any comparison within and between classes (groups of drugs) must be evaluated beyond a simple acceptance of belonging to a particular group.
- Narrative treatment recommendations should be replaced by structured ones that include clear questions, identified management options and outcomes, justifications based on systematic reviews of evidence, and application of value judgments and preferences in decision-making[183]. Unstructured recommendations unfounded by some kind of a systematic review of evidence should be scrutinized for their potential limited value.

9.2.6 Further considerations

The classical evaluation of treatment and care must be expanded to respond to specific conditions of various medical specialties, information technology developments and advances in medical and general technology.

9.2.6.1 Clinical trials in special circumstances: surgery and general medicine

Clinical trials in surgery represent a special challenge. The need for controlled, randomized clinical trials in surgery was stressed as early as in the 1970s[184,185]. More recently, their specific methodology was reviewed in series of articles in the *World Journal of Surgery*[186–189]. Surgical treatment has its own inherent limitations and specific characteristics that render randomized controlled clinical trials less feasible:

1. Given the radical character of surgery, it is often reserved for cases with poorer prognosis, thus randomization may be less ethical;
2. It is more difficult to preserve equipoise when considering radical or conservative treatment;
3. Randomization is more apt to be suitable when comparing two competing surgical procedures in patients having comparable indications for each procedure;
4. Surgical acts often have a more powerful placebo effect than conservative therapies (drugs)[185];
5. Surgery is irreversible; patients do not subsequently have access to alternative procedures[190];
6. Identical maneuvers may be performed with various skills by different surgeons[190];
7. There is no direct transfer of experience from animals to humans, thus there is no Phase I of a surgical trial: a surgeon cannot see how a healthy individual would tolerate a heart transplant or a Whipple's procedure;
8. Blinding is often impossible;
9. As in orthopedics[190], long-term effects require a long follow-up;
10. Randomization may jeopardize a surgeon's credibility in the patient's eyes by making the surgeon appear unsure and indecisive[190].

These shortcomings and limitations, however, may be overcome[191]. For example, Zelen's method of randomization[56] may be considered; or, since surgeons often believe that one particular procedure is superior to its alternatives, and they master and prefer to perform this procedure, **surgeons instead of surgical procedures may be randomized** as proposed by Van den Linden[192]. Patients must, however, agree to sometimes leave 'their' surgeon and accept another. The expanding field of controlled trials in surgery brings more thorough and richer information, such as in the assessment of surgery for breast cancer[193] or coronary bypass[194]. More innovative approaches and modifications as alternatives to classical randomized clinical trials will certainly be developed with respect to radical interventions.

In general practice, other special circumstances make challenging both the transfer of information from clinical trials into practice[195] and the running of clinical trials in a general practice setting[196]. Clinical and demographic characteristics of patients are different from those of the hospital population and the setting of general practice is most often different from the setting of hospital-based clinical trials. Patients' judgment and values may also differ from those of hospital-based trial participants. Hence, the ubiquitous EBM question 'Does this apply to my patient(s)?' (i.e. transfer of information), becomes more challenging to answer. Conducting randomized trials in general practice means facing additional challenges compared to a hospital setting. Patients may prefer a particular treatment. They may less easily accept randomization. Patient compliance may be more limited. Trials may require several sites and may then be subject to the rules of multicenter trials. (See Section 9.2.6.3 in this chapter.) Clinical trials in general practice will subsequently be more pragmatic than explanatory[51].

9.2.6.2 Pharmacoepidemiology

Pharmacoepidemiology has become an additional tool in the study of drug effects. Pharmacoepidemiology is currently defined as *'the study of the distribution and determinants of drug-related events in populations, and the application of this study to efficaceous drug treatment'*[3].

A monograph is devoted to this topic[197] and research in this field is expanding[198]. The primary focus of pharmacoepidemiology is the study of what controlled trials cannot do, such as the study of secondary adverse effects of drugs. Hence, pharmacoepidemiology currently focuses mostly on:

1. The epidemiological surveillance of secondary drug effects, or pharmaco-surveillance (including drug incompatibilities). These must be defined in operational terms[199]. Adverse reactions or side effects are defined as *'any undesirable or unwanted consequence of a preventive, diagnostic, or therapeutic procedure'*[3]. In pharmacoepidemiology, it should be *'any response to a drug that is noxious and unintended and that occurs at doses used in man for prophylaxis, diagnosis, or therapy, excluding failure to accomplish the intended purpose'*[200]. An algorithm for the assessment of adverse drug reactions has been developed[201] and tested[202,203]. Descriptive methods in the follow-up of such reactions are used first.

2. Observational analytical studies focus on establishing causal relationships between a particular drug and its undesirable effects[199]. The case–control approach is often used.

3. The process of information on drugs, drug distribution and utilization is also studied[204].

Pharmacoepidemiology has developed well beyond its original function as a complement to clinical trials and its traditional field[205,206]. It has now even its proper terminology and vocabulary[207]. It may evolve progressively into the *'study of conditions determining drug use and of various impacts of drug use on patients' health and disease outcomes'* in conformity with the basic definition of epidemiology beyond this field. Drugs may and must be studied as independent and dependent variables for their role in cause–effect relationships (NB Strictly speaking, clinical trials are, by this definition, an integral part of pharmacoepidemiology). A classical example of drug surveillance in pharmacoepidemiology is the surveillance of side effects of vaccines[208]. Findings may focus on regional differences, major culprits, or on the most often observed secondary effects. Such descriptive findings are powerful stimuli for hypotheses on causes of differences found: regional differences in vaccine storage, transport and application; specific components of different vaccines; components of vaccines causing specific reactions; different target populations, etc. Explanatory research and control of these problems may follow.

9.2.6.3 *Multicenter clinical trials*

Readers of this text may be involved in multicenter trials as important providers of data and information or researchers. Very often, new medical technologies or procedures are used infrequently at the beginning, and in few hospitals or other centers. They are costly and require special skills, which have not yet been mastered by all. Disease cases under diagnostic work-up or treatment may be less frequent. To build studies of diagnostic validity or treatment effectiveness, enough patients are needed to add power to the findings. This was the primary reason (and it remains so) to involve more than one hospital, research center or primary care institution in the same research project by pooling patients from these places. Coronary artery bypass surgery (CASS)[209], cancer treatment, or pharmacopsychiatric interventions[210] are just a few examples of fields where multicenter studies are not only useful but necessary to obtain valid findings within a reasonable time frame. Hence, trials may be classified as follows:

1. **Single center trials.** Single center trials are easier to prepare, run, and evaluate. Participants are motivated, patient and investigator compliance is good;

2. **Multiple independent trials.** Sometimes, a common problem may be shared between several investigating institutions. Patients from different prognostic groups or at different stages of disease may be preferably treated at different places, various diagnostic or therapeutic procedures may be performed preferentially in one institution versus another. These studies, however, must have a common protocol and central coordination. They are not necessarily parallel in time but their components 'stand on their own feet'[211]. Consequently, multiple independent trials are methodologically less strong than multicenter trials. Research integration of findings (meta-analysis) of these trials may be considered. This kind of trial was proposed for the study of migraine control[211].

3. **Multicenter trials** represent 'one trial at several places'. Their methodology is well established and described in more detail elsewhere[8,11]. The great advantage of multicenter trials is that they give findings more statistical power. They may reach a broader pool of patients (a more representative sample of an often wider spectrum and gradient of disease). The external validity (extrapolation to the whole population) may be enhanced[8]. Not only may an increase in the standards of the trial itself be expected, but a positive impact on routine medical practices in participating institutions may be expected as well. Multicenter trials are better suited to the study of short-term effects of treatments. They are not often 'scientifically innovative'[212] and they tend to bring conservative results. Obviously, they are expensive and more difficult to coordinate and administer. Compliance, data collection and processing require a more complex quality control[8]. Participating physicians may be less motivated. A strong leadership (an imposing principal investigator) may enhance the scientific innovation and quality of the study and its findings[8]. Also, website data management may further simplify technical aspects, quality and complexity of data gathered from several sites. Despite these shortcomings, only multicenter trials can answer many questions. They may also strongly enhance negative findings, which would be doubted on the basis of a single center trial. Such is the case with multiple intervention programs to prevent and control cardiovascular diseases[213]. Costly multicenter trials such as the Lipid Research Clinics Trial, MRFIT, or the North Karelia Project in Finland, which bring negative or inconclusive results leading some[214] to doubt the outcome, would be unjustified if the results of a single center trial were considered as good.

It must be remembered that findings leading to the abandonment of ineffective preventive or curative measures are as valid as those bringing more convincing arguments for the adoption of effective measures elsewhere. Further developments may be expected in the way multicenter trials are analyzed and their findings interpreted. More emphasis is necessary **to evaluate and interpret the heterogeneity of findings** from one participating center to another. Discrepancies are not always due to quality control. Differences found may and should act, wherever relevant, as powerful hypothesis generators. Are differences in treatment results due to the state of patients, to different maneuvers, or are new causal associations worthy of further study, etc.? Component results produced by participating centers in multicenter trials or in multiple independent trials are worthy of analysis by methodology developed in qualitative and quantitative meta-analysis (see Chapter 11). Participating centers and the results they provide may be seen as an ensemble of studies of the same topic, their heterogeneity assessed and the synthesis of their findings done by pooling not only individual observations in patients, but also local results. In essence, multiple independent studies should complement findings, and multicenter studies should duplicate efforts to strengthen a particular finding.

9.2.6.4 Medical technology assessment

Evaluation of new medical technologies (treatments) is now a continuous endeavor strengthened by stable human and material resources given the fact that the development of new medical technology is increasing and accelerating. Professional and public expectations are high – people want to know as soon as possible how and if a technology works. New antibiotics, genetically engineered vaccines, automatic external defibrillators, lithotripsy, prosthetic or microsurgical equipment are just a few examples of topics of interest. The epidemiological aspects of their evaluation are of increasing importance. **Medical technology** is defined by the US Congress' Office of Technology Assessment as '*techniques, drugs, equipment, and procedures used by health care professionals in delivering medical care to individuals, and the systems within which such a care is delivered*'[215].

Any medical technology may be considered **new** if its safety, efficacy and effectiveness, cost–effect and cost–benefit ratios, ethical, legal and social impacts are unknown. Hence, even traditional medical practices, tools and their fields of application like components of bedside clinical examination, care or herbal remedies may be considered 'new' if they still have not been evaluated as rigorously as 'truly new' technologies are. Its assessment has been defined as follows[215]: '*Assessment of a medical technology denotes any process of examining and reporting properties of a medical technology used in health care, such as safety, efficacy, feasibility, and indications for use, cost, and cost-effectiveness, as well as social, economic, and ethical consequences, whether intended or unintended. Technology assessment ideally would be comprehensive and include evaluation not only of the immediate results of the technology but also of its long-term consequences. A comprehensive assessment of a medical technology – after assessment of its immediate effects – may also include an appraisal of problems of personnel training and licensure, new capital expenditures for equipment and buildings, and possible consequences for the health insurance industry and the social security system . . . Not all technologies warrant the full assessment, nor is it feasible to provide comprehensive assessments for all technologies.*'

Epidemiological methods and techniques used in this field do not differ substantially from the methods and techniques described in this text[216]. Observational methods are used in studying the safety of preventive and curative interventions (surveillance); clinical trials or observational analytical methods are used in the study of efficacy and effectiveness of technologies. Efficiency is assessed by way of cost–effect ratios, such that knowledge of the impact of the treatment modality is necessary. Nonetheless, it is felt[215,216] that a comprehensive assessment varies from one sector of interest to another. The most comprehensive evaluations are currently done on drugs, medical devices, equipment and supplies and less comprehensive ones focus on medical, surgical procedures, support systems and organizational/administrative measures. The assessment of medical technologies must take place in two ways: 1) by studying the factors of implantation and use; and 2) by evaluating the impact on individuals and society. The greatest challenge remains to balance the clinical and economical aspects of new technology evaluation[218].

The surveillance of new technologies should provide basic information for the assessment of their effectiveness, complications and adverse effects. Thacker and Berkelman[218] warn against premature conclusions on the value of new technologies without proper surveillance and subsequent evaluation, citing such procedures as surgical sterilization (tubal ligation), subcutaneous, continuous-infusion insulin pumps (associated deaths), or the prevention of stroke by carotid endarterectomy (effectiveness, safety, audit). Besides the evaluation of treatment impact (outcomes), epidemiological methods are useful for the study of the prevalence of technology related outcomes (secondary effects), the prevalence of health problems to determine potential demand for new technologies (bypasses, organ transplants, etc.), for the occurrence of use of new technologies and their economic aspects. Time limitations to prepare such studies, limited available information and the cost of good epidemiological studies will require innovative approaches in the future.

Together with original studies, technology assessment by using meta-analytical methods and systematic reviews will increase (see also Chapter 11). Social and political pressure to accelerate assessments is sometimes enormous, such as in the development and use of new drugs to control AIDS. However, the time taken for evaluation cannot be shorter than the natural and clinical course of the disease to properly grasp the whole impact on risk and prognosis of this serious problem. A consequent *'festina lente'* approach often appears unacceptable to many decision-makers and pressure groups, for which epidemiology is not a compulsory part of wisdom. The evaluation of new diagnostic technologies by meta-analysis will be discussed in Chapter 11.

9.3 Evaluation of health promotion programs and interventions

At any level of prevention, interventions are centered on a well-defined health problem or group of problems. Illness and disease as well as their causes, consequences and treatment are thus a common focus. Another emerging focus is health itself and the approaches and activities to maintain and enhance its existing level. **Health promotion** is currently defined as *'the process of enabling individuals and communities to increase control over the determinants of health and thereby improve their health'*[219]. As Tables 9.7 and 9.8 illustrate, health promotion and disease prevention differ in their concepts as well as in their methods to address the problem, where to focus it, how to implement it and how to evaluate the results[220]. Contrary to disease prevention, health promotion is a way of intervention that addresses less well-defined populations, uses medical and non-medical means, and involves not only health professionals but also administrative, social, cultural and other resources in communities. Soft data may represent some maneuvers and outcomes. For these reasons, health promotion interventions are becoming an increasing component of activities to improve a population's health and decrease health costs. On the other hand, despite remarkable efforts to improve

Table 9.7 Health promotion versus disease prevention – Prevalent differences in concept

Health promotion	Disease prevention
Health = positive and multidimensional concept	Health = absence of disease
Participatory model of health	Medical model
Aimed at the population in its total environment	Aimed mainly at high-risk groups in the population
Concerns a network of health issues	Concerns a specific pathology
Diverse and complementary strategies	One short strategy
Facilitating and enabling approaches	Directive and persuasive strategies
Incentive measures are offered to the population	Directive measures are enforced in target groups
Changes in man's status and environment are sought by the program	Programs focusing mostly on individuals and groups of subjects
Non-professional organizations, civic groups, local, municipal, regional and national governments are necessary for achieving the goal of health promotion	Preventive programs are the affair of professional groups from health disciplines

Source: Ref. 220, reproduced with permission of the *Canadian Journal of Public Health*

Table 9.8 Health promotion versus disease prevention. Main differences challenging the epidemiological approach to health promotion

Health promotion	Disease prevention
Population at large	Groups at high risk
'Webs of causes, webs of consequences' situations	Simple cause–effect relationships (e.g. immunization–disease incidence)
General, non-specific states of subjects are studied (well-being, healthy behavior, etc.)	Specific states of subjects are measured (e.g. HIV status, lead in blood, etc.)
Independent and dependent variables under study are often soft data (persuasion, public awareness, behavior, attitudes, etc.)	Independent and dependent variables are most often hard data (drug intake, blood pressure, cholesterol levels, incidence of infection, etc.)
Focus on the state of individuals before exposure to noxious agents	State of subjects in relation to exposure to specific agent(s)
Means of intervention are those with the best chance to act upon webs of consequences	Means of intervention which are best for a specific, expected effect are chosen
Long-term results (in ten years or more)	Expected results immediate or in a time feasible for a single health program
Uncertain compliance of subjects	Compliance of participants may be monitored and controlled
Uncertainty about having similar information gathered by comparable methods at the beginning and end of the program	Comparable information is available at the beginning and end of a health program (initial and subsequent states comparable)
The main subject of interest is the status of individuals or proportions of given characteristics of subjects in the community, or rates of non-events	The main subject deals with rates of events (incidence, mortality, etc.)
Object of evaluation is mainly process evaluation	Object of evaluation is endpoint effect evaluation
Complex evaluation of cost/benefit, cost/effectiveness ratios	Better evaluability of cost/benefit, cost/effectiveness ratios

Source: Ref. 220, reproduced with permission of the *Canadian Journal of Public Health*

health promotion methodology[221], it remains an epidemiologist's nightmare to properly evaluate the effectiveness of health promotion programs. Consequently, most of the evaluation of health promotion focuses on the assessment of its process rather than on its effect.

9.4 Conclusions

Health care can devour up to 10–12% of a nation's gross national product and along with diagnostic procedures, preventive and curative interventions are the most costly areas of health care. For that price, they must work at a reasonable cost without making major concessions to human, ethical, universal, or comprehensive medicine. New treatments must be tested and only the acceptable ones put into practice. Moreover, many treatments already traditionally entrenched in medical practice must be periodically re-evaluated and removed from daily practice if proved ineffective or inefficient. The assessment of efficacy and effectiveness is now an integral part of basic professional curricula. Clinical economics and evaluation of the efficiency of medical intervention education follows[222]. Clinical trials themselves appear cost-effective and worth funding from this point of view[223]. A pragmatic approach to the evaluation of medical interventions does not mean another dehumanizing act of medicine. On the contrary, it would be professionally unethical to give ineffective treatment. On the other hand, how unethical would it be to prefer an effective but costly treatment for one individual over cheaper treatments of equal total cost for many individuals, thus saving several lives? The decision to treat or not to treat, prevent or not prevent, alleviate or not alleviate is often complex and based on the sum of medical, clinical and epidemiological expertise. The last chapter (Chapter 13) of this text deals with this topic.

Readers interested in methodology will be interested in the following periodicals devoted to the topic of this chapter: *Controlled Clinical Trials* (a more medical approach) and *Statistics in Medicine* (a more statistical approach). As for the assessment of new technologies, the *International Journal of Technology Assessment in Health Care* is devoted to this field. *ACP Journal, Evidence-Based Medicine, Evidence-Based Mental Health,* and *Evidence-Based Nursing* offer readers critically abstracted information on recent findings in treatment, as well as systematic reviews of currently available evidence.

One of the great challenges in preventive medicine will be the decision to put into practice large-scale community interventions based on multiple preventive and/or curative measures (no smoking, no drinking, treating blood pressure, lowering cholesterol, educating the population, etc.). The bigger and more comprehensive these programs and the bigger their health promotion component, the more difficult they will be to evaluate. These programs, however, are often fuelled by important political pressures (from concerned physicians and non-physicians alike) as alternative choices that should lower the cost of health care. Conclusions on this subject remain controversial[214,224,225]. Part of the daily work of any health professional should be to ensure that the treatment and care provided works to the greatest benefit of individual patients. This chapter has offered several elements to help make these decisions.

One simple fact remains: without knowing cause–effect relationships linking possible risk factors and disease incidence, there are no specific intervention modalities in primary prevention. Without a proven cause–effect relationship between a treatment modality and a shortened duration (lowering disease prevalence) of cases or the control of disease progression, secondary and tertiary prevention remain a 'shot in the dark' approach. What methodological developments can be expected in the near future?

- A possible duel between '**probability fraternity**' and '**likelihood brotherhood**'. Customary inferential statistics and *P* value uses are recently questioned given their deductive nature. Many practitioners use inductive methods such as differential diagnosis. Protagonists of the Bayes factor propose likeli-

hood ratio uses as a better alternative to evaluate strength of associations in a biostatistical sense (not in terms of the strength of causal association)[226,227]. The well-established inferential statistics may be progressively complemented by much younger Bayes factor users.

- Reality, availability of data, medical ethics, time, and material and personal resources do not allow rigorous clinical trials as experiments in all situations. Observational studies, either descriptive or analytical (case–control, cohort) fall into the area labeled in EBM as **outcome research**, i.e. research on outcomes of interventions[3]. Outcomes have a very broad sense: '*All the possible results that may stem from exposure to a causal factor, or from preventive or therapeutic interventions; all identified changes in health status arising as consequence of the handling of the health problem.*'[3] In addition to well-established rules of observational research, outcome research pays particular attention to factors arising from medical services themselves[218,219]. We may understand it as a kind of 'webs of consequences' research.

- **Economic analysis** of medical and other health interventions and services already has well-established foundations[229], and applications in evidence-based medicine were also defined[230,231]. However, this domain is beyond the scope of this text.

- The effectiveness of prevention and cure evaluation[232,233] will increasingly **combine** methods and techniques **from quantitative field methods** (biostatistics, epidemiology, decision analysis, economic analysis, systematic reviews) **and from qualitative research methods** focusing on the distributional, legal, ethical and social effects of interventions.

- The assessment of the quality of life (see Chapter 5) as a measure of success or failure of treatment is methodologically considerably improved[234]. Moreover, its choice as an outcome measure means bringing treatment choices to patient preferences. An aging patient is much more interested in keeping and improving his or her autonomy than in a paraclinical demonstration showing that his or her osteoporosis or osteoarthritis does not advance.

- The use of **fuzzy logic** in health intervention decision-making has only just begun. However, strategies of measles control have been developed using fuzzy logic techniques[235].

The next chapter will discuss how to apply epidemiological and evidence-based reasoning in the area of prognosis.

REFERENCES

1. McCance RA. The practice of experimental medicine. President's Address. *Proc Roy Soc Med*, 1951;**44**:189–94
2. Kim JH, Gallis HA. Observations on spiraling empiricism: Its causes, allure, and perils, with particular reference to antibiotic therapy. *Am J Med*, 1989; **87**:201–6
3. Last JM (ed.). *A Dictionary of Epidemiology*. 2nd Edition. New York: Oxford University Press, 1988 (see also 4th Edition, 2001)
4. Colombo F, Shapiro S, Slone D, Tognoni G (eds). *Epidemiological Evaluation of Drugs*. Littleton: PSG Publishing, 1977
5. Rothman KJ. Epidemiologic methods in clinical trials. *Cancer*, 1977;**39**:1771–5
6. Kewitz H, Roots I, Voigt K (eds). *Epidemiological Concepts in Clinical Pharmacology*. Berlin: Springer Verlag, 1987
7. Good CS (ed.). *The Principles and Practice of Clinical Trials*. Edinburgh: Churchill Livingstone, 1976
8. Pocock SJ. *Clinical Trials. A practical approach*. Chichester: J. Wiley & Sons, 1983
9. Friedman LM, Furberg CD, DeMets DL. *Fundamental of Clinical Trials*. 2nd Edition. Littleton: PSG Publishing, 1985
10. Fleiss JL. *The Design and Analysis of Clinical Experiments*. New York: John Wiley & Sons, 1986
11. Meinert CL, Tonascia S. *Clinical Trials. Design, Conduct, and Analysis*. New York: Oxford University Press, 1986
12. Louis TA, Shapiro SH. Critical issues in the conduct and interpretation of clinical trials. *Ann Rev Public Health*, 1983;**4**:25–46
13. Shapiro SH, Louis TA (eds). *ClinicalTrials. Issues and Approaches*. New York: Marcel Dekker Inc., 1983
14. Chaput de Saintonge DM, Vere DW (eds). *Current Problems in Clinical Trials*. Oxford: Blackwell, Scientific, 1984
15. Lawrence Jr W. Some problems with clinical trials. James Ewing lecture. *Arch Surg*, 1991;**126**:370–8
16. *The Bible. The Old Testament*. Book of Daniel, Chapter 1
17. Lind J. *Treatise on Scurvy*. Edinburgh: Kinkaid and Donaldson, 1753
18. Szmuness W, Stevens CE, Harley EJ, et al. Hepatitis B vaccine. Demonstration of efficacy in a controlled clinical trial in a high-risk population in the United States. *N Engl J Med*, 1980;**303**:833–41
19. Ware JH, Mosteller F, Ingelfinger JA. P values. In: Bailar JC III Mosteller F eds. *Medical Uses of Statistics*. Waltham, MA: NEJM Books, 1986:149–69
20. Orenstein WA, Bernier RH, Hinman AR. Assessing vaccine efficacy in the field. Further observations. *Epidemiol Rev*, 1988;**10**:212–41
21. Hatton P. The use of the screening technique as a method of rapidly estimating vaccine efficacy. *Public Health*, 1990;**104**:21–5
22. Farrington CP. Estimation of vaccine effectiveness using the screening method. *Int J Epidemiol*, 1993; **22**:742–6
23. Jenicek M, Cléroux R. Epidémiologie. *Principes, techniques, applications. (Epidemiology. Principles, techniques, applications)*. St. Hyacinthe and Paris: EDISEM and Maloine, 1982
24. Anon. Glossary. Terms used in therapeutics. *ACP Journal Club*, 2002, 4 p. online: http://www.acpjc.org/shared/glossary.htm
25. Laupacis A, Sackett DL, Roberts RS. An assessment of clinically useful measures of the consequences of treatment. *N Engl J Med*, 1988;**318**:1728–33
26. Cook RJ, Sackett DL. The number needed to treat: a clinically useful measure of treatment effect. *Br Med J*, 1995;**310**:452–4
27. Chatellier G, Zapletal E, Lemaitre D, et al. The number needed to treat: a clinically useful nomogram in its proper context. *Br Med J*, 1996;**312**:426–9
28. Ebrahim S, Smith GD. The 'number needed to treat': does it help clinical decision-making? *J Hum Hypertension*, 1999;**13**:721–4
29. Sackett DL, Straus SE, Richardson WS, et al. *Evidence-Based Medicine. How to Practice and Teach EBM*. Edinburgh: Churchill Livingstone, 2000
30. Sinclair JC, Cook RJ, Guyatt GH, et al. When should an effective treatment be used? Derivation of the threshold number needed to treat and the minimum event rate for treatment. *J Clin Epidemiol*, 2001;**54**: 253–62
31. Wu LA, Kottke TE. Number needed to treat: Caveat emptor. *J Clin Epidemiol*, 2001;**54**:111–6
32. Lesaffre E, Boon P, Pledger GW. The value of the number needed-to-treat method in antiepileptic drug trials. *Epilepsia*, 2000;**41**:440–6
33. Anon. Glossary. *ACP Journal Club*; 2000;**133**:A–20
34. Anon. Glossary. *EBM*.2001;**6**: interior back page.

35. Anon. Glossary. *ACP Journal Club*, 2001;134:a–23

36. Anon. Glossary. *EBM Mental Health*, 2001;4: interior back page

37. James IM. Volunteer studies and human pharmacology – Phase I. In: Good CS ed. *The Principles and Practice of Clinical Trials*. Edinburgh: Churchill Livingstone, 1976:17–22

38. Smith RB. Clinical Trials – Phases II, III, and IV. In: Good CS ed. *The Principles and Practice of Clinical Trials*. Edinburgh: Churchill Livingstone, 1976: 23–35

39. Naranjo CA, Janecek E. Drug development and regulations. In: Kalant H, Rochelau WHE eds. *Principles of Pharmacology*. 5th Edition. Toronto: BC Decker Inc., 1989:723–30

40. Jones WR, Judd SJ, Ing RMY, et al. Phase I clinical trial of a World Health Organization birth control vaccine. *Lancet*, 1988;1:1295–8

41. Gustavson LE, Carrigan PJ. The clinical pharmacokinetics of estazolam. *Am J Med*, 1990;88 (Suppl 3A):2S–5S

42. Kantarjian HM, Keating MJ, Walters RS, et al. Phase II study of low-dose continuous infusion of homoharringtonine in refractory acute myelogenous leukemia. *Cancer*, 1989;63:813–7

43. Bland KI, Kimura AK, Brenner DE, Basinger MA, et al. A phase II study of the efficacy of diamminedichlorplatinum (Cisplatin) for the control of locally recurrent and in transit malignant melanoma of the extremities using tourniquet outflow-occlusion techniques. *Ann Surg*, 1989;209:73–80

44. Foon KA, Bottino GC, Abrams PG, et al. Phase II trial of recombinant leucocyte A interferon in patients with advanced chronic lymphocytic leukemia. *Am J Med*, 1985;78:216–20

45. The Anturane Reinfarction Trial Research Group. Sulfinpyrazone in the prevention of sudden death after myocardial infarction. *N Engl J Med*, 1980; 302:250–6

46. Pierce MW, Shu VS. Efficacy of estazolam. The United States clinical experience. *Am J Med*, 1990; 88(Suppl 3A):6S–11S

47. Pierce MW, Shu VS, Groves LJ. Safety of estazolam. The United States experience. *Am J Med*, 1990;88 (Suppl 3A):12S–17S

48. Strom BL, Melmon KL, Miettinen OS. Postmarketing studies of drug efficacy. *Arch Intern Med*, 1985;145:1791–4

49. Strom BL, Miettinen OS, Melmon KL. Postmarketing studies of drug efficacy: How? *Am J Med*, 1984;77:703–8

50. Feinstein AR. Current problems and future challenges in randomized clinical trials. *Circulation*, 1984;70:767–74

51. Schwartz D, Lellouch J. Explanatory and pragmatic attitudes in therapeutic trials. *J Chron Dis*, 1967;20: 637–48

52. Freedman LS. Evaluating and comparing imaging techniques: a review and classification of study designs. *Br J Radiol*, 1987;60:1071–81

53. Nierenberg AA, Feinstein AR. How to evaluate a diagnostic maker test. Lessons from the rise and fall of dexamethasone suppression test. *JAMA*, 1988; 259:1699–702

54. Gore SM, Altman DG. *Statistics in Practice* (From articles published in the British Medical Journal). London: British Medical Association, 1982

55. Fleiss JL. How to randomise. *Statistical Methods for Rates and Proportions*. 2nd Edition. New York: J Wiley & Sons, 1981;4:50–5

56. Zelen M. A new design for randomized clinical trials. *N Engl J Med*, 1979;300:1242–5

57. Chang RW, Falconer J, Stulberg SD, et al. Prerandomization: An alternative to classic randomization. *J Bone Joint Surg*, 1990;72–A:1451–5

58. Feinstein AR. An additional basic science for clinical medicine: III. The challenges of comparison and measurement. *Ann Intern Med*, 1983;99:705–12

59. Feinstein AR. *Clinical Epidemiology. The Architecture of Clinical Research*. Philadelphia: WB Saunders, 1985

60. Greenland S. Randomization, statistics, and causal inference. *Epidemiology*, 1990;1:421–9

61. Byar DP, Simon RM, Friedewald WT, et al. Randomized clinical trials. Perspectives on some recent ideas. *N Engl J Med*,1976;295:74–80

62. Horwitz RI, Feinstein AR. Improved observational method for studying therapeutic efficacy. Suggestive evidence that lidocaine prophylaxis prevents death from acute myocardial infarction. *JAMA*, 1981;246: 2455–9

63. Chalmers TC. The challenges of clinical measurement. *The Mount Sinai J Med*, 1983;50:138–40

64. Kaptchuk TJ. The double-blind, randomized, placebo-controlled trial: Gold standard or golden calf? *J Clin Epidemiol*, 2001;54:541–9

65. Wall P. The placebo response. In: Pain. *The Science of Suffering*. New York: Columbia University Press, 2000:125–40

66. Hrobjartsson A. What are the main methodological problems in the estimation of placebo effects? *J Clin Epidemiol*, 2002;55:430–5

67. Wolf S. Effect of suggestion and conditioning on action of chemical agents in human subjects – pharmacology of placebos. *J Clin Invest*, 1950;29:100–9

68. Couch JR Jr. Placebo effect and clinical trials in migraine therapy. *Neuroepidemiology*, 1987;6: 178–85

69. Brody H. The lie that heals: the ethics of giving placebos. *Ann Intern Med*, 1982;97:112–8

70. Turner JA, Deyo RA, Loeser JD, et al. The importance of placebo effects in pain treatment and research. *JAMA*, 1994;271:1609–14

71. Kiene GS, Kiene H. The powerful placebo effect: Fact or fiction? *J Clin Epidemiol*, 1997;**50**:1311–8

72. Wynder EL. Introduction. The American Health Foundation's Nocebo Conference. *Prev Med*, 1997;**26**:605–6

73. Hahn RA. The nocebo phenomenon: Concept, evidence, and implications for public health. *Prev Med*, 1997;**26**:607–11

74. Spiegel H. Nocebo: The power of suggestibility. *Prev Med*, 1997;**26**:616–21

75. Benson H. The nocebo effect: History and physiology. *Prev Med*, 1997;**26**:612–5

76. Louis TA, Lavori PW, Bailar III JC, Polanski M. Crossover and self-controlled design in clinical research. *N Engl J Med*, 1984;**310**:24–31

77. Woods JR, Williams JG, Tavel M. The two-period crossover design in medical research. *Ann Intern Med*, 1989;**110**:560–6

78. Armitage P, Berry G. *Statistical Methods in Medical Research*. 2nd Edition. Oxford: Blackwell Scientific, 1987

79. Lewis JA. Migraine trials: Crossover or parallel group. *Neuroepidemiology*, 1987;**6**:198–208

80. Knipschild P, Leffers P, Feinstein AR. The qualification period. *J Clin Epidemiol*, 1991;**44**:461–4

81. Kunkel RS. Clinical trials in migraine: Parallel versus crossover studies. *Neuroepidemiology*, 1987;**6**:209–13

82. Johnston DL, Gebhardt VA, Donald A, Kostuk WJ. Comparative effects of propranolol and verapamil alone and in combination on left ventricular function and volumes in patients with chronic exertional angina: a double blind, placebo-controlled, randomized crossover study with radionuclide ventriculography. *Circulation*, 1983;**68**:1280–9

83. Bowles MJ, Subramanian VB, Davies AB, Raftery EB. Double-blind randomized crossover trial of verapamil and propranolol in chronic stable angina. *Am Heart J*, 1983;**106**:1297–306

84. Guyatt G, Sackett D, Taylor DW, et al. Determining optimal therapy – randomized trials in individual patients. *N Engl J Med*, 1986;**314**:889–92

85. Guyatt G, Sackett D, Adachi J, et al. A clinician's guide for conducting randomized trials in individual patients. *Can Med Ass J*, 1988;**139**:497–503

86. Petersen E (ed.). Single Case Studies. Proceedings from a Symposium in Oslo, 14–15 March 1987. *Scand J Gastroenterol*, 1988;**23**(Suppl 147):1–48

87. Guyatt GH, Keller JL, Jaeschke R, et al. The n-of-1 randomized controlled clinical trial: Clinical usefulness. Our three-year experience. *Ann Intern Med*, 1990;**112**:293–9

88. McLeod RS, Cohen Z, Taylor DW, Cullen JB. Single patient randomized clinical trial. Use of determining optimum treatment for patient with inflammation of Kock continent ileostomy reservoir. *Lancet*, 1986;**1**:726–8

89. Controlled trials in single subjects. 1. Value in clinical medicine (Johanessen T). 2. Limitations of use (Louis JA). *Br Med J*, 1991;**303**:173–6

90. Rochon J. A statistical model for 'N-of-1' study. *J Clin Epidemiol*, 1990;**43**:499–508

91. Wald A. Sequential Analysis. New York: John Wiley, 1947

92. Bross I. Sequential medical plans. Biometrics, 1952;**8**:188–205

93. Armitage P. Sequential Medical Trials. 2nd Edition. New York: John Wiley, 1975

94. Lewis DH, Davis JW, Archibald DG, et al. Protective effects of aspirin against acute myocardial infarction and death in men with unstable angina. Results of Veterans Administration Cooperative Study. *N Engl J Med*, 1983;**309**:396–403

95. Hamilton M. Methodology of Clinical Research. Edinburgh: Churchill Livingstone, 1974

96. Halloran ME, Longini IM Jr, Struchiner CJ. Design and interpretation of vaccine field studies. *Epidemiol Rev*, 1999;**21**:73–88

97. 97. Gehan EA. The evaluation of therapies: Historical control studies. *Stat Med*, 1984;**3**:315–24

98. 98. Black N. Why we need observational studies to evaluate effectiveness of health care. *Br Med J*, 1997;**312**:1215–8

99. Rodrigues LC, Smith PG. Use of case–control approach in vaccine evaluation: Efficacy and adverse effects. *Epidemiol Rev*, 1999;**21**:56–72

100. Hulley SH, Cummings SR (eds). *Designing Clinical Research*. Baltimore: Williams & Wilkins, 1988

101. Kurtzke JF. On the role of clinicians in the use of drug trial data. *Neuroepidemiology*, 1982;**1**:124–36

102. Jenicek M, Cléroux R. *Epidémiologie clinique. Clinimétrie. (Clinical Epidemiology. Clinimetrics)*. St. Hyacinthe et Paris: EDISEM et Maloine,1985

103. The Lipid Research Clinics Program. The coronary primary prevention trial: Design and implementation. *J Chron Dis*, 1979;**32**:609–31

104. Friedman GD, Cutter GR, Donahue RP, et al. CARDIA: Study design, recruitment, and some characteristics of the examined subjects. *J Clin Epidemiol*, 1988;**41**:1105–16

105. Shapiro SH, Macklem PT, Gray-Donald K, et al. A randomized clinical trial of negative pressure ventilation in severe chronic obstructive pulmonary disease: Design and methods. *J Clin Epidemiol*, 1991;**44**:483–96

106. Manson JAE, Buring JE, Satterfield S, Hennekens CH. Baseline characteristics of participants in the Physicians' Health Study: A randomized trial of aspirin and beta-carotene in U.S. physicians. *Am J Prev Med*, 1991;**7**:150–4

107. Steering Committee of the Physicians' Health Study Research Group. Final report on the aspirin component of the ongoing Physicians' Health Study. *N Engl J Med*, 1989;**321**:129–35

108. Lipid Research Clinics Program. The Lipid Research Clinics Coronary Primary Prevention Trial Results. I. Reduction in incidence of coronary heart disease. *JAMA*, 1984;**251**:351–64. II. The relationship of reduction in incidence of coronary heart disease to cholesterol lowering. *Idem*:365–74

109. Feinstein AR. An additional basic science for clinical medicine: II. The limitations of randomized trials. *Ann Intern Med*, 1983;**99**:544–50

110. Horwitz RI, Feinstein AR. Improved observational method for studying therapeutic efficacy. Suggestive evidence that lidocaine prophylaxis prevents death in acute myocardial infarction. *JAMA*, 1981;**246**: 2455–9

111. Solomon S. Selection of patients for clinical drug trials in migraine. *Neuroepidemiology*, 1987;**6**: 164–71

112. Kroenke K, Arrington ME, Mangelsdorff AD. The prevalence of symptoms in medical outpatients and the adequacy of therapy. *Arch Intern Med*, 1990;**150**:1685–9

113. Lemmer B (ed.). *Chronopharmacology: Cellular and Biochemical Interactions*. New York: Marcel Dekker Inc., 1989

114. Reinberg A, Labrecque G, Smolensky G. *Chronobiologie – Chronopharmacologie*. Paris: Flammarion Médecine-Sciences, 1991

115. Lachin JM. Introduction to sample size determination and power analysis for clinical trials. *Contr Clin Trials*, 1981;**2**:93–113

116. Hallstrom AP, Trobaugh GB. Specificity, sensitivity, and prevalence in the design of randomized trials: A univariate analysis. *Contr Clin Trials*, 1985;**6**: 128–35

117. Hennekens C, Buring JE. Need for large sample sizes in randomized trials. *Pediatrics*, 1987;**79**:569–71

118. Tfelt-Hansen P, Nielsen SL. Patient numbers needed in prophylactic migraine trials. *Neuroepidemiology*, 1987:**6**:214–9

119. Schafer A. The ethics of the randomized clinical trial. *N Engl J Med*, 1982;**307**:719–24

120. Ad Hoc Committee on Medical Ethics, American College of Physicians. American College of Physicians Ethics Manual. Part I. History of medical ethics, the physician and the patient, the physician's relationship to other physicians, the physician and society. *Ann Intern Med*, 1984;**101**:129–37. Part II. Research, other ethical issues. Recommended reading. *Idem*:263–74

121. Herxheimer A. The rights of the patient in clinical research. *Lancet*, 1988;**2**:**1128**–30

122. Hoffenberg R (Chairman) Working Party of the Royal College of Physicians. Research involving patients. Summary and Recommendations of a Report of the Royal College of Physicians. *J Roy Coll Phys Lond*, 1990;**24**:10–4

123. Freedman B. Equipoise and the ethics of clinical trials. *N Engl J Med*, 1987;**317**:141–5

124. Schneiderman LJ, Jecker N, Jonsen AR. Medical futility: Its meaning and ethical implications. *Ann Intern Med*, 1990;**112**:949–54

125. Lantos JD, Singer PA, Walker RM, et al.The illusion of futility in clinical practice. *Am J Med*, 1989; **87**:81–4

126. Soskolne CL. Epidemiology: Questions of science, ethics, morality, and law. *Am J Epidemiol*, 1989; **129**:1–18

127. Beauchamp TL, Cook RR, Fayerweather WE, et al. Ethical guidelines for epidemiologists. In: Fayerweather WE, Higginson J, Beauchamp TL (Guest eds). Industrial Epidemiology Forum's Conference on Ethics in Epidemiology. *J Clin Epidemiol*, 1991;**44**(Suppl 1):151S–69S

128. Friedman M, Thoresen CE, Gill JJ, et al. Alternation of type A behavior and reduction in cardiac recurrences in postmyocardial infarction patients. *Am Heart J*, 1984;**108**:237–48

129. Saigal S, Watts J, Campbell D. Randomized clinical trial of an oscillating air mattress in preterm infants: Effect on apnea, growth, and development. *J Pediatr*, 1986;**109**:857–64

130. Nolan T, Zvagulis I, Pless B. Controlled trial of social work in childhood chronic illness *Lancet*, 1987;**2**:411–5

131. Deyo RA, Diehl AK, Rosenthal M. How many days of bed rest for acute low back pain? *N Engl J Med*, 1986;**315**:1064–70

132. Spitzer WO, Feinstein AR, Sackett DL. What is a health care trial? *JAMA*, 1975;**233**:161–3

133. Gerson LW, Collins JF. A randomized controlled trial of home care: Clinical outcome for five surgical procedures. *Can J Surg*, 1976;**19**:519–23

134. Battista RN, Guibert RL. L'évaluation des médecines douces. Problématique et paradigme. (Evaluation of alternative medicines. Problems and paradigm). *Un Méd Canada*, 1986;**115**:704–6

135. Skrabanek P. Paranormal health claims. *Experientia*, 1988;**44**:303–9

136. Beyerstein BL. Alternative medicine and common errors of reasoning. *Acad Med*, 2001;**76**:230–7

137. Mar C, Bent S. An evidence-based review of the 10 most commonly used herbs. *WJM*, 1999;**171**: 168–71

138. Feinstein AR. The need for humanized science in evaluating medication. *Lancet*, 972;**2**:421–3

139. Feinstein AR. Iatrotherapy. *Clin Pharmacol Therap*, 1986;**10**:568–70

140. Enel P, Jenicek M. Iatrothérapie ou pouvoir guérisseur du médecin. Méta-analyse qualitative (Iatrotherapy or physician's healing power. Qualitative meta-analysis). *Psychol Méd*, 1989;**21**:56–60

141. Reiser DE, Rosen DH. *Medicine as a Human Experience*. Baltimore: University Park Press, 1984

142. Lakshmanan MC, Hershey CO. Hospital admissions caused by iatrogenic disease. *Arch Intern Med*, 1986;**146**:1931–4

143. Meador CK (ed.). *A Little Book of Doctors' Rules II. A Compilation*. Philadelphia: Hanley & Belfus, 1999

144. Byington RP, Curb DJ, Mattson ME for the Beta-blocker Heart Attack Trial Research Group. Assessment of double-blindness at the conclusion of the beta-blocker heart attack trial. *JAMA*, 1985;**253**:1733–6

145. Vietti TJ. Evaluation of toxicity: Clinical issues. *Canc Treatment Rep*, 1980;**64**:457–61

146. Department of Clinical Epidemiology and Bio-statistics, McMaster University Health Sciences Centre. How to read clinical journals: VI. To learn about the quality of clinical care. *Can Med Assoc J*, 1984;**130**:377–81

147. Donabedian A. *A Guide to Medical Care Administration* (Vol. 2). New York: American Public Health Association, 1969

148. Secretaries of State for Health, Wales, Northern Ireland and Scotland. Medical Audit. Working Paper No 6 of White Paper (Cmnd 555). London: HMSO, 1989

149. Batstone GF. Medical Audit. Proceedings of a meeting. 3 November 1989. *Postgrad Med J*, 1990;**66** (Suppl 3):S1–S47

150. Stone DH. Proposed taxonomy of audit and related activities. *J Roy Coll Phys Lond*, 1990;**24**:30–1

151. Rutstein DD, Berenberg W, Chalmers TC, et al. Measuring the quality of medical care. A clinical method. *N Engl J Med*, 1976;**294**:582–8

152. Dixon N. Practical principles of medical audit. *Postgrad Med J*, 1990;**66**:S17–S20

153. Detsky AS, Sackett DL. When was a 'negative' clinical trial big enough? How many patients you needed depends on what you found. *Arch Intern Med*, 1985;**145**:709–12

154. Browner WS, Newman TB. Are all significant P values created equal? The analogy between diagnostic tests and clinical research. *JAMA*, 1987;**257**:2459–63

155. Leddin D. Alpha errors, beta errors and negative trials. *Can J Gastroenterol*, 1988;**4**:147–50

156. Young MJ, Bresnitz EA, Strom BL. Sample size nomograms for interpreting negative clinical studies. *Ann Intern Med*, 1983;**99**:248–51

157. Weinstein MC, Stason WB. Foundations of cost-effectiveness analysis for health and medical practices. *N Engl J Med*, 1977;**296**:716–21

158. Riddiough MA, Sisk JE, Bell JC. Influenza vaccination. Cost-effectiveness and public policy. *JAMA*, 1983;**249**:3189–95

159. Stason WB, Weinstein MC. Allocation of resources to manage hypertension. *N Engl J Med*, 1977;**96**:732–9

160. Weinstein MC. Cost-effective priorities for cancer prevention. *Science*, 1983;**221**:17–23

161. Stason WB. Costs and benefits of risk factor reduction for coronary heart disease: Insights from screening and treatment of serum cholesterol. *Am Heart J*, 1990;**119**:718–24

162. Goldman L. Cost-effectiveness perspectives in coronary heart disease. *Am Heart J*, 1990;**119**:733–40

163. O'Brien B, Rushby J. Outcome assessment in cardiovascular cost–benefit studies. *Am Heart J*, 1990;**119**:740–8

164. Edelson JT, Tosteson ANA, Sax P. Cost-effectiveness of misoprostol for prophylaxis against non-steroidal anti-inflammatory drug-induced gastro-intestinal bleeding. *JAMA*, 1990;**264**:41–7

165. Lindgren B. The cost–benefit approach to pricing new medicines: Doxazosin versus beta-blocker treatment in Sweden. *Am Heart J*, 1990;**119**:748–53

166. Hollenberg JP, Subak LL, Ferry Jr JJ, Bussel JB. Cost-effectiveness of splenectomy versus intravenous gamma globulin in treatment of chronic immune thrombocytopenic purpura in childhood. *J Pediatr*, 1988;**112**:530–9

167. Detsky AS, Naglie IG. A clinician's guide to cost-effectiveness analysis. *Ann Intern Med*, 1990;**113**:147–54

168. Eisenberg JM. Clinical economics: Economic analysis in medical care. In: Asawapokee N, Lilasarami A eds. *Symposium on Clinical Decision Analysis and Clinical Economics*. Pattaya, March 11–13. Bangkok: Medical Media Press, 1987:78–120

169. Padgett D, Mumford E, Hynes M, Carter R. Meta-analysis of the effects of educational and psychological interventions on management of diabetes mellitus. *J Clin Epidemiol*, 1988;**41**:1007–30

170. DerSimonian R, Charette LJ, McPeek B, Mosteller F. Reporting methods in clinical trials. *N Engl J Med*, 1982;**306**:1332–7

171. Chalmers TC, Smith Jr H, Blackburn B, et al. A method for assessing the quality of a randomized control trial. *Contr Clin Trials*, 1981;**2**:31–49

172. Nicolucci A, Grilli R, Alexanian AA, et al. Quality, evolution, and clinical implications of randomized, controlled trials on the treatment of lung cancer. *JAMA*, 1989;**262**:2101–7

173. The Standards of Reporting Trials Group. A proposal for structured reporting of randomized controlled trials. *JAMA*, 1994;**272**:1926–31

174. The Asilomar Working Group on Recommendations for reporting of Clinical trials in the Biomedical Literature. Checklist of information for inclusion in

reports of clinical trials. *Ann Intern Med*, 1996;**124**: 741–3

175. Anon. Purpose and Procedure. *ACP Journal Club*, 1999 (July/August):A15–A16

176. Anon. Purpose and Procedure. *Evidence-Based Med*, 2001;**6**:65

177. Anon. Purpose and procedure. *EBMH*, 2001;**4**:34–5

178. Guyatt GH, Sackett DL, Cook DJ for the Evidence-Based Medicine Working Group. Users' guides to the medical literature. II. How to use an article about therapy or prevention. A. Are the results valid? *JAMA*, 1993;**270**:2598–601

179. Guyatt GH, Sackett DL, Cook DJ. Users' guides to the medical literature. II. How to use an article about therapy or prevention. B. What were the results and will they help me in caring for my patients? *JAMA*, 1994;**271**:59–63

180. Dans AL, Dans LF, Guyatt GH, Richardson S for the Evidence-Based Medicine Working Group. Users' guides to the medical literature. XIV. How to decide on the applicability of clinical trials results to your patient? *JAMA*, 1998;**279**:545–9

181. Bucher HC, Guyatt GH, Cook DJ, et al. for the Evidence-Based Medicine Working Group. Users' guides to the medical literature. XIX. Applying clinical trial results. A. How to use an article measuring the effect of an intervention on surrogate end points. *JAMA*, 1999;**282**:771–8

182. McAlister FA, Laupacis A, Wells GA, et al. for the Evidence-Based Medicine Working Group. Users' guides to the medical literature. XIX. Applying clinical trial results. B. Guidelines to determining whether a drug is exerting (more than) a class effect. *JAMA*, 1999;**282**:1371–7

183. Guyatt GH, Sinclair J, Cook DJ, Glasziou P for the Evidence-Based Medicine Working Group and the Cochrane Applicability Methods Working Group. Users' guides to the medical literature. XVI. How to use a treatment recommendation. *JAMA*, 1999;**281**: 1836–43

184. Spodick DH. The surgical mystique and the double standard. Controlled trials of medical and surgical therapy for cardiac disease: Analysis, hypothesis, proposal. *Am Heart J*, 1973;**85**:579–83

185. Stolley PD, Kuller LH. The need for epidemiologists and surgeons to cooperate in the evaluation of surgical therapies. *Surgery*, 1975;**78**:123–5

186. Kestle JRW. Clinical trials. *World J Surg*, 1999;**23**: 1205–9

187. McLeod RS. Issues in surgical randomized controlled trials. *World J Surg*, 1999;**23**:1210–14

188. Etchels E. Informed consent in surgical trials. *World J Surg*, 1999;**23**:1215–19

189. Krahn M. Principles of economic evaluation in surgery. *World J Surg*, 1999;**23**:1242–8

190. Rudicel S, Esdaile J. The randomized clinical trial in orthopaedics: Obligation or option? *J Bone Joint Surg*, 1985;**67A**:1284–93

191. Salzman EW. Is surgery worthwhile? Presidential address. *Arch Surg*, 1985;**120**:771–6

192. Van den Linden W. Pitfalls in randomized surgical trials. *Surgery*, 1980;**87**:258–62

193. Donegan WL. Surgical clinical trials. *Cancer*, 1984; **53**:691–9

194. Killip T, Ryan TJ. Randomized trials in coronary bypass surgery. *Circulation*, 1985;**71**:418–21

195. Fahey T. Applying the results of clinical trials to patients in general practice: perceived problems, strengths, assumptions, and challenges for the future. *Br J Gen Pract*, 1998;**48**:1173–8

196. Ward E, King M, Lloyd M, et al. Conducting randomized trials in general practice: methodological and practical issues. *Br J Gen Pract*, 1999;**49**:919–22

197. Strom BL. *Pharmacoepidemiology*. New York: Churchill Livingstone, 1989

198. Kewitz H, Roots I, Voigt K (eds). *Epidemiological Concepts in Clinical Pharmacology*. Berlin: Springer-Verlag, 1987

199. Karch FE, Lasagna L. Toward the operational identification of adverse drug reactions. *Clin Pharmacol Ther*, 1977;**21**:247–54

200. Karch FE, Lasagna L. Adverse drug reactions – A critical review. *JAMA*, 1975;**234**:236–41

201. Kramer MS, Leventhal JM, Hutchinson TA, Feinstein AR. An algorithm for the operational assessment of adverse drug reactions. I. Background, description, and instructions for use. *JAMA*, 1979; **242**:623–32

202. Hutchinson TA, Leventhal JM, Kramer MS, et al. An algorithm for the operational assessment of adverse drug reactions. II. Demonstration of reproducibility and validity. *JAMA*, 1979;**242**:633–9

203. Leventhal JM, Hutchinson TA, Kramer MS, Feinstein AR. An algorithm for the operational assessment of adverse drug reactions. III. Results of tests among clinicians. *JAMA*, 1979;**242**:1991–4

204. Kunin CM (Guest ed.). Pharmacoepidemiology in developing countries. *J Clin Epidemiol*, 1991;**44** (Suppl II):IS–105S

205. Guess HA, Stephenson WP, Sacks ST, Gardner JS. Beyond pharmacoepidemiology: The larger role of epidemiology in drug development. *J Clin Epidemiol*, 988;**41**:995–6

206. Inman WHW. Beyond pharmacoepidemiology. *J Clin Epidemiol*, 1988;**41**:997–8

207. Cobert BL, Biron P. Pharmacovigilance from A to Z. *Adverse Drug Event Surveillance*. Malden: Blackwell Science, 2002

208. Duclos P, Koch J, Hardy M, et al. Adverse effects temporally associated with immunizing agents –

1989 report. *Canada Diseases Weekly Rep*, 1991; **17–29**:147–58

209. CASS Principal Investigators and their Associates. Coronary Artery Surgery Study (CASS): a randomized trial of coronary artery bypass surgery. *Circulation*, 1983;**68**:939–50 (Survival data); 1983;**68**:951–60 (Quality of life in patients randomly assigned to treatment groups)

210. Sartorius N, Helmchen H. Multicentre Trials. In: *Modern Problems in Pharmacopsychiatry*, no 16. Basel: S Karger, 1981

211. Hedman C, Andersen AR, Olesen J. Multi-centre versus single-centre trials on migraine. *Neuroepidemiology*, 1987;**6**:190–7

212. Rahimtoola SH. Some unexpected lessons from large multicenter randomized clinical trials. *Circulation*, 1985;**72**:449–55

213. Stamler J, Liu K. The benefits of prevention. In: Kaplan NM, Stamler J eds. *Prevention of Coronary Heart Disease. Practical Management of the Risk Factors*. Philadelphia: WB Saunders Co., 1983: 188–207

214. McCormick J, Skrabanek P. Coronary heart disease is not preventable by population interventions. *Lancet*, 1988;**2**:839–41

215. Goodman CS. The scope of US medical technology assessment. In: Mosteller F, Chairman, Committee for Evaluating Medical Technologies in Clinical Use (Institute of Medicine). *Assessing Medical Technologies*. Washington: National Academy Press, 1985: 32–69

216. Brorsson B, Wall S. *Assessment of Medical Technology – Problems and Methods*. Stockholm: Swedish Medical Research Council, 1985

217. Laupacis A, Feeny D, Detsky AS, Tugwell PX. How attractive does a new technology have to be to warrant adoption and utilization? Tentative guidelines for using clinical and economical evaluations. *Can Med Assoc J*, 1992;**146**:473–81

218. Thacker SB, Berkelman RL. Surveillance of medical technologies. *J Public Health Policy*, 1986;**7**:363–77

219. Epp J. *Achieving Health for All: A Framework for Health Promotion*. Ottawa: Supply and Services Canada, 1986 (H 39 102/1986 E)

220. Stachtchenko S, Jenicek M. Conceptual differences between prevention and health promotion: Research implications for community health programs. *Can J Public Health*, 1990;**81**:53–9

221. Abelin T, Brzezinski ZJ, Carstairs VDL (eds). *Measurement in Health Promotion and Protection*. Copenhagen: World Health Organization Regional Office for Europe, WHO Regional Publications, European Series No 22, 1987

222. Eisenberg JM, Freud D, Glick H, et al., INCLEN Economics Faculty. Clinical economics education in the International Epidemiological Network. *J Clin Epidemiol*, 1989;**42**:689–95

223. Detsky AS. Are clinical trials a cost-effective investment? *JAMA*, 1989;**262**:1795–800

224. Gunning-Schepers LJ, Barendregt JJ, van der Maas PJ. Population intervention reassessed. *Lancet*, 1989; **1**:479–81

225. Fries JF, Green LW, Levine S. Health promotion and the compression of morbidity. *Lancet*, 1989;**1**:481–3

226. Goodman SN. Towards Evidence-Based Medical Statistics: The P value fallacy. *Ann Intern Med*, 1999; **130**:995–1004

227. Goodman SN. Towards Evidence-Based medical Statistics: The Bayes factor. *Ann Intern Med*, 1999; **130**:1005–13

228. Naylor CD, Guyatt GH, for the Evidence-Based medicine Working Group. Users'guides to the medical literature. X. How to use an article reporting variations in the outcomes of health services. *JAMA*, 1996;**275**:554–8

229. Drummond MF, O'Brien BJ, Stoddart GL, Torrance GW. *Methods for the Economic Evaluation of Health Care Programmes*. 2nd Edition. Oxford: Oxford University Press, 1997

230. Drummond MF, Richardson SW, O'Brien BJ, et al. for the Evidence-Based Medicine Working Group. Users' guides to the medical literature. XIII. How to use an article on economic analysis of clinical practice. A. Are the results of the study valid? *JAMA*, 1997;**277**:1552–7

231. O'Brien BJ, Heyland D, Richardson WS, et al. for the Evidence-Based medicine Working Group. Users' guides to the medical literature. XIII. How to use an article on economic analysis of clinical practice. B. What are the results and will they help me in caring for my patients? *JAMA*, 1997;**277**:1802–6

232. Teutsch SM. A framework for assessing the effectiveness of disease and injury prevention. *MMWR* (Recommendations and Reports), 1992;**41**(RR–3): 1–12

233. Haddix AC, Teutsch SM, Shaffer PA, Dunet DO (eds). *Prevention Effectiveness. A Guide to Decision Analysis and Economic Evaluation*. New York and Oxford: Oxford University Press, 1996

234. Special Section: Health-Related Quality of Life in Clinical Studies. Series of papers. *Ann Med*, 2001; **33**:323–84

235. Massad E, Burattini MN, Siqueira NRS. Fuzzy logic and measles vaccination: designing a control strategy. *Int J Epidemiol*, 1999;**28**:550–7

Chapter 10

Prognosis. Studies of disease course and outcomes

The physician who cannot inform his patient what would be the probable issue of his complaint if allowed to follow its natural course, is not qualified to prescribe any rational treatment for its cure.
Hippocrates (460–373 BC)[1]

Prognoses are the disliked stepchildren of medicine. . . . The more the prognoses refer to the future, the more they resemble prophecies. . . . Individual prognoses are necessary in every medical decision, and, beyond that, they even legitimize every medical act. If there is no prognostic relevance, no intervention can be justified. The methodology of prognosis forms the core of medical practice and a humane medicine.
Claudia Wieseman (1998)[2]

A woman in her fifties complains of meno- and metrorrhagia, and a subsequent biopsy confirms endometrial cancer. Her attending physician suggests a hysterectomy, and other treatments, as needed. The patient may ask: *'Doctor, is this operation absolutely necessary? What would happen to me if I decided not to have an operation? . . . How beneficial will this operation be? . . . Will it stop my bleeding? . . . What other problems might the operation cause? . . . Is my disease serious? How probable is it that I will die from it? . . . How probable is it that I might die on the operating table? . . . What other treatments can I expect? . . .'* In many cultures around the world, where the patient's attitude is generally fatalistic, these questions would not be asked and the physician accepting these questions could be perceived as incompetent. The patient might say, *'Doctor, you are the specialist, you are university-trained, I pay you to decide for me, you must know . . .'* Elsewhere, an intelligent and curious patient will demand intelligent and competent answers since he or she expects the best possible estimation of his(her) chances and not a guess or an impression. Making a prognosis is another example of a logical discourse whose validity relies heavily on the best evidence available. For example, bronchial cancer is diagnosed in a fifty-year-old male patient who has been smoking since his teens:

Clinical practice	Logical discourse	Evidence
'We both know that smoking cigarettes caused your lung cancer.'	Smoking tobacco causes lung cancer. (*Premise A*)	Extensive **analytical observational research**.
'Unfortunately, your life expectancy is now very short.'	The life expectancy of such patients is two years at maximum. (*Premise B*)	**Prognostic studies**.

'You must stop smoking immediately and never smoke again!'	Smoking must stop if the patient's survival is to be improved. **(Conclusion C)**	Do the results of clinical **trials** and other analytical studies **show** that stopping smoking at that stage of bronchial cancer improves the **survival** of these patients? If not, this advice to the patient is unsubstantiated.

Astute readers will note right away that two of several valid premises are available. Each premise is supported by extensive etiological research (premise A) and survival studies (premise B). Is conclusion C a natural corollary of premises A and B, which are supposed to support and lead to that conclusion? Conclusions in this example do not follow from other, equally solid evidence that tobacco smoking is not only a predominant etiological (risk) factor of bronchial cancer, but also a prognostic one. Are there studies, particularly clinical trials, which show that if lung cancer patients stop smoking, their life expectancies will increase? Or does quitting smoking merely offer a chance to improve some symptoms? **Neither focus, nor premises or evidence, are interchangeable. (Not only do they not 'travel well', they do not travel at all!) This explains why logical discourse and supporting evidence are more challenging in the area of prognosis than in the area of risk.** Current experience is still, in general, much richer in the area of risk than in that of prognosis.

10.1 Conceptual considerations

A patient wants to know what to expect regarding the outcome of the health problem for which he is being treated. Foreseeing what **may** happen to a disease sufferer is the substance of prognosis. This part of a physician's work must be as solid and professional as the ability to assess risks, make a diagnosis, or treat. In community health, physicians must foresee the future of disease occurrence and spread.

10.1.1 Definition of prognosis

Prognosis (from the Greek 'foreknowledge') is traditionally defined as *'the act or art of foretelling the course of disease'*, or better, *'the prospect of survival and recovery from a disease as anticipated from the usual course of that disease or indicated by special features of the case in question'*[3]. Such a conceptual definition of prognosis as stated above is found in many dictionaries but requires precision.

1. Contemporary prognosis is not a guess or a product of clinical flair. It is an estimation of probabilities, as is the evaluation of risk. The basic epidemiological approach is the same. In risk assessment, probabilities of developing disease are estimated according to the characteristics of the individual and his general environment. In prognostic assessment, probabilities of various good **and** bad events as well as outcomes in the already diseased individual are assessed.
2. While risk is usually related to one event (falling ill), prognostic studies are multidimensional in that they deal with several outcomes, not just death.
3. Whereas risk depends mostly on non-medical factors, prognosis is largely determined by clinical factors, human biology and pathology.

With these considerations in mind, we may define prognosis as *'an assessment of the patient's future (based on probabilistic considerations of various beneficial and detrimental clinical outcomes as causally or otherwise determined by various clinical factors, biological and social characteristics of the patient), and of the pathology under study (disease course) itself. Its main purpose is to prevent undesirable events and to intervene precociously to modify disease course and drive it to its best possible outcome'*. Hence, prognosis is an important element of medical decision-making that goes well beyond reassurance of the patient as part of good bedside manners. It is a professional act like any other, be it diagnosis, surgery or medication.

Field epidemiology and public health are the first disciplines to eliminate uncertainty about what will happen in the community (immunized or not) if an infectious disease appears. Disease incidence is studied, prevalence of population time and place characteristics are determined, and time trends of past events are studied, as well as how these characteristics will change in time, such that realistic estimates of disease incidence can be made for the future. A contemporary clinician must proceed with the same rigor when evaluating what will happen to an individual patient. The clinician must know, and will use, all relevant information from community and clinical epidemiology findings to assess the probability of the worst possible events in order to prevent or alleviate them. In these terms, Fries and Ehrlich[4] see prognosis as a probabilistic prediction that is multidimensional, qualitative and quantitative, as well as well defined in time, with emphasis on variability from one disease gradient and spectrum to another, and its dependence on clinical intervention. To make a realistic prognosis for a patient or for a disease as a whole, high-quality data from high-quality studies of prognosis are needed. According to Armitage and Gehan, findings from these sources provide valuable information for practice and research[5]:

1. They provide insight into the mechanism of disease (course);
2. They are necessary for better planning of clinical studies (for example, patients in clinical trials are assembled in different prognostic groups);
3. They are necessary to better evaluate the findings from clinical research (for example, when comparing treatment outcomes);
4. They are important considerations in deciding what treatment to give patients; and
5. Causes of poor prognosis (prognostic factors) may be modified to ensure patients' recovery.

Despite the relevance of a rigorous approach to prognosis, physicians in general (not just researchers[6]) have only recently been introduced to this approach through overviews[7–10] or specialized chapters in textbooks of clinical epidemiology[11–15], in an *ad hoc* book[4], or from writings focusing more on the methodology of survival studies[16–19]. This chapter is an overview of the field of prognosis – basic concepts, principles, special methods used, considerations allowing for the adoption or rejection of prognostic studies and their findings in relation to clinical decisions, as well as directions for further research.

10.1.2 Prognosis as opposed to risk

As predicted by the above-mentioned considerations, making a prognosis is more complicated than assessing risk. In risk assessment, as explained in Chapter 8, various risk markers and factors must be evaluated separately[20-21]. Similarly, **prognostic characteristics** fall into two categories: **prognostic markers** (which cannot be modified and upon which disease course is dependent); and **prognostic factors** (which can be modified; consequently disease course can also be modified). Knowledge of both is necessary to make a good prognosis. In addition, methodological aspects of prognosis depend on different individuals under study, the duration of events, different causal factors, and the main topics under study, all differing from risk assessment. Figure 10.1 and Table 10.1 summarizes these differences. Traditionally, knowledge of risk factors in medicine was automatically extrapolated to the field of prognostic factors. Doing so, however, is often quite misleading. For example,

smoking is a powerful risk factor for lung cancer, but is it justified for a clinician to suggest that a lung cancer patient stop smoking? Is it wise to suggest that an octogenarian with a small facial basocellular lesion minimize exposure to the sun in order to avoid skin cancer, even if the patient is carefully followed up, screened and surgically treated in time?

Some risk factors lose their power as prognostic factors, and some are important at both levels. For example, alcohol abuse is a powerful risk factor for chronic hepatitis and liver cirrhosis. These patients will also further deteriorate if they continue to drink. Thus, alcohol is a powerful prognostic factor as well. An alcoholic, cirrhotic patient should stop drinking, but a lung cancer patient whose life expectancy is two years at best might possibly continue smoking without greatly altering the disease's course, even though smoking caused the fatal neoplasia in the first place. Table 10.2 illustrates selected risk and prognostic characteristics as identified for pancreatic cancer and stable angina. These characteristics are different for each disease entity. Variability from one pathology to another may be considerable and ultimately will determine medical counseling and treatment.

Finally, risk remains the focus of primary prevention, whereas prognosis and ensuing clinical decisions fall into the field of secondary and tertiary prevention. Consequently, effective secondary and tertiary prevention will depend on a knowledge of prognostic markers and factors in their best qualitative and quantitative terms. Table 10.3 shows that the relationship between risk characteristics and disease occurrence is simpler than relationships in the field of prognosis. In the case of risk, one or several risk factors may lead to disease occurrence. In the case of prognostic factors, as independent variables, these may result in worsening of the disease gradient. Elsewhere, certain states, already being consequences of other prognostic factors, lead to the diversification and aggravation of the disease spectrum and ultimately its gradient.

Finally, prognostic factors arise not only from the web of causes of principal disease outcomes, but also from concurrent diseases or newly appearing co-morbid states (such as cross-infections, metabolic imbalances, etc.). Indeed, all may act upon the

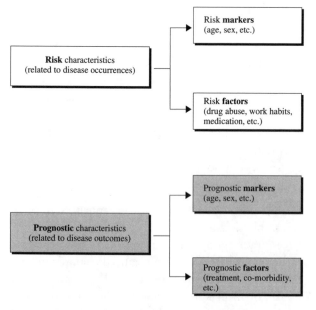

Figure 10.1 Classification of risk and prognostic characteristics: markers and factors

Table 10.1 Basic characteristics of prognosis as opposed to risk

Topic of interest	Risk	Prognosis
Individual	Healthy subjects	Subjects already have disease under study
Occurrence of expected effects	Less frequent or rare	Frequent
Controllability of independent variable	Risk characteristics: – Uncontrollable: risk markers – Controllable: risk factors	Prognostic characteristics: – Uncontrollable: prognostic markers – Controllable: prognostic factors
Aim of study	Primary prevention Better assessment of individuals	Secondary and tertiary prevention Better clinical decisions
Population size	Many subjects are often studied (large size of studies)	Few patients are often available for the study (small size of studies)
Major focus of interest	Often: – Causes – Non-medical factors – Risk factors	Often: – Consequences – Medical factors – Prognostic markers
Time factor	Occurrence of events towards a given moment (incidence, mortality, etc.)	Occurrence of events evolving in time ("survival" curves)
Target population	Mainly community at large	Hospital-bound individuals (bedridden patients, clinics, etc.)
Accessibility and compliance of participants	Poor or variable	Usually good
Interest and motivation of investigators	Variable	Usually high
Cost of study	Usually higher	Usually lower
Competence of investigators to do study	Usually better	Variable

Source: Partially from Ref. 12

Table 10.2 Risk characteristics versus prognostic characteristics

Disease	Characteristics		
	Risk marker	**Prognostic marker**	**Both***
Angina pectoris (stable)	Heredity	Recent myocardial infarction	Age
	Risk factor	**Prognostic factor**	**Both***
	Physical inactivity	Uncontrolled high blood pressure	Smoking
	Risk marker	**Prognostic marker**	**Both***
Cancer of the pancreas	Heredity	Pre-operative comorbidity, (cardiopathies, hypertension, etc.) Tumor characteristics (size, location, stage, etc.)	Age
	Risk factor	**Prognostic factor**	**Both***
	Smoking	Surgeon's experience	Not yet well understood

* Equally important before and after the onset of disease. Source: Examples selected from Refs. 22 and 23

Table 10.3	Characteristics of risk and prognosis
Definition	*Related to*
Risk characteristics (factors, markers)	Probability of disease in healthy individuals (the characteristic is an independent variable, i.e. drug abuse, sexual practices, etc.)
Prognostic gradient characteristics (factors or markers)	Probability of a modified, hastened, or aggravated outcome of an already sick individual (the characteristic is the independent variable), e.g. additional infections in AIDS sufferers reduce life expectancy (multihit theory)
Prognostic spectrum characteristics • also 'late risk' characteristics (markers or factors) • or 'additional burden' characteristics • or 'double-decker factors'	Probability of additional events (dependent variables) which by themselves produce modified and/or additional outcome, i.e. once established, it may become a new prognostic factor, e.g. AIDS: immunodeficiency increases the risk of additional infections in AIDS seroconverters (outcome); Once established, they may modify probabilities of cancer, survival, etc.

outcome of the disease of main interest and/or on any other comorbidity or additional new disease or health problem.

10.1.3 Classification of prognosis according to interactions under study

Table 10.4 illustrates that compared to a single cause–effect (risk factor–disease occurrence) relationship in the field of risk, at least 15 categories of prognostic associations and studies must be recognized. Such a classification is not only conceptual and gnostic, but it is also necessary in practice. What does saying that a patient's prognosis is good or bad mean? Will the patient live or die, or might something else happen too? The prognosis must be specific in relation to one or more of the categories in Table 10.4. For example, continuing to smoke will not significantly affect a lung cancer patient's survival (category I). In a hemophiliac patient, the

transfusion of contaminated blood will lead to HIV infection (poor prognosis in category VI). It will not change the prognosis of hemophilia (category VII); the patient will remain hemophiliac.

The concept of a 'good' or 'bad' prognosis depends on which category of prognosis is being discussed and what measures of outcome are used (see the lower portion of the table). Therapeutic decisions will also vary from one case to another.

10.1.4 Objectives of prognosis and prognostic studies

There are three major objectives of prognosis.

1. For the patient, the *best possible estimation of the disease's future course and outcome* gives either reassurance and improvement of mental well-being, or (if the prognosis is poor) allows for timely considerations for the best possible quality of life remaining.
2. For physicians and nurses, good prognostic information allows the *best therapies and care* to be planned for the patient.
3. For social services, good prognostic information allows a *timely and optimal re-integration of the patient* into the family, occupation and environment to an extent and degree corresponding to foreseeable health status.

Given the considerable human and material resources involved, prognostic studies must arrive at conclusions that are as close to the future reality as possible.

10.1.5 Basic expressions (measures) of prognosis. Events and outcomes

A good or bad (qualitative) prognosis also requires quantification in terms of probabilities. A probabilistic prognosis can be expressed many different ways, such as:

• By establishing a **survival rate** after five years of observation, as is usually done in studies of cancer patients;
• By determining a **case fatality rate** at any moment (NB Mortality may also be a measure of risk and

Table 10.4 Classification of prognostic studies according to various cause–effect relationships

	Outcome (altered course)		
	1. *Clinical (a) or natural (b)* *course of the principal* *pathology (disease)*	*2.* *Clinical (a) or natural (b) course* *of already existing comorbid* *states (other diseases)*	*3.* *Clinical (a) or natural* *(b) course of a new* *disease*
Prognostic factor			
A. Re-exposure to an 'old' risk factor (becoming a prognostic factor)	I	II	III
B. Exposure to a new factor	IV	V	VI
C. Exposure to a new clinical factor (maneuvers)	VII	VIII	IX
D. Occurrence of a complicating outcome of the principal disease	X	XI	XII
E. Occurrence of a complicating outcome a) of an already existing or b) new comorbidity(ies)	XIII	XIV	XV

In terms of death, survival, occurrence or disappearance of signs, symptoms, clinimetric indexes, cure, alleviation, improvement of function and capacity, quality of life, choice of treatment or health services, social impact (family, workplace).

Independent variable   *Dependent variable*

prognosis since it is the product of incidence density and case fatality rate as explained in Chapter 5);

- By detecting a **response rate to treatment** at any moment of a follow-up period (such as an improvement rate after treatment of leukemia patients);

- As a **remission rate** following a defined treatment (provided that a remission period and its criteria are well-defined);

- As a **relapse rate** (with the same conditions as above); and finally

- By establishing a **longitudinal picture of events during the natural or clinical course of disease**, known as **survival curves.**

A **survival curve** is essentially a sequence of rates (proportions) of events of interest in time. Originally, a proportion of patients (usually cancer sufferers) surviving or dying at a given moment were the subject of study. Today, the terms 'survival' or 'survival studies' are rather awkward or misleading, because any event appearing during the natural or clinical course of disease may be the subject of 'survival' analysis. The methodology of studying survival also applies to outcomes of disease other than death: development of complications; another spell of disease such as a migraine attack or an epilepsy 'mal'; surgical complications after an operation; adverse effects of treatment; and others. During the last two decades, a new term, **time-to-event analysis,**[33–36] has been applied to these studies of morbid events. In studies of treatment effectiveness, time-to-event analysis may be even more specific. For example, in such studies of migraine treatment, time-to-event analysis becomes **'time-to-relief analysis'**[37]; or, elsewhere, it may become **'time-to-effect analysis'**. Both 'survival analysis' and 'time-to-event analysis' or 'survival curves' and 'time-to-event curves' are used interchangeably in this text. For example, Balfour et al[29] studied various outcomes of a herpes zoster infection. These authors established **'survival curves', i.e. time-to-event curves** for the occurrence of new lesions, positive virus cultures from lesions, lesions not scabbed and pain occurrence, as illustrated in Figure 10.2. As may be seen, a survival curve is a special form of graph in which time units of follow-up are on the X-axis and the proportion of patients surviving (i.e. still not having the

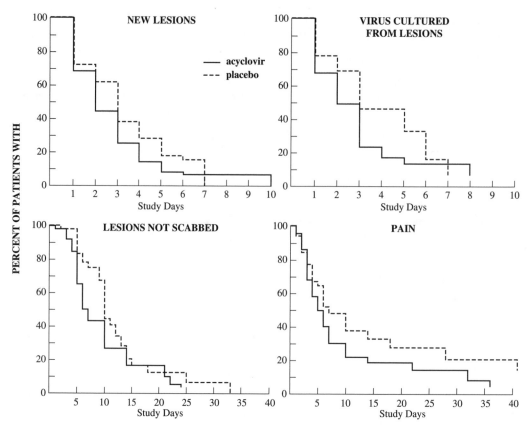

Figure 10.2 Kaplan–Meier time-to-event graphs for 52 patients receiving Acyclovir as compared with 42 placebo recipients. Source: Ref. 29, reproduced with permission from the Massachusetts Medical Society (*N Engl J Med*)

measure of prognosis, such as attack, remissions, relapses, etc.) are on the Y-axis from one moment of study to another (NB Reverse pictures of survival are also presented as increasing proportions of patients developing a prognostic event with time).

10.2 General methodology of prognostic studies

Like studies of risk, studies of prognosis may be either descriptive, observational analytical, or experimental and most are longitudinal cohort studies by nature. This methodology has already been described *ad hoc* in previous chapters.

10.2.1 Descriptive studies of prognosis

As in descriptive studies of risk, descriptive studies of prognosis serve several purposes:

- To generate hypotheses on probable causes of a good or bad prognosis in patients;

- To identify patients at high probability of a bad prognosis; and

- To give arguments (components) necessary for clinical decision analysis and clinical decisions themselves.

For example, Froehling et al[30] established a descriptive picture of incidence and prognosis of positional vertigo in a community study. In this historical prospective study (retrolective study), vertigo rates (incidence as a measure of risk), and stroke and death occurrence in vertigo sufferers (as measures of prognosis) were established. Jones and Ratnoff[31] made a prognostic study of mortality and median life expectancy of hemophiliac patients (factor VIII deficiency) during the last two decades. They attributed the worsening prognosis to AIDS. These kinds of descriptive studies are most often large case series studies, as outlined in Chapter 7. Descriptive studies often have an analytical component. Inductively, groups of patients bearing different characteristics are

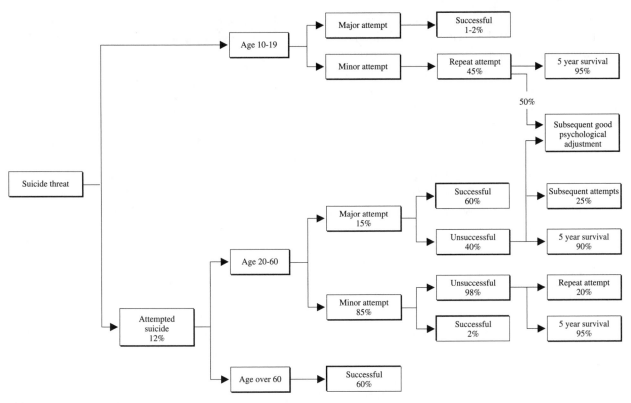

Figure 10.3   Prognostic tree (descriptive data) for a suicidal patient. Source: Adapted from Ref. 34

compared to identify possible prognostic factors and markers. McElwee et al[32] prospectively studied 329 cases of ibuprofen overdose. By analyzing the drug's concentration, the serum, and correlating this information with gastrointestinal and life-threatening manifestations, serum concentrations of the drug did not prove to be good predictors of patient outcome or an indicator for clinical decisions. Westling et al[33] carried out a survival study of 438 stroke patients, in an effort to establish prognosis of survival in relation to patient age, subtype, severity, and occurrence of stroke diagnosis. Based on descriptive findings, subsequent regression analysis identified the patient's age and severity of stroke as the prognostic marker and factor respectively.

The end product of a descriptive prognostic study is a portrait of the patient's possible future in terms of alternatives and their probabilities. Such a '**prognostic tree**' can be created for obvious medical and psychiatric problems as well. Figure 10.3 illustrates such a description of prognosis and possible

outcomes in suicidal patients[34]. Contrary to algorithms and decision trees, as explained in Chapter 13, 'prognostic trees' do not give an indication of what to do; neither do they review alternative options with their outcomes and utilities (values). The quality of descriptive studies of prognosis relies heavily on their representativity (target population, gradient, spectrum, and course of disease) and interval validity given by the respect of rigorous clinimetric criteria for an acceptable description of disease course.

10.2.2 *Observational analytical studies of prognosis*

Besides fundamental descriptive studies, analytical observational (cohort and case–control studies) research can take place through comparative studies of 'survival' in time. Analytical studies of prognosis can be either inductive or deductive. Many studies in this area are based on an inductive approach to data (information already exists in clinical charts). In a carefully designed and executed study of possible prognostic markers and factors related to the survival of compensated silicotic patients, Infante-Rivard et al[35] reviewed a registry of silicosis sufferers in Quebec, their clinical and paraclinical findings, as well as additional exposure to undesirable factors such as smoking. In the analytical part of their studies, a Cox proportional hazard analysis (see Section 10.3.2.4) showed several clinical (dyspnea, expectoration, etc.) and paraclinical (opacities on chest radiograph) or behavioral (smoking) findings as predictors and characteristics related to patient survival. In this type of 'retrospectively' conducted study, conclusions on 'causes' or 'predictors' of a good or bad prognosis must be taken only at face, i.e. inductive, value. In cohort studies of prognosis, where hypotheses are constructed deductively and study designs built *ad hoc*, conclusions can be more solid.

10.2.3 *Experimental studies of prognosis or clinical trials*

Finally, intervention studies, such as clinical trials, may be based on comparison of survival curves (or prognostic curves) in different groups of patients subjected to different treatment modalities, such as in the above-mentioned study by Balfour et al[29] on the efficacy of acyclovir in herpes zoster in immuno-compromised patients. A simple comparison of frequency of outcomes in treatment groups usually represents the assessment of treatment impact in the short term. A comparison of prognostic (survival) curves represents an important method of evaluation of a treatment's long-term impact. In these studies, the natural (placebo) and clinical course are compared, or various clinical courses (under various treatment modalities) are assessed with regard to their best efficacy and effectiveness. Comparative studies of disease course represent yet another type of study dealing with cause–effect relationships between various non-clinical and clinical events and disease outcomes. Besides special statistical techniques, the principles of which are outlined below, they are subject to the same clinimetric rigor and causal reasoning as any other study in clinical epidemiology.

10.3 Special methodology of prognostic studies. Survival or time-to-event analysis

10.3.1 *Describing disease course and outcomes by establishing survival or time-to-event curves*

Making a prognosis based simply on knowing how many patients will survive a certain time period (e.g. five years following the detection of a cancer or any other disease) would rely on very poor information since the exact timing (moment of occurrence) of the events in **this five-year period** would be ignored. As shown by Fletcher et al[11], several diseases may show a comparable survival rate at a given moment, 10% for example. Such a prognosis can be made for a rapidly dissecting aortic aneurysm: subjects mainly die within the first one or two years following its discovery. A similar five-year survival rate can be observed in chronic granulocytic leukemia, but more patients survive beyond the first year and years after within the same five-year period. Similarly, Figure 10.4 represents two survival curves for glioma patients[36]. If, for example, only survival rates at 25 or 30 months of study were compared, both groups would look quite similar. However, more patients having frontal lobe tumors survive longer than patients having parietal lobe and/or deep-seated tumors throughout the 25-month period under study, i.e. they die in the later months of the study. This information would be lost if only survival rates at 25 or 30 months were compared between the groups.

Hence, to describe and analyze disease course and outcomes, it is necessary to first position disease events in time. Such occurrences of events are represented by life tables and survival curves[10,14–16,18,19]. First, survival curves for groups of patients must be established. Then, different groups of patients can be compared in terms of survival.

10.3.1.1 *Basic vocabulary*

A **life table** is a summarizing technique used to describe the pattern of mortality (or of any other event of clinical interest) and survival (i.e. non-event) in populations. The **clinical life table** '*describes the outcome experience of a group or cohort of individuals classified according to their exposure or treatment history*[37]'.

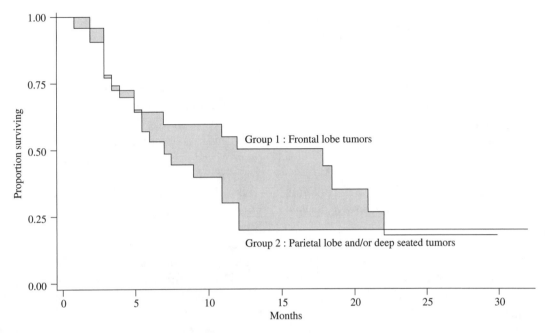

Figure 10.4 Survival curves for two groups of patients with high-grade gliomas. Source: Ref. 45, reproduced and adapted with permission from the ACP-ASIM (*Ann Intern Med*)

A **survival curve** is '*a curve that starts with 100% of the study population and shows the percentage of the population surviving at successive times for as long a period as information is available*[37]'. As already mentioned, '**survival**' is not merely 'avoiding death', when death represents the disease outcome of interest. It is a state until the occurrence of some event or outcome of interest. *It can be any discrete event such as a relapse, recovery, disease spell (well-defined), or any other change of disease course. The term 'survival' is chosen here because of its persisting use, although it represents 'time-to-event', 'survival time' or any 'prognostic' function of interest.* If the endpoint in 'true' survival studies is too difficult or expensive to detect, some other '**surrogate**' point, more readily measurable, but well-correlated with the former, and biologically well-justified for substitution, may be selected and analyzed. In survival studies of cancer, surrogates for tumor response may be its progression, reappearance of the disease, or the pre-defined particular value change of carcinoembryonic antigen[38].

In the statistical literature, establishing a survival curve is called a '**survivorship study**', which is currently defined as the '*use of a cohort life table to provide the probability that an event, such as death,*

will occur in successive intervals of time after diagnosis (or other time point defined a priori), and conversely, the probability of surviving each interval. The multiplication of these probabilities of survival for each time interval for those alive at the beginning of that interval yields a cumulative probability of surviving for the total period under study[37]. In these studies, estimation of 'survival' is based on information available about **all** patients including cases of incomplete follow-up for reasons unrelated to the outcome of interest such as patients dropping out, moving away, dying from other causes, etc. Only principles of survival analysis are outlined in this chapter. Numerical examples abound in the medical literature[10,18 and elsewhere]. Quantitative methodology of survival analysis is described in the statistical literature and is nowadays available in standard statistical analysis computer software such as SPSS[39] or SAS [40]. However, all clinicians should know what information they need to provide for such an analysis and how to understand its findings. They are the final users of prognostic findings and decision-makers.

To describe and properly analyze prognostic events, a life table[43,44, see also 14,16,18] (a kind of summary of moments and events of interest) must first be established, and then a survival curve must be estimated from it. Once survival curves are established through an appropriate survivorship study, a survival analysis, i.e. comparison of curves, can be carried out. **Survival analysis** is a '*class of statistical procedures for estimating the survival function and for making inferences about the effects of treatments, prognostic factors, exposures, and other covariates*'[37]. Consider how such an outcome experience might be described.

10.3.1.2 *Describing what happens. Building survival tables and establishing a survival or time-to-event curve*

Two methods of assessing survival (i.e. an 'event-free' interval or period) are most often used in clinical research on prognosis today: They are the Kaplan–Meier or product limit method[41] and the actuarial or life table method[42,43]. The **Kaplan–Meier method** often serves in clinical situations when dates of events are known and when fewer patients are available. The probability of surviving beyond a given time **t** is estimated and denoted by **S(t)**. The survivorship function S(t) is estimated for all successive time intervals. These intervals are irregular since they are determined by the observed times (moments) of occurrence of events. For example, if death by cancer appears in the fifth month after the entry of one patient into the study, the first interval is five months. If another death occurs eight months after the death of the first patient, the next interval will cover the period from the fifth month of the study to the thirteenth, etc. Hence, the survivorship function changes (i.e. decreases) only at the moments when deaths occur.

The **actuarial** or **life table method** operates with fixed regular intervals being determined in advance, for example from one year, month, or week to another. This method is used for large data sets like those in with which life and health insurance companies are interested. Both methods use all the information available, that is, they take into account events called '**censored' data**. For a given patient, survival or time-to-event is said to be censored when the event of interest has not been observed for some reason. Outcomes of interest may remain unknown at the time of analysis: patients lost to follow-up, other events (outcomes) occurring such as deaths by another cause

(outcome) than that due to the disease under study, etc. Also, staggered entry of patients into clinical trials means that some patients have a shorter follow-up period, thus are more likely to have censored data. Estimation of **S(t)** is based on the assumption of non-informative censoring which means that censoring occurs randomly, and that the patients with censored observations are not different from the 'uncensored ones', i.e. those experiencing an outcome event of interest.

Both curves, Kaplan–Meier and actuarial, give an illustration of similar trends: Visually speaking, the Kaplan–Meier curve in an irregular step pattern reflects observed times of occurrence of events (irregular steps); the actuarial (life table) method based on uniform periods of observation gives a smoother pattern. Coldman and Elwood's introductory paper on survival analysis for physicians[18] applies both methods to the same data set and gives a good concurrent illustration of both methods.

10.3.2 *Comparison (analysis) of two or more curves. Explanation of what happens*

Several statistical methods are available for comparison of survival curves. Only their principles will be outlined here; computational details may be found in the literature quoted.

10.3.2.1 *An 'eye' test: simple visual comparison of survival rates using confidence intervals*

All survival rates described above were point estimates of proportions of patients surviving. Standard errors (SE) and confidence intervals (usually given in prognostic studies as a point estimate ± 2 SE) are calculated for each point of interest[44,45]. Non-overlapping confidence intervals indicate significant differences in survival trends. Such a simple, however inexact impression of findings, obtained just by looking at graphic or numerical data is called teasingly by some an '**eye test**'. Such an instant and first impression never replaces any more rigorous analysis of data. For example, a surgeon may find a five-year survival after a new surgical method three times better than after the standard procedure. His 'eye test' must be confirmed by a more rigorous quantitative analysis. For example, Jass et al[46] evaluated a

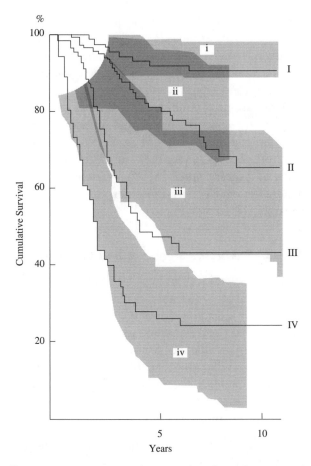

Figure 10.5 Four prognostic categories of rectal cancer and their prognostic curves (point estimates and confidence intervals). Dented lines: Point estimates of survival curves for categories I – IV; Shaded areas: Confidence intervals for survival curves. Source: Ref. 46, reproduced and adapted with permission from Elsevier Science (*The Lancet*)

new prognostic classification of rectal cancer. Two sets of patients were involved, falling into four prognostic categories – excellent (I), good (II), fair (III), and poor (IV). Survival of scored and classified patients was established, the first data set yielding confidence interval estimates of survival as illustrated in Figure 10.5. Point estimates of the survival curves of the second data set fit well within the 95% confidence bands for the first data set. The scoring system was thereby considered reproducible by the authors.

10.3.2.2 *Establishing relative survival or time-to-event rates*

In a sense, the relative survival rate is a misnomer since it is a survival ratio, i.e.

$$\text{Relative survival rate} = \frac{\text{Observed survival rate}}{\text{Expected survival rate}}$$

Observed rates are obtained from the survival study itself. (In other applications, expected rates can be obtained outside the study, such as from survival rates in a population bearing similar characteristics, such as age, sex, etc., to those of the patients in the study.)

The relative survival rate (or ratio) would then be an indication of the difference between the two curves. The exact computations of relative survival rates are, however, more complex[47,18]. When interpreting relative survival rates compared to observed survival rates, their meanings will be different although both are expressed in percent form. These rates give the percentage of individuals surviving **from those who would normally survive during the period under study**. Obviously, values under 100% indicate poorer survival than that of the reference population (i.e. subjects in the community in general).

10.3.2.3 *Statistical comparison of surviving groups (rates). Log-rank test*

In another approach, expected survival rates are derived from **within** the study. Observed and expected rates (like observed and expected frequencies) are treated with a chi-square test to see whether the difference between two or more survival curves is likely due to chance (random factors or events) only, or whether observations reflect a systematic difference in survival. One frequently used test is the Mantel–Cox **log-rank test**[48], a modification of the Mantel–Haenszel chi-squared test; it is a nonparametric test based on analysis of orders of outcomes (deaths) as they appear from one moment to another in different groups under comparison. Appropriate detailed computations can be found in Coldman and Elwood's[18] or Young et al's[10] review articles. Good (and health professional friendly) textbooks like those on biostatistics[49] or epidemiology[50] offer essentials of statistical techniques in the domain of prognosis. Again, several statistical packages like SPSS[39] or SAS[40] include such computational programs.

The log-rank test involves counting in each stratum the number of deaths observed in each group (0) and comparing this with the number of expected events (E) that would otherwise occur in each group under the null hypothesis of equivalence in survival in both groups. *p*-values can be estimated by comparing the sum of $(0 - E)^2/E$ with an appropriate chi-square distribution. Readers interested in obtaining more information on this topic should consult the article written by Peto et al[17]. The wide acceptance of the log-rank test is due to its capacity to compare entire survival curves instead of survival rates at selected unique points in time.

10.3.2.4 *Evaluating several causes of survival simultaneously. Cox regression analysis*

As in the 'web of causes' view and subsequent multivariable risk analysis, several prognostic factors and markers determine disease prognosis. When clinicians want to determine how a variety of prognostic characteristics (factors and markers) determine the rate of prognostic events, a multivariable approach is used, most often the **Cox regression analysis**[51,52]. Multiple logistic regression evaluates the effect of several factors on disease risk simultaneously, and for a single point in time. The Cox procedure analyses values for the entire survivorship curve.

Biostatisticians have introduced the concept of 'hazard' with regard to this field. Put simply, *risk is the probability of disease occurrence, in terms of incidence or mortality densities, while 'hazard' is probability in the field of prognosis, usually as a function of mortality, although any outcome other than death can also apply.* More precisely, a hazard function h(t) of survival time T gives the *conditional failure rate*. The hazard function is synonymous in the literature with *instantaneous failure rate, force of mortality, conditional mortality rate,* or *age-specific failure rate*[53]. Hence the Cox survivorship model, also called '**proportional hazards model**', allows the analysis of the role of different factors in determining survivorship. For example, emergency medicine specialists might be interested in the most important prognostic factors and markers of cardiac arrest survival in pre-hospital emergency care: bystander cardio-pulmonary resuscitation (CPR), the initial ECG rhythm, or age of the patient[10]. From these analyses of several prognostic characteristics at once, an individual probability of prognosis (**individual**

'risk' or '**hazard**') for a patient of interest or for the group can be determined, as well as prognostic ratios (**relative** 'risks' or '**hazards**'), while taking into account the contribution of each prognostic characteristic introduced to the model (study).

Applications of multivariable analysis of prognosis and its contributing factors in clinical trials and observational analytical studies abound in the literature. For example, they can be found in such fields as cancer surgery[46,52,54], multiple sclerosis[55], ophthalmology[52,56], cardiosurgery[57], cardiology[58], hepatology[59] or pulmonology[35].

10.3.3 *Predicting a good or bad prognosis*

As already mentioned in Chapter 6, one of the most important aspects of a good diagnosis is its prognostic value. If a diagnosis does not indicate whether a patient will do better or worse than other individuals, appropriate therapeutic decisions cannot be made. Prognostic studies and their results give meaning to diagnostic methods. Matthew et al[60] summarize their critical review of biostatistical methodology in the domain of prognosis as follows:

- Survival analysis should be carried-out by the Kaplan–Meier method;
- Median survival time should be reported;
- Confidence intervals should be provided as measure of variability;
- A log-rank test should be used to compare two or more survival curves;
- Stratified analysis and the Cox model should be used to define the impact of multiple prognostic factors on survival.

This chapter outlines only the principles, meaning and relevance of these recommended methods and techniques.

10.4 Lessons for clinical research from experience gained in prognostic studies

10.4.1 *Prognostic stratification*

Even randomized clinical trials are not absolute indicators of irrefutable results corresponding to clinical reality. Prognostic disparities may appear in a

Table 10.5 An example of prognostic stratification and its effect on results. Lidocaine use and death by ventricular arrhythmia

Overall results before quasi-experimental precautions and prognostic stratification

	Survivors	Fatalities				
			Odds ratio	$CI_{95\%}$	χ^2	p
Lidocaine prophylaxis	55 (36%)	50 (33%)	1.16	0.72–1.88	0.36	> 0.5
No lidocaine prophylaxis	96	101				
Total	151	151				

Results after taking quasi-experimental precautions and prognostic stratification

Patients with a prognostically good infarction
   (Killip class 1)

	Survivors	Fatalities				
			Odds ratio	$CI_{95\%}$	χ^2	p
Lidocaine prophylaxis	18 (25%)	2 (12%)	2.55	0.55–11.89	1.44	> 0.5
No lidocaine prophylaxis	53	15				
Total	71	17				

Patients with a prognostically poor infarction
   (Killip class 2, 3, and 4)

	Survivors	Fatalities				
			Odds ratio	$CI_{95\%}$	χ^2	p
Lidocaine prophylaxis	29 (45%)	3 (17%)	4.03	1.14–14.17	4.65	< 0.05
No lidocaine prophylaxis	36	15				
Total	65	18				

Source: Rewritten and reconstructed from data in Ref. 65

randomized design, at an alpha level of 0.05 in about one out of every 20 randomization schedules[61]. Patients selected for clinical trials are often those who are eligible for randomization, thus excluding (by definition) serious cases where surgical or other radical treatment is mandatory, such as in cancer or coronary artery disease. Treatment effect may work differently in different prognostic subgroups. A prevailing opinion in the literature is the need to partition data from observational etiological research or clinical trials into prognostic subgroups, defined on a sound pathological and clinical basis[62–70]. Such a **prognostic stratification** often contributes to more objective conclusions on treatment effectiveness. Table 10.5 illustrates the usefulness of prognostic stratification as evaluated by Horwitz and Feinstein[65] in the assessment of effectiveness of lidocaine treatment following myocardial infarction. If lidocaine effectiveness to prevent death after infarction were to be evaluated (by a case–control approach) in an overall study, lidocaine would appear ineffective (see the upper portion of Table 10.5). The study's authors made two refined arrangements. First, patients were enrolled in this evaluation only if they were eligible for randomization in a controlled clinical trial (for example, patients who died before routine clinical orders could be made, or patients with a strong indication for lidocaine use were excluded). Second, patients were divided into two distinct prognostic subgroups according to their Killip classification (as quoted in Chapter 6). The lower portion of Table 10.5 illustrates this division. In this example, prognostic stratification shows that the efficacy of lidocaine prophylaxis to control poor outcome (death) after myocardial infarction depends on the clinical severity of cases. Lidocaine is shown to be effective in cases with poorer prognosis (Killip grades 2 to 4). Feinstein suggests stratified or block randomization as a remedy[61,66]. Prognostic subgroups are identified before the trial protocol preparation, and treatments are randomized separately within each prognostic subgroup.

10.4.2 Prognostic migration in time

Often, treatment effectiveness is evaluated on the basis of clinical data collected over a long period of time (one or more decades). This may result in recent cases subjected to a lead-time bias (see section 6.6) particularly if staging (and prognostic classification) of the disease depends on new medical technologies, such as diagnostic methods to detect early stages and spread of cancer. Better and earlier detection of cases may lead to classification of cases into different prognostic categories (stages) depending on their occurrence in time. 'Contemporary' cases, subject to better diagnostic methods and new treatments, may thus bias the study in favor of the new treatments. Feinstein et al[67] called this prognostic or stage migration the '*Will Rogers phenomenon*'. In stage migration, better cases can migrate from a prognostically poorer group into a better one. The American humorist Will Rogers commented on the migration of people from one state to another during the Depression years as an act raising the average intelligence level in all states concerned at once. The same happens in stage migration – one stage suddenly shows a better prognosis, while the other worsens. Hence, it is necessary to classify subjects in prognostic studies by methods that remain unaltered by changes in diagnostic techniques.

10.5 Outcomes research

Outcomes research, as briefly outlined in Chapter 9, focuses not only on short-term effects of medical care but also on its longer-term impact. To do so, outcomes researchers use a variety of methods including observational analytical research, clinical trials, and ultimately prognostic methodology. Outcomes research is not new. Its history covers almost the entire last century since Ernest Codman's interest and initiatives in Boston at the beginning of the twentieth century[71,72]. Outcomes research does not differ substantially from other bedside-oriented clinical research except with respect to focus. Its basic characteristics are:

- From the web of causes of various disease outcomes like premature death, chronicity, handicap, disease complications and spread or uses of care, outcomes research focuses on the potential **impact of medical care**[73,74]. To do this, a '**risk adjustment**' is made in multivariate analyses by controlling for the effects of other relevant possible causes of outcomes like disease severity, comorbidity or sociodemographic characteristics of the patient[75]. The role of medical care is 'extracted' and visualized from other factors of interest.

- A **starting point of analysis** is not necessarily some moment in the natural or clinical course of disease, but rather a moment when some **care is implemented**. For example, in an emergency medical care study of the effectiveness of cardiopulmonary resuscitation[76], patients and pre-hospital and hospital services may be evaluated from their first on-site contact with paramedics or admission at the hospital emergency room. Causes of cardiac arrest and its underlying pathology are studied only as an additional part of the web of causes of a patient's condition and its evolution.

- The **web of outcomes** under study may include classical **clinical** findings such as bringing cardiac rhythm or blood pressure under control and **paraclinical** findings such as acid–base balance, but outcome research focuses particularly on '**patient-centered**' outcomes such as various indicators and indexes of well-being, functioning, independency and other patient-valued issues[77]. Williams et al[78] identify predictors of post-stroke quality of life to illustrate uses of patient-centered outcomes.

- Outcomes researchers are interested in the **evolution in time of medical care and its consequences** by using methodology proper to prognostic studies. However, **periods of follow-up are often shorter**, such as minutes, hours or days in emergency care and services evaluation, not years such as in large-scale health statistics.

- Outcomes analyses using **hazard function methodology** as proposed by Blackstone[79], or **time-to-event methodology** used by Clark and

Ryan[80] to evaluate injury outcomes, belong to the classical field of survival analysis methodology.

- **Health economic evaluation** is an important part of outcomes research. It focuses on **cost minimization** (which equally effective intervention is less expensive), **cost–benefit analysis** (economic trade-offs of competing strategies of care), **cost-effectiveness analysis** (outcome costs of types of care with different effectiveness), and **cost–utility analysis** (cost effectiveness as valued by the patient)[81].
- The **type and quality of care** are variables of interest[82]: service provided, by whom, where and when.
- **Important prognostic factors**, reproducible and accurate, as well as comparable prognostic characteristics of patients[82] will help in the analysis and interpretation of medical care – outcomes studies.

Overall, just as probabilistic research produces probabilities, outcomes research is motivated by a desire for certainty; it rationalizes the health care delivery system[70].

10.6 Clinical prediction rules

Clinical prediction rules (syn. Clinical decision rules) are tools that assist practitioners by estimating the probability either of a diagnostic outcome or of a prognostic outcome[83]. A clinical prediction rule is defined as a '*decision-making tool for clinicians that includes three or more variables obtained from the history, physical examination, or simple diagnostic tests and that either provided the probability of an outcome or suggested a diagnostic or therapeutic course of action*' [84]. Clinical prediction tools belong therefore to both diagnosis and prognosis[85]. For example the Ottawa Ankle Rules[86] is a prediction tool that should help clinicians decide if a patient with an ankle injury evaluated in an emergency department needs ankle X-ray series or not: '*An ankle X-ray series is required only if there is any pain in the malleolar zone and any of these findings:*

1. *Bone tenderness at the posterior edge or tip of the lateral malleolus,*

or

2. *Bone tenderness at the posterior edge or tip of medial malleolus,*

or

3. *Inability to bear weight both immediately and in emergency department*'[85,86].

When such rules are developed, diagnostic properties (validity) of each component and their combinations must be determined. Prospective studies focus on outcomes in these patients with or without diagnostic and therapeutic maneuvers. Statistical analyses determine which predictors should be included in prediction rules. Patients with a high probability of a serious problem and its poor outcome (prognosis) are a priority for special care. Clinical prediction rules are then put into practice to assess their effectiveness and their authors' other expectations. Prognostic studies are a crucial contribution to clinical prediction rules. For example, Silver et al[87] developed a clinical rule to predict preserved left ventricular ejection fraction in patients after myocardial infarction. First, prognostic studies must demonstrate that left ventricular function is an important prognostic factor with specific therapeutic implications. Then, clinical prediction rules showing patients with preserved left ventricular systolic function allow clinicians to focus on those patients who need special care. Clinical prediction rules may be presented in terms of scores or as algorithms. Clinical prediction rules are not, however, exclusively based on variables that are possible causal factors of good or bad prognosis. Prognostic markers may also be relevant.

10.7 Prognostic studies as subject of systematic reviews

The field of research on prognosis also requires systematic reviewing and research integration. The methodological heterogeneity of studies of prognosis, as well as the heterogeneity of their results, is also of interest. For example, meta-analysis, or a systematic review of the methodology of prognostic studies, was attempted by Marx and Marx[88] in the area of idiopathic membranous nephropathy. Meta-analyses of outcomes in prognostic studies as reported in observational analytical research or clinical trials represent a considerable methodological challenge[89]. Chapter 11 is devoted to this topic in literature reviewing and integration.

10.8   How to construct a study on prognosis

Prognostic studies do not differ from other studies in terms of general criteria for clinical research as detailed in previous chapters. If a descriptive study of prognosis is under consideration, clinimetric rigor (operational criteria), representativity (disease, target population, exposure to prognostic factors, clinical practices, etc.), validity of follow-up (diagnostic) methods, etc. are equally applicable. If an etiological (analytical) observational study is of interest, a step-by-step evaluation of the quality and completeness of all its phases and steps (see Figures 4.2 and 9.1) is mandatory. If the prognostic study is experimental, i.e. a clinical trial requiring evaluation of treatment impact in the long term, the following applies: the selection of a randomized or non-randomized design with parallel, internal or external, or historical groups. The prognostic study is performed and analyzed and its results interpreted according to the requirements reviewed in Chapter 9. In addition to these common criteria, specific criteria and precautions apply to prognostic studies.

10.8.1   *A priori precautions, components, and criteria proper to prognostic studies*

The length and other inherent characteristics of prognostic studies require particular attention with regard to the following:

1. As in any other study, the **objectives, hypothesis, research question, and practical expectations** are well formulated in advance[90]. Clearly formulated questions are *conditio sine qua non* (necessary condition).
2. Both **independent variables** (possible prognostic factors) and **dependent variables** (outcomes of interest) are well defined according to clear inclusion and exclusion criteria. The choice of relevant dependent and independent variables is becoming more and more relevant for clinical decision-making. For example, surgeons were recently evaluated as a prognostic factor of colorectal cancer[91]. Another example may be studies focusing on comorbidity as a prognostic factor[92].
3. Comparability of patients at the beginning of the study is necessary. A **zero time** or **inception moment,** i.e. the moment of a patient's entry into the prognostic follow-up, requires particular attention as it must correspond to a precise moment in the natural or clinical course of disease. For example, according to Tugwell et al[68], a study of the prognosis of myocardial infarction would yield unrealistic results if it were based on emergency cases only, i.e. on patients 'who made it to the hospital' (the worst cases often die before reaching the hospital). Incomplete cohorts should be avoided, or complementary corrective measures should be considered.
4. The **inception cohort** consists of persons **initially free of the outcome** of interest[93,94].
5. The **inception cohort** assembles individuals **at a uniform point of disease development**[95].
6. The **follow-up of a cohort should not be biased** by accessibility to medical services, and consequently equal maneuvers (treatments) and follow-up must be available.
7. **Enough time** (duration of the study) must be allowed to cover whatever may happen during the disease course. If metastases of cancer can occur during the five years after surgical removal of the primary lesion, the prognostic study of the cancer's metastatic spread must cover at least five years.
8. One of the greatest challenges of prognostic studies is to ensure the **stability of patients participating**. At least 80% of enrolled patients must participate until a major study end point occurs or the study ends[93–95]. Corrective measures for dropouts must be foreseen in advance and incorporated into the study design. **Statistical considerations** of sample size must be adapted to prognostic studies as suggested in the *ad hoc* literature[69,70,96].

NB   Statistical note. A clinician wanting to study prognosis and its causes (by doing an analytical study) must first determine how many patients are needed. The statistician may ask the following questions[69,70], and the clinician must be prepared to give the most accurate answers possible:

1. *What alpha error would be acceptable?*
2. *What power of the study (1-beta error) is desirable?*

3. *What is the median survival rate of the control group?*

4. *What accrual rate may be expected in the study (e.g. how many patients per month will come to a clinician's attention and enter the study)?*

5. *How many prognostic events of interest (called 'failures', such as deaths, in terms of rates) may be expected in the control group?*

6. *What ratio of failure rates in the experimental and control group may be expected in the study?*

Such estimations should be as close as possible to clinical reality, allowing for the determination of an equally realistic sample size. They represent the basic elements or 'clinical ingredients' necessary for a proper computation of the number of patients needed, i.e. the size of the study of prognosis. Also, similar information may be found by any reader in an article on prognosis, i.e. what considerations, for example, led the authors to study 200 patients instead of 50, and how valid their study might be from a biostatistical point of view.

9. It is necessary to maintain a uniform use and respect of **well-defined criteria of prognostic variables and their impact (outcomes)** over a considerable period of time especially with regard to soft data. Soft data (psychiatry) and/or harder data, such as physiological variables (like blood cell count, neurologic deficit, arterial oxygen tension, hematocrit, or serum albumin level in the recent prognostic staging of AIDS[97]) are used more and more often as prognostic variables. The occurrence of 'non-specific' signs or symptoms is hardly acceptable.

10. The **quality control of data** production during a long-term study is mandatory.

11. Whenever relevant, studies of prognosis must be performed using the proper degree of **blinding**, as with any other kind of clinical trial or etiological observational study (see Chapters 8 and 9).

12. **Confounding** the role of a particular prognostic factor with other possible prognosis determining ('confounding') factors should be avoided, preferably *a priori* by careful biological formulations of the problem and interactions under study. This should eventually be reviewed by more sophisti-

cated multivariate statistical methods of analysis once the study is completed.

13. **Causal associations** between prognostic factors and disease outcomes must be submitted to a criteria analysis similar to the etiological evaluation of causal association in the field of risk: assessment of individual or group prognosis; evaluation of contrasts between groups; assessment of impact; and evaluation of imputability of outcomes to the prognostic variables under study.

14. **Conclusions** regarding a good or bad prognosis should not be generalized without specifying the kind of prognosis being dealt with (see Section 10.1.3).

General and specific precautions for prognostic studies can be translated into a 'how to' proposal for a good prognostic study, as detailed in Table 10.6.

10.8.2 A posteriori evaluation. Was the study good?

10.8.2.1 General acceptability of the study of prognosis

The assessment of a prognostic study[98] follows the same logical path and components as mentioned above. Infante-Rivard et al[99] have suggested criteria to evaluate and conduct prognostic studies and outlined four important components: design; usefulness; validity and precision of information; statistical analysis. These should be determined when reading articles on prognosis. The quoted study[99] also shows, through an example of liver cirrhosis prognosis, that all these criteria are not entirely respected from one prognostic study to another.

10.8.2.2 Applicability of a prognostic study to the individual patient

General applicability of research evidence to individual patients[100] and its integration with care[101] is equally valid in the domain of prognosis. The applicability of a prognostic study to an individual patient under a physician's care falls under the criteria outlined in Section 4.2.3 of this text. It may be summarized in just a few questions: **Would my patient be eligible for a study of prognosis whose results should**

Table 10.6   Recommendations for clinicians interested in running a study of prognosis

1. Acquire the best and most complete **information** possible on the natural and clinical course of the disease under study. This information must be clinimetrically explicit, such as: frequency, sequence, and chronology of events (clinical spectrum) and its evolution (progress) or data on disease auxometry (evolution of clinical gradient).

2. Know as much as possible on clinical **maneuvers and exposures** to other prognostic factors relevant to the problem under study.

3. Define and evaluate all relevant associated troubles (**comorbidity**) and **cotreatments** which might affect (in addition to the treatment of interest) the disease course and outcome(s), i.e. 'extraneous prognostic factors'.

4. Specify the **reason** (scientific, practical) for the study. Justify the endeavor.

5. State the principal **research question** and other relevant (additional and/or alternative) questions to be scrutinized in the study.

6. Define the problem in terms of **dependent** (point 1) **and independent variables** (point 2) to evaluate. Does the study focus on prognostic factors or markers?

7. Choose the type and **category of prognostic study** (descriptive, etiological, or clinical trial) and the type(s) of interaction (category(ies) of Table 10.4).

8. Assess whether the proposed study will fulfill the **criteria of a good study** on prognosis.

9. Fix the **zero time** (inception moment) for disease follow-up, and the **initial state** of patients.

10. Specify how patients will be **enrolled** in the study. Compare with the referral pattern in routine hospital practice at the end of the study to specify to whom the results will apply.

11. Define **outcome (endpoints)** of interest. Allow for a long enough period of follow-up to cover a 'complete' time interval during which prognostic phenomena may occur.

12. Anticipate what can be an **expected effect** (prognosis) in the study in quantitative terms.

13. Define the **sample size**.

14. Create **documents** for the study (data sheets, coding, procedures, descriptions, etc.).

15. Prepare a plan for the **statistical analysis** of results (description and comparison of survival curves, etc.).

16. Control the quality and stability of **data production** (collection, follow-up), such as blinding, compliance, drop-outs, non-responses, replacements, filling out data sheets, their transfer into a computerized data bank, etc.

17. Correct and complete any **error or omission** occurring during data acquisition if possible.

18. Perform biostatistical, epidemiological, and clinical **analysis and assessment of results**.

19. **Interpret results** and give their relevance from all three standpoints (biostatistical, epidemiological and clinical).

20. Supply **answers to questions** raised at the onset (point 5); specify what was not answered and why.

21. **Draw conclusions** as to the applicability of the results of the study – disease, patients, community, medical practices.

22. Critically **assess the study**, its strengths, weaknesses, objectivity, etc.

23. Give **recommendations** for decisions to be made in clinical practice and for further research.

24. **Anticipate** that the above-mentioned points will be scrutinized by those to whom the study is addressed (medical journal reviewers first, then readers).

apply to him or her? Would my patient finish such a study? And, would my patient finish in the 'winning group', i.e. those ending with a good prognosis? Needless to say, the third question is more difficult to answer than the first two. Neither socio-demographic comparability nor clinical and paraclinical characteristics of the disease in the patient are adequate. The clinician must also ensure that the clinical setting and care, its accessibility and coverage, as well as human and material resources needed for such a care, are compatible. In other terms, **does the patient evolve in a similar environment of care** (primary care, hospital, long-term care, social services, living conditions)?

10.9 Conclusions. Considerations for further work in the area of prognosis

Despite the considerable development of a conceptual and methodological basis of prognosis, this field remains 'young'. Thousands of survival and other prognostic studies have taken place, but once published, their results are still less often used in practice than information obtained from the areas of diagnosis and treatment. However, prognostic information that goes beyond educated guesswork is necessary for patient counseling. Moreover, it is crucial when deciding what problem is worthy of prevention (secondary and tertiary prevention in particular).

Table 10.7   A review of prerequisites and information necessary for decision-making regarding preventive measures

Primary prevention
- Risk factors (causes) are known and quantified.
- Data on risk are available (or will be) before ('baseline' data) and after (impact data) a prevention program. Information on both numerators and denominators of rates are necessary.
- Natural history of the disease to prevent is known.
- An effective intervention (prevention modality) is available.
- Meta-analysis* confirms that the program under consideration is effective.
- Decision analysis** indicates that the program under consideration is a priority among others (competing programs, other diseases to prevent).

Secondary prevention
- **Same as for primary prevention, plus**:
- Risk markers are known.
- Prognostic markers are known.
- Prognostic factors are known.
- Natural history of the disease under consideration is known.
- Clinical course of the disease is known.
- An effective outcome modifying intervention modality is available and known.
- Baseline clinical data are available.
- Outcome data will be available.
- Meta-analysis* confirms that the program under consideration is effective.
- Decision analysis** indicates that this secondary prevention program and this disease is a preferred option among other major alternative choices.

Tertiary prevention
- **Same as for secondary prevention, plus**:
- Disease auxometry (measured evolution of disease gradient and spectrum) is known and its methods of follow-up are available for the program.
- Meta-analysis* confirms that the program under consideration is effective.
- Decision analysis** indicates that tertiary prevention programs for this disease are preferred choices among other treatment modalities and other diseases to control at this level.

* Meta-analysis is discussed in Chapter 11; ** Decision analysis is discussed in Chapter 13.

Table 10.7 summarizes the necessary factual information for decision-making regarding preventive measures. It can be noted that in secondary and tertiary prevention, more attention is paid to risk markers and prognostic factors. Such a consideration is necessary for the identification of individuals and groups in which a high occurrence of problems worthy of intervention can be expected.

Prognostic scoring systems are now increasingly the subject of pragmatic evaluation. Hussain et al's[102] study of such systems in the field of gastrointestinal bleeding is an excellent example of such initiatives. It is still necessary to know if the structured approach to prognosis (called 'actuarial judgement'[103]) or the clinical approach supports the preference of actuarial judgment based on experience in psychiatry and medicine. The prognostic performance of physicians may vary considerably from one physician to another and adversely affect care in emergency situations and in critical care. In cardiology, inter-physician variability may be substantial. In coronary artery disease, statistical predictions based, for example, on the Cox model explained in this chapter, can provide better predictions than the 'expert' clinical judgment of individual cardiologists[104]. Such conclusions, however, come from the rather fragmented experience and bibliography represented here by pinpoint studies of isolated topics, rather than from a systematic evaluation of prognostic activities from one medical specialty to another. The following perspective may emerge from the field of prognosis as described in this chapter:

- A more structured approach to prognosis in terms of its causes, outcomes and types of associations (categories of prognosis).
- Separation, in research and practice, of risk factors and markers from prognostic factors and markers.
- It should be better known if differences in causes of individual cases and causes of disease incidence, as stressed by Rose[105,106] in the field of risk and

Table 10.8 Epidemiological prerequisites for setting priorities in health programs

Priority	= *Occurrence* ×	*Clinical importance* ×	*Controllability (in proportional terms)*	*Operational considerations* × *of health programs (target population)*
Level of prevention				
Primary (control of disease incidence)	Incidence	Disease severity (case fatality rate, severity score, etc.)	Etiological (attributable) fraction of risk	General population proportion reached by the disease prevention program
Secondary (control of disease prevalence by controlling the duration of cases)	Prevalence	Disease severity (case fatality rate, severity score, etc.)	Etiological (attributable) fraction of prognosis (survival, or duration of disease)*	Group of patients reached by the health care program
Tertiary (control of disease spectrum and/or gradient without affecting its duration)	Clinical events	Disease severity (case fatality rate, severity score, etc.)	Etiological (attributable) fraction of prognosis (outcomes occurrence timing and duration in terms of disease spectrum and/or gradient)**	Group of patients reached by the health care program

All components may be considered in terms of absolute frequencies, rates, or proportional rates, depending on the view of importance.
* From observational analytical studies, more desirable from clinical and community trials; ** Mainly from clinical trials.

primary prevention, should be considered for the field of prognosis. If such a distinction also exists in the field of prognosis, what are its implications for use in clinical decisions?

- The reality of life today is that medical practice in a given social and health care system leads, according to Pochin, to a certain 'acceptance of risk'[107]. What this means in terms of 'acceptance of prognosis' remains to be better understood.

In summary, when setting priorities for primary, secondary and tertiary prevention, the lessons of disease etiology (Chapter 8), controllability and course control (Chapter 9) should be taken into account. Table 10.8 summarizes the epidemiological pre-requisites for setting priorities in health programs. At this point, it would be misleading to confound etiological fractions from the field of risk with those from the field of prognosis. An additional challenge remains the choice of expression of clinical importance of disease competing for priority in the decision process.

Returning to this chapter's introductory example, the attending physician advising a patient to get a hysterectomy should, on the basis of the above-mentioned considerations, give the patient the second half of the answer: 'You will be fine, **because**. . . In other words, the physician is telling the patient that specific prognostic data from description, research of causes and clinical trials or other types of outcomes research speak in her favor (her situation being similar to other patients in these studies). The physician can conclude by telling her: 'But, given your specific characteristics, here is how sure you can be . . .'.

REFERENCES

1. Adams F (ed.). *The Genuine Works of Hippocrates*. Birmingham, AL: Classics of Medicine Library, 1985
2. Wiesemann C. The significance of prognosis for a theory of medical practice. *Theor Med Bioethics*, 1998;b:253–61
3. *Dorland's Illustrated Medical Dictionary*. 27th Edition. Philadelphia: WB Saunders, 1988
4. Fries JF, Ehrlich GE (eds). *Prognosis. Contemporary Outcomes of Disease*. Bowie, MD: The Charles Press, 1981
5. Armitage P, Gehan EA. Statistical methods for the identification and use of prognostic factors. *Int J Cancer*, 1974;**13**:16–36
6. Peto R, Pike MC, Armitage P, et al. Design and analysis of randomized clinical trials requiring prolonged observation of each patient. II. Analysis and examples. *Br J Cancer*, 1977;**35**:1–39
7. Rose G, Barker DJP. Prognosis and outcome. *Br Med J*, 1978;**2**:1355–6
8. Chastang CL, Auquier A. Prognostic et décision médicale (Prognosis and medical decision). *Rev Prat*, 1983;**33**:1067–83
9. Jenicek M. Risque et pronostic en décision médicale préventive et thérapeutique (Risk and prognosis in preventive and therapeutic decisions in medicine). *Un Méd Canada*, 1986;**115**:451–6, 462
10. Young KD, Menegazzi JJ, Lewis RJ. Statistical methodology: IX. Survival analysis. *Acad Emerg Med*, 1999;**6**:244–9
11. Prognosis. In: Fletcher RH, Fletcher SW, Wagner EH. *Clinical Epidemiology. The Essentials*. Baltimore and London: Williams & Wilkins, 1982: 106–28
12. Pronostic (Prognosis). In: Jenicek M, Cléroux R. *Epidémiologie clinique. Clinimétrie (Clinical Epidemiology. Clinimetrics)*. St. Hyacinthe et Paris: EDISEM et Maloine, 1985:167–90
13. Sackett DL, Haynes RB, Guyatt GH, Tugwell P. *Clinical Epidemiology. A Basic Science for Clinical Medicine*. 2nd Edition. Boston: Little, Brown, 1991
14. Life table (survival) analysis. In: Kramer MS. *Clinical Epidemiology and Biostatistics. A Primer for Clinical Investigators and Decision-Makers*. Berlin: Springer Verlag, 1988:236–53
15. Prognosis. Studies of disease course and outcomes. In: Jenicek M. *Epidemiology. The Logic of Modern Medicine*. Montreal: EPIMED International, 1995; 8:241–65
16. Irwin AC. Survivorship: The estimation and interpretation of survival experience. *Can Med Assoc J*, 1971;**105**:489–7
17. Fleiss JL, Dunner DL, Fieve RR. The life table: A method for analyzing longitudinal studies. *Arch Gen Psychiatry*, 1976;**33**:107–12
18. Coldman AJ, Elwood MJ. Examining survival data. *Can Med Assoc J*, 1979;**121**:1065–71
19. Gore SM. Statistics in question. Assessing methods – survival. *Br Med J*, 1981;**283**:840–3
20. Grundy PF. A rational approach to the 'at risk' concept. *Lancet*, 1973;**1**:1489
21. Anon. Risk Factors – A Misleading Concept. *J Soc Commun Med*, 1983;**97**:(title page)

22. Andrén-Sandberg A, Ihse I. Factors influencing survival after total pancreatectomy in patients with pancreatic cancer. *Ann Surg*, 1983;**198**:605–10

23. Friesinger GC. Angina pectoris. In: Fries JF, Ehrlich GE eds. *Prognosis. Contemporary Outcomes of Disease*. Bowie, MD: The Charles Press, 1981: 268–74

24. Allgulander C, Fisher LD. Survival analysis (or time to an event analysis), and the Cox regression methods for longitudinal psychiatric research. *Acta Psychiatr Scand*, 1986;**74**:529–35

25. Anderson JR, Crowley JJ, Propert KJ. Interpretation of survival data in clinical trials. *Oncology* (Huntingt.), 1991;**5**:113–4

26. Korn EL, Graubard BI, Midthune D. Time-to-event analysis of longitudinal follow-up of a survey: Choice of time-scale. *Am J Epidemiol*, 1997;**145**: 72–80

27. Cristaldi M, Sampietro GM, Danelli P, et al. Long-term results and multivariate analysis of prognostic factors in 138 consecutive patients operated on for Crohn's disease using 'Bowel-sparing' techniques. *Am J Surg*, 2000;**179**:266–70

28. Allen C, Jiang K, Malbecq W, Goadsby PJ. Time-to-event analysis, or who gets better sooner? An emerging concept in headache study methodology. *Cephalgia*, 1999;**19**:552–6

29. Balfour HH, Bean B, Laskin OL, et al., Burroughs Wellcome Collaborative Acyclovir Study Group. Acyclovir halts progression of herpes zoster in immunocompromised patients. *N Engl J Med*, 1983; **308**:1448–53

30. Froehling DA, Silverstein MD, Mohr DN, et al. Benign positional vertigo: Incidence and prognosis in a population-study in Olmsted County, Minnesota. *Mayo Clin Proc*, 1991;**66**:596–601

31. Jones PK, Ratnoff OD. The changing prognosis of classic hemophilia (factor VIII 'deficiency'). *Ann Inter Med*, 1991;**114**:641–8

32. McElwee NE, Veltri JC, Bradford DC, Rollins DE. A prospective, population-based study of acute ibuprofen overdose: Complications are rare and routine serum levels not warranted. *Ann Emerg Med*, 1990;**19**:657–62

33. Westling B, Norrving B, Thorngren M. Survival following stroke. A prospective population-based study of 438 hospitalized cases with prediction according to subtype, severity and age. *Acta Neurol Scand*, 1990;**81**:457–63

34. Eiseman B. *What Are My Chances?* Philadelphia: WB Saunders, 1980

35. Infante-Rivard C. Armstrong B, Ernst P, et al. Descriptive study of prognostic factors influencing survival of compensated silicotic patients. *Am Rev Respir Dis*, 1991;**144**:1070–4

36. Patronas NJ, Di Chiro G, Kufta C, et al. Prediction of survival in glioma patients by means of positron emission tomography. *J Neurosurg*, 1985; **62**:816–22

37. Last JM, for the International Epidemiological Association. *A Dictionary of Epidemiology*. 2nd Edition. New York: Oxford University Press, 1988 (see also 4th Edition, 2001)

38. Ellenberg SS, Hamilton JM. Surrogate endpoints in clinical trials: *Cancer*. Stat Med, 1989;**8**:405–13

39. SPSS Inc. *SPSS for Windows*. Version 11.0.1. Chicago: SPSS Inc., 2002

40. SAS® Institute. *SAS® System*. Version 8.2. Cary, NC: SAS® Institute Inc., 2000

41. Kaplan EL, Meier P. Nonparametric estimation from incomplete observations. *J Am Stat Ass*, 1958;**53**: 457–81

42. Cutler SJ, Ederer F. Maximum utilization of the life table method in analyzing survival. *J Chronic Dis*, 1958;**8**:699–712

43. Fleiss JL, Dunner DL, Stallone F, Fieve RR. The life table. A method for analysing longitudinal studies. *Arch Gen Psychiatry*, 1976;**33**:107–12

44. Hall WJ, Wellner JA. Confidence bands for a survival curve from censored data. *Biometrika*, 1980; **67**:133–43

45. Simon R. Confidence intervals for reporting results in clinical trials. *Ann Intern Med*, 1986;**105**:429–35

46. Jass JR, Love SB, Northover JMA. A new prognostic classification of rectal cancer. *Lancet*, 1987;**1**: 1303–7

47. Ederer F, Axtell LM, Cutler SJ. The relative survival rate: a statistical methodology. *Natl Cancer Inst Monogr*, 1961;**6**:101–21

48. Mantel N. Evaluation of survival data and two new rank order statistics arising in its consideration. *Canc Chemother Rep*, 1966;**50**:163–70

49. Norman GR, Streiner DL. *Biostatistics. The Bare Essentials*. 2nd Edition. Hamilton and London: BC Decker Inc., 2000

50. Gordis L. *Epidemiology*. 2nd Edition. Philadelphia: WB Saunders Co., 2000

51. Cox DR. Regression models and life-tables. *J R Stat Soc*, 1972;**B34**:187–202

52. Seigel DG. Cox regression analysis in clinical research. *Arch Ophthalmol*, 1990;**108**:888–9

53. Lee ET. Statistical Methods for Survival Data Analysis. New York: John Wiley & Sons, Inc., 1992

54. Wiggers T, Arends JW, Schutte B, et al. A multivariate analysis of pathologic prognostic indicators in large bowel cancer. *Cancer*, 1988;**61**: 386–95

55. Riise T, Gronning M, Aarli JA, et al. Prognostic factors for life expectancy in multiple sclerosis analysed by Cox-models. *J Clin Epidemiol*, 1988;**41**: 1031–6

56. Gass JDM. Comparison of prognosis after enucleation vs cobalt 60 irradiation of melanomas. *Arch Ophthalmol*, 1985;**103**:916–23

57. Schaff HV, Gersh BJ, Pluth JR, et al. Survival and functional status after coronary artery bypass grafting: Results 10 to 12 years after surgery in 500 patients. *Circulation*, 1983;**68**(Suppl II):11/200–11/204

58. Case RB, Heller SS, Case NB, Moss AJ, and the Multicenter Post-infarction Research Group. Type A behavior and survival after myocardial infarction. *N Engl J Med*, 1985;**312**:737–41

59. Infante-Rivard C, Esnaola S, Villeneuve J-P. Clinical and statistical validity of conventional prognostic factors in predicting short-term survival among cirrhotics. *Hepatology*, 1987;**7**:660–4

60. Matthew A, Pandey M, Murthy NS. Survival analysis: caveats and pitfalls. *Eur J Surg Oncol*, 1999;**25**:321–9

61. Feinstein AR, Landis RJ. The role of prognostic stratification in preventing the bias permitted by random allocation of treatment. *J Chronic Dis*, 1976;**29**:277–84

62. Gehan EA, Smith TL, Buzdar AU. Use of prognostic factors in analysis of historical control studies. *Canc Treat Rep*, 1980;**64**:373–9

63. Simon R. Patient heterogeneity in clinical trials. *Canc Treat Rep*, 1980;**64**:405–10

64. Sather HN. The use of prognostic factors in clinical trials. *Cancer*, 1986;**58**:461–7

65. Horwitz RI, Feinstein AR. Improved observational method for studying therapeutic efficacy. Suggestive evidence that lidocaine prophylaxis prevents death in acute myocardial infarction. *JAMA*, 1981;**246**:2455–9

66. Feinstein AR. An additional basic science for clinical medicine: III. The challenges of comparison and measurement. *Ann Intern Med*, 1983;**99**:705–12

67. Feinstein AR, Sosin DM, Wells CK. The Will Rogers phenomenon. Stage migration and new diagnostic techniques as a source of misleading statistics for survival in cancer. *N Engl J Med*, 1985;**312**:1604–8

68. Department of Clinical Epidemiology and Biostatistics. McMaster University Health Sciences Centre (P.X. Tugwell). How to read clinical journals: III. To learn the clinical course and prognosis of disease. *Can Med Assoc J*, 1981;**124**:869–72

69. Lachin JM, Foulkes MA. Evaluation of samples size and power for analyses of survival with allowance for non-uniform patient entry, losses to follow-up, non-compliance, and stratification. *Biometrics*, 1986;**42**:507–19

70. Dixon DO, Simon R. Sample size considerations for studies comparing survival curves using historical controls. *J Clin Epidemiol*, 1988;**41**:1209–13

71. Kaska SC. Ernest Amory Codman, 1869–1940. A pioneer of Evidence-Based Medicine: The end result idea. *Spine*, 1999;**23**:629–33

72. Tanenbaum SJ. Evidence and expertise: The challenge of the outcomes movement to medical professionalism. *Acad Med*, 1999;**74**:757–63

73. Wright JG. Outcomes research: What to measure. *World J Surg*, 1999;**23**:1224–6

74. Brenneman FD, Wright JG, Kennedy ED, McLeod RS. Outcomes research in surgery. *World J Surg*, 1999;**23**:1220–3

75. Kane RL (ed.). *Understanding Health Care Outcomes Research*. Gainsburg, MD: Aspen Publishers Inc., 1997

76. Spaite DW, Maio R, Garrison HG, et al. Emergency Medical Services Outcomes Project (EMSOP) II: Developing the foundation and conceptual models for out-of-hospital outcomes research. *Ann Emerg Med*, 2001;**37**:657–63

77. Lorenz W, Troidl H, Solomkin JS, et al. Second step: Testing outcome measurements. *World J Surg*, 1999;**23**:768–80

78. Williams LS, Weinberger M, Harris LE, Biller J. Measuring quality of life in a way that is meaningful to stroke patients. *Neurology*, 1999;**53**:1839–43

79. Blackstone EH. Outcome analysis using hazard function methodology. *Ann Thorac Surg*, 1996;**61**:52–7

80. Clark DE, Ryan LM. Modeling injury outcomes using time-to-events methods. *J Trauma Inj Inf Crit Care*, 1997;**42**:1129–34

81. Epstein RS, Sherwood LM. From outcomes research to disease management: A guide for the perplexed. *Ann Intern Med*, 1996;**124**:832–7

82. Naylor CD, Guyatt GH for the Evidence-Based Medicine Working Group. Users' guides to the medical literature. X. How to use an article reporting variations in the outcomes of health services. *JAMA*, 1996;**275**:554–8

83. Wasson JH, Sox HC, Neff RK, Goldman L. Clinical prediction rules. Applications and methodological standards. *N Engl J Med*, 1985;**313**:793–9

84. Laupacis A, Sekar N, Stiell IG. Clinical prediction rules. A review and suggested modifications of methodological standards. *JAMA*, 1997;**277**:488–94

85. McGinn TG, Guyatt GH, Wyer PC, et al. Users' guides to the medical literature. XXII. How to use articles about clinical decision rules. *JAMA*, 2000;**284**:79–84

86. Stiell IG, Greenberg GH, McKnight RD, et al. Decision rules for the use of radiography in acute ankle injuries; refinement and prospective validation. *JAMA*, 1993;**269**:1127–32

87. Silver MT, Rose GA, Paul SD, et al. A clinical rule to predict preserved left ventricular ejection fraction in patients after myocardial infarction. *Ann Intern Med*, 1994;**121**:750–6

88. Marx BE, Marx M. Prognosis of idiopathic membranous nephropathy: A methodologic meta-analysis. *Kidney International*, 1997;**51**:873–9

89. Simon R, Altman DG. Statistical aspects of prognostic factor studies in oncology. *Br J Cancer*, 1994;**69**: 979–85

90. Hall PA, Going JJ. Predicting the future: a critical appraisal of cancer prognosis studies. *Histopathology*, 1999;**35**:489–94

91. Maegher AP. Colorectal cancer: is the surgeon a prognostic factor? A systematic review. *MJA*, 1999; **171**:308–10

92. Gijsen R, Hoeymans N, Schellevis FG, et al. Causes and consequences of comorbidity: A review. *J Clin Epidemiol*, 2001;**54**:661–74

93. Anon. Purpose and procedure. *Evidence-Based Medicine*, 2001;**6**:66

94. Anon. Purpose and procedure. *ACP Journal Club*, 1999;(July/August):A15– A16

95. Anon. Purpose and procedure. *EBM Mental Health*, 2001;**4**:34–5

96. Cantor AB. Sample size calculations for the log rank test: A Gompertz model approach. *J Clin Epidemiol*, 1992;**45**:1131–6

97. Justice AC, Feinstein AR, Wells CK. A new prognostic staging system for the acquired immunodeficiency syndrome. *N Engl J Med*, 1989;**320**:1388–93

98. Laupacis A, Wells G, Richardson WS, Tugwell P for the Evidence-based Medicine Working Group. Users' guides to the medical literature. V. How to use an article about prognosis. *JAMA*, 1994;**272**:234–7

99. Infante-Rivard C, Villeneuve J-P, Esnaola S. A framework for evaluating and conducting prognostic studies: An application to cirrhosis of the liver. *J Clin Epidemiol*, 1989;**42**:791–805

100. Guyatt GH, Haynes RB, Jaeschke RZ, et al. for the Evidence-Based Medicine Working Group. Users' guides to the medical literature. XXV. Evidence-Based Medicine: Principles for applying the users' guides to patient care. *JAMA*, 2000;**284**:1290–6

101. McAlister FA, Straus SE, Guyatt GH, Haynes RB for the Evidence-Based Medicine Working Group. Users' guides to the medical literature. XX. Integrating research evidence with the care of the individual patient. *JAMA*, 2000;**283**:2829–36

102. Hussain H, Lapin S, Cappell MS. Clinical scoring systems for determining the prognosis of gastrointestinal bleeding. *Gastroenterol Clin North Amer*, 2000;**29** (June, No 2):445–64

103. Dawes RM, Faust D, Meehl PE. Clinical versus actuarial judgement. *Science*, 1989;**243**:1668–74

104. Lee KL, Pryor DB, Harrell FE Jr, et al. Predicting outcome in coronary disease. Statistical models versus expert clinicians. *Am J Med*, 1986;**80**:553–60

105. Rose G. Sick individuals and sick populations. *Int J Epidemiol*, 1985;**14**:32–8

106. Rose G. *The Strategy of Preventive Medicine*. Oxford: Oxford University Press, 1992

107. Pochin EE. The acceptance of risk. *Br Med Bull*, 1975;**31**:184–90

Putting Experiences Together
and Making Decisions in Medicine

Structured uses of evidence

Analyzing and integrating a body of knowledge. Systematic reviews and meta-analysis of evidence

. . . it became requisite to exhibit a full and impartial view of what had hitherto been published on the scurvy, and that in a chronological order, by which the sources of these mistakes may be detected.
James Lind, *A Treatise of the Scurvy, 1753*

Systematic reviews of evidence should not bestow the confidence to perpetrate other people's mistakes. Rather, they should encourage the search for new, better and richer evidence.

Moreover:
- *The evidence you have is not always what you want.*
- *The evidence you want is not always what you need.*
- *The evidence you need is not always what you can obtain.*
Paraphrasing Fenagle (1977)[1]

A single, even epidemiologically impeccable study, does not always answer all of the important questions in a particular area of medical work. Does jogging do more harm than good? Is diethylstilbestrol a predominant cause of clear cell vaginal carcinoma? Do beta-blockers prevent death after myocardial infarction? Is the BCG vaccine equally effective around the world? Chapter 8 stresses consistency of findings as one of the criteria of causality. Systematic reviews of evidence are meant to uncover whether findings about a health problem are consistent across the body of available original studies and valid information in the literature. Readers of medical journals quickly realize how complicated and diversified information becomes. Original studies multiply fast and exponentially, especially in such crucial fields as cardiovascular disease and cancer, among others. These studies, as comprehensive as they may be, do not give homogeneous results across often enormous bodies of accumulated knowledge on a single subject. These studies are followed by 'review articles', 'position papers', 'consensus on . . .' with recommendations to practitioners as to what and how to diagnose, what treatment to choose, etc. To accept or refute such recommendations and translate them into office decisions or further research is crucial for patient well being, for institutional budgets, and for good medicine and/or research. By analyzing and summarizing bodies of evidence, clinicians seek new and better premises and conclusions for logical arguments, supported by the best available evidence. Consider what can happen while treating a patient:

Clinical practice:	Logical discourse:	Evidence:
'. . . Doctor, you are worried about my high cholesterol. You have told me that I am not eating well. . . .'	There are a considerable number of original studies establishing links between what you eat and serum cholesterol. **(Premise A)**	**Systematic review** of a body of evidence on the effect of diet on blood cholesterol levels.
'. . . I have heard that eating a lot of garlic might help, in addition to your treatment plan. . . .'	Yes, I have read several studies which concluded that adding more garlic to the diet helps to lower serum cholesterol levels, but some were not too convincing. **(Premise B)**	**Systematic review** of evidence that garlic supplements in the diet lower blood cholesterol levels.
'. . . You can try adding a clove of garlic to your daily diet. It will help. . . .'	Eating garlic reduces total serum cholesterol levels by about 9% in patients studied. This also applies to my patient and it should work. **(Conclusion C)**	The evidence from **systematic reviews** and its **applicability** to this patient justifies its trial.

However, if the patient asks whether garlic will reduce the risk of myocardial infarction, blood cholesterol must be considered as a surrogate point in this discussion and further evidence focusing on garlic's preventive role in myocardial infarction should be assessed. Concluding that 'garlic reduces the risk of myocardial infarction' (Conclusion C) is justified only if the relation between the surrogate point and the outcome of primary clinical interest, i.e. not having a heart attack, is as clearly understood as possible in this situation. Additional evidence in this sense would be mandatory. Otherwise, such a resolution of a logical discourse should be refuted. In this fictitious discussion, ignoring evidence would lead the physician to make recommendations based solely on hearsay, faith and goodwill. This is what distinguishes health professionals from charlatans, well-intentioned lay persons and health gurus. Is there a more reliable clinical argumentation than the opinion of a respected medical professional, coming from an equally respectable institution and published in a reputable medical journal? This question was first tackled by authors in the fields of psychology and education. They were the first to develop a structured and systematic way of analyzing and synthesizing independent studies on the same topic. This method should allow the best possible conclusions to be reached by reflecting reality across the different studies under consideration.

The best possible synthesis of available information is essential for all decision-makers. This information is necessary in clinical medicine when treating a patient or establishing common strategies for groups of similar patients; the effectiveness of a treatment must be established. It is valuable in medical research, where new hypotheses should follow reliable information. It is necessary in health planning and in administration, where the most efficient and effective programs and policies have to be established. In addition, classical or field epidemiology requires such a synthetic view for a better etiological study of disease and for a better control of disease spread. **Narrative reviews** have existed since the dawn of medicine. In essay form or in a structured paper, the author(s) explain a problem and how to resolve it.

Narrative reviews:

- Are subjective in nature;
- Rely on individual knowledge and experience (always limited);
- Frequently confirm authors' wishful thinking and preconceived ideas;
- Are very often based on references selectively chosen from the available body of evidence;
- Are powerful generators of new ideas (if well done).

For Cook et al[2], narrative reviews:

- Are appropriate for describing the development and management of a given problem;
- May be better reporters of cutting-edge developments and other topics with limited and imperfect evidence;
- Examine the problem in light of underlying theories and concepts;
- Draw analogies between and integrate two or more independent fields of research, such as infection and cancer.

For other types of reviews, more organized and structured approaches are necessary.

11.1 Definitions and objectives of meta-analysis, reviews and summaries of evidence

Any body of evidence may be analyzed and interpreted in different ways. Figure 11.1 represents a classification of various methods to evaluate a body of evidence. Some confusion still exists pertaining to the use of basic terms such as quantitative or qualitative meta-analysis, systematic review, overview, research synthesis, and research integration. These terms are sometimes used interchangeably in the medical literature. However, they should be interpreted in light of the definitions included in this section. Any work with a body of knowledge includes **research analysis,** i.e. *the resolution of a whole into its parts or elements; a method of determining or describing the nature of the thing by resolving it into its parts*[3]. It also involves **research synthesis,** which is *the assembling of separate and subordinate parts into a new form; also a new complex whole resulting from this*[3]. In logic, this means a *combination of separate elements into a whole, as a species into gender*[3]. Even these terms are sometimes unnecessarily confused. The current edition of *The Dictionary of Epidemiology*[4] defines **meta-analysis** as a '*statistical synthesis of the data from separate, but similar, i.e. comparable, studies, leading to a quantitative summary of the pooled results.*' (The rest of the definition follows the ideas presented here as originally stated, including quantitative and qualitative components[5,6]). The **systematic review** represents '*the application of strategies that limit bias in the assembly, critical appraisal, and synthesis of all relevant studies on a specific topic. Meta-analysis may be, but is not necessarily, used as part of this process*'[4]. More exact distinctions are currently rather indistinct. Readers of today's medical literature may expect elements of meta-analysis and systematic review, as defined above, to support any analysis and reporting of a given body of knowledge.

11.2 Original field of meta-analysis

Originally, in psychology and education, meta-analysis was defined by Glass[7] as a statistical integration of **results** (not of individual observations) of

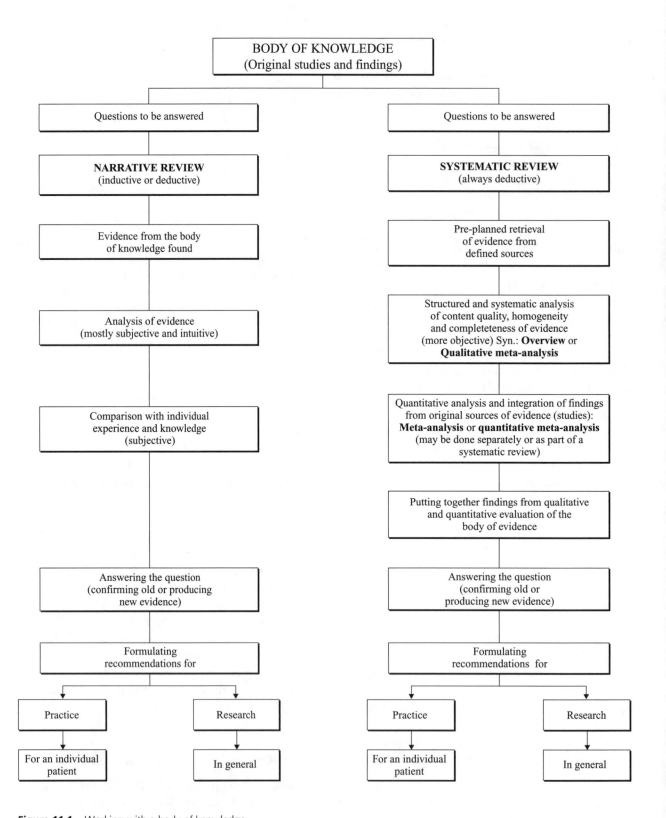

Figure 11.1 Working with a body of knowledge

independent studies of the same topic and more precisely, as a '*statistical analysis of a large collection of analyses resulting from individual studies for the purpose of integrating the findings*'. For example, do psychoactive drugs such as Ritalin control hyperactivity in children[8,9]? Does diet work[10,11]? Does psychotherapy work[12,13]? Does a full moon affect mental health[14]? (NB It does not; only the hypothesis of the effect of light remains plausible). The procedure differs from the integration of individual observations, such as in multicenter clinical trials, which increase the statistical power of the study. In meta-analysis, results from individual studies such as statistical parameters (t, F, chi-square, or r values) or categorical data (frequencies of responses from contingency tables) become units of observation, evaluation and synthesis. From its original field[15], meta-analysis migrated into such various fields as marketing, meteorology, and medicine[16]. 'Authoritative' articles have been replaced by 'structured review' articles for which uniform rules and requirements have been formulated by medical journals[17,18]. These are largely inspired by meta-analysis. Several introductory articles were originally offered to the general medical public[2,17–20], to clinical epidemiologists[6], and researchers[21], to practitioners of clinical trials[22,23] (the field from which meta-analysis in medicine originated), and applied to practically all major medical specialties. Meta-analysis was also anchored in a first textbook covering this topic in medicine[5] and structured together with decision analysis and cost-effectiveness analysis[24].

11.2.1 Definition of meta-analysis

In its original field, meta-analysis evolved independently. Lipsey and Wilson[25] recently discussed its content, orientation and methodology. In summary, meta-analysis today can be defined as follows: **In psychology and education, where it originates, *meta-analysis is the process of using statistical methods to combine results from different studies.*** The original procedure did not pay much attention to the different characteristics or quality of the original studies. **In medicine and its allied health sciences, *meta-analysis is a systematic, organized and structured evaluation and synthesis of a problem of interest based on the***

results of many independent studies of that problem (disease cause, treatment effect, diagnostic method, prognosis, etc.). Meta-analysis in medicine requires two components:

1. **Qualitative meta-analysis,** which is a systematic and uniform application of predetermined criteria of quality (such as completeness of data, absence of biases, random errors, adequate statistical analysis and adequacy of interpretation).
2. **Quantitative meta-analysis** is, in its original sense, a statistical integration of numerical information on a given subject, as reflected by results of several independent studies. The homogeneity of findings or the assessment of effect size (e.g. the best assessment of relative risk or of preventable fraction across studies, etc.) are some of its main features.

In the epidemiological sense, results of different studies become a new unit of observation, and the subject of study is a new cluster of data similar to groups of subjects in the original studies. It is a '**study of studies**' or '**epidemiology of their results**'.

The third element of meta-analysis in medicine is the **integration of its qualitative and quantitative findings.** For example, the quality of a randomized clinical trial may be scored and a subsequent quantitative assessment of the efficacy (or effectiveness) of treatment determined across several trials by weighting the results of each study using its quality score or some other measure. **Its objectives are:**

- To confirm information;
- To find errors;
- To search for additional findings (induction); and
- To find new ideas for further research (deduction).

After a slow start[26], meta-analysis is now considered an integral part of medical thinking and encouraged as a way to arrive at better decisions in practice and research[27,28]. Other critiques[29] focus mainly on faults in meta-analysis and remaining imperfections and gaps in its still-evolving methodology. Besides the *ad hoc* monographs already quoted, special chapters in other monographs[30–31] have appeared in increasing numbers. Clinicians are currently trained, and train others, to conduct original research studies, but have not been instructed on how to evaluate information from several studies or on how to make a valid synthesis of original results on a topic of interest. This, however, is essential in research as well as in practice (clinical medicine practitioners, community medicine and public health practitioners), and for decision-making (in governments and companies, for lawyers and judges). Consider now how meta-analysis worked in its original field, and how it subsequently expanded and adapted to medicine. **Why is it important to learn the basics of traditional meta-analysis?**

- *Both quantitative variables and findings such as biochemical or hematological values or quantitative variables, or binary data such as risk or survival, may be subject to systematic review and integration.*
- *To integrate quantitative findings, meta-analysis relies on its fundamental quantitative methodology, a description of which follows.*
- *To integrate epidemiological findings, such as variables studied in the field of risk or prognosis, additional methodology is needed (see Section 11.3).*

The purpose of a quantitative, 'classical' meta-analysis is usually to assess the effectiveness of treatments, health programs and interventions, and less often to assess other cause–effect relationships. For instance, is there a relationship between intelligence and schizophrenia in young subjects? Does a full moon affect mental health and behavior? Is psychotherapy effective? Can hyperactivity in children be controlled pharmacologically or by dietary regimens? 'Classical' or quantitative meta-analysis addresses two basic questions:

- How is one variable related to another?
- How strong is the evidence for the relationship?

To obtain adequate answers, meta-analysts gathered as many published and unpublished studies as possible. The quality of the studies was not taken into consideration; this was later criticized. In the seventies, researchers in psychology and education, as in other fields, were increasingly unhappy with the traditional methods of synthesis and integration of findings. Historically, such endeavors were represented by narrative reviews, secondary replicative analysis or box-score analysis, each having inherent flaws of their own[13].

11.2.2 Narrative reviews

Narrative reviews[32], as already commented[2], express the personal opinions of their authors and depend heavily on the perspicacity and personal experience of the reviewer. At one extreme, literature overviews are conducted by inexperienced individuals as sequences of 'who said what', ornated by a bibliography. At the other extreme, remarkably rich and objective overviews can be found, such as McDonald and McDonald's overview of mesothelioma epidemiology[33], or Yusuf et al's overview of results of randomized clinical trials in heart disease[34]. However, after a careful and systematic review of the literature, conclusions are made without any quantitative manipulation and integration of findings. High-quality discussion, conclusions and recommendations rely solely on the authors' outstanding experience – not all writers possess such experience.

Light and Smith[35] gave the name **box-score analysis or voting method** to essentially simple comparisons of how many studies confirm or reject the hypothesis under scrutiny. As in ice hockey, goals by both competing teams are confronted. The procedure can be risky. This example (not conclusions) comes from Frishman et al's[36] overview of the efficacy of beta-blockers in preventing death after myocardial infarction. Table 11.1 gives mortality rates in experimental and control groups in 14 studies of this problem (A – N). A simple voting method would show four studies with some effect (D, G, H, and I), and 10 showing no effect. However, closer examination (see bold-face data) reveals that only larger-sized studies with more statistical power (1 – beta) show some effect. 'Small' studies show no effect. Hence, **box-score analysis**, or the vote-counting method[37] as in sports statistics, compares the number of studies that confirm a hypothesis under study to the number of studies that reject it.

In **secondary replicated analysis**, researchers re-analyze original individual data in a study to reconfirm the primary findings, or to verify some new hypothesis by proceeding by induction. Similarly, observations **in individual patients** in several trials or other studies may be combined and re-analyzed with more statistical power. **Secondary replicative or**

Table 11.1 An example of research synthesis of selected studies on the effect of beta-blockers after myocardial infarction

	Experimental group		Control group		
Trial	Number of subjects	Case fatality rate (%)	Number of subjects	Case fatality rate (%)	p
A	114	6.1	116	12.1	0.18
B	69	7.2	93	11.8	0.48
C	151	27.2	147	31.3	0.51
D	**1,533**	**6.3**	**1,520**	**8.2**	**0.051***
E	238	25.2	242	26.2	0.92
F	355	7.9	365	7.4	0.91
G	**945**	**10.4**	**939**	**16.2**	**0.0003***
H	**1,916**	**7.2**	**1,921**	**9.8**	**0.005***
I	**698**	**5.7**	**697**	**8.9**	**0.03***
J	278	9.0	282	13.1	0.16
K	873	7.3	583	8.9	0.32
L	632	9.5	471	10.2	0.78
M	263	17.1	266	17.7	0.36
N	861	6.6	880	5.1	0.14

Source: Modified from Ref: 36. Reproduced with permission
* Studies rejecting null hypothesis.

replicated analysis[38] is based on the return to original data gathered on individuals in various studies; individual record linkage allows for greater statistical power. **A 'true' meta-analysis** does not return to individual data, but it deals with end-point findings as units of observation, such as occurrence rates or proportions, or various statistical parameters produced by inferential analysis, such as *p* or **chi** values, correlation coefficients, etc.

11.2.3 'Classical' meta-analysis

In the early seventies, researchers in academic institutions in Boston and Denver called for better decisions in research and practice. Light and Smith[35] traced the field, Glass defined meta-analysis as quoted above[7], and Rosenthal gave initial methodological encouragement[39]. These opening papers

were followed by many other papers as well as several monographs, such as Light and Pillemer's classic[40], or more methodological volumes such as Lipsey and Wilson's[25]. From these remarkable foundations, only the most fundamental principles are quoted here in a defined context. The quality of studies was not originally questioned, because research (especially experimental) in psychology and education is more standardized and uniform than clinical research in medicine and public health. Experimental conditions may be more easily used, compared groups have fixed sizes, etc. Qualitative considerations in the integration of studies in medicine are far more important.

11.2.3.1 The effect size in an original study

The first studies focused on such an effect in experimental or other conditions assessing various interventions such as psychotherapy, drugs, diet, etc. The original effect size, mark of the efficacy of intervention, was based on the concept of Z scores, 'allowing to compare the incomparable'. For example, as shown in Table 11.2, a medical student must choose between taking specialty training in surgery or psychiatry. The student's Z score in surgery, in terms of a fraction of the standard deviation of the student's grades compared to the class mean, is higher than the score in psychiatry. Would the student become a better surgeon? In the same vein, 'successes' or 'effect sizes' (**ES** or **d**) in an experiment were proposed as follows:

For a quantitative variable (performance score, anxiety or hyperactivity score, blood pressure, etc.):

$$\text{ES (or } \mathbf{d}) = (\overline{X}_e - \overline{X}_c) / S_c$$

Where
$\overline{X}_e$ = mean score (value) for the experimental group

For a qualitative variable[41] (occurrence of falling ill, improving, dying, etc.):

$$\text{ES (or } \mathbf{d}) = (P_e - P_c) / \sqrt{P_c(1 - P_c)}$$

Where
P_e = proportion of events in an experimental group

$\overline{X}_c$ = mean value for the control group

S_c = standard deviation of the control group (or reasonable substitute, such as a pooled S of experimental and control group)[42]

P_c = proportion of events in a control group

Table 11.2   Z Scores: An example

	Surgery	*Psychiatry*
Student:	X = 84	X = 90
Class average:	$\overline{X}$ = 76	$\overline{X}$ = 82
	S = 10	S = 16

$$Z = (X - \overline{X})/S$$

Z score in surgery   Z score in psychiatry
= (84 − 76)/10 = 0.8   = (90 − 82)/16 = 0.5

$\overline{X}$ = Average score (grade) for students' class
S = Standard deviation of student grades
Scores: 1 to 100, 0.1 to 1.0

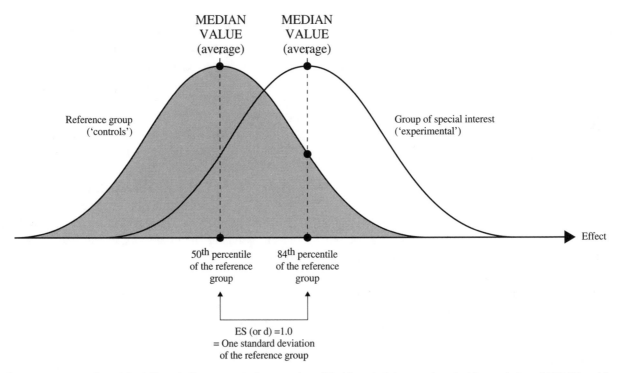

Figure 11.2   Meaning of the 'effect size'*. Source: Redrawn and modified from Ref. 9, reproduced with permission of PRO-ED and the *Journal of Learning Disabilities*

Interpretation:

- A median subject (i.e. at the 50th percentile) of the control group would be expected to rise to P_{84} of the control group if treated[31].
- The average treated subject was better off than 84% of the placebo group, while only 16% of the placebo group was improved when compared to the average subject treated by the drug under study[23].
- The average drug-treated subject would reveal a 34% gain on the outcome measured (dependent variable under study[31]).

Importance (Cohen[52]):

- 0.2 = "small"
- 0.5 = "medium"
- 0.8 = "large"

Figure 11.2 shows how results of the effect size[43] estimation might be interpreted if an effect size of 1.0 (i.e. one standard deviation distance) were found. (NB Remember the number of subjects between intervals by standard deviation around the mean or between a given percentile distribution. The ES statistics are interpreted similarly to the Z score providing a normal distribution of data.) Cohen's consideration of the importance of the effect size[43] might concern practitioners. It is a statistical consideration that says nothing about the clinical importance of the impact under study. The clinical or practical importance or magnitude of effect is still the subject of discussion in the original domain of meta-analysis[44] and in evaluation research[45]. Greenland[21] also warns that by expressing effects in standard deviation units, one can force studies with identical results to appear to yield different results. Once point estimates of effect size are obtained, their confidence intervals are determined by simple computations[46]. Such interval estimates are then used in the graphical presentation of findings in meta-analysis (see later in this chapter) and to identify 'outlying studies' or outliers (see also Section 7.3.2).

11.2.3.2 Average effect size across studies

A simple averaging of effect sizes from original studies is most often replaced by various weighted averages, such as point estimates weighted by study sizes. For example[41], each point estimate of **d** (i.e. ES) can be multiplied by n_i/N, where n_i is the size of the study and N is the overall number of subjects from all studies that are the subject of meta-analysis. Other ways of weighing are also possible, as outlined later in this chapter. Point and confidence interval estimates can also be obtained.

11.2.3.3 Other ways to assess the effect

The originators of meta-analysis used almost all available statistical parameters to assess the effect size. Computational formulas were proposed to convert t, F, chi-square into r values and subsequently into **d** values. These methods are found in several references[5,40,41,46]. More important, however, is the use of epidemiological measures of impact.

11.2.3.4 Assessment of homogeneity or heterogeneity of individual studies

Rosenthal's methodology allows for the assessment of homogeneity of findings across studies and the subsequent integration of as few as two or three studies[39,47]. If study results are heterogeneous, the reason for this heterogeneity must be found – different study designs, different patients, clinical methods, statistical descriptive and/or analytical methods, etc.? Consequently, the question becomes 'should findings be better stratified or analyzed otherwise?'

11.2.3.5 File drawer problem and fail-safe number of studies

Rosenthal[48] also drew attention to the potentially considerable problem of unpublished studies. Some studies are not finished for various reasons – editorial boards refuse them or authors themselves decide not to publish[56]. How might this affect meta-analysis? Should these unpublished studies be taken into account? In psychology and education, unpublished studies were assumed mostly to confirm the null hypothesis (negative results). In medicine, this situation is not clear. According to the formula[47,48] $X = (\Sigma Z/1,645)^2 - 1$ where ΣZ = the sum of d_i from the studies (effect sizes), and N = the total number of studies, then X gives a number of unpublished studies whose average effect would be contrary (or none) to the effect size based only on published studies, which would be necessary to reverse conclusions from meta-analysis of published studies. (NB 5N + 10 studies are suggested as a cut-off point[48,49].) If only a few unpublished studies (X) were necessary to reverse the conclusions from a meta-analysis, the evidence is weak. If, on the other hand, a large number of unpublished studies were necessary, the published evidence is strong. Such a computation of a '**fail-safe number**' will not uncover 'lost' studies. Its greatest value is in the assessment of the solidity of available evidence.

If unpublished studies exist, it is almost impossible to submit them to similar selection criteria as meta-analysis, which deals with already published studies. Such a search for unpublished studies would most often not add significant information to that already produced by meta-analysis of the published material only. Many clinicians have been preoccupied by the publication bias concerning studies reporting 'no effect', i.e. confirming a null hypothesis. If, for example, studies mostly confirming that a particular treatment works are published, practitioners risk adopting treatments that may be ineffective or even hazardous (i.e. if a drug's side effects are important or if an ineffective drug is preferred over another effective, competing medication). In the field of perinatology, Hetherington et al[50] have found that it is very difficult to retrieve unpublished studies retrospectively. As a remedy, they propose a prospective registration of clinical trials. Eastbrook et al[51] found that 487 studies approved by the Central Oxford Research Ethics Committee yielded 285 actual studies, of which only 52% were published. Bias towards significant results was found especially in laboratory-based experimental studies as well as in observational ones (years 1984–7, as of May 1990). **All in all, one must be very careful when evaluating unpublished studies. They are of uneven quality. It is generally impossible to submit these studies to the same criteria of acceptability as those of studies that have not been rejected (and non-submitted) by a peer review.**

11.3 Meta-analytic procedures, methods and techniques in medicine

Experimental studies in fields other than medicine, such as psychology and education, may be more uniform in design and execution; target populations may be less heterogeneous. Medical research is much more heterogeneous – one must adapt meta-analysis to this heterogeneity[8]. Table 11.3 defines some of the sources of such heterogeneity. Consider which strategies might be adopted first in quantitative meta-analysis and second in qualitative meta-analysis. Finally, consider an appropriate synthesis of both.

11.3.1 *Measurement of effect or quantitative meta-analysis*

First, **quantitative meta-analysis in medicine may be defined as a general, systematic and uniform evaluation of dimensions.** These dimensions may occur across studies dealing with the following:

Table 11.3 Some important sources of 'internal' heterogeneity of studies in medicine

Approach to the problem + hypothesis testing:
- Induction (data → hypothesis → evaluation)
- Deduction (hypothesis → data → evaluation)

Study architecture:
- Observational (case–control, cohort, etc.)
- Experimental (clinical trial)

Intellectual quality:
- Rigor in the formulation of a problem and execution of an *ad hoc* study
- Unbiased interpretation of results in terms of qualitative and quantitative information

Also:
- Biases, blunders, obscurantism, missing information, demagoguery, megalomania, etc.

- *The magnitude of a health problem;*
- *The strength and specificity of a causal relationship in etiological research;*
- *The strength and specificity of the impact of a preventive (contrapathic) or therapeutic (contratrophic) intervention (= 'effect size');*
- *The internal and external validity of clinical tools (e.g. diagnostic methods);*
- *The costs and benefits of diagnostic methods and treatments.*

Hence, the subject should not be only the effect of an interesting treatment. Other topics mentioned above can also be studied. The study of causal relationships between independent and dependent variables is based on logic and measurement. This applies just as well to the study of undesirable factors causing disease as to the beneficial effect of treatment on outcome.

In classical epidemiology, the effect size or the quantitative dimension of the strength and specificity of causal relationships is given by risk ratios (relative risk or **RR**), risk differences (attributable risk, **AR** or **RD**) or by the proportional expression of the latter relative to exposed subjects or to the target population (etiological fraction, **EF**), or attributable risk percent, (**AR %**)). In clinical epidemiology and EBM, indices summarized in Table 9.1 are worthy of consideration, **number needed to treat** [52] giving the additional practical meaning to treatment effectiveness. An alternative methodology based on Efron and Morris' empirical Bayes approach was proposed and used by Gilbert, McPeek and Mosteller[53] to evaluate benefits and risks in surgery and anesthesia. Despite this, different epidemiological expressions of 'risk' are most often used in the etiological research of noxious factors and less often in the assessment of causal relationships between intervention and cure, where sole statistical significance still prevails in many studies. There are three possible approaches to the estimation of the effect size across studies:

1. A simple averaging of results of original studies. This may be a rather simplistic approach, even if studies are stratified and/or weighted according to some preselected criteria;
2. The characteristic effect across studies is recalculated from cell frequencies of events in two-by-two tables (or their extensions) for original studies[54–56]. This approach, developed by British authors, stems from the original Mantel–Haenszel approach to stratified observations in case–control studies[57]. Conceptually, strata are replaced by original studies[58]. The resulting **relative risk (risks ratio) across studies**[56] and **typical odds ratio**[53,54] represent another assessment of effect size;
3. Cochran's guidelines (REVMAN or systematic REView MANual)[59] for combining rates from individual trials or Epi Meta software from the US Centers for Disease Control and Prevention are also used[60].

Although the following text concerns clinical trials, the same concepts apply to any assessment of causality by either analytical (etiological) studies, or observational or experimental studies based on comparisons of two or more groups of patients or individuals in the community.

11.3.1.1 Typical odds ratio or odds ratio across studies

A typical odds ratio across studies is not a simple average or a somehow weighted average of odds ratios from original studies. The same applies to relative or other measures of risk across studies. To illustrate the computational approach, here is how Yusuf et al[55] evaluated the across studies effect of beta

blockade during and after myocardial infarction: In the search for a typical odds ratio across studies, categorical data must be retrieved from each trial (or etiological study), for example from a basic two-by-two table (example of beta blockers, (BB) in prevention of death after myocardial infarction (MI)):

	Death after MI	Survival after MI	
Patients treated by BB	O		n
Patients treated by another modality (no BB)			c
	d		N

Where[55]:

N = Total number of patients in the trial

n = Number of patients treated by the modality (drug under study)

d = Number of outcomes (expected events such as deaths, etc.) in the whole trial (both groups – BB and non-BB)

c = Number of patients treated by a control intervention (no treatment, placebo, another active drug, etc.)

O = Number of outcomes (events under study) in patients receiving treatment modality of interest

E = Number of events (outcomes) expected in patients receiving treatment modality of interest, i.e. n.d/N

If the treatment under study had no effect, an (O – E) value would differ only randomly from zero. If some undesirable outcome is a measure of effect (such as death in this example), this value will be negative (fewer deaths will occur).

V_{O-E} = E·(1 – n/N)(N – d)/(N – 1) as in Ref. 55
or   E·(1 – d/N)/(N – 1)   as in Ref. 56

From these basic components provided by original studies, the following information is obtained across studies:

GT = Grand total of (O − E) values from each trial

VT = Sum of the variances (ΣV_{O-E}) from individual trials

TOR = Point estimate of 'Typical Odds Ratio',

$$= \exp(GT/VT)$$

(log odds ratio = GT/VT)

$\overline{TOR}$, $\overline{TOR}_{95\%}$ = Confidence interval estimate (95%) of TOR, i.e.

$$= \exp(GT / VT \pm 1.96 / \sqrt{VT})$$

Finally, a chi-square test for heterogeneity is performed[55] (i.e. 'do all studies come from the same batch?' or 'do they yield results going in the same direction? Hence, can results be integrated?'). Heterogeneous ensembles of studies should be stratified, i.e. grouped into more homogenous subgroups, subject to subsequent integration or other ways of reassessment.

$$\chi^2 = \Sigma[(O_i - E_i)^2 V_{O_i-E_i}] - [\Sigma(O_i - E_i)^2 / \Sigma V_{O_i-E_i}]$$

More detailed quantitative methodology may be found in Yusuf et al's[55] and Collins and Langman's[56] original papers.

Graphically, results of such a meta-analysis are usually presented as a group of point estimates of TORs (or of any other measure of risk, see later in this chapter) represented by 'dots', with their confidence intervals represented by 'lines' and the TOR across all studies represented by 'diamonds', as well as eventually similar findings in various strata, if subgroups of studies are of interest.

Stratification can be done in several ways, contrasting (for example):

- Inductive vs deductive studies;
- Case–control vs cohort studies;
- Randomized vs non-randomized trials;
- Persons, time, place characteristics;
- Different measurements of outcome (outcome variables);
- Stages of natural or clinical course of disease;
- Other.

Figure 11.3 illustrates our findings from a meta-analysis of the effectiveness of antacids in preventing gastrointestinal bleeding in intensive care units (cimetidine or antacids)[61]: odds ratios with 95% confidence interval limits and typical odds ratio of studies on the prophylaxis of upper gastrointestinal

bleeding acquired in the intensive care units (ICU) are presented here. Odds ratios less than 1 mean that cimetidine or antacids prevented bleeding. Results were considered of interest if the 95% confidence interval did not override the ratio of 1. Results show a comparable effect of antacids and cimetidine across studies, and that both drugs seem effective in preventing upper gastrointestinal bleeding. However, when the quality of original studies was assessed by qualitative meta-analysis (see the *ad hoc* section later in this chapter), the numerical findings of meta-analysis are shown to lose some of their importance[62]. Thus, methodological failures and missing information in the original studies can be found, risking invalidation of the quantitative findings.

11.3.1.2 Relative risk, attributable risk and etiological fraction across studies

Additional methodological developments allow the computation of other measures across studies:

- **Relative risk across studies**[54] or
- **Attributable risk across studies**[63–65]
- As for the **etiological fraction across studies**, the methodology requires further improvement.

As yet, there is no good methodology dealing with the integration of etiological fraction across studies. Despite this, the question remains crucial in practice. Can the overall protective efficacy of a vaccine or chemotherapeutical agent or antibiotic ever be established? On the other hand, an overdone integration of heterogeneous findings from various studies focusing on different populations or groups at risk may mask inherent differences, which should ideally be explained rather than mixed into an entity which encompasses everything but explains and represents nothing. For example, BCG vaccination programs in different parts of the world were presented by Clemens et al[66]. Such naturally and biologically heterogeneous findings should be properly interpreted on their own (why such differences?) rather than integrated into a larger entity. (In this overview, studies with more statistical power and less bias point to the effectiveness of BCG.)

Some proportional expression, conceptually close to etiological fraction or protective efficacy ratio, is represented by Einarson et al's [41] formula for

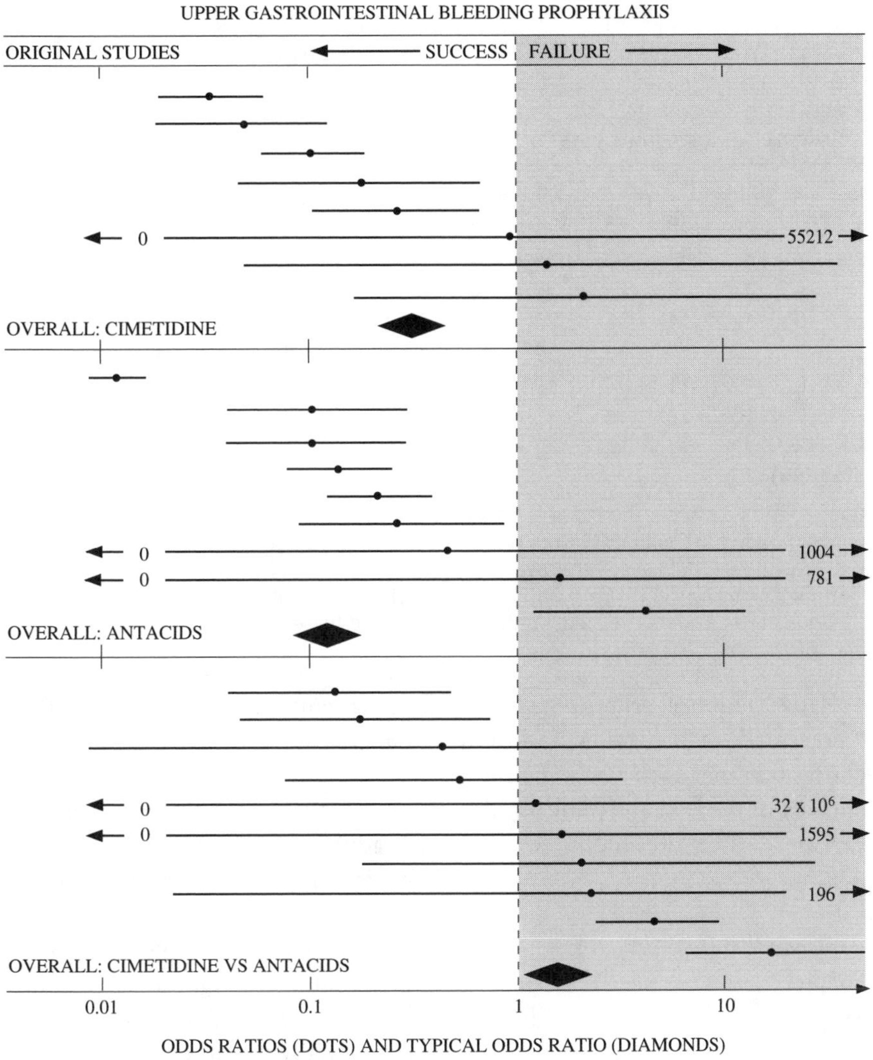

UPPER GASTROINTESTINAL BLEEDING PROPHYLAXIS

Figure 11.3 Graphical presentation of basic quantitative information from meta-analysis. Source: Ref. 61, reproduced with the authors' permission

computation of the effect size from the frequencies of outcomes (qualitative data) as already quoted in Section 11.3. They evaluated therapeutic efficacy of intradiscally-injected chymopapain in herniated lumbar disc sufferers. Elsewhere, Wortman and Yeaton[67] evaluated the effectiveness of coronary artery bypass graft surgery by comparing numbers of angina-free subjects in surgically and medically treated patients. An angina-free period represented a 'quality-of-life benefit' in their study. Their formula for calculating the quality-of-life benefit (QLB) was:

$$QLB = \frac{X_2 - X_1}{N_1} - \frac{Y_2 - Y_1}{N_2}$$

Where:

N_1 = Number of patients assigned to surgery less those not receiving surgery

N_2 = Number of patients assigned to medical treatment

X_2 = Number of surgical patients remaining angina-free, longest follow-up

X_1 = Number of surgical patients free of angina at entry

Y_2 = Number of angina-free medical patients, longest follow-up

Y_1 = Number of angina-free medical patients at entry

Table 11.4 Odds Ratio

	Odds ratio																	
	Preventive Intervention								Treatment									
CER	0.5	0.55	0.6	0.65	0.7	0.75	0.8	0.85	0.9	1.5	2	2.5	3	3.5	4	4.5	5	10
0.05	41	46	52	59	69	83	104	139	209	43	22	15	12	9	8	7	6	3
0.1	21	24	27	31	36	43	54	73	110	23	12	9	7	6	5	4	4	2
0.2	11	13	14	17	20	24	30	40	61	14	8	5	4	4	3	3	3	2
0.3	8	9	10	12	14	18	22	30	46	11	6	5	4	3	3	3	3	2
0.4	7	8	9	10	12	15	19	26	40	10	6	4	4	3	3	3	3	2
0.5	6	7	8	9	11	14	18	25	38	10	6	5	4	4	3	3	3	2
0.7	6	7	9	10	13	16	20	28	44	13	8	7	6	5	5	5	5	4
0.9	12	15	18	22	27	34	46	64	101	32	21	17	16	14	14	13	13	11

^ **Control Event Rate (CER)**

Calculation of the number needed to treat (NNT) from odds ratios. Tables for estimating the NNT when the odds ratio (OR) and control event rate (CER) are known, published for preventive interventions. The formula for determining the NNT for preventive interventions is $\{1 - [CER \times (1 - OR)]\}/[1 - CER) \times CER \times (1 - OR)]$. For treatment, the formula is $[CER(OR - 1) + 1]/[CER(OR - 1) \times (1 - CER)]$. Source: Ref. 52, reproduced with permission from the ACP-ASIM (*Ann Intern Med*)

The absolute or relative number or proportion of lives saved, cases prevented, or prognoses improved remains the most important means to assess the clinical relevance and impact of medical and public health interventions at various levels of prevention.

11.3.1.3 Number needed to treat across studies

As explained in Chapter 9, **number needed to treat** or NNT is a reciprocal of the absolute risk reduction (ARR); in other words, of risk difference or attributable risk. Given the fact that relative risk reduction can also be calculated as 1 – relative risk or 1 – odds ratio, NNTs can be derived from odds ratios or relative risks provided by systematic reviews. McQuay and Moore[52] give formulas for the calculation of the number needed to treat from odds ratios and control event rates for preventive interventions as well as for treatment (Table 11.4). An NNT of 1, ideal but mostly unseen in practice, indicates an ideal effectiveness of treatment. An NNT of 2 or 3 shows that treatment is quite effective, and an NNT of 20 to 40 suggests that treatment may still be effective[52]. The issue is the application of NNTs from systematic reviews to decisions in individual patients. The body of studies entering a systematic review may represent a more rather than a less heterogeneous population of patients, too 'ecumenical', different, or omitting patients at a particular risk.

11.3.1.4 Cumulative meta-analysis

Traditionally, meta-analysis is performed on all eligible studies as a whole. Lau et al[62] and Antman et al[68] proposed and put into practice an additional approach called **cumulative meta-analysis**. In this procedure, original studies are first put in chronological order, then a meta-analysis is performed sequentially from one study addition to another. Figure 11.4 illustrates both traditional and cumulative meta-analysis of clinical trials of beta-blockers as preventive treatment after myocardial infarction. The left portion of the figure represents point-and-interval estimates of original studies' odds ratios, as well as an overall odds ratio from the ensemble. The right portion is a sequence of **overall cumulative odds ratios** from one study addition to another. Cumulative meta-analysis provides additional useful information. For example, the first sequence, indicating that the treatment works, identifies the moment at which a convincing piece of evidence is available. Economy of research and speedier approval of new drugs are at stake. This example (Figure 11.4) shows that the usefulness of beta-blockers became evident in 1977. However, attempts to refine this study lasted

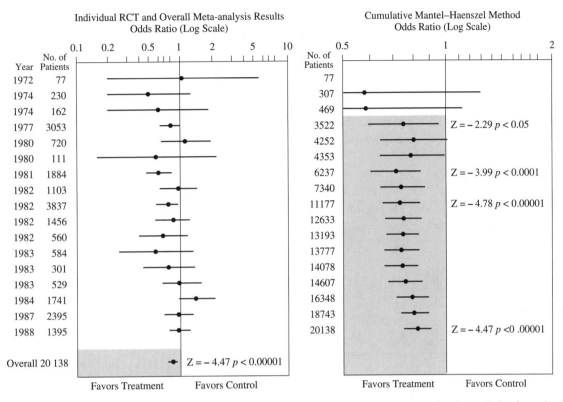

Figure 11.4 Example of overall (classical) and cumulative meta-analysis. Source: Ref. 68, reproduced with permission from the Massachusetts Medical Society (*N Engl J Med*)

until 1988 at which time a similar conclusion was reached. In the future, results off clinical trials may be meta-analyzed prospectively (as soon as they are published, they are sequentially synthesized) to arrive to the point at which evidence is obtained.

11.3.1.5 More advanced quantitative and graphical methods

Statistical methods in meta-analysis focusing on the evaluation of heterogeneity of studies and their results are based on two models: **fixed-effect models** assume that an intervention has a single true effect, i.e. results of different studies vary around some true common effect; **random-effect models** assume that an effect may vary across studies. Lau et al propose more information about the evaluation of these models in their comprehensive *ad hoc* paper[69]. An evaluation of various causes of impact may be further strengthened using **regression models**. The possibility of performing a meta-analysis on these findings is reviewed in depth in an excellent article by Greenland[21]. A regression analysis in which

individual sets of data are used as the unit of observation is called **meta-regression**[69,70]. Various **graphical methods to describe and analyze findings** such as 'funnel plot'[42], 'odd man out'[71], 'box plot'[72] or time trends of prevalent effects (including also outliers)[73] help to better visualize findings from meta-analyses.

11.3.2 Qualitative meta-analysis – the core of systematic reviews

In medicine, contrary to other fields of research, variables of interest such as methodology, health problems, target populations and etiological factors are considerably diversified and heterogeneous. In such a situation, an adequate assessment of the quality of original studies must be made before a quantitative meta-analysis is performed. Unacceptable studies must be rejected. Some weighting of studies according to quality (score) or some other stratification based on quality may be attempted. The effect size may be evaluated in different strata or across studies with appropriate attention to quality.

Such an approach currently represents one of the greatest challenges of meta-analysis in medicine: to find a good integration of the qualitative and quantitative aspects of meta-analysis in the synthesis of research. Until now, the question of which studies to include and how to weigh them has not been settled. **Qualitative meta-analysis in medicine** can be **defined as** '*a method of assessment of the importance and relevance of medical information coming from several independent sources through (by) a general, systematic and uniform application of pre-established criteria of acceptability of original studies representing the body of knowledge of a given health problem or question*'[5]. The objectives of qualitative meta-analysis are:

- To determine the prevalence, homogeneity and distribution of quality attributes;
- To expand the knowledge of missing and/or imperfect data; and
- To evaluate and interpret 'outliers' (e.g. observations beyond a customary range).

There is no universal system, method or procedure to evaluate the quality of any kind of study, be it a diagnostic method, descriptive, analytical observational, experimental (clinical trial) study, or a study of prognosis. For example, Feinstein's qualitative criteria for case–control studies[74] represent a structured guideline in the assessment of an 'initial state → maneuver → subsequent state' model. However, in many cases, scoring for quality of the study would be useless if, for example, the presence of an important protopathic or susceptibility bias were to invalidate the interpretation of the quantitative results of the study. Elsewhere, Lichtenstein et al[75] use 34 criteria to assess the quality of case–control studies. Twenty items such as methods of data collection, sources of cases and controls, blinding of interviewers, description of sampling and analytic methods, diagnostic procedures and criteria, information on exposure etc., are considered essential. A quality score is not given.

In their assessment of the quality of clinical trials, DerSimonian et al[76] seek 11 components which should figure in a good clinical trial: eligibility criteria; admission before allocation; random allocation; method of randomization; patient blindness to treatment; blind assessment of outcome; treatment complications; loss to follow-up; statistical analyses; statistical methods; and statistical power of the trial. Detsky et al's[77] list of quality assessment questions covers 14 similar concerns. Such criteria for a clinical trial must often be adapted to reflect specific characteristics of the pathology and treatment modality under investigation. In their assessment of the benefit of oral corticosteroid therapy in the treatment of stable chronic obstructive pulmonary disease, Callahan et al[78] also translate general criteria as above to specific measures of pulmonary function.

The fundamental components of qualitative meta-analysis are **evidence tables**. In such tables, all relevant characteristics, components and numerical results of original studies are compiled. They allow for first-hand assessment of homogeneity of studies and missing information. A recent study of adverse (or secondary) effects of oral contraceptives[79] is a good example of qualitative meta-analysis and uses of evidence tables. (NB Authors, however, did not score studies for quality.) Assessment of heterogeneity of studies often provides more important information than typical effects or other descriptions across studies.

11.3.2.1 Scoring of studies for quality

In many cases, simply listing attributes as being present or absent in each study may not be enough. An appropriate dimension must be given to these facts where necessary. Scoring of quality is of particular interest. As mentioned in Chapter 7, Chalmers et al[80] proposed a qualitative assessment of clinical trials in which, from a total score of 100, a maximum of 60 points is given to the database, design and 'protocol' with emphasis on blinding, 30 points are given to statistical analysis, and 10 points to the study's presentation. The McMaster group used another type of scoring to evaluate the quality of compliance research reports[81,82]. The highest score was given to studies with good internal and external validity (e.g. a randomized trial based on a random population sample, in which replicable diagnostic inclusion and exclusion criteria are clearly stated, where direct longitudinal measures of compliance are taken and where compliance and therapeutic regimens are completely described to the reader and replicable by others). Obviously, as with any original method or technique, methods of study quality assessment are progressively validated. Oxman and Guyatt's[83] study is a good example of this validation.

There is a substantial difference between the scoring of studies to be done (research proposals and study protocols and designs) and the scoring of studies already done. The former, especially, is hotly debated. Granting agencies are occasionally tempted to score research proposals. Good scores, however, may hide some major error, which would invalidate the study despite an acceptable overall score (the study's 'death knell'). This must always be checked. For example, what would a study of diabetes be worth if diabetic cases were not properly defined in operational terms, with clear inclusion and exclusion criteria? Unfortunately, the published literature does not contain an equivalent method of undertaking the quality assessment of observational analytical studies, giving some 'quantitative assessment of quality' that might be used in the meta-analysis of a given problem, where both qualitative and quantitative aspects of evaluation are integrated. Only checklists are available[84] to accomplish this objective. Detsky et al[77] propose plotting effect size against quality score and sequentially combining trial results according to quality scores.

In meta-analysis, the quality of studies can be considered in two ways. First, quality can be viewed as an independent variable, and one may examine whether study results depend on good or bad quality. Second, study results may be weighted **if and only if** there is a pre-established association between these results and the quality of the study. Would such scoring be necessary if there were not such an association? Should the effect size observed in each study be weighted by the study's quality score and the overall effect size across studies determined thereafter? Fleiss and Gross[85] propose two ways to weigh results of quantitative meta-analysis based on the original studies' quality:

1. If large studies yield more statistical power ('more patients in the study means a better study'), any effect size across studies (ES, typical odds ratio,

relative risk etc.) weighted by quality would be

Quality weighted average effect size = $e = \Sigma\, we_i / \Sigma\, w$

Where:

w = Total number of patients in the study (approximation; see [88])

e_i = Effect size found in an original study

2. Wherever an acceptable measure of study quality is available (scoring system etc.), giving a value (q = quality value of an original study graded from 0.0 to 1.0), quality weighted average effect size would be

$$e = \Sigma\, (qw)\, e_i / \Sigma\, (qw)$$

An alternative to scoring of quality is to analyze subgroups of studies according to their qualitative characteristics.

11.3.2.2 Best evidence synthesis

Slavin[86] proposed an alternative to the challenge of quality heterogeneity of studies: to evaluate and integrate the best evidence only. In an assessment of causal relationship, the quality of evidence progresses from case studies across observational etiological research to an experimental well controlled proof, such as all phases of clinical trials. (See also Section 4.2.2 of this text.) Should experimental studies of a causal relationship of interest be the only ones retained for meta-analysis if evidence is also available from observational cohort and/or case–control research? In their guidelines for meta-analyzing clinical trials, Gerbarg and Horwitz[87] stress as the first step the conduct of a structured and consistent **methodological analysis** of all available clinical trials, and consider pooling only those that adhere to current standards of methodologic rigor.

The best type of study giving the strongest evidence (nature of the problem permitting) may be chosen for meta-analysis, such as controlled clinical trials only in the assessment of treatment impact, as was done by Hayes et al[88] to evaluate the therapeutic effectiveness of propranolol. Another approach is to score or otherwise evaluate the inherent quality of the original studies and to integrate only the best ones. Spitzer et al[89] adopted this second approach in their assessment of the link between passive smoking and outcomes of various health problems. In the above-mentioned approaches, an appropriate sequence appears to be the qualitative assessment of studies first, followed by a selection of acceptable studies and quantitative meta-analysis of the latter.

11.3.3 Beyond clinical trials; meta-analysis in other fields of medical research

Up until now, the main purpose of meta-analysis was to integrate information from preventive or curative intervention work. Meta-analysis is thus well established in the domain of clinical trials and public health programs, but it is also used in other fields. There are already some meta-analytical forays into the areas of normative (reference) values, description of disease occurrence, analytical observational studies, diagnosis, and prognosis. Hence, meta-analysis is much more omnipresent now than when it began.

11.3.3.1 Diagnosis and 'diagnosimetrics'[90,91]

In the field of **diagnosis** and its quantitative evaluation (i.e. diagnosimetrics), meta-analyses are still scarce. It would not always be appropriate to integrate studies in order to find the overall sensitivity or specificity of a diagnostic test (see Koch et al's[92] methodology). It is often more interesting to know how meta-analysis works in subgroups of patients[93] bearing different characteristics. On the other hand, diagnostic test properties may be integrated to assess their differential diagnostic value, such as was done by Arana et al[94] in the assessment of the dexamethasone suppression test for the diagnosis and prognosis of various affective and psychotic disorders. Encouragingly, authors pay increasing attention not only to new technologies, but also to diagnostic methods based on physical examination in clinical practice[95,96].

11.3.3.2 Descriptive studies of risk

In the area of **descriptive studies of risk**, a similar approach, i.e. making a mosaic of complementing original studies, may be attempted[97]. Mahoney and Michalek[98] published a meta-analysis of cancer incidence in US and Canadian native populations. Their study shows an uneven point estimate of standardized incidence ratio of cervical cancer (with

overlapping confidence interval) across studies in native women. In this case, meta-analysis is used in a more classical way to assess the magnitude of occurrence (cancer incidence) and its heterogeneity across various studies. In another example, Gray Davis et al[99] integrated several hepatitis B seroprevalence studies to better understand the various ways of horizontal transmission in developed and developing countries (variable endemicity).

11.3.3.3 Analytical observational studies of causality

In **analytical observational studies of causality**, meta-analysis is used in two ways. First, it can focus on the consistency and plausibility of a causal relationship across various studies (their design, different target populations, quality of studies, etc.). Schlesselman et al's[100] study of oral contraceptives in relation to breast cancer showed inconsistency of such a cause–effect relationship. Meta-analysis can also be used to combine a mosaic of studies to assess if a given causal relationship confirms various criteria of causality (see Chapter 8). This approach was used in the assessment of adrenocorticosteroid treatment and osteoporosis[101], social support and well-being[102], gastric colonization by Gram-negative bacilli and nosocomial pneumonia[103], and in another, more recent verdict on smoking and health[104]. The association of neonatal survival depending on a child's being born at a hospital with neonatal intensive care units, or being born elsewhere and being transferred to these units, was assessed across observational studies by Ozminkowski et al[105].

If studies are stratified according to different study designs, patient groups, treatment, diagnostic, or prognostic subgroups, one may ask if these strata or subgroups give the same information through meta-analysis. L'Abbé et al[19] named this assessment **sensitivity analysis** (i.e. 'of meta-analysis')[see also 69]. The same can be done on the basis of analytical observational studies of other causal relationships. For these kind of studies, Stroup et al[84] propose a checklist useful in meta-analysis research proposals or reports, prerequisites of good meta-analysis of observational studies. As with any other research protocol and report, they should include:

- The background of the study with problem definition;
- A search strategy to find original studies including selection criteria;
- Methods of evaluation (including qualitative assessment) and integration of studies;
- Manners in which results of meta-analysis will be reported and discussed;
- Conclusions with guidelines for further use and research.

Second, according to Fleiss and Gross[85], meta-analysis of observational analytical studies may be used with a 'guarded yes' to integrate the strength of associations (magnitude of effect).

11.3.3.4 *Studies of prognosis*

In the meta-analysis of studies of **prognosis**, two strategies can be adopted. Either relapse-free survival rates, or overall survival rates, or any other measure of outcome can be analyzed for heterogeneity and integrated, such as in Himel et al's[65] study of adjuvant chemotherapy for breast cancer, or Cuzick

et al's[106] study of a similar effect of adjuvant radiotherapy. On the other hand, adjuvant tamoxifen and cytotoxic therapy effect on mortality in early breast cancer[107] was assessed by log-rank survival analysis as an example of integration and comparison of trends. Shore et al[108] used proportional hazard analysis to analyze the impact of radiotherapy and chemotherapy on Stage I and II Hodgkin's disease.

11.4 Components and attributes of a good meta-analytic study

Meta-analysis of any topic in medicine must be conducted along similar rigorous guidelines as used in the studies of origin. As already mentioned, meta-analysis is performed similarly to any original research, but instead of individual patients as units of observation, findings from original studies become such units. Throughout this general philosophy, several key recommendations corroborate what should be desirable components and attributes of meta-analysis[109,110]. Table 11.5 compares some of

---

Table 11.5   A comparison of desired components and criteria of original studies and meta-analysis

Basic criteria of a good original study	*Basic criteria of a good meta-analytic study*
<ul><li>The problem is clearly identified</li><li>The hypothesis is clearly formulated</li><li>The topic is well documented</li><li>The design <u>and</u> the protocol are worked up before the study begins</li><li>All variables under study are well defined by operational criteria</li><li>Quality data are collected</li><li>A proper quantitative analysis of data is made</li><li>Critical evaluation of results is done</li><li>Results are interpreted in relation to the initially stated problem and hypothesis</li><li>The relevance of results is addressed before putting them into practice</li></ul>	<ul><li>What question(s) should be answered?</li><li>Sources of studies (meticulous retrieval) are identified</li><li>Selection criteria of studies are defined</li><li>An assessment of publication bias is made</li><li>A clear description of the 'architecture' of meta-analysis (type, steps, chronology, etc.) is presented</li><li>Methods and quantitative techniques used are described</li><li>Reasons for variability of studies are identified</li><li>Assessment of data <u>both</u> within and between studies is carried out</li><li>Results and their practical relevance are proposed</li><li>A bibliography is present (methods, reference data)</li><li>A list of studies - subject of meta-analysis is given</li></ul>

For both[122]

- Solidity and validity of evidence
- Generalizability of findings
- Applicability to particular settings and patients
- Results answer relevant clinical questions
- Results have an important effect on clinical practice (keep it or change it)

the most important components of an original study with those of meta-analysis. A meta-analytic study should answer a problem or question that was clearly formulated at the beginning of the study. Such a deductive approach to the subject of interest is far superior to an inductive one. The results of a meta-analytic study should not be awaited. Deductive and inductive approaches are iterative in research, but a meta-analytic study should be developed to answer a specific question first. The logical sequence of meta-analysis is qualitative assessment first, then quantitative assessment. Both should be integrated in a logical sequence and frame. Our flow chart in Figure 11.5 sums up one possible kind of procedure. This model also assumes that the typical or overall effect is not the only subject of interest. The homogeneity of results should also be tested[46] and an additional examination of results carried out. Are there any outliers[111,112]? Are there some strata of particular interest? Such questions may be at the origin of new hypotheses for further studies and research. Light and Pillemer[40] and Greenland[21] are correct in stating that **an analysis of the heterogeneity of studies is more likely to reveal important information than some 'typical' or 'average' effect.**

Most probably, the best and most comprehensive summary of the major steps in a meta-analysis and the relevant issues at each step was given by Durlak and Lipsey[113]. These authors, and others, focus mainly on six components of meta-analysis: research question; literature search; coding procedures, i.e. handling of data; assessment of effects; statistical analyses; and ways of interpreting the findings as well as the conclusions reached. These components listed below are well reflected in many recent reports on prevention and treatment effectiveness, such as BCG immunization in community medicine[114], shortened antibiotic treatment of otitis media in medicine[115], or outcomes following knee replacement in surgery[116], to name a few:

- Objective;
- Data sources;
- Study selection;
- Data extraction;
- Data synthesis; and
- Conclusion.

Table 11.6 Questions based on the new Canadian Medical Association Journal form for reviewers of review articles

Abstract:
- Is the specific purpose of the review stated?
- Are the search methods clearly described?
- Are the important findings clearly summarized?
- Are the major conclusions and recommendations clearly outlined?

Introduction:
- Is the specific purpose of the review clearly stated?
- Were the sources and the methods for identifying the relevant sources clearly described?
- Were the guidelines for including and excluding articles clearly identified?

Findings:
- Was the validity of the included articles assessed objectively?
- Were limitations of the results of the relevant studies identified?
- Was variation in the findings of relevant studies critically analyzed?
- Were the findings of the relevant studies combined appropriately?

Conclusions:
- Was a clear summary of pertinent findings provided?
- Were the reviewers' conclusions supported by the evidence provided?
- Were specific directives for new research initiatives proposed?

Source: Ref. 117, reprinted with permission of the Canadian Medical Association

---

These components direct the reader's attention and search for answers.

Meta-analysis is, in a way, the review of a problem of interest. Hence, any review article identified as a meta-analysis should bear its principal components and philosophy, as was recently proposed (Table 11.6) to Canadian authors[117]. From a clinical point of view, additional attention must be paid in meta-analysis to findings in subgroups[118], be they different prognostic subgroups, various combinations of treatments, or types of original studies[87]. Hasselblad and McCrory[119] propose a flow chart to facilitate the choice of quantitative meta-analysis according to the nature of data (dichotomous, other)

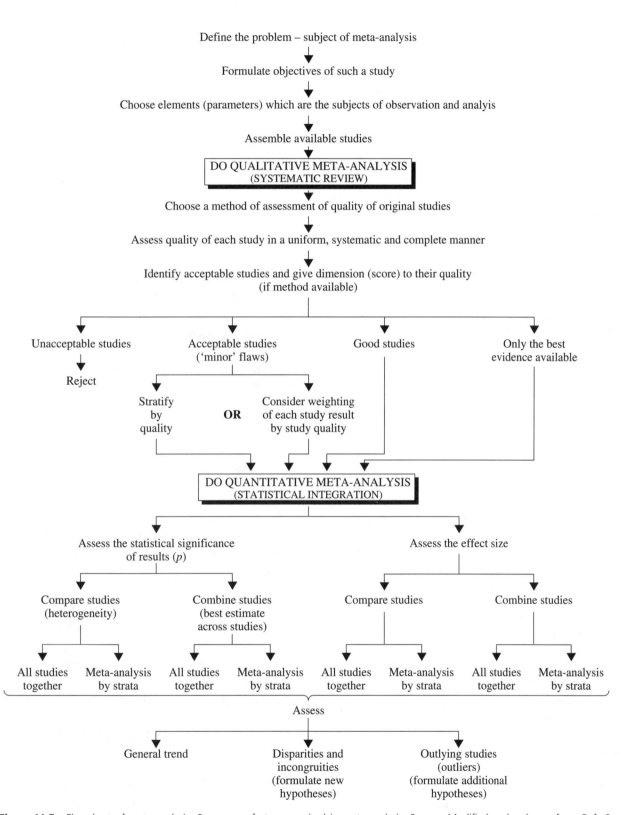

Figure 11.5 Flowchart of meta-analysis. Sequence of steps required in meta-analysis. Source: Modified and redrawn from Ref. 6, with permission from Elsevier Science (*J Clin Epidemiol*)

and fields of application such as diagnosis, cause–effect studies and others.

Finally, validity of currently available evidence, generalization of findings, answers to important clinical questions, and the effect of results on clinical practice must be clarified by meta-analysis. Such relevant findings were originally expected from clinical trials, but they apply to any original study or meta-analysis[120]. At present, there is no scoring system to assess the quality of meta-analysis itself, unlike the system for original studies. Guidelines for research protocols for systematic reviews of randomized control trials require[109,121] the coverage of:

- Protocol development for the systematic review;
- Search strategy;
- Study selection;
- Methodology quality assessment;
- Data extraction;
- Analysis;
- Evaluation of heterogeneity;
- Subgroup analyses;
- Sensitivity analyses;
- Presentation of results;
- Interpretation;
- Dissemination and updating;
- Conduct of trials in the future; and
- Conduct of systematic reviews in the future.

Once the systematic review is finished and ready for publication, it must include the following major elements, which will be easier to do if the above-mentioned requirements for systematic reviews protocols have been respected:

- Structured abstract;
- Background of the problem and systematic review objectives;
- Study selection criteria, search strategy, and quality assessment;
- Methods of data synthesis;
- Results giving evidence tables, quality evaluation results, findings;
- Discussion including limitations and future questions;
- Implications for practice and research;
- Tables, figures and references including excluded studies, unassessed completed studies, and ongoing studies.

Gallagher's paper[122] offers more detailed guidance on how to structure these elements. Understanding desirable components of review articles will enable readers of medical literature to comprehend the meaning of these articles. Very often, readers feel that they do not have enough knowledge to understand the author or authors' meaning. The fault is not always the reader's. Research synthesis must be clear and explicit, according to the following summarized criteria for meta-analyses and research reviews.

11.5 Conclusions and recommendations for the future

Expectations from meta-analysis and systematic reviews are high. All health professionals are expected to understand their principles and their core and use it in their practices. In the meantime, the methodology in this field develops rapidly beyond the universal grasp, yielding specialized methodologists who call themselves 'meta-analysts'. Both should develop common language and understanding.

11.5.1 *Information that should be contained in systematic reviews and meta-analysis*

The following problems, which have been at least partly covered in this chapter, should be better clarified in the future:

- What subjects (topics) and questions are a priority and worthy of systematic review and meta-analysis?
- How does one determine which studies should be combined? (Some ideas have been given here.)
- How can meta-analysis (or meta-analysts') biases be minimized?
- Which quantitative and qualitative techniques are most appropriate?
- What should be done about unpublished studies?
- What is the relevance of findings from meta-analysis for medical practice in prevention and cure? How should such clinical decisions change?
- What is the relevance of findings from meta-analysis for research conclusions and for further orientation of scientific studies?

The notion of the 'importance' of analytic and meta-analytic findings is ambiguous. What is statistically important merits epidemiological analysis, and what is epidemiologically important is not necessarily clinically important. Such scientific importance does not necessarily change clinical decisions. This is equally true for an original study and for a meta-analytic study. Meta-analysis is still presented mainly as a method of evaluating whether a particular treatment works. It should be more than that. Indeed, meta-analysis should be developed and used far beyond randomized clinical trials. Observational descriptive and analytic studies and the evaluation of diagnostic methods are also domains of interest. Meta-analysis in these fields should be further developed.

The analysis of the heterogeneity of studies should not be sacrificed for some global encompassing average or 'typical' value. Both should be analyzed. The pooling of results is sometimes inappropriate, as the results of some studies may be very heterogeneous. This requires analysis rather than a search for some overall picture that would be hard to interpret. As an example, the preventable fraction and effectiveness of a new vaccine may be evaluated in separate trials in developed and developing countries, in healthy subjects, in malnourished subjects or in individuals suffering from an important comorbidity. In such an instance, it is better to analyze differences and to draw new hypotheses and test them, rather than to try to obtain some universal protective ratio which applies to neither group in the original studies.

11.5.2 Projections (fields of application) of meta-analysis and systematic reviews

Meta-analysis should not be seen exclusively as a new tool in etiological and intervention research. An even more important field may be **health policies and health programs,** tactics and strategies at the hospital and in the community. In national politics, meta-analysis may become an important tool to assess effectiveness of interventions in the health field, in order to choose the best ones and thus help control escalating health costs. Available studies of medical care[123,124], of process[125] or of the impact of medical decisions confirm this. The cost-effectiveness of interventions is also open to meta-analysis[126,127]. Indeed, meta-analysis has been used in several distinct and very different fields of applications. For example:

○ In the assessment of already **well-established medical practices** and 'unshakable' paradigms, such as the effectiveness of physical activity in the prevention of coronary heart disease[128], digoxin therapy in congestive heart failure[129], ascorbic acid in the common cold[130], aminophyline in acute severe asthma[131], antibiotic treatment of urinary tract infections[132], progesterone support for normal pregnancy[133–135], psychological and social interventions on outcomes of diabetes[136], aspirin in the prevention of coronary heart disease[137], diuretics in the prevention of pre-eclampsia[138], intracoronary versus intravenous thrombolytic therapy of acute myocardial infarction[139].

○ **Innovative treatments in surgery**[140], new technologies and their effectiveness and impact such as fetal monitoring[73], magnetic resonance imaging[141], transrectal ultrasonography in prostatic cancer[142]. or

○ Other **new technology assessment,** such as the validity of the enzyme immunosorbent assay human immunodeficiency virus antibody test[143].

○ **Alternative medicines** such as acupuncture[144,145].

○ **Administrative measures** such as de-institutionalization in mental health[146].

In a more general sense, the meta-analytical approach is used by the Canadian Task Force in the assessment of various components of the periodic health examination by a systematic and structured approach described in the basic reference[147] and numerous *ad hoc* updates. Several national health technology evaluation agencies use it as well. Uses of systematic reviews in decision analysis and decision-making will be discussed in Chapter 13. At an international level, meta-analysis becomes an important tool in the continuous surveillance and evaluation of the effectiveness and efficiency of medical interventions, coordinated by the Cochrane Collaboration[148,149].

11.6 Advantages and disadvantages of meta-analysis

Despite these extensive applications, as for any other method of work and technique, meta-analysis bears its own advantages and disadvantages summarized in Table 11.7. However, when properly used, it has established itself as a new and integral part of medical reasoning and decision-making. The limitations and advantages of meta-analysis have been widely discussed in the literature. A main challenge remains the risk that the meta-analytic methodology, impressive and at the same time understood by a larger professional audience, will be used indiscriminately, inductively, and without precise operational criteria and guidelines. A very hard look at the data must first occur.

One important and justified reason for critique is that some meta-analysts try to integrate studies (mostly clinical trials) into large sets, expecting that they will obtain a substitute of a large trial with more satisfactory statistical power. The linkage of study results, however, is not linkage of records or another type of multicenter clinical trial. Original trials are heterogeneous in terms of patients, treatments, care and methods of evaluations. Multicenter groups are not. This is not a purpose of meta-analysis, and has not been proposed and accepted into the mainstream of systematic review movement. For a practicing clinician, **it is most often impossible to apply results of meta-analysis to an individual patient.** The most important reason may be overly broad characteristics of patients in integrated studies, demographically and clinically.

11.7 What next?

Medical journals, such as the *Canadian Medical Association Journal*, *Annals of Internal Medicine* or the *New England Journal of Medicine*[150], encourage good meta-analysis of important topics, which cannot be better understood otherwise. In their review, Dickersin and Berlin[151] quote an important rise in the number of meta-analyses published, from 21 in 1986 to 431 in 1991[151], over 500 in 1996[70] and counting. Even critics of meta-analysis should take notice. It is no surprise that systematic reviews have become a critical link in the chain of evidence[152]. They are one of medical training's most important experiences[52,153]. Systematic reviews and meta-analysis are useful well beyond the scope of new drugs or new medical technologies. However, they particularly apply to four specific fields:

Table 11.7 Advantages and disadvantages of meta-analysis in medicine

Advantages of meta-analysis	Disadvantages of meta-analysis
• Its principles are simple and easy to understand even for non-statisticians. • Systematic, structured, and reproducible procedure. • Studies of different types, architecture, and quality (conditional) may be grouped, stratified, evaluated, and integrated. • Integration of several studies increases statistical power of analysis and findings. • May be used in the analysis and integration of findings from multicenter trials. • Additional information, which would never be available from a single study, can be obtained from meta-analysis. • Further development of informatics will allow an even better return to original (individual) data and findings. • Possibility of identifying 'outliers' as an important source of new hypotheses, and giving an additional possibility of identifying and correcting errors.	• Temptation to integrate all studies regardless of their quality. • Meta-analysis works with studies' results; nothing can be changed. The ensemble of good and bad attributes must be accepted. • Main attention is often driven to the effect of main interest. Other effects may be omitted, neglected, or not analyzed. Additional, potentially interesting interactions may be omitted. • It is difficult to integrate studies encompassing various outcomes, measures of impact (dependent variables). • Still unresolved problem of how far the integration should go if studies are too heterogeneous as to different types and groups of patients, treatments, and outcomes. • Difficulty establishing criteria for eligibility of original studies for meta-analysis that are either too restrictive, or too lenient. • Not all authors fully discuss relevance, limitations, misses, and errors of findings from meta-analysis.

1. New drugs and new medical technologies.
2. Treatments and other medical interventions already in use[154].
3. Herbal medicines and other natural alternatives to main stream treatment[155].
4. Biologically still unsubstantiated treatments, circumventing the currently available body of evidence[156].

Beyerstein[157] outlines the reasons for the public's often uncritical acceptance of alternative medicine:

- Anti-intellectualism and anti-scientific attitudes piggy-backing on New Age mysticism.
- Vigorous marketing and extravagant claims.
- Inadequate media scrutiny and attack on critics.
- Social malaise and mistrust of traditional authority figures.
- Anti-doctor backlash.
- Dislike of delivery of scientific biomedicine.
- Myth of safety and less important side effects.

Moreover, logical errors and shortcomings of judgment, missing control groups, wishful thinking, diseases having run their natural course, placebo effects, spontaneous remissions, somatizations, fears of loosing 'wellness', hedging of bets (replacing 'alternative' by 'complementary' or 'integrative' in the qualification of the proposal of alternative care), misdiagnoses, derivative benefits (produced by enthusiasm for and by charismatic healers themselves) compound to form the uncritical appeal of laics and consumers at large[157].

Secondary only to its use in the experimental and clinical field is the use of meta-analysis in public health and health administration. It is becoming an important tool in health planning, allocation of resources and the setting of priorities between various health programs and policies[123,148,150] or clinical strategies[150,151]. Meta-analysis may also be increasingly used by health policy decision-makers in developing countries, where all necessary original research cannot be done, but best decisions must be made given limited resources. Hence, even if they are not involved in original medical and community health research, decision-makers should be trained in the most objective methods allowing for the best decisions in given circumstances.

There are always decisions to be made about whether to do another, better study on the same subject, or whether to remember the childhood lesson 'stop, look and listen' for crossing a road. In other words, it is necessary from time to time to reassess currently available medical knowledge. Such a meta-analytic approach is even more important for decision-makers in governments and institutions, that is, wherever health policies are decided, proposed, and evaluated. Institutions seldom produce first-hand information; however, they are responsible for the best possible evaluation of current information and for the best possible implementation of adequate health policies and programs. This should not be the subject of improvisation or solely a matter of serendipity and flair. Even if political decisions finally override recommendations, well-organized research is needed. Better political decisions will follow[20].

Perhaps meta-analysis and systematic reviews in medicine should not be considered fairly recent or new. Winkelstein[158] examines whether the first 'meta-analyst' in medicine was Joseph Goldberger (of pellagra fame) who, in 1907, reported a systematic review and pooled data from 47 studies conducted between 1881–1907 on the origin and prevalence of typhoid fever in the District of Columbia. Does this complete a full circle, or was James Lind[159] the first 'meta-analyst'? Of course, meta-analysis dates back to the beginning of time – Gordis[160] points to the first program evaluation found in the first chapter of the Book of Genesis:

' 1. *In the beginning, God created heaven and the earth . . .*

 . . .

31. *And God saw every thing that he made, and, behold, it was very good. And the evening and the morning were the sixth day.*'

Peer reviews, consensus, clinical trials and systematic reviews of evidence came only later, after this *n*-of-1 expert opinion evaluation.

Chapter 12 gives an overview of some uses of evidence in logical thinking and Chapter 13 examines how precepts from this and previous chapters are used and integrated in medical decision-making and its products, such as clinical and public health guidelines and recommendations.

REFERENCES

1. Matz R. Principles of medicine. *NY State J Med*, 1977;**77**:99–101

2. Cook DJ, Mulrow CD, Haynes RB. Systematic reviews: Synthesis of best evidence for clinical decisions. *Ann Intern Med*, 1977;**126**:376–80

3. *New Illustrated Webster's Dictionary of The English Language. Thesaurus.* New York: PAMCO Publishing, 1992

4. Last JM (ed.). *A Dictionary of Epidemiology.* 4th Edition. Oxford and New York: Oxford University Press, 2001

5. Jenicek M. *Méta-analyse en médecine. Évaluation et synthèse de l'information clinique et épidémiologique. (Meta-Analysis in Medicine. Evaluation and Synthesis of Clinical and Epidemiological Information.)* St. Hyacinthe and Paris: EDISEM and Maloine, 1987

6. Jenicek M. Meta-analysis in medicine. Where we are and where we want to go. *J Clin Epidemiol*, 1989; **42**:35–44

7. Glass GV. Primary, secondary, and meta-analysis of research. *Educ Res*, 1976;**5**:3–8

8. Thurber S, Walker CE. Medication and hyperactivity: A meta-analysis. *J Gen Psychol*, 1983;**108**: 79–86

9. Kavale K. The efficacy of stimulant drug treatment for hyperactivity: A meta-analysis. *J Learn Disabil*, 1982;**15**:280–9

10. Kavale KA, Forness SR. Hyperactivity and diet treatment: A meta-analysis of the Feingold hypothesis. *J Learn Disabil*, 1983;**16**:324–30

11. Mattes J. The Feingold diet: A current reappraisal. *J Learn Disabil*, 1983;**16**:319–23

12. Steinbrueck SM, Maxwell SE, Howard GS. A meta-analysis of psychotherapy and drug therapy in the treatment of unipolar depression with adults. *J Consult Clin Psychol*, 1983;**51**:856–63

13. Smith ML, Glass GV. Meta-analysis of psychotherapy outcome studies. *Am Psychol*, 1977;**37**: 752–60

14. Rotton J, Kelly IW. Much ado about full moon: A meta-analysis of lunar-lunacy research. *Psychol Bull*, 1985;**97**:286–306

15. Kavale KA, Glass GV. Meta-analysis and the integration of research in special education. *J Learn Disabil*, 1981;**14**:531–8

16. Mann C. Meta-analysis in the breech. *Science*, 1990;**249**:476–80

17. Mulrow CD. The medical review article: State of the science. *Ann Intern Med*, 1987;**106**:485–8

18. Haynes RB, Mulrow CD, Huth EJ, et al. More informative abstracts revisited. *Ann Intern Med*, 1990; **113**:69–76

19. L'Abbé KA, Detsky AS, O'Rourke K. Meta-analysis in clinical research. *Ann Intern Med*, 1987;**107**: 224–33

20. Thacker SB. Meta-analysis. A quantitative approach to research integration. *JAMA*, 1988;**259**:1685–9

21. Greenland S. Quantitative methods in the review of epidemiologic literature. *Epidemiologic Reviews*, 1987;**9**:1-30

22. Sacks HS, Berrier J, Reitman D, et al. Meta-analyses of randomized clinical trials. *N Engl J Med*, 1987; **316**:450–5

23. Colton T, Friedman LS, Johnson AL (eds). Proceedings of the Workshop on Methodologic Issues in Overviews of Randomized Clinical Trials, May 1986. *Stat Med*, 1987;**6**:217–410

24. Petitti DB. *Meta-Analysis, Decision-Analysis and Cost-Effectiveness Analysis. Methods for Quantitative Synthesis in Medicine.* 2nd Edition. Monographs in Epidemiology and Biostatistics. Volume 31. New York and Oxford: Oxford University Press, 2000

25. Lipsey MW, Wilson DB. *Practical Meta-Analysis.* Applied Social Research Methods Series, Volume 49. Thousand Oaks, CA: Sage Publications, 2001

26. Goldman L, Feinstein AR. Anticoagulants and myocardial infarction. The problems of pooling, drowning, and floating. *Ann Intern Med*, 1989;**90**:92–4

27. Naylor CD. Two cheers for meta-analysis: problems and opportunities in aggregating results of clinical trials. *Can Med Ass J*, 1988;**138**:891–5

28. Goodman SN. Have you ever meta-analysis you didn't like? *Ann Intern Med*, 1991;**114**:244–6

29. Feinstein AR. Meta-analysis: Statistical alchemy for the 21st century. *J Clin Epidemiol*, 1995;**48**:71–9

30. Summing up. In: Fletcher RH, Fletcher SW, Wagner EH. *Clinical Epidemiology. The Essentials.* 2nd Edition. Baltimore: Williams & Wilkins, 1988: 226–40

31. Meta-analysis in medicine. Putting experiences together. In: Jenicek M. *Epidemiology. The Logic of Modern Medicine.* Montreal: EPIMED International, 1995:267–95

32. Zautra A, Hempel A. Subjective well-being and physical health: A narrative literature review with suggestions for future research. *Int J Aging Hum Dev*, 1984;**19**:95–110

33. McDonald JC, McDonald AD. Epidemiology of mesothelioma from estimated incidence. *Prev Med*, 1977;**6**:426–46

34. Yusuf S, Wittes J, Friedman L. Overview of results of randomized clinical trials in heart disease. I. Treatments following myocardial infarction. *JAMA*, 1988;**260**:2088–93. II. Unstable angina, heart failure, primary prevention with aspirin, and risk factor modification. *Idem*:2259–63

35. Light RJ, Smith PV. Accumulating evidence: Procedures for resolving contradictions among different research studies. *Harvard Educ Rev*, 1971;**41**: 429–71

36. Frishman WH, Charlap S, Rotmensch HH, Furberg DC. Beta-adrenergic blockade in patients with myocardial infarction. Treatment and prevention. In: Frishman WH. *Clinical Pharmacology of the Beta-Adrenoceptor Blocking Drugs*. 2nd Edition. Norwalk, CN: Appleton-Century-Crofts, 1984;**10**: 299–340

37. Hedges LV, Olkin I. Vote-counting methods in research synthesis. *Psychol Bull*, 1980;**88**:359–69

38. George LK, Landerman R. Health and subjective well-being: A replicated secondary data analysis. *Int J Aging Hum Dev*, 1984;**19**:133–56

39. Rosenthal R. Assessing the statistical and social importance of the effects of psychotherapy. *J Consult Clin Psychol*, 1983;**51**:4–13

40. Light RJ, Pillemer DB. *Summing-Up. The Science of Reviewing Research*. Cambridge, MA: Harvard University Press, 1984

41. Einarson TR, McGhan WF, Bootman J, Sabers DL. Meta-analysis: Quantitative integration of independent results. *Am J Hosp Pharm*, 1985;**42**:1957–64

42. Glass GV, McGaw B, Smith ML. *Meta-Analysis of Social Research*. Beverly Hills, CA: Sage Publications, 1981

43. Cohen J. *Statistical Power Analysis For the Behavioral Sciences*. New York: Academic Press, 1977

44. Jacobson NS (ed.). Defining Clinically Significant Change. *Behav Ass* (Special Issue), 1988;**10**:131–223

45. Light RJ (ed.). Evaluation Studies Review Annual, 1983. Beverly Hills: Sage Publications, 1983;**8**

46. Hedges LV, Olkin I. *Statistical Methods for Meta-Analysis*. New York: Academic Press, 1985

47. Rosenthal R. Meta-analysis: A review. *Psychosom Med*, 1991;**53**:247–71

48. Rosenthal R. The 'File Drawer Problem' and tolerance for null results. *Psychol Bull*, 1979;**86**:638–41

49. Friedman H. Magnitude of experimental effect and a table for its rapid estimation. *Psychol Bull*, 1968;**70**:245–51

50. Hetherington J, Dickersin K, Chalmers I, Meinert CL. Retrospective and prospective identification of unpublished controlled trials: Lessons from a survey of obstetricians and pediatricians. *Pediatrics*, 1989; **84**:374–80

51. Eastbrook PJ, Berlin JA, Gopalan R, Matthews DR. Publication bias in clinical research. *Lancet*, 1991;**337**:867–72

52. McQuay HJ, Moore RA. Using numerical results from systematic reviews in clinical practice. *Ann Intern Med*, 1997;**126**:712–20

53. Gilbert JP, McPeek B, Mosteller F. Progress in surgery and anesthesia: Benefits and risks of innovative therapy. In: Bunker JP, Barnes BA, Mosteller F eds. *Costs, Risks, and Benefits of Surgery*. New York: Oxford University Press, 1977:156–61

54. Stampfer MJ, Goldhaber SZ, Yusuf S, et al. Effect of intravenous streptokinase on acute myocardial infarction. Pooled results from randomized trials. *N Engl J Med*, 1982;**307**:1180–2

55. Yusuf S, Peto R, Lewis J, et al. Beta blockade during and after myocardial infarction: An overview of the randomized trails. *Prog Cardiovasc Dis*, 1985;**27**: 335–71

56. Collins R, Langman M. Treatment with histamine H2 antagonists in acute upper gastrointestinal haemorrhage. *N Engl J Med*, 1985;**313**:660–6

57. Mantel N, Haenzsel W. Statistical aspects of the analysis of data from retrospective studies of disease. *J Nat Cancer Inst*, 1959;**22**:719–48

58. Janicak PG, Davis JM, Gibbons RD, et al. Efficacy of ECT: A meta-analysis. *Am J Psychiatry*, 1985;**142**: 297–302

59. The Cochrane Collaboration. *Review Manager (RevMan)* 4.1. [Computer Program]. Version 4.1 for Windows. Oxford, England: The Cochrane Collaboration. 2000: http://www.cochrane.org/cochrane/revman.htm

60. Centres for Disease Control and Prevention. *Epi Meta* (software). Atlanta: CDC, 2001. http://www.cdc.gov/epo/dpram/epimeta/epimeta.htm

61. Lacroix J, Infante-Rivard C, Jenicek M, Gauthier M. Prophylaxis of upper gastrointestinal bleeding in intensive care units: A meta-analysis. *Crit Care Med*, 1989;**17**:862–9

62. Lau J, Antman EM, Jimenez-Silva J, Kupelnick B, et al. Cumulative meta-analysis of therapeutic trials for myocardial infarction. *N Engl J Med*, 1992;**327**: 248–54

63. DerSimonian R, Laird N. Meta-analysis and clinical trials. *Contr Clin Trials*, 1986;**7**:177–88

64. Cochran WG. The combination of estimates from different experiments. *Biometrics*, 1954;**10**:101–29

65. Himel HN, Liberati A, Gelber RD, Chalmers TC. Adjuvant chemotherapy for breast cancer. A pooled estimate based on published randomized control trials. *JAMA*, 1986;**256**:1148–59

66. Clemens JD, Chong JJH, Feinstein AR. The BCG controversy. A methodological and statistical reappraisal. *JAMA*, 1983;**249**:2362–9

67. Wortman PM, Yeaton WH. Cumulating quality of life results in controlled trials of coronary artery bypass graft surgery. *Contr Clin Trials*, 1985;**6**: 289–305

68. Antman EM, Lau J, Kupelnick B, et al. A comparison of results of meta-analyses of randomized control trials and recommendations of clinical experts. Treatments for myocardial infarction. *JAMA*, 1992; **268**:240–8

69. Lau J, Ioannidis JPA, Schmid CH. Quantitative synthesis in systematic reviews. *Ann Intern Med*, 1997;**127**:820–6

70. Lau J, Ioannidis JPA, Schmid CH. Summing up evidence: one answer is not always enough. *Lancet*, 1998;**351**:123–7

71. Walker AM, Martin–Moreno JM, Rodriguez Artelejo F. Odd Man Out: A graphical approach to meta-analysis. *Am J Public Health*, 1988;**78**:961–6

72. Williamson DF, Parker RA, Kendrick JS. The Box Plot: A simple visual method to interpret data. *Ann Intern Med*, 1989;**110**:916–21

73. Le Coutour X, Jenicek M. Plus de monitoring foetal, plus de césariennes? Essai de la méta-analyse du problème. (Does more fetal monitoring mean more cesarean sections? Attempting meta-analysis of the problem). *Rev Épidém et Santé Publ*, 1989;**37**:61–72

74. Feinstein AR. *Clinical Epidemiology. The Architecture of Clinical Research*. Twenty scientific principles for trohoc research, pp. 543–7. Scientific standards in an excellent study, pp. 552–3. Philadelphia: WB Saunders, 1985

75. Lichtenstein MJ, Mulrow CD, Elwood PC. Guidelines for reading case–control studies. *J Chron Dis*, 1987;**40**:893–903

76. DerSimonian R, Charette J, McPeek B, Mosteller F. Reporting on methods in clinical trials. *N Engl J Med*, 1982;**306**:1332–7

77. Detsky AS, Naylor CD, O'Rourke K, et al. Incorporating variations in the quality of individual randomized trials into meta-analysis. *J Clin Epidemiol*, 1992;**45**:255–65

78. Callahan CM, Dittus RS, Katz BP. Oral corticosteroid therapy for patients with stable chronic obstructive pulmonary disease. A meta-analysis. *Ann Intern Med*, 1991;**114**:216–23

79. Realini JP, Goldzieher JW. Oral contraceptives and cardio-vascular disease: A critique of the epidemiologic studies. *Am J Obstet Gynecol*, 1985;**152**:729–98

80. Chalmers TC, Smith Jr H, Blackburn B, et al. A method for assessing the quality of a randomized clinical trial. *Contr Clin Trials*, 1981;**2**:31–49

81. Haynes RB, Sackett DL in collaboration with Taylor DW, et al. Appendix I: An annotated bibliography (including notes on methodological standards for compliance research). In: Sackett DL, Haynes RB eds. *Compliance with Therapeutic Regimens*. Baltimore and London: The Johns Hopkins University Press, 1976:193–9

82. Haynes RB, Taylor DW, Snow JC, Sackett DL in collaboration with Tugwell PJ, et al. Appendix I: Annotated and indexed bibliography on compliance with therapeutic and preventive regimens. In: Haynes RB, Taylor DW, Sackett DL eds. *Compliance in Health Care*. Baltimore and London: The Johns Hopkins University Press, 1979:337–43

83. Oxman AD, Guyatt GH. Validation of an index of the quality of review articles. *J Clin Epidemiol*, 1991;**44**:1271–8

84. Stroup DF, Berlin JA, Morton SC, et al. for the Meta-analysis of Observational Studies in Epidemiology (MOOSE) Group. Meta-analysis of observational studies in epidemiology. A proposal for reporting. *JAMA*, 2000;**283**:2008–12

85. Fleiss JL, Gross AJ. Meta-analysis in epidemiology, with special reference to studies of the association between exposure to environmental tobacco smoke and lung cancer: A critique. *J Clin Epidemiol*, 1991;**44**:127–39

86. Slavin RE. Best-evidence synthesis: an alternative to meta-analytic and traditional reviews. *Educ Res*, 1986;**15**:5–11 (Reprinted in: *Eval Stud Rev Ann*, 1987;**12**:667–73)

87. Gerberg ZB, Horwitz RI. Resolving conflicting clinical trials: guidelines for meta-analysis. *J Clin Epidemiol*, 1988;**41**:503–9

88. Hayes PC, Davis JM, Lewis JA, Bouchier IAD. Meta-analysis of value of propranolol in prevention of variceal haemorrhage. *Lancet*, 1990;**336**:153–6

89. Spitzer WO, Lawrence V, Dapes R, et al. Links between passive smoking and disease: A best evidence synthesis. A report of the Working Group on Passive Smoking. *Clin Invest Med*, 1990;**13**:17–42

90. Midgette AS, Stukel TA, Littenberg B. A meta-analytic method for summarizing diagnostic test performances: receiver-operating-characteristic-summary point estimates. *Med Decis Making*, 1993;**13**:253–7

91. Irwig L, Tosteson NA, Gatsonis C, Lau J, et al. Guidelines for meta-analyses evaluating diagnostic tests. *Ann Intern Med*, 1994;**120**:667–76

92. Koch M, Capurso L, Llewelyn H. Analysing the discriminating power of individual symptoms, signs and test results. In: Llewelyn H, Hopkins A eds. *Analysing How We Reach Clinical Decisions*. London: Royal College of Physicians of London, 1993:51–67

93. Oxman AD, Guyatt GH. A consumer's guide to subgroup analyses. *Ann Intern Med*, 1992;**116**:78–84

94. Arana GW, Baldesarini RJ, Ornsteen M. The dexamethasone suppression test for diagnosis and prognosis in psychiatry. *Arch Gen Psychiatry*, 1985;**42**:1193–204

95. Vroomen PCAJ, de Krom MCTFM, Knottnerus JA. Diagnostic value of history and physical examination in patients suspected of sciatica due to disc herniation: a systematic review. *J Neurol*, 1999;**246**:899–906

96. Craig JV, Lancaster GA, Williamson PR, Smyth RL. Temperature measured at the axilla compared with

rectum in children and young people; systematic review. *Br Med J*, 2000;**320**:1174–8

97. Jones DR. Meta-analysis of observational epidemiological studies: a review. *J Roy Soc Med*, 1992; **85**:165–8

98. Mahoney MC, Michalek AM. A meta-analysis of cancer incidence in United States and Canadian native populations. *Int J Epidemiol*, 1991;**20**:323–7

99. Gray Davis L, Weber DJ, Lemon SM. Horizontal transmission of hepatitis B virus. *Lancet*, 1989;**1**: 889–93

100. 100. Schlesselman JJ, Stadel BV, Murray P, et al. Consistency and plausibility in epidemiologic analysis: Application to breast cancer in relation to use of oral contraceptives. *J Chron Dis*, 1987;**40**:1033–9

101. Guyatt GH, Weber CE, Mewa AA, Sackett DL. Determining causation – a case study: adrenocorticosteroids and osteoporosis. Should the fear of inducing clinically important oesteoporosis influence the decision to prescribe adrenocorticosteroids? *J Chron Dis*, 1984;**37**:343–52

102. Broadhead WE, Kaplan BH, James SA, et al. The epidemiological evidence for a relationship between social support and health. *Am J Epidemiol*, 1983; **117**:521–37

103. Heyland D, Mandell LA. Gastric colonization by Gram-negative bacilli and nosocomial pneumonia in the intensive care unit patient. Evidence for causation. *Chest*, 1992;**101**:187–93

104. Surgeon General's Advisory Committee on Smoking and Health. *Smoking and Health*. Washington: Public Health Service Publ., No 1103, 1973

105. Ozminkowski RJ, Wortman PM, Roloff DW. Inborn/outborn status and neonatal survival: A meta-analysis of non-randomized studies. *Stat Med*, 1988;**7**:1207–21

106. Cuzick J, Stewart H, Peto R, et al. Overview of randomized trials of postoperative adjuvant radiotherapy in breast cancer. *Cancer Treat Rep*, 1987; **71**:15–29

107. Early Breast Cancer Trialists' Collaborative Group. Effect of adjuvant tamoxifen and of cytotoxic therapy on mortality in early breast cancer. An overview of 61 randomized trials among 28,896 women. *N Engl J Med*, 1988;**319**:1681–92

108. Shore T, Nelson N, Weinerman B. A meta-analysis of stages I and II Hodgkin's disease. *Cancer*, 1990;**65**: 1155–60

109. Oxman AD, Cook DJ, Guyatt GH for the Evidence-Based Medicine Working Group. Users' guides to the medical literature. VI. How to use an overview. *JAMA*, 1994;**272**:1367–71

110. Mulrow C, Cook D (eds). *Systematic Reviews. Synthesis of the Best Evidence for Health Care Decisions*. Philadelphia: American College of Physicians, 1998

111. Bolton S. Outliers. In: *Pharmaceutical Statistics. Practical and Clinical Applications*. New York: Marcel Dekker Inc., 1984:294–300 and 485

112. Canner PL, Huang YB, Meinert CL. On the detection of outlier clinics in medical and surgical trials. I. Practical considerations. *Contr Clin Trials*, 1981;**2**: 231–40. II. Theoretical considerations. *Idem*:241–52

113. Durlak JAS, Lipsey MW. A practitioner's guide to meta-analysis. *Am J Comm Psychol*, 1991;**19**:291–332

114. Colditz GA, Brewer TF, Berkey CS, et al. Efficacy of BCG vaccine in the prevention of tuberculosis. Meta-analysis of published literature. *JAMA*, 1994; **271**:698–702

115. Kozyrskij AL, Hildes-Ripstein GE, Longstaffe SEA, et al. Treatment of acute otitis media with a shortened course of antibiotics. *JAMA*, 1998;**279**: 1736–42

116. Callahan CM, Drake BG, Heck DA, Dittus RS. Patient outcomes following tricompartmental total knee replacement. A meta-analysis. *JAMA*, 1994; **271**:1349–57

117. Squires BP. Biomedical review articles: What editors want from authors and peer reviewers. *Can Med Ass J*, 1989;**141**:195–7

118. Oxman AD, Guyatt GH. A consumer's guide to subgroup analyses. *Ann Intern Med*, 1992;**116**:78–84

119. Hasselblad V, McCrory DC. Meta-analytic tools for medical decision-making: A practical guide. *Med Decis Making*, 1995;**15**:81–96

120. Laupacis A, Conolly SJ, Gent M, et al. for the CAFA Study Group. How should results from completed studies influence ongoing clinical trials? The CAFA Study experience. *Ann Intern Med*, 1991;**115**:818–22

121. Cook DJ, Sackett DL, Spitzer WO. Methodologic guidelines for systematic reviews of randomized control trials in health care from the Potsdam consultation on meta-analysis. *J Clin Epidemiol*, 1995;**48**: 167–71

122. Gallagher EJ. Systematic reviews: A logical methodological extension of evidence-based medicine. *Acad Emerg Med*, 1999;**6**:1255–60

123. Silberman G, Droitcour JA, Scullin EW. Cross Design Synthesis. *A New Strategy for Medical Effectiveness Research. Report to Congressional Requesters*. Washington: United States General Accounting Office, Publ No GAO/PEMD-92-18, March 1992

124. Droitcour J, Silberman G, Chelimsky E. Cross-design synthesis. A new form of meta-analysis for combining results from randomized clinical trials and medical-practice databases. *Int J Technol Ass Health Care*, 1993;**9**:440–9

125. Posavac EJ, Sinacore JM, Brotherton SE, et al. Increasing compliance with medical treatment regimens. A meta-analysis of program evaluation. *Eval Health Prof*, 1985;**8**:7–22

126. Oster G, Huse DM, Delea TE, Colditz GA. Cost-effectiveness of nicotine gum as an adjunct to physician's advice against cigarette smoking. *JAMA*, 1986;**256**:1315–18

127. Udvarhelyi S, Colditz GA, Rai A, Epstein AM. Cost-effectiveness and cost-benefit analysis in the medical literature. Are the methods being used correctly? *Ann Intern Med*, 1992;**116**:238–44

128. Berlin JA, Colditz GA. A meta-analysis of physical activity in the prevention of coronary heart disease. *Am J Epidemiol*, 1990;**132**:612–28

129. Jaeschke R, Oxman AD, Guyatt GH. To what extent do congestive heart failure patients in sinus rhythm benefit from digoxin therapy? A systematic overview and meta-analysis. *Am J Med*, 1990;**88**:279–86

130. Chalmers TC. Effects of ascorbic acid on the common cold. An evaluation of the evidence. *Am J Med*, 1975;**58**:532–6

131. Littenberg B. Aminophyline treatment in severe, acute asthma. *JAMA*, 1988;**259**:1678–84

132. Philbrick JT, Bracikowski JP. Single-dose antibiotic treatment of uncomplicated urinary tract infections. Less for less? *Arch Intern Med*, 1985;**145**:1672–8

133. Macdonald RR. Does treatment with progesterone prevent miscarriage? *Br J Obstet Gynaecol*, 1989;**96**:257–64

134. Goldstein P, Berrier J, Rosen S, et al. A meta-analysis of randomized control trials of progestational agents in pregnancy. *Br J Obstet Gynaecol*, 1989;**96**:265–74

135. Daya S. Efficacy of progesterone support for pregnancy in women with recurrent miscarriage. A meta-analysis of controlled trials. *Br J Obstet Gynaecol*, 1989;**96**:275–80

136. Padgett D, Mumford E, Hynes M, Carter R. Meta-analysis of the effects of educational and psycho-social interventions on management of diabetes mellitus. *J Clin Epidemiol*, 1988;**41**:1007–30

137. Canner PL. An overview of six clinical trials of aspirin in coronary heart disease. *Stat Med*, 1987;**6**:255–63.

138. Collins R, Yusuf S, Peto R. Overview of randomized trials of diuretics in pregnancy. *Br Med J*, 1985;**290**:17–23

139. Marder VJ, Francis CW. Thrombolytic therapy for acute transmural myocardial infarction. Intra-coronary versus intravenous. *Am J Med*, 1984;**77**:921–8

140. Gilbert JP, McPeek, Mosteller F. Progress in surgery and anesthesia: Benefits and risks of innovative therapy. In: Bunker JP, Barnes BA, Mosteller F eds. *Costs, Risks, and Benefits of Surgery*. New York: Oxford University Press, 1977:124–69

141. Cooper LS, Chalmers TC, McCally M, et al. The poor quality of early evaluations of magnetic resonance imaging. *JAMA*, 1988;**259**:3277–80

142. Diagnostic and Therapeutic Technology Assessment (DATA). Transrectal ultrasonography in prostatic cancer. *JAMA*, 1988;**259**:2757–60

143. Philips KA. The use of meta-analysis in technology assessment: A meta-analysis of the enzyme immuno-absorbent assay human immunodeficiency virus antibody test. *J Clin Epidemiol*, 1991;**44**:925–31

144. Patel M, Gutzwiller F, Paccaud F, Marazzi A. A meta-analysis of acupuncture for chronic pain. *Int J Epidemiol*, 1989;**18**:900–6

145. ter Riet G, Klejnen J, Knipschild P. Acupuncture and chronic pain: A criteria-based meta-analysis. *J Clin Epidemiol*, 1990;**43**:1191–9

146. Straw RB. Deinstitutionalization in mental health. A meta-analysis. In: *Evaluation Studies Review Annual*. Volume 8. Beverly Hills: Sage Publications, 1983:253–78

147. The Canadian Task Force on the Periodic Health Examination. *The Canadian Guide to Clinical Preventive Health Care*. Ottawa: Health Canada, 1994

148. The Cochrane Collaboration. Preparing, maintaining and disseminating systematic reviews of the effects of health care. Oxford: The UK Cochrane Centre, 1994:12 pp

149. Chalmers I, Haynes B. Reporting, updating, and correcting systematic reviews of the effects of heath care. *Br Med J*, 1994;**309**:862–5

150. Kassirer JP. Clinical trials and meta-analysis. What do they do for us? *N Engl J Med*, 1992;**327**:273–4

151. Dickersin K, Berlin JA. Meta-analysis: State-of-the-science. *Epidemiol Rev*, 1992;**14**:154–76

152. Mulrow CD, Cook DJ, Davidoff F. Systematic reviews: Critical links in the great chain of evidence. *Ann Intern Med*, 1997;**126**:389–91

153. Badgett RG, O'Keefe M, Henderson MC. Using systematic reviews in clinical education. *Ann Intern Med*, 1997;**126**:886–91

154. Thomas M, Del Mar C, Glasziou P. How effective are treatments of other than antibiotics for acute sore throat? *Br J Gen Pract*, 2000;**50**:817–20

155. Vogler BK, Ernst E. Aloe vera: a systematic review of its clinical effectiveness. *Br J Gen Pract*, 1999;**49**:823–8

156. Cooke B, Ernst E. Aromatherapy: a systematic review. *Br J Gen Pract*, 2000;**50**:493–6

157. Beyerstein BL. Alternative medicine and common errors of reasoning. *Acad Med*, 2001;**76**:230–7

158. Winkelstein W Jr. The first use of meta-analysis? *Am J Epidemiol*, 1998;**147**:717

159. Hampton JR. The end of medical history? *J Roy Coll Physic Lond*, 1998;**32**:366–75

160. Gordis L. *Epidemiology*. 2nd Edition. Philadelphia: WB Saunders, 2000

Using evidence and logic in everyday clinical reasoning, communication, and legal and scientific argumentation

'. . . You know, I had those aches, coughs and sneezes for a whole week! Then, I asked my Doc to give me some really strong stuff like antibiotics. In two days, all my troubles disappeared! His pills really worked! Boy, this Doc is a pretty smart guy! . . .'
Overheard in a local watering hole.

'. . . Don't tell anyone, but to get rid of my flu, I went to see a homeopath. She prescribed me powdered pieces of the Berlin Wall. People say it doesn't work. But look, no one has proved that it doesn't and my case shows that it does. . . .'
Overheard during a coffee break at a downtown office.

Fuzzy premises lead to fuzzy conclusions. However, final decisions in medicine must always be clear and precise. Or must they?

Good medicine relies not only on good evidence, but also on the ways evidence is used. Besides evidence itself, the second key factor then, is how evidence is integrated within our reasoning and how we convey our conclusions to their intended recipients. Any good evidence, such as a valid diagnostic test or the effectiveness of a new vaccine demonstrated in an impeccable clinical trial, is useful and beneficial only when applied critically. In other terms, it can be used well or poorly depending on how we introduce it in our reasoning about the health problem under scrutiny. Did we properly assess the risks and benefits of an intervention? Did we properly choose the individuals who would benefit the most from a new treatment? And so on. **Critical thinking** can be defined as *the process of evaluating a claim for the purpose of deciding whether to accept, reject, or perhaps suspend judgment about it . . . or as . . . reasonable reflective thinking that is focused on deciding what to believe or do*[1]. A simpler definition was proposed by Ennis[2,3]: '. . . *Reasonable reflective thinking that is focused on deciding what to believe or do . . . .*' For Harrison[4], **rational thought** means . . . *to analyze reasons given for different statements and to determine how these reasons are related in justifying and/or understanding other statements.*

As we will see further in this chapter, critical use of evidence is necessary not only at the patient's bedside, but also equally in research and in health policies and programs. In public health, critical thinking is vital in properly presenting to governmental bodies, decision-makers, and other stakeholders, the soundness and relevance of health programs and policies that we propose, implement and evaluate. Critical thinking in medicine is about deciding and conveying well to others what we are doing or what we intend to do, not for our personal intellectual satisfaction, but for the full benefit of the patient or the community.

12.1 Introducing evidence into the process of logic

Obtaining evidence is only the first, important step of our work. The next step is to use this evidence correctly. Defending our ideas and putting them into practice is based on arguments, not in the colloquial confrontational sense of the term, but rather as they are defined in logic and briefly outlined in Chapter 3. Uses of logic are expected to sharpen reasoning, to improve the analysis of arguments, to develop the capacity to evaluate arguments as good or bad or better or worse[5], as well as to assess the real value of their conclusions.

12.2 Clinical rounds, reports, papers, testimonies, and health policies as arguments

As already briefly mentioned in Chapter 3, the practice of medicine itself (not only research) relies heavily on logic and critical thinking:

- In the clinical management of **individual patients** in daily hospital and family practice, we want our patients to understand our decisions and recommendations and explain to them what lead us to the treatment plan.
- At **clinical rounds**, we try to find the best possible common ground with our peers for the clinical work-up of a patient including treatment plans.
- At **scientific gatherings**, we must convincingly explain our findings.
- At business **meetings on health programs and policies**, we must justify health interventions and human and material resources involved.
- In **legal litigations** involving occupational and environmental health issues for individual patients or whole communities, our arguments must be understood not only by health professionals, but by all other decision-makers.
- At any other gathering focusing on **decision-making**.
- In our **research papers**, discussion of our findings and our recommendations rely not only on the 'hard' evidence of the results themselves, but also and mainly on their critical analysis.

The practice of good medicine relies as well on our ability to properly explain the reasoning which leads to our conclusions and which is translated into clinical orders, health programs and policy implementation decisions, as well as into our legal views of individuals or situations under scrutiny. Some patients will accept our orders ('take this pill twice a day after meals!' . . . 'between you and me, I would definitely operate!') without comment. They expect that the physician will think and decide for them. Others will rightfully ask 'why?' Explaining and justifying our decisions is a learned experience, as is our volume of acquired knowledge or practical clinical skills. With the exception of unfortunate dogmatic and/or unsubstantiated decisions and declarations, health policy makers, planners, funding agencies, administrators and politicians will always ask 'why?' The more important the expected impact of our interpretations and decisions, the more solid the evidence and its uses in decision-related reasoning should be. Using and 'selling' evidence is also a learned skill. Needless to say, our argumentation must be flawless, realistic, and correct. To ensure this, let us add to the fundamentals of reasoning from Chapter 3 some additional considerations and examples to keep in mind and/or avoid.

12.3 Logical argumentation in medicine

Valid argumentation in any medical discourse relies not only on the validity of evidence, but also on the way in which it is incorporated and interpreted in our reasoning. (We shouldn't forget that 'Reasoning is thinking enlightened by logic.'[6]) Any orders for diagnostic work-up, treatment, follow-up, or research proposals are the result of some kind of logical argument as defined in logic, whether purely Aristotelian as briefly outlined in Chapter 3, modified, correct or flawed.

12.4 Argument and argumentation the Aristotelian way

How can an **argument** be defined? In light of this term's definitions in Chapter 3, for Weston[7], '. . . to give an argument means to offer a set of reasons of evidence in support of a conclusion . . .'. For Copi[5], an argument is '. . . any group of propositions of which one is claimed to follow from the others, which are regarded as providing support or grounds for the truth of that one . . .'. An argument is expected to yield a better view of a problem and to support such a view. Sometimes, we use classical categorical syllogisms: one or more categorical

premises supporting and leading to some categorical conclusion. However, in daily life, the conclusion is presented first ('my patient must get antibiotics') and premises follow ('because he or she has a bacterial infection proven sensitive to antibiotics') in the reverse order of a classical syllogism.

In medical practice, syllogisms may look truncated by keeping one of the premises tacit: 'my patient must get antibiotics', because 'he has a bacterial infection'. This tacitly admits the premise that the infection responds well to antibiotics. An argument is called an **enthymeme** when one of the premises of the conclusion is not expressed[8]. For Hitchcock[9,10 and pers. comm.] however, 'such arguments generally do not have tacit premises. Rather, they should be evaluated as they stand to see whether there is a justified general principle (universal or probabilistic – 'most', 'usually'), presumptive 'presumably' or possibilistic ('sometimes') in accordance with which the conclusion follows non-trivially from the premises.' In this case, only a qualified principle 'most patients with a bacterial infection must receive antibiotics' is justified given exceptions: some agents may be resistant to antibiotics.

The solidity and value of an argument for medical decision-making rely on:

- The best evidence representing the desired body of each premise, and
- The way premises really lead to proposed conclusions.

For example, a randomized double-blind controlled trial may be the best evidence of effectiveness of drug control of arthritis in elderly patients. In our office, we have to decide how to treat an elderly arthritis sufferer seeking some relief from pain and dysfunction. We can reason in the following way:

Premise A: Many controlled clinical trials, as well as their systematic review, produce corroborating results showing that drug M has been proven effective in controlling the symptoms of chronic degenerative arthritis diagnosed according to a set of inclusion and exclusion criteria.

Premise B: My patient is an elderly sufferer whose arthritis was diagnosed the same way (by a set of stringent inclusion and exclusion criteria used in patients enrolled in clinical trials of the new drug and whose clinical and other characteristics are similar to those found in the literature (trials)).

Conclusion C: 1. Drug M will be effective in controlling the symptoms in my patient.
2. My patient is a good candidate for treatment by drug M.
3. I should prescribe drug M to my patient.

It should be noted that although inference (conclusion) 1 is formally valid, neither inference (conclusion) 2, nor inference (conclusion) 3 is formally valid. In each case they follow only presumptively. There might be exceptions to conclusion 2: Contraindications, or cheaper and equally effective drugs to choose from. Conclusion C is right provided that my patient complies well with the treatment regimen; he might comply better with other treatments. These considerations are in addition to those in premises A and B, however sound they render Conclusions 2 and 3 presumptive only and limit their formal validity. As we can see from the above-mentioned examples of syllogisms and their uses, correct argumentation is vital to all decisions in prevention and care. The application of general logic is necessary to purge medicine of numerous flaws of reasoning threatening decisions, not so much to please formal logicians, but rather to put to the best use, the best available evidence for the best benefit to the patient.

In medicine, fortunately, we are much less inclined to appeal to emotions, but we are still tempted to rely on opinions of specific persons and authorities, less substantiated claims, political or economical pressures, cultural traditions, religion, parental attitudes, etc. We continue to be tempted by ambiguity, *non sequitur* (a conclusion that does not follow from the premises), circular reasoning (a chain of arguments whose final conclusion is the same as the starting premise) or deficiencies in causal reasoning like *post hoc ergo propter hoc* (if it follows something, it must be because of that which preceded it). On **floor rounds**, we discuss how we made a diagnosis in a patient, what speaks for it and what pleads against it.

We propose our treatment plan, balancing its benefits and risks. We try to establish a realistic prognosis. In our **specialty reports (consults)**, we usually go beyond one case, but in both situations, uses of evidence must be logical, i.e. as good as evidence itself.

In the area of **cause–effect relationships**, like causes of disease or improvements in health and disease due to treatment and/or care, we must necessarily go beyond the classical canons of causality as outlined in philosophy by John Stuart Mill (1806–1873)[12,14]: agreement, difference, agreement and difference, residues, concomitant variation[5,11,12]. This is due to the fact that classical philosophers and logicians were mostly observers, but not experimenters skilled in trials. As previously mentioned in Chapter 8, we are already well aware that correlated events are not necessarily related, that they may have a 'third' common cause (another event), that one may be a cause of another and that causes may be multiple and complex[7]. Analytical methods in epidemiology and biostatistics take these realities into account.

A third instance of the use of evidence falls within the realm of **social relationships and law**[8,12]. Claims of compensation for injury and work-related chronic problems are presented by patients, their doctors and ultimately lawyers for various bodies: employers, trade unions, compensation boards, and courts. They are all interested in decisions on whether some tort was inflicted on an individual or a community, by whom it was inflicted and how. Cases must be logically explained on the basis of relevant evidence. Both lawyers and decision-makers, as well as presenters of cases, must 'be on the same wavelength'. They must all know not only the solidity and weight of evidence, but also ways to use it properly in argumentation and in reaching conclusions[12]. Unfortunately, heath professionals are often much better prepared for producing and evaluating evidence itself than for its logical uses. It is possible for proponents of the problem to arrive at false conclusions when using good evidence (premises), to arrive at correct conclusions despite inadequate evidence (premises) or, in the best case, to arrive at correct conclusions based on the right evidence. Needless to say that the last instance remains an ideal to strive for.

There are specifics to human biology and medicine, but neither human biology, nor medicine escapes the fundamental rules of thought, reasoning and decision-making in general. Basic medical paradigms from the first three chapters of this book and basics of good evidence covered in the second part of this reading must now be brought together to form an organic entity.

12.4.1 Architecture and basic validity rules of arguments (syllogisms)

Reasoning means directing thinking towards a conclusion. Reasons are called premises. What they support is a 'conclusion'. Reasons and their pathway to a conclusion (included) form an argument. Logic should help us distinguish between good and bad arguments and arguments should be free of fallacies, i.e. any error in reasoning. This applies not only to a classical Aristotelian argumentation through syllogisms, but to any other form of argument. As already mentioned, thinking, in relation to speech, is a matter of combining words in propositions[13]. Three categorical propositions (two premises and one conclusion) form an argument (syllogism). (NB Logicians may study arguments consisting of less or more than two premises.) The conclusion of an argument must be a statement correctly supported by solid evidence. Logical analysis focuses on the relationship between conclusions and evidence that support it[15]. Three terms are used in a syllogism[15]:

- The **major term** (symbolized by the letter **P**, i.e. *predicate*) is the predicate of the conclusion. It appears in the major premise.
- The **minor term** (symbolized by the letter **S**, i.e. *subject*) is the subject of the conclusion. It also appears in the **minor** premise.
- The **middle term** (symbolized by the letter **M**) appears in each premise, but not in the conclusion.

In everyday life, premises are presented in any order. Sometimes, one premise is presented (A), and the other (B) may be tacit (although it must be known to the conclusion users!). For example:

Premise A – major: Anyone with a streptococcal infection (**M**) must be treated with antibiotics (**P**).

Premise B – minor: My patient (**S**) has a streptococcal infection (**M**).

Conclusion C: My patient (**S**) must be treated with antibiotics (**P**).

NB In practice, a clinician may consider Premise B first (my patient has an infection), then weigh its consequences and risks (premise A), leading to his or her therapeutic decision (Conclusion C).

In expanding our reasoning about the problem, some linking or chaining of ideas can occur: The proposition that a streptococcal infection not treated by antibiotics may lead to serious complications could be the premise of another argument in support of premise A. This new argument could be made into a valid categorical syllogism by adding the premise that 'anyone must be treated with antibiotics if they have a condition which may lead to serious complications if not treated with antibiotics'. This premise in turn should be justified by a more general principle such as 'do whatever is necessary to prevent serious complications in a patient'. In fact, clinical reasoning is a kind of 'bricklaying of arguments'.

In the literature on logic, relationships between **P**, **S**, and **M** are often visualized by Venn diagrams. Clinicians are already familiar with these diagrams from the field of diagnosis (see Chapter 6, Fig 6.9) and sport fans see them visually as 'Olympic circles'. They can be used as a pictorial representation of the extent to which various entities (sets) of interest are mutually inclusive or exclusive[16]. A **Venn diagram** is a diagram of circles. Each area displayed by these circles represents a distinct class. It is used to picture all possible relations holding between those classes[4]. Figure 6.9 in this book, illustrating relationships between different subcategories of juvenile arthritis, can serve as an example. Other examples, from the fields of psychiatric diagnosis of subtypes of depression[17] or relationships between suicide, attempted suicide and relapse rates in depression[18] are visualized and understood better through circular diagramming. In argumentation, premises, conclusions, and their components are also pictured as overlapping or disjoint circles, but they are used and analyzed in a different way. By looking at what is in each set alone, jointly contained, or contained in neither, we can better understand how logical terms are valid for conclusions[5] (do they lead to them interrelatedly or independently), how useful various manifestations of disease are in differential diagnosis, and so on.

For a logician, a syllogism is valid if **S**, **P** and **M** are correctly combined. Venn diagrams graphically represent and analyze syllogisms through to some degree of overlapping circles that position **S**, **P**, and **M** according to their use in premises and conclusion. Detailed instructions on how to construct and read Venn diagrams are given by Seech[16] and many others. A physician must also make sure that all propositions are correct. Let us consider the following syllogism:

Premise A: All sore throats are caused by streptococci.

Premise B: Streptococcal infections respond well to antibiotics.

Conclusion C: All sore throats must be treated with antibiotics.

No competent logician would regard this argument as formally correct. Instead, what follows formally from premises is this:

Conclusion C: The cause of all sore throats responds well to antibiotics. (NB It does not.)

Hence, in some situations, although S, P, and M may be correctly combined, they can lead to incorrect conclusions. Such syllogisms are not medically valid (true) either: All sore throats are not caused by streptococci (Premise A is untrue). The conclusion might be true (though in fact it is not!), but the syllogism above does not prove it. Elsewhere, both premises may be untrue and the conclusion may be incorrect.

Premise A: All sore throats are caused by streptococci.

Premise B: Streptococcal infections are a contraindication to treatment with antibiotics.

Conclusion C: No sore throat should be treated with antibiotics.

Finally, if a syllogism can be formally correct and its premises are true and based on solid evidence, then the conclusion must be true:

Premise A: Some sore throats are caused by streptococci.

Premise B: Laboratory confirmed streptococcal infections must be treated with antibiotics to prevent potentially serious late complications.

Conclusion C: Some sore throats must be treated with antibiotics.

Let us take another example of deductively invalid reasoning in surgery:

Premise A: The patient has a tender abdomen.

Premise B: Patients with a tender abdomen may have appendicitis.

Conclusion C: The patient must have his appendix removed right away. (NB No other considerations are taken into account.)

Thus, clinical reasoning must use the most appropriate evidence as a basis for each proposition. Also, all propositions must be linked in a way, which is logically valid. This is a necessary part of the art of medicine as defined in Chapter 1. Correct premises based on good evidence are driven to equally correct and valid conclusions, which themselves become new evidence in the next argument (syllogism) and so on, in our chain of reasoning and problem solving. Errors sometimes cause an unexpected snowball effect.

The validity of our views of a question to be answered relies on two aspects of truth. Any proposition may be deductively valid, inductively strong, or neither. Consequently, several situations can arise:

- **One or more of the premises are false (untrue) and the conclusion of a deductively valid argument is false:** 'All physicians wear a white coat; all psychiatrists are physicians; therefore, all psychiatrists wear a white coat'. (NB They don't.)

- **A deductively doubtful argument may by chance have a correct (truthful) conclusion:** 'Some people who wear a white coat are physicians; all psychiatrists wear a white coat; all psychiatrists are physicians.' (NB Not all psychiatrists wear a white coat.)

Formal deductive validity depends on the form of the argument[19], not on its content. Good medical decisions mean using arguments which are both truthful (propositions based on good evidence) and valid (used correctly). 'All physicians are health professionals; George is a physician; therefore, George is a health professional' is a valid inference based on truthful premises. 'All physicians are health professionals; George is a health professional; therefore, George is a physician' is a deductively invalid inference, despite the fact that George is a health professional. (He may be a pharmacist, microbiologist, laboratory technician, or physiotherapist, etc.) Damer[1] proposes three general criteria of a good argument under a mnemonic 'ARG':

- Its premises must be true or *acceptable* (A)
- Premises must be *relevant* to the truth of the conclusion (R)
- Premises together constitute good or adequate *grounds* for the truth of the conclusion (G).

Fallacies, as any error in our reasoning, may also be classified according to whether they violate acceptability (A), relevance (R) or grounds for the truth (G) of an argument. However, there is no single classification of fallacies in argumentation, as we will see later.

12.4.1.1 Classification and examples of fallacies

A **fallacy** is '*any mistaken idea or false belief, or error in reasoning or in argument*'[4]. A fallacy is also generally defined as a *flaw in reasoning*; anything that diverts the mind or eye; or any reasoning, exposition, argument, etc. contravening the canons of logic[20]. Again, the application of general logic is necessary to purge medicine from numerous fallacies threatening reasoning and decisions, not so much to please formal logicians, but rather to put to the best use, the best available evidence for the best benefit to the patient.

A **fallacy** is a term used in logic to characterize some mistake in reasoning, e.g. in the transition from premises to conclusion. By contrast, a **falsity** refers to a single statement (or evidence, as outlined above)[21]. Our reasoning may then be **fallacious** because our arguments do not respect the rules of formal validity. Moreover, our propositions, interpretations and decisions may be **false**, because of uses of inappropriate evidence. Hence, good medicine means correctly

using good evidence. A fallacy in logical discourse does not mean that the conclusion is false. It simply means that better evidence is needed in order to show that the conclusion is true. Fallacies may be based on illicit assumptions, ambiguity, irrelevance or faulty causal reasoning.

Some fallacies, such as the **ecological fallacy**[22] (where some associations applicable to groups are inappropriately applied to individuals), are already known to epidemiologists. However, logical thinking in medicine is still poorly taught. **Biases**, defined as any systematic deviation of results or inferences from the truth[22] and their extent[23], are now better known to epidemiologists. In fact, the list of biases in medicine is ever-expanding[24]. As in any endeavor, proper reasoning to avoid fallacies should be the subject of more formal and structured training for every health professional, not only for those directly involved in medical research. **Formal fallacies**, from which logicians protect us so well, do not arise from the specific matter of the argument. The physicians must keep an eye on these matters. They arise *from a structural pattern of reasoning that is generically incorrect*[25].

Classification of fallacies

Fallacies can be divided into three types: material, formal, and verbal[25]. These are more extensively reviewed and enumerated elsewhere[4,15,16,20,25], but some are particularly important in the practice of medicine. The classification of fallacies across the literature is not uniform and the list of fallacies is perhaps still not complete. The following classification[25] will suffice in the context of this reading:

Material fallacies (or non-logical fallacies) are also called *fallacies of presumption* because the premises 'presume' too much[25]. They covertly assume the conclusion or avoid the issue of interest. Uses of poor evidence for premises also fall into this category. Facts are misstated.

Formal fallacies (or logical fallacies) occur when the fault is in the very process of reasoning. An improper process of inference is at the root of formal fallacies[25]. They represent wrong connections between premises and conclusions, hence deficiencies in the process of logical thinking[28].

Verbal fallacies occur in arguments whose ambiguous words shift the meaning within the course of an argument[4]. The incorrect use of terms is a culprit[25].

For medical decision-making, two other categories[28] must be considered:

Substantive fallacies (we can also call them **content fallacies**) arise from overly general premises leading to inappropriate conclusions. Inadequate evidence supporting premises results in conclusions as new poor evidence. **Causal fallacies** are mistaken inferences about the cause(s) of something. Both these categories depend on how good the evidence supporting premises is and on how well the cause–effect criteria (see Chapter 8) are fulfilled. *Post hoc ergo propter hoc,* taking correlation for causation, inverting cause and effect, appealing to ignorance (because no evidence exists, it must or it must not exist), or taking a belief for knowledge[28] are fallacies falling into this latter category. For these authors[28], a **belief** is not necessarily the **truth**. Any kind of **assertion** (belief) is speaker-relative. Hence, we may conclude that truth is a belief based on the best available evidence.

Even the best of our **knowledge**, i.e. justified true belief (the 'scientific knowledge') is dependent on dominating paradigms of the time and evidences occurring within the framework of such a paradigm[29]. Beliefs, sometimes accepted as true may change within new paradigms. For example, the paradigm of a peptic ulcer as a disease related to stress, diet and other non-infectious factors is replaced by the paradigm of a peptic ulcer as an infectious disease related to exposure to *Helicobacter pylori*. Hence, finding, categorizing and correcting fallacies is a never-ending endeavor.

Examples of fallacies

To avoid fallacious practice and research in medicine, we must be aware of several traps. Only a few fallacies from their much wider spectrum will be quoted here:

1. A *fallacy of accident* stems from the application by an argument of a general rule to a particular case in which some special circumstance ('accident') makes the rule inapplicable[25]. This occurs when a general proposition is used as the premise for an argument without attention to the (tacit) restrictions and qualifications that govern it and invalidate its application in the manner at issue[25]. For example, in a clinical trial of a new drug, a prognostic staging of patients remains unknown for some reason. The drug proves beneficial. To conclude that this drug is beneficial for a particular prognostic subgroup would be fallacious.

2. A *converse fallacy of accident* occurs when one incorrectly argues from a special case or situation to a general rule[25]. For example, a certain drug is proved beneficial for patients at advanced stages of cancer. It would be fallacious to conclude that all cancer patients, regardless of the stage of their cancer, would benefit from the treatment. This situation can arise if prognostic stratification and its analysis are not considered in clinical trials and interpretation of their results.

3. A *fallacy of irrelevant conclusion* occurs when a conclusion changes the point that is at issue in the premises[25]. *Fallacies of relevance* sometimes prevail in law or politics when persons, rather than issues are attacked. This type of fallacy can originate from any individual or organization interested in the results of clinical trials, public health programs and policies. Health promotion programs merit particular attention from this point of view.

4. A *fallacy of circular argument* ('begging the question') occurs when premises presume, openly or covertly, the very conclusion that has to be demonstrated[25]. Patient Newbury always follows the treatments prescribed. How do we know? He (she) always takes his (her) non-steroidal anti-inflammatory drug (NSAID) according to his (her) physician's orders.

5. A *vicious circle fallacy* can be considered a special case of the previous fallacy, where premise A is used to prove premise B, premise B is used to prove premise C etc. and finally, premise Z is used to prove premise A. For example: 'NSAIDs are the best form of arthritis treatment because of the ability of ibuprofen, diclofenac, or celecoxib to control pain and inflammation based on several trials, one comparing ibuprofen to dicolofenac, another comparing diclofenac to celexoxib, yet another comparing celexocib to . . ., etc. Hence, we can conclude that arthritis should be treated

based on research from the field of NSAIDs.' This kind of *petitio principii* illustrates inept argumentation. The argument from A – Z as a premise for Z – A as a conclusion is not deductively invalid[25] but lacks any power of conviction, since no one questioning the conclusion could concede the premise.

6. A *fallacy of false cause* occurs when mere sequence or correlation is taken to prove a causal connection. This situation is already known to epidemiologists and other scientists as *post hoc ergo propter hoc*, i.e. 'after which, hence by which' (or event B which follows event A is due to A). A simple temporal sequence becomes a cause–effect sequence. For example, hyperacidity was caused by the meal, which preceded its occurrence; an embolism was caused by a trans-oceanic flight because the victim was fine on boarding the plane; epilepsy or autism are due to immunization, because they occurred after the child was immunized, etc.

7. A *fallacy of many questions* occurs when a single answer is required for a question that might have several possible answers such as: 'Are the two patients in Room 26 sick? Patient A is sick and patient B is not.' In this situation, an answer can be refused altogether when a mistaken presupposition is involved. For example: Have you stopped taking detailed patient histories? This frightens your patients. (Detailed scrutinizing makes some patients uncomfortable.)

8. A *fallacy of non sequitur* ('it does not follow') occurs when there is not even a deceptively plausible appearance of valid reasoning because there is virtually a complete lack of connection between the given premises and the conclusion drawn from them. For example:

Premise A: The computerized axial tomography of the patient's right kidney shows a suspicious lesion.
Premise B: This hospital and its department of surgery have an outstanding reputation in the field of abdominal surgery.
Conclusion C: This patient should have his right kidney removed.

9. Some other fallacies are caused by improper *content* or by improper content and its improper uses. In an **'if . . . then' form of reasoning**, fallacies may occur due to an improper handling of **antecedent(s)**, i.e. sentences after '*if . . .*', or **consequents** (sentences that follow '*then . . .*').

10. A *fallacy of affirming the consequent*[30] asserts that because the consequent is true, the antecedent is also true:

Premise A: **If** this patient has diabetes, his blood sugar will be high.
Premise B: His blood sugar is high.
Conclusion C: **Then** (**therefore**), this patient has diabetes.

In this kind of reasoning, the web of causes of high blood sugar is simply ignored. However, diabetes is not the only cause of high blood sugar.

11. A *fallacy of denying the antecedent*[30] occurs when arguing that because the antecedent is false, the consequent must necessarily be false too:

Premise A: **If** this patient has diabetes, his blood sugar will be abnormally high.
Premise B: But this patient does not have diabetes.
Conclusion C: **Then** (**therefore**) his blood sugar should be normal.

A more complete compilation of a numerically open-ended list of fallacies in medical reasoning still must be worked up.

12.4.2 Ways to improve arguments and argumentation

Arguments in everyday medical communication are mostly 'hidden' in the flow of the message, which is only rarely an obvious structured syllogism or any other well-defined form of argument. Discussion and conclusions of research findings do not always necessarily follow the above-mentioned canons of proper argumentation. If arguments are already satisfactorily structured, they may be submitted to direct scrutiny for their structure and content. If they are not, a 'real argument' must be 'deciphered, extracted, unearthed' from the flow of words and messages or '**reconstructed**', as logicians say. A clinical microbiology resident may inform the Chief Resident of the following: '. . . Our nurse on call told me that the elderly immunocompromised patient in Room 20 is distressed and disoriented. It looks to me like he is developing a sepsis. Before ordering blood cultures, we started treatment with a combination of antibiotics, given that a delay in treatment might be hazardous for the patient. As soon as we get the results of the blood cultures, we will adjust treatment accordingly . . .'

Premise or argument **indicators** may be identified first by words such as '*for, since, because, assuming that, seeing that, granted that, in view of, given that, in as much as*', among others. **Conclusion indicators** are words like '*therefore, thus, hence, so, for this reason, accordingly, consequently, which proves that, which means that, as a result, in conclusion*'[31], among others. The above-mentioned resident's message can be reconstructed into a corresponding syllogism:

- Premise A: The patient in Room 20 is distressed and disoriented; he may have sepsis.
- Premise B: Delay in treatment may be hazardous for this patient if he effectively has sepsis.
- Conclusion C: This patient must receive antibiotics without delay. His treatment will be adjusted according to the forthcoming laboratory results and monitoring of the patient.

Arguments may then be scrutinized for fallacies related to the already mentioned Damer's mnemonic 'ARG' [1]: Acceptability of premises (A), relevance of the premises to the truth of the conclusion (R), and premises constituting together good or adequate grounds for the truth of the conclusion (G). All discovered fallacies must be corrected. Detailed ways of reconstruction of arguments[28] and correction of fallacies[1] are well beyond this introductory chapter and may be found in these excellent original references[28,1] and others.

12.5 Possible uses of evidence and argumentation in the area of fuzzy logic applications

For many novices, fuzzy theory and fuzzy logic have quickly become ubiquitous, often interchangeable terms. For the purpose of this reading, a clearer distinction must be made between these 'buzz-words' of today:

- **Fuzzy theory**, like any other body of basic principles underlying the fundamentals and application of science, stresses the continuity and transitionality of our observations of fuzzy sets and their interpretation.
- **Fuzzy logic**, like any other kind of logic, refers to the principles of valid reasoning fuelled by information provided by fuzzy sets and information from the historically 'excluded middle'.

12.5.1 *Paradigm of fuzziness in medicine*

Proponents of fuzzy theory and fuzzy logic argue that classical logic in daily reasoning may be further away from the reality of overall human thinking and communication[32]. As already mentioned in Chapter 3, classical logic works with an 'excluded middle'. One has a disease or one does not, one smokes or one does not. Protagonists of fuzzy logic point out that a patient is not simply sick or not, but also might be 'a little sick', 'moderately sick' or 'severely sick'. In extremis though, a woman might not be pregnant, 'a little pregnant', 'moderately pregnant', or 'very pregnant', if not 'definitely pregnant'. This might be valid from the point of view of fuzzy theory, but it is not supported by the biological reality of pregnancy. Provided that we also have convincing evidence for the 'excluded middle' (a little, moderately, or very pregnant), do we first need some additional and perhaps special evidence for the excluded middle? Should we know how to apply it as correctly as we already use evidence in classical argumentation?

Despite all our attention to clinimetrically valid and well-defined observations, our daily life and communication is full of 'excluded middles' and fuzzy terms. We might hear on the radio that 'it will be *partly* cloudy tomorrow, with *occasional* showers and *some heavy* rain by the end of the day'. Similarly, an intern may report that 'we have admitted a diabetic, insulin receiving patient with a history of *recent* surgery, showing a *worrisome* hyperglycemia, *advanced decompensation* of his (her) acid–basic balance and acting *considerably* confused'. (NB All fuzzy terms are in italics.) Such a message may mean either that our intern does not know exactly what is he talking about or that we have at hand (and that we know and understand all) stringent operational clinimetric criteria defining which hyperglycemia is *worrisome*, which metabolic decompensation is *advanced* (ketoacidosis requiring insulin, fluid, electrolyte and mineral replacement?) and what degree of mental confusion is *considerable* (is the patient sending everybody around him or her to hell?). Some staff-person may suggest to the intern: 'Your treatment and follow-up orders are *fine, watch* him *closely*, and do not forget to *give him (her) some* potassium! It is *unlikely* that we will be obliged to do *more* than that'. (NB Presumably, the intern will not consider such orders as 'fuzzy' and will correctly calculate potassium requirements for this patient and choose the right manner by which potassium should be given while also knowing about the full array of diagnostic and therapeutic options in this case.)

Another good example of fuzzy communication is given by Asbury and Tzabar[33]: '*If the arterial pressure is **slightly** above the **desired** range, increase the infusion rate **a little**. If the arterial pressure falls **catastrophically**, stop the infusion **temporarily**.*' Zadeh[34] calls the above highlighted assertions **fuzzy predicates**, **fuzzy quantifiers** and **fuzzy probabilities**. He concludes then, that the classical probability theory and logic do not well represent common sense knowledge and uses. Fuzzy logic focuses on such kinds of uncertainty and lexical imprecision. Values of observations (statements, evidence) are directional and progressive between the existent and the non-existent.

Propositions from Sadegh-Zadeh[35] stating that nosology, diagnosis or treatment are fuzzy, specific to the available information and its context or that somebody may be ill or not[21] do not facilitate practical decision-making in clinical life. For the moment, clinicians have two ways of dealing with such uncertainty:

- Either they may attempt some kind of **hardening of soft data,** as outlined in Chapter 6, and use this 'sharper' information for sharp conclusions and decisions, or
- They may leave fuzzy terms as they are and submit them to the process of fuzzy logic.

12.5.2 *Essentials of fuzzy argumentation*

Contrary to sharp Aristotelian logic, fuzzy logic means approximate reasoning where everything is a matter of degree[34]:

- While appreciating **truth** of information, things may not only be true or false, but also *very true* or *not quite true.*
- **Predicates** (propositions stated about subjects) are not sharp either. The patient *feels ill*, the uterus of an expectant mother is *much larger than usual.*
- A single **predicate modifier** in classical systems, negation or *not* is introduced into a larger set of considerations such as *very, more or less, quite, rather* or *extremely.*
- **Quantifiers** are also more numerous than universal and existential: *few, several, usually, most, almost always, frequently, about 10 cm.*
- Numerical or interval-valued **probabilities** are replaced by entities qualified as *likely, unlikely, very likely, by the end of the day* and so on.
- Bivalent **possibilities** like *possible* or *impossible* are expanded by such degrees as *quite possible, almost impossible* and others.

Fuzzy logic is used in four kinds of reasoning[34]:

- In **categorical reasoning,** there are no fuzzy quantifiers and/or probabilities in premises. If premises are fuzzy, conclusions are also fuzzy: This patient has anemia; this patient is malnourished; hence, this patient is anemic and malnourished. (The conclusion is a sum of premises here.)

- In **syllogistic reasoning,** the inference may be made from premises containing fuzzy quantifiers: *Most* patients suffering from ketoacidosis have poorly controlled insulin-dependent diabetes; *Most* patients suffering from ketoacidosis have recently undergone a pathologically and physiologically challenging event like myocardial infarction or extensive surgery; Hence, most patients suffering from ketoacidosis suffer from poorly controlled insulin-dependent diabetes and have recently had a serious acute and radical clinical condition.

The classical argument (syllogism) is replaced by a **fuzzy argument,** which may be based then, on one or more fuzzy premises and its conclusion will necessarily be fuzzy. It may lead to a deductively invalid argument such as:

Premise A: *Many* North Americans are becoming *increasingly obese*.

Premise B: *Many* North Americans are not *physically active enough*.

Conclusion C: *Many* North Americans are *increasingly obese* because they are not *physically active enough*.

- In **dispositional reasoning**, propositions are not necessarily always true; *Heavy* alcohol drinking is a *leading cause* of liver cirrhosis. To avoid liver cirrhosis, avoid *heavy* drinking of alcohol.

- In **qualitative reasoning**, the input–output is expressed as a collection of fuzzy if-then rules in which the antecedents (premises) and consequents (conclusions) involve linguistic variables. This kind of reasoning bears some similarity to the if-then reasoning in the artificial intelligence domain[30].

For the moment, routine or 'scientific' clinical reasoning is still not studied and understood enough from the point of view of fuzzy logic theory. Let us remember though that classical logic has been studied, understood and applied for many centuries and that fuzzy logic is only a few decades old. Providing a logical structure and rules of logical reasoning for daily life and using daily life terms and information (evidence) properly are both necessary. They are a reality of everyday clinical practice. So far, some foundations of evidence and its uses have been traced, mainly in logic itself and in medical research. Their integrated uses in daily clinical practice will certainly not be quickly forgotten. An additional challenge emerges: The use of fuzzy logic requires the availability of valid 'fuzzy' evidence, which fits 'fuzzy' premises (antecedents) and 'fuzzy' conclusions (consequents). For the moment, our understanding of 'not-fuzzy' evidence appears better and more complete than our mastery of evidence of the fuzzy kind. Let us see if logic can be brought to the individual patient's bedside. Patients, in fact, should all benefit from its proper use.

12.6 Conclusions

Logic is not a field exclusively reserved for advanced areas of research in medicine such as artificial intelligence development and applications, computer modeling, or fuzzy logic. Let us again stress, it is equally, if not more important, in the daily life of a physician:

- When writing down clinical orders and making decisions about an individual patient.
- When advising patients, answering their questions and explaining decisions to be made about the diagnostic process or treatment.
- When presenting patients and discussing, during clinical rounds, solutions to their problems.
- When giving expert advice through specialty consults.
- When writing down various reports and research papers.
- When explaining and defending clinical guidelines, programs and strategies at various levels of prevention.
- When offering expert opinions and giving testimonies to various civic bodies and defending cases at courts of law[8,12,36].
- When defending community medicine health programs and policies in public health.

Correct reasoning and logical argumentation is a learned experience like any other intellectual endeavor. Nonetheless, the history and uses of medicine and the application of logic to medicine is still more limited[37] than it should be. Introductions to it are still exceptional[30] and fragmented. Although logic is widely used in the area of artificial intelligence and its applications to medicine[34], logic in the daily life of a physician requires equal, if not greater attention. It must be taught and learned. Reasoning logically in medicine is truly a learned experience just like suturing wounds or understanding and treating an acutely depressed or delusional patient. All of our arguments must be valid, strong, and truthful. All these terms have their specific meaning in informal logic[13]:

Truth is embedded in propositions. It is supported by the best evidence, as defined in Chapter 2. Hence, evidence-based medicine contributes to the building of truthful propositions.

Validity, by contrast, is a property of the deductively valid argument as a whole: True premises lead to a true conclusion. Validity gives us the overall value of an argument in a logical discourse. It gives us certainty. This is a rather rarely attained ideal for medical decisions.

Strength is also a property of an inductively strong argument and its overall characteristic: If the premises are true, the conclusion is probably also true. It gives us a measure of probability under uncertainty. Strength, as well, reflects the overall solidity of an argument. It contributes to the realism and reality of medical decisions.

To make medicine successful, we must know how to find the best available arguments and their conclusions, how to build them properly, and how to use them in practice and research. Dispositions of a good medical critical thinker may be borrowed with some modifications from Ennis[38]. This author expects, among others, the following virtues in his disciples:

- Clarity on the intended meaning of what is communicated.
- Being able to determine and maintain focus on a question and its conclusion.
- Taking into account the situation in its entirety.
- Being able to seek, find and offer reasons.
- Being well informed.
- Looking for alternatives.
- Being precise according to the requirement of the situation.
- Being aware of own beliefs, but also being open to others' views.

- **Withholding judgment when the evidence and reason are insufficient.** NB However, physicians must exert judgment and make decisions even under uncertainty.
- **Taking or changing position when the evidence and reasons are sufficient** to do so.

For this author[38], the above-mentioned virtues may be learned through a FRISCO approach. FRISCO is an anagram encompassing focus, reasons, inference, situation, clarity and overview (looking back to what was done). His entire monograph is devoted to this paradigm of learning and practicing critical thinking. Bowell and Kemp's guide[28] is also a good companion to the former. Chapters 4 to 11 were about truth. Chapter 3, the present chapter, and Chapter 13 are about validity and strength. Let us now see in the next chapter how to obtain the best possible evidence from our overall experience in order to produce the best possible premises and how to make our decision more 'logical', beyond intuition, guts, and flair. We must always ask ourselves:

- Is our argumentation logical? In other words, is the evidence used logically in the concept, interpretation and recommendations concerning the problem of interest?
- Do we have satisfactory evidence to support any premise and conclusion of logical arguments, whatever their structure might be?

For the moment, the balance speaks more in favor of evidence itself rather than its uses. But let us never forget that an uncritical adoption of faulty arguments may be disastrous for the patient.

The way we use evidence itself through our reasoning may be seen as a kind of intervention itself. We are still far from evaluation, if the logically correct use of evidence through critical thinking works better for our patients than its spontaneous uses. Can we foresee a kind of clinical trial to answer such questions? Evaluating our critical thinking and using evidence as a kind of maneuver instead of counting the number of pills ingested by the patient will be a challenge in itself.

REFERENCES

1. Damer TE. *Attacking Faulty Reasoning*. 2nd Edition. Belmont, CA: Wadsworth Publ. Co., 1987

2. Ennis RH. A taxonomy of critical thinking dispositions and abilitIes. In: Baron JB, Sternberg RJ eds. *Testing Thinking Skills: Theory and Practice*. New York: WH Freeman and Co., 1987:9–26

3. Ennis R. Critical thinking: A streamlined conception. *Teach Phil*, 1991;**14**:5–24

4. Harrison FR III. *Logic and Rational Thought*. St. Paul: West Publishing Co., 1992

5. Copi IM. *Informal Logic*. New York: Macmillan, 1986

6. Johnson DM. Reasoning and logic. In: Sills DL ed. *International Encyclopedia of the Social Sciences*. New York and Toronto: The Macmillan Co. & The Free Press, 1968:344–9

7. Weston A. *A Rulebook for Arguments*. Cambridge. Indianapolis: Hackett Publishing Co., 1987

8. Aldisert RJ. *Logic for Lawyers. A Guide to Clear Legal Thinking*. 3rd Edition. Notre Dame: National Institute for Trial Advocacy, 1997

9. Hitchcock D. Enthymatic arguments. *Informal Logic*, 1998;**VII 2&3**:83–96

10. Hitchcock D. Does the traditional treatment of enthymemes rest on mistake? *Argumentation*, 1998: **12**:15–37

11. Mill JS. System of Logic. In: Robson JM ed. *Mill JS. Collected Works of John Stuart Mill*. Toronto: University of Toronto Press, 1963;**7–8**

12. Waller BN. *Critical Thinking. Consider the Verdict*. Englewood Cliffs: Prentice-Hall, 1998

13. Department of Philosophy, University of Guelph. *Logic Outline*. 7th Edition, revised. Guelph: University of Guelph. November 2000 (22p. mimeographed)

14. Salmon WC. *Logic*. Englewood Cliffs: Prentice-Hall, 1963

15. Engel SM. *The Chain of Logic*. Englewood Cliffs: Prentice-Hall, 1987

16. Seech Z. *Logic in Everyday Life. Practical Reasoning Skills*. Belmont, CA: Wadsworth Publishing Co., 1987

17. Leckman JF, Weissman MM, Prusoff BA, et al. Subtypes of depression. Family study perspective. *Arch Gen Psychiatry*, 1984;**41**:833–8

18. Avery D, Winokour D. Suicide, attempted suicide and relapse rates in depression. *Arch Gen Psychiatry*, 1978;**35**:749–53

19. West HR. Logic. *Microsoft® Encarta® Encyclopedia*. © 1993–1997, Microsoft Corp. (Electronic Edition)

20. Michalos AC. *Improving Your Reasoning*. 2nd Edition. Englewood Cliffs: Prentice-Hall, 1986

21. *The Columbia Encyclopedia*. 6th Edition (electronic) 2001 www.bartleby.com

22. Last JM (ed.). *A Dictionary of Epidemiology*. 4th Edition. New York: Oxford University Press, 2001

23. Sackett DL. Bias in analytical research. *J Chronic Dis*, 1979;**32**:51–63

24. Les biais. In: Jenicek M, Cléroux R. *Épidémiologie. Principes, techniques applications. (Epidemiology. Principles, Techniques, Applications)*. St. Hyacinthe and Paris: EDISEM and Maloine Éditeurs, 1982: 236–41

25. Hughes GE, Wang H, Roscher N. The History and Kinds of Logic. In: McHenry R, ed. *The New Encyclopaedia Britannica. Macropaedia/Knowledge in Depth*. Chicago: Encyclopaedia Britannica, Inc., 1992;**23**:226–82

26. Hansen HV, Pinto RC (eds). *Fallacies. Classical and Contemporary Readings*. University Park, Pa: The Pennsylvania State University Press, 1995

27. Whately R. Of fallacies. In: Sills DL ed. *International Encyclopedia of the Social Sciences*. New York and Toronto: The Macmillan Co. & The Free Press, 1968:67–84

28. Bowell T, Kemp G. *Critical Thinking. A Concise Guide*. London and New York: Routledge, 2002

29. Crofton I (ed.). *Instant Reference Philosophy*. London: Hodder Headline, 2000

30. Albert DA, Munson R, Resnik MD. Deductive inference. In: *Reasoning in Medicine. An introduction to Clinical Inference*. Baltimore and London: The Johns Hopkins University Press, 1988;**5**:97–111

31. Nolt J, Rohatyn D, Varzi A. *Logic*. 2nd Edition. Schaum's Outline Series. New York: McGraw-Hill, 1998

32. Sadegh-Zadeh K. Fuzzy health, illness, and disease. *J Med Phil*, 2000;**25**:605–38

33. Asbury AJ, Tzabar Y. Fuzzy logic: New ways of thinking in anaesthesia. *Br J Anaesthesia*, 1995;**75**: 1–2

34. Zadeh LA. Knowledge representation in fuzzy logic. In: Yager RR, Zadeh LA eds. *An Introduction to Fuzzy Logic Applications in Intelligent Systems*. Boston/ Dordrecht/London: Kluwer Academic Publishers, 1992:1–26

35. Sadegh-Zadeh K. Fundamentals of clinical methodology: 1. Differential indication. *Artif Intell Med*, 1994;**6**:83–102

36. McCall Smith A. Legal reasoning and medical practice. In: Phillips CI ed. *Logic in Medicine*. London: BMJ Publishing Group, 1995:133–53

37. Tomassi P. Logic and medicine.1–29. Logic and scientific method, 30–58. In: Phillips CI ed. *Logic in Medicine*. London: BMJ Publishing Group, 1995

38. Ennis RH. *Critical Thinking*. Upper Saddle River, NJ: Prentice Hall, 1996

Decision analysis and decision-making in medicine. Beyond intuition, guts, and flair

*Nothing is more difficult,
and therefore more precious,
than to be able to decide.*
Napoléon Bonaparte, *Maxims* (1804–1815)

*A physician who is 90 per cent 'certain'
about any decision will always seek additional
information in the hope that it will increase
the 'confidence' with which he makes such a
decision. The decision . . . will be either correct
or incorrect, and the outcome is independent of
the confidence with which the decision is reached.
When additional information cannot possibly alter
the decision, but only gives rise to a greater sense
of comfort on the part of the physician, such
additional information is of no benefit to the patient.
Its only benefit is in reducing the discomfort
of the physician.*
Harold M. Schoolman[1], 1977

Good evidence is not necessarily a high priority for intervention. In fact, a high priority for intervention, may lack good evidence. An evidence of priority is not a priority of evidence. It is additional evidence. Evidence surrounding a single question and covering the same problem must be brought together in a logical way, as seen in Chapters 11 and 12. Also, evidence supporting different questions in the chain of medical reasoning must be organized as organically as possible in the process of medical decision-making. This chapter will discuss how to build, interpret and evaluate the chain of evidence supporting each link in choosing the best options for diagnosis and treatment.

Making correct decisions may be challenging not only when working with new, advanced, expensive and sophisticated technologies, but also in daily clinical practice when dealing with everyday problems. The latter, due to their sheer number, also require the best possible decisions to benefit an important number of patients and to minimize the costs and risks of less appropriate decisions. A boy arrives at a family medical practice complaining of a mild fever, fatigue and sore throat. His nasopharynx is cherry-red, and his tonsils are plum-sized with whitish patchy spots not adhering to the surface and not overlying the tonsils. Lymphatic nodes are palpable below his ears and under his chin. The boy's mother stresses how much he is suffering and insists that the doctor do something to relieve his symptoms. The physician has four choices:

1. Immediately prescribe antibiotics for a streptococcal infection of the throat;
2. Take throat swabs and send them to the laboratory to identify the infectious agent, and eventually prescribe an appropriate antibiotic;
3. Prescribe antibiotics immediately and wait for the laboratory results, which indicate whether to continue or withhold the treatment;
4. Reassure the mother that the illness is not serious and that simple 'fever medication' and pain killers will suffice.

New laboratory techniques are constantly appearing. As an example, patients with suspected Zollinger-Ellison syndrome should be evaluated either by an initial gastric analysis (elevated serum gastrin values) alone, or by an added secretion infusion test. Is such a costly addition worth it? Does it improve clinical decision-making? More importantly, how will it affect the patient's health and outcome? Should gastric analysis first be performed, followed by a secretin infusion test? Would such testing obviate unnecessary hospitalization and medical costs[2,3]? In the above-mentioned cases, the patient's health and life are at stake. Additional tests are usually costly, thus the best possible and most cost-effective decisions should be made given the circumstances.

These examples illustrate what may be at stake if decisions are made based on a simple gut feeling, the simple authority of a senior physician (the 'mandarin attitude'), or based on a more structured approach, integrating in as organized a way as possible clinical options (decisions), the probabilities of their impact (outcomes), values of the latter, and the validity of procedures (such as paraclinical tests). The latter alternative and option in clinical decision-making represents the basis of clinical decisions today. Again, structured decision-making requires a sequence of evidence supporting logical discourses like this one:

Clinical situation	Logical discourse	Evidence
'Mrs Smith, your son has a serious sore throat.'	This is a case of beta-hemolytic group A streptococcal infection of the throat. **(Premise A)**	Clinical picture completed and confirmed in laboratory (agent isolated).
'You will give him these pills every day.'	Penicillin is the treatment of choice. **(Premise B)**	Test for sensitivity to antibiotics shows that penicillin is the best choice of treatment in this patient.
'You will avoid serious complications, which your son might get without such treatment.'	Treatment by antibiotics reduces the prognosis of complications. **(Conclusion C)**	Observational studies *and* **decision analysis** both confirm that treatment by antibiotics is preferred to symptomatic treatment only.

This example shows that one possible way to reach Conclusion C is decision analysis. An explanation of decision analysis follows.

13.1 How decisions in medicine are made. General concepts

There is no uniform way to make decisions in medicine. In the past, the rational basis of medical practice was often blended, to various degrees, with several irrational attitudes, steering an often correct decision in the wrong direction:

- **Teachers and older colleagues are often the objects of blind confidence and idolization** – 'they are never wrong'.
- Clinicians are often **emotionally attached to what has been laboriously learned,** and afraid that years spent perfecting skills will be found irrelevant and not useful anymore. It is hard to stop performing a surgical procedure that took 10 years to master.
- Sometimes, **clinical ritualism** is *'de rigueur'*. If a given diagnostic maneuver is a part of the 'complete examination', it is done whether it is proven useful or not in a given situation. Ortolani's maneuver 'must' be done right at the first newborn examination, even if a short delay may be more useful[2].
- Sometimes, decisions are dictated by the **defensive practice of medicine.** If physicians risk lawsuits for neglecting to perform cesarean sections in some cases, they **do not take risks,** and they choose a surgical means of delivery. If a significant wound is treated, an anti-tetanus booster dose is given even if it has only been a short time since the patient was completely immunized against this disease.
- Clinicians want to treat patients well, even if it is uncertain that a treatment works or if a diagnostic method is truly proven valid. Especially in interventionist medicine, as it is practiced in North America, 'something must be done'. This unidirectional thinking ignores the 'art of doing nothing' and the 'art of waiting'. An old surgical saying holds that 'it takes two years to get into the abdomen and 20 years to learn to stay out'. **Medicinal negation, denial and humanitarian irrational activism** often prevail.

- Sometimes decisions are made while **ignoring epidemiological information and methods.** A positive result of a diagnostic test is not interpreted in its context, for example a positive test result for AIDS in a heterosexual and sexually inactive subject who is not an intravenous drug user, who is in good health and who has not had a single blood transfusion.
- Sometimes **decisions are dictated by an extraneous power** and/or justified socially or culturally. This is especially true when decision-makers are short of arguments. Therapeutic abortions, refusal of transfusions by some patients or interruption of per oral treatment by fasting patients fall into this category of decision problems and implementation.

Fortunately for physicians and patients, **most medical decisions are correct.** We are learning more and more not only the important facts and information in medicine, but also the right means, principles, methods and techniques leading to valuable findings and, ultimately, correct decisions.

Decisions in medicine can be based on different ways and means:

1. Knowledge of facts, experience, 'intuition', 'common sense' and 'gut feeling' are the components of what is called today **distilled clinical judgment.** Decisions are made on the basis of hypothetic-deductive thinking, from major *a priori* formulated clues to the most probable diagnosis and treatment of possible problems. If a patient develops a fever after a kidney transplant, it may be equally due to an infection or to rejection of the organ. In the case of an erroneous diagnosis, antibiotics would not prevent organ rejection with its possible fatal consequences for the patient, but immunosuppression would not help in the case of an infection. In such situations, a 'steepest ascent type of thinking'[2] is mandatory.

2. The **Gestalt** or **pattern recognition** method is useful in other situations and allows for appropriate 'right' decision-making. A patient with nocturnal distress and dyspnea, who sleeps on several pillows and holds the bed frame with both hands 'to breathe better', exhibits a pattern of cardiac insufficiency which is easily recognized by the physician.

3. When competing health conditions are at stake, two decisions can be considered. In a 'minimax' approach, a solution is sought which would give a minimum probability of a maximum loss. In a situation of a possible streptococcal infection of the throat, without the possibility of laboratory testing, a clinician may decide to prescribe antibiotics to prevent any late systemic complications (maximum loss) of this infection. In a 'maximin' or 'Las Vegas approach', decisions are made to reach a maximum probability of a minimal loss. In cancer medicine, a chemotherapeutic or physical agent leading to fewer secondary effects in cases of competent efficacy is often chosen for treatment.

4. Decisions made on the basis of the **magic of numbers** (what is statistically significant must be better!) are most often among the worst.

5. Finally, accumulation of data and information and their handling through an organized intellectual process may best be achieved on the basis of **clinical decision analysis,** as described in this chapter.

Most medical textbooks and many teachers in the past concentrated on the building blocks of clinical decision-making: knowledge of abnormal values and manifestations; diagnostic entities; pharmacology of drugs; etc. Using building blocks to construct a valuable clinical decision (to treat or not to treat) must be learned too. In these terms, we can agree with Sox[4] that decision analysis is a fundamental clinical skill to be learned and put into practice. It will, however, complement the intuitive component of clinical practice, which will remain its integrate part[5].

Information in medicine is never complete, never entirely true, because of patient and physician human nature. Decisions are always probabilistic, no matter how confident the attitude of senior colleagues; they are always made in situations with a variable degree of uncertainty. This does not mean that such decisions are inevitably made in a disorganized and chaotic way – they may be structured. This chapter is about a structured approach to medical decision-making in which all clinical information is integrated: knowledge about risk; diagnosis and its validity; treatment and its possible results; and the values which disease outcomes produce in the eyes of the patient, the health professional, or a decision-maker

who provide the means for all this through the contribution of the whole community. Such a structured approach to reaching the best possible medical decisions is accomplished through a process called **decision analysis**. It is already used in finance, business, military affairs, industry and economics. Why not in medicine, provided human nature is involved and that the patient's opinion and decision prevails? The patient must have the last word as to whether a leg is amputated, a breast removed, or a colostomy opened. Zarin and Pauker[6] believe that structured decision-making through decision analysis will improve dealings with the complexity and uncertainty around clinical cases, and will also allow for patient participation in shared clinical decision-making. Clinicians must learn not only how to auscultate the heart, count blood cells, or remove an appendix, but also how to arrive at this decision.

More objective decisions may be reached in different ways. First, some agreement may be reached between several specialists and experienced professionals in the field. A **consensus** of the group is produced, representing either a unanimous or a prevalent agreement by its members[7]. This kind of decision may be made in an even more organized and structured manner. For example, in the so-called Delphi method, the least important (or frequent) opinions are progressively removed from the array of choices. Such a reduced set is re-evaluated, additional deletions are made, and the whole process is repeated until the group reaches the best possible option. Decisions may also be rated[8]. Second, **computer-assisted decision-making** facilitates the use of structured approaches to medical decisions as explained in this chapter, and allows decisions to be made on the basis of a wider body of information, data, and premises, which go well beyond the capacity of a single deciding individual or group[9,10]. Third, clinical thinking may be understood and organized in a structured way, which represents the basis of **decision analysis** in medicine. The present chapter is devoted to this topic. Finally, any of the above-mentioned approaches to clinical decisions provide the best possible information that should be incorporated in a similarly organized way into the physician's practice. Clinical algorithms or clinical practice guidelines are the most frequently used of such tools. The second part of this chapter is devoted to this topic. Thus, two practical problems will be examined:

1. How to arrive at the best decision – by decision analysis, or by some other means? What evidence is needed? How can it be integrated in an understandable way to reach the best possible decision?

2. How to use the decision in practice? What is the best way to make the right strategic or tactical decisions when dealing with clinical problems? Should its result be introduced as a component(s) of clinical algorithms, and their indications be followed in clinical practice, or should something else be done? Is it possible to develop and use evidence-based clinical practice guidelines efficiently?

13.2 Basic vocabulary and reference readings

There is no medicine without decisions, which are made at every step of clinical work. Should a patient be prohibited from smoking? What treatment should be chosen to control migraine pain? Should a clinically silent hernia be surgically repaired now, later or not at all? Will physical activity after myocardial infarction improve a patient's prognosis? Such decisions are most often made with a variable degree of uncertainty: clinical data and information are missing or are incomplete; characteristics of patients; exposure to various factors; treatments; their possible outcomes; or patients' comorbidity; these are all changeable.

Conceptually, the **medical decision** represents the choice of the best option in assessing risk (explanatory decisions), in treating patients (managerial decisions), or in making prognosis (both explanatory and managerial, if treatment decisions are involved). **Medical decision-making** is a process by which one arrives at a given medical decision, the latter being the result or endpoint of such a process. **Decision analysis** tackles precisely such situations. It is a systematic approach to decision-making under conditions of uncertainty[11]. It has also been defined as a '*derivative of operations research and game theory that involves identifying all available choices and potential outcomes of each, in a series of decisions that have to be made*', in medicine, '*about aspects of*

patient care – diagnostic procedures, therapeutic regimens, prognostic expectations . . . Epidemiological data play a large part in determining the probabilities of outcomes following each choice that has to be made . . .'[12]. In the above-mentioned, wider sense, **clinical decision analysis** is considered as an '*application of decision analysis in a clinical setting with the aim of applying epidemiological and other data to the probability of outcomes, when alternative decisions can be made*'[12]:

- It represents any activity;
- It systematizes (organizes) decision-making;
- It clarifies decision-making;
- It leads to the 'correctness' of decisions.

Using the above definition, such a field in medicine dates back to Lusted's original writings at the University of Chicago, Kassirer and Pauker's at Tufts, Weinstein et al's at Harvard, and Sox's at Stanford University. Principles of decision-making in general[13] and in medicine for the uninitiated[14] were followed by several introductory papers in medicine[15–22], surgery[23–26], gynecology and obstetrics[27–29], pediatrics[30], emergency medicine[31], clinical microbiology (infectious diseases)[32], public health[33–36], quality assessment[37] and medical technology assessment[38]. Nursing[39], dentistry[40], veterinary medicine[41] and other fields in the health sciences followed the trend. These are just a few examples of the many fields of application of decision analysis. Kassirer et al[42] reviewed them more extensively in their *ad hoc* paper. Updated topics may be found in the *Medical Decision Making* journal. Recent monographs and other *ad hoc* writings focus either on methodology and content[43–45], or on how to teach clinical decision analysis and decision-making[46–49]. Finally, indications are given on not only on how to use clinical decision analysis as a tool to identify general clinical strategies for selected problems, but also on how to use it in the care of individual patients[50–54], i.e. not only deciding if coronary bypass surgery is the best choice at a given stage of coronary heart disease in male or female patients, but also if diabetic, hypertensive Mr X, aged 65 years with a history of silent myocardial infarctions, should or should not have a coronary bypass given his recent complaints and coronary angiogram results. The following sections describe in more detail how decision analysis and decision-making work in general, as well as the direction-searching methodology and direction-giving methods in clinical decision-making.

13.3 Direction-searching tools in decision-making

Decision analysis is based on several mathematical models, such as decision trees, Markov models, Monte Carlo simulation, survival analysis and the hazard function, fuzzy logic, or sensitivity analysis[55]. Only decision analysis will be discussed here. Reproducing on paper the visual and graphical structuring of a multidimensional problem in two dimensional form, is used in various fields: path analysis[56] (see Chapter 8); prognostic trees (see Chapter 10); concept mapping in medical education[57]; and finally in decision and chagrin analysis or clinical algorithms as outlined in this chapter. However, beginners should be aware that not everything that has branches is a decision tree.

13.3.1 Decision trees and their analysis. Outline of the decision analysis process

The obvious objective of decision analysis is to find, among all options in a given clinical situation, the decision or way that would be the most beneficial to the patient. As paradoxical as it may appear, the approach described here, which is full of probabilities, values and computations, contributes much to the humanitarian aspect of medicine. It helps find by objective means a better clinical procedure or a choice of treatment for a given patient or for particular disease sufferers in general, than a method based on declarations of 'tender loving care', and/or indiscriminate use of new diagnostic and therapeutic technologies, even if all of the above are sometimes necessary in certain clinical situations. This should lead to the best primary, secondary, or tertiary prevention. As will be seen, patients have their own opinions, they express their preferred values of disease outcomes, and the physician takes this into account and introduces it into the decision-making process.

Modern medicine may appear dehumanized and technicized when based on the undesirable behavior of some clinicians, but if properly used in its substance, principles, and values, it is quite the opposite. It combines patient and physician contributions in order to reach a mutual agreement, which represents the best solution in a given clinical situation. It emphasizes the patient's opinion about an operation or its alternatives in terms of conservative (medical) treatment, after being thoroughly informed of the consequences. It represents an alternative to an impulsive, but unorganized way of decision-making, and allows for an integrated and organized approach to the problem and its subjective aspects. Clinical decision analysis does this by proceeding through stages of finding the best decision possible, where the patient's expectations are taken into account and where the physician is at ease with the decision, being as sure as possible that all means of diagnosis and treatment and their outcomes have been taken into account.

Decisions and their outcomes and values are a part of daily life. Consider how they might be made more concrete and applicable to a few clinical situations. First, consider the following situation between spouses. At a moment of tension, a spouse arrives home expecting a possible hostile welcome. He or she may decide to speak to the other spouse right away and produce a better situation (establish peace) or no change, or in fact make things worse (violent conflict). He or she may also decide not to speak right away, to 'let things cool down' and speak later. Similar possible outcomes as before, perhaps in different proportions, will occur, depending if the situation improves, does not change, or worsens. At each moment of decision, three outcomes may appear: spousal harmony will be re-established; tension will continue as before; or things will worsen in terms of immediate conflict. Figure 13.1 illustrates such a situation as described by a graphical representation called a 'decision tree'. (NB The tree 'grows from left to right', with squares representing decision points and circles indicating possible outcomes of preceding decisions.) It might be first thought that decisions should be made in the direction consistent with the greatest proportion of spousal harmony. However, if spouses want to separate, the conflict and ensuing disintegration of the relationship would have the greatest desirable value. Hence, the value of each outcome depends on what final outcome is desired. This situation has a more serious parallel in medicine. Figure 13.2 illustrates the case of a patient in an emergency room with acute abdominal pain. The attending physician may decide to do an exploratory operation right away, looking for appendicitis, mesenterial infarction, volvulus, intussusception, ruptured aneurysm, trauma, or other source of intra-abdominal bleeding, ectopic pregnancy, etc., or 'to get out' in the case of an infectious mesenteritis 'without doing anything' and closing the surgical wound. Or, the physician may decide to observe the patient for some time, do a further diagnostic work-up (e.g. laboratory tests, etc.), and decide later to operate or not, as often occurs in such situations. Is such an attitude of expectation a virtue of a seasoned clinician, or a serious error, which might be detrimental

to the patient's health and/or survival? Similarly, an organized structure may be given to any clinical decision process, which may then be analysed and the best possible solution found.

13.3.1.1 Stages of decision analysis, or 'growing, blooming, pruning, and harvesting' decision trees

Good decision-making should proceed through several stages as presented in Table 13.1. Many texts have been written on how to navigate these steps[15,46,58,59]. Consider the application of the above-mentioned steps of clinical decision analysis to the following example, which is a modified situation as discussed by Sisson et al[60] in another context.

Definition and position of the problem

In oncology, cancers *in situ*, localized and well delineated without any lymphatic or multi-organ

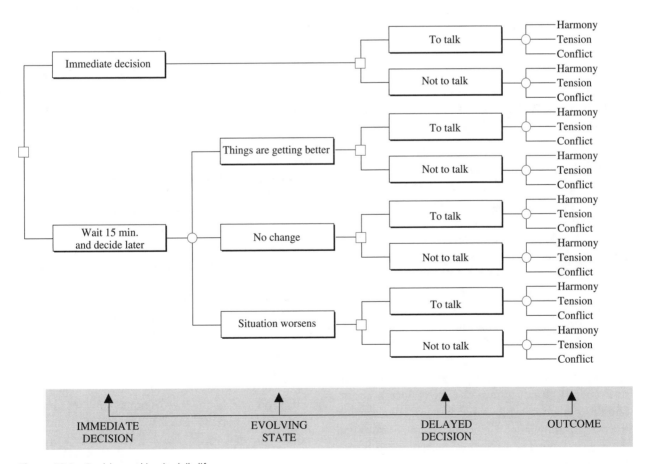

Figure 13.1   Decision-making in daily life

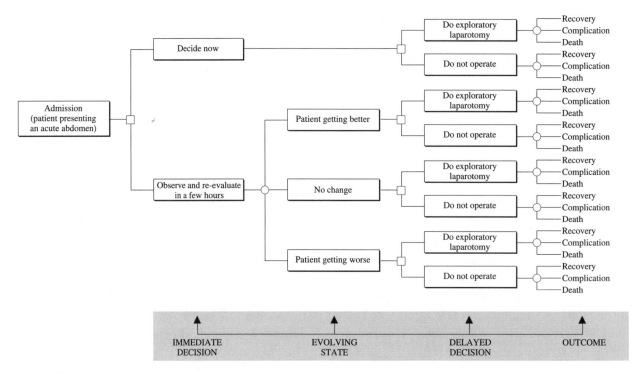

Figure 13.2 Example of a decision tree for the evaluation of an acute abdomen: Operate now or wait?

involvement and metastases are operated on and possibly treated with additional chemotherapy and/or radiotherapy. If the cancer has spread beyond the original site, these interventions are usually less successful.

What is the question to be answered?

A new radiological imaging procedure becomes available, and oncologists may reflect on whether such an additional diagnostic procedure to find metastases should be added to the battery of diagnostic tests already in use. However, the new radiodiagnostic imagery, in terms of its internal validity, may have an imperfect sensitivity and specificity, leading to wrong decisions to operate or not and to subsequent undesirable outcomes having their own acceptable or unacceptable values (utilities). True positive and negative results, as well as false negative or positive results and ensuing erroneous surgical decisions, their outcomes, and values must be taken into account. Should patients be operated on without further testing, or only after the result of the additional diagnostic test? The following discussion addresses this last question.

Structuring the problem, or 'growing and pruning' decision trees

First, **the starting point of the decision process should be recognized.** In this case, after the initial diagnostic work-up for cancer, the decision to operate or not must be made. Second, **a basic structure or 'maze' leading to the best clinical decision must be constructed.** To find the best clinical decision among many, all options must be defined along with possible outcomes of choosing one of these options. A **decision tree** is a picture or graphical expression of such a situation. It is a temporal and spatial representation, in a proper clinical sequence of options, offered to the clinician (to add a diagnostic method or not, to treat or not to treat, to choose different treatments, etc.) at moments of clinical work, represented as **decision nodes** of a decision tree (conventionally identified by squares).

Wherever possible, and without abandoning reality, preferably only two options should be attached to each decision node. However, more options do exist in the real world. For example, in the introductory example in this chapter, a physician must decide

---

Table 13.1 Stages of decision analysis

---

1. **DEFINE THE PROBLEM ('choose the seed')**

2. **WHAT IS THE QUESTION TO BE ANSWERED BY DECISION ANALYSIS? ('plant the seed')**

3. **STRUCTURE THE PROBLEM OVER TIME AND SPACE ('grow a decision tree')**
    - Recognize the starting decision point;
    - Make an overview of possible decision options (choices) and their outcomes;
    - Establish a temporo-spatial sequence if more than one pair of 'decision(s) – option(s)' – is involved, i.e. when ensuing outcomes of initial decisions engender other subsequent decisions, etc.;
    - Delete unrealistic, technically and ethically rare, and/or impossible or irrelevant options ('prune the tree').

4. **GIVE DIMENSION TO ALL RELEVANT COMPONENTS OF THE PROBLEM**
    ('foliate and let the tree bloom')
    - By obtaining available data to figure out probabilities of each outcome at any moment of the sequence of decisions and outcomes to be decided;
    - By obtaining the best and most objective data reflecting values ('utilities' in decision-making vocabulary) of each possible relevant outcome.

5. **ANALYZE THE PROBLEM ('examine the tree's branches')**
    - Choose the best way through the available decision paths;
    - Evaluate the sensitivity of the preferred decision (path), i.e. what would happen if conditions of the decision were to change?

6. **SOLVE THE PROBLEM ('choose what to pick')**
    - Choose the preferred decision (path), and

7. **ACT ACCORDING TO THE RESULT OF THE ANALYSIS ('enjoy the harvest')**

---

whether to treat a sore throat by antibiotics right away, not give antibiotics at all, or give antibiotics later depending on the result of a throat culture. In the treatment of herpes simplex encephalitis, a physician may decide to use an antiviral agent (vidarabine) while taking into consideration both its side effects and its benefits if disease is present or absent[61]. Clinical decisions incorporated into the decision tree are not only decisions to treat or not to treat. They may also concern whether or not to add another (presumably more modern and better) diagnostic method in serial or parallel testing in the clinical process preceding treatment decisions, additional medical or nursing care following an operation, social support and home care to convalescent patients, etc.

The next element, or sequence of the procedure, is a listing of what will happen to the patient if one or another decision is made. Such results or options are represented graphically (in examples which will follow and in the literature in general) by circles, as **chance** or **probability nodes**. Each event (outcome of the disease following a decision) has a probability ranging from 0.0 to 1.0. Since branches are exhaustive and mutually exclusive (for example, after surgery a patient recovers, develops a complication, or dies, but not a combination of the above), the sum of their probabilities must equal the whole, i.e. 1.0. Figure 13.3 illustrates how a basic decision tree might be constructed using the above-mentioned cancer surgery decision problem. The 'decision maze' is worked up or 'the decision tree is grown'. Next, the whole clinical situation is reviewed to see if it adequately reflects the most essential and prevalent (and relevant) components of the clinical situation and if their important outcomes have been retained. The superfluous or less frequent decisions with more negligible outcomes are deleted. This procedure of simplification is called '**pruning the decision tree**'. It would be useless to incorporate into a decision tree any procedure, however available, which would be highly risky for the patient or whose price would be prohibitive in a given clinical setting. The decision tree is consequently simplified to contain only essential, realistic components.

Giving dimensions to the decision tree, or 'blooming'
To let the decision tree 'foliate' or 'bloom', two basic dimensions must be found:

- A proportional distribution of outcomes following each decision (probabilities are assigned to any result of every decision); and
- A value, called '**utility**' in terms of decision analysis, must be given to each good or bad outcome.

Assigning utility to outcome is a question of judgment and we already know that judgment means attributing a value to something. In fact, the assignment of utility is one of the greatest challenges of decision analysis. Should the outcome be some monetary value (such as the cost of subsequent cure and care), some measure of pain and/or suffering, patient's quality of life, impact on a patient's surrounding, a physician's measure of therapeutic success or failure, or a score based on some or all of the above elements? There is no clear-cut answer to this problem. Decision analysis and its solution are valid only in the context of pre-established probabilities and utilities. These values are given to each outcome by the patient in the first place, by a physician in terms of a desired realistic result, or by an administrator or community health policy decision-maker in terms of economic (monetary), social, or political gains. These utilities can express a patient's

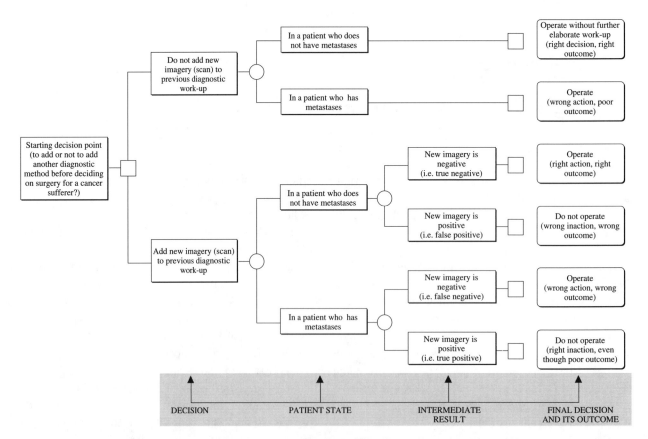

Figure 13.3 Example of a decision tree for a diagnostic work-up and surgery for cancer and its basic architecture. Source: Ref. 60, redrawn and reproduced with permission of the American Medical Association (*JAMA*)

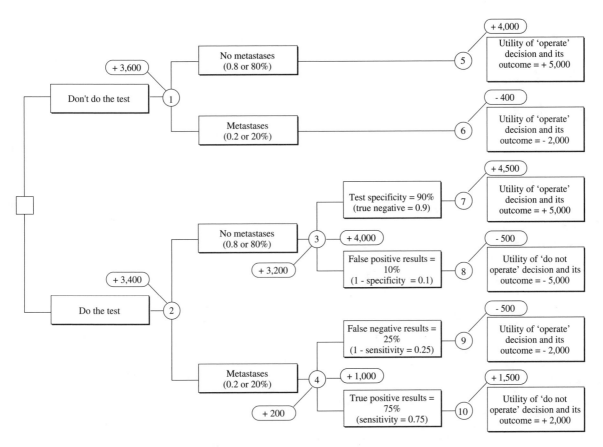

Figure 13.4 A fully 'blooming' or 'foliated' decision tree. Source: Ref. 60, redrawn and reproduced with permission of the American Medical Association (*JAMA*)

preferences (yes or no, or on a scale, for example, from 0 to 10, etc.), physician's preferences in terms of the chance of survival, or probability (prognosis) of complications, economist's preferences in terms of monetary value or savings of each outcome, etc. (NB This is the most difficult and delicate step in decision analysis. Will the patient's preferences satisfy the economist or administrator, or will monetary savings be acceptable to the patient, who should have the last word in terms of medical ethics?) In this example, a proportion of true or false positive and negative results of the new imaging method should be introduced in this model, as well as the value (utility) of all surgical decisions and their outcomes facing a given problem. In this example, utilities of each outcome are scored *ad hoc*. Such a score should reflect survival, patient preferences, money saved, or any combination of the above. This is the strength and also

the weakness and challenge of decision analysis, to find the best evaluation of the outcome's value.

Figure 13.4 illustrates the same decision tree, 'decorated as a Christmas tree' by probabilities of outcome and values that might be given to each outcome. In this case, a scoring system was chosen (taken from Sisson et al[60]) for each right and wrong decision. The greatest gain in terms of an expected good result is given the highest score, i.e. 5,000 positive points, if a primary cancerous lesion without metastases is excised, leading to the patient's cure or longer-term survival. A lesser utility but a positive one nonetheless, i.e. 2000 positive points, is attained when a surgeon decides not to operate when multisystemic cancerous involvement is present. 'Do not operate', a wrong decision in the case of false positive results (i.e. allowing a primary cancer to run its course without treating it before it metastizes), would have the least utility, i.e. 5,000 negative points. A decision not to operate in the presence of metastases would be a valid one. Its lesser value reflects that it would not influence the outcome of an already metastasized cancer case, i.e. a small gain of 2,000 positive points in this example. In the same way, the risk of operation to patients who already have metastatic cancer spread would be related to the risk of the operation only, i.e. scored by 2,000 negative points only.

Analyzing the problem through the decision tree, or 'choosing the best decision pathway'

At this stage of the decision analysis, a decision–outcome–utility pathway leading to the highest expected overall value (utility) of the pathway is chosen first. Utilities and probabilities are combined retroactively from each outcome in a procedure called 'folding back'. The **'folding back procedure'**, or following the sap 'from tips to roots', is based on the progressive multiplication of utilities (scores) by probabilities of outcomes following each decision point, starting with the final situation and going back to the original question point, i.e. adding or not adding the new imagery technique before therapeutic decisions are made. In this example (Figure 13.4), the value of a decision and of its outcome at point 5 would be $0.8 \times 5,000$, i.e. + 4,000, and – 400 points at point 6. Both of these values added give a value of + 3,600 to the outcome point 1. The same procedure, started at decision–outcome points 7, 8, 9 and 10, going through points 3 and 4, gives the value of + 3,400 at the point 2. Point 1 shows a higher value (3,600 compared to 3,400). Consequently, it can be concluded, on the basis of the premises of this example, that it is of no benefit to add the new imagery to a cancer patient's clinical work-up. The new imagery would not improve upon the clinical decision in the above-mentioned conditions.

Sensitivity analysis, or 'fertilizing and grafting' decision trees

In this final step, the decision analyst looks at how a decision would change if probabilities, reference values, and/or probabilities of outcomes and their values were to change. Such a procedure is called **'robustness'** in statistics (will different methods of analysis give similar results?), and is represented here

using the terminology **'sensitivity analysis'**, i.e. the assessment of how conclusions would change if the 'rules of the game' (i.e. probabilities of outcomes and/or their values) were to change.

Pauker and Kassirer[51] give an example of a young man for whom coronary arteriography might be considered given the patient's ventricular ectopic beats and an abnormal stress test. Figure 13.5 (redrawn from their paper) shows how the decision would change if the utility of coronary arteriography were to improve life expectancy after this invasive diagnostic method and subsequent surgery for left main coronary artery disease, compared to the expected 'baseline' utility, i.e. life expectancy without coronary angiogram. Available software for personal computers makes sensitivity analysis, based on numerous recalculations of decision analysis, fast and affordable in practice for an experienced decision analyst[51,62]. Based on sensitivity analysis represented in this figure, comparisons can be made between option A (perform the angiogram and surgery if necessary) and B (do not perform it). If life expectancy were less than 15 years after surgery, expected utilities for not performing the angiogram and surgery are better than those of a radical approach. If life expectancy after surgery were greater than 15 years, the radical option (invasive diagnostic method followed by surgery) would be preferable. If life expectancy after surgery reaches 15 years, both options give a comparable utility. Such situations often occur in clinical practice, making the clinician appear undecided. Kassirer and Pauker[63] identified these situations as a **'toss up'** or 'six of one, half a dozen of the other'. Such a point in decision-making allows the clinician to go beyond the initial premises of the decision. The clinician can now focus on other factors that may be important in making a right choice, such as the patient's attitude towards pain, complications, hospitalization, isolation from family and friends, etc[63]. Hence, decisions can be further refined to the best benefit and preferences of the patient once the 'big questions' such as survival are clarified.

Figure 13.6, from Barza and Pauker's study[61] of the therapeutic approach to herpes encephalitis, illustrates results of sensitivity analysis, related this time to expected utilities in relation to the clinical

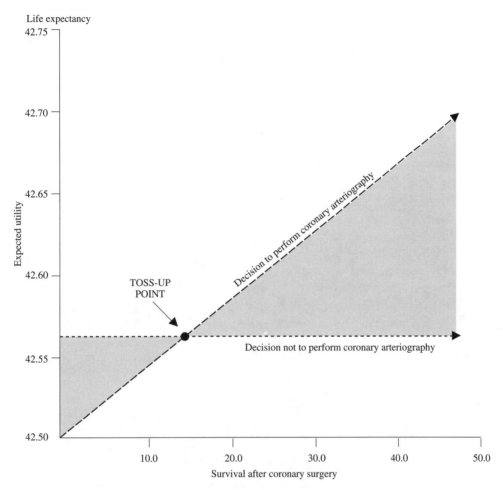

Figure 13.5 Graphical representation of sensitivity analysis results in considering coronary arteriography before performing surgery. Source: Ref. 51, redrawn and reproduced with permission of the American Medical Association (*Arch Intern Med*)

likelihood of disease (herpes encephalitis) before brain biopsy (which is not without risk of complications). Three toss-up points are noted here between various diagnostic–therapeutic options. Wherever the likelihood of disease is very low, i.e. less than 3%, neither treatment nor biopsy should be considered. Between 3 and 42%, doing the biopsy is the preferred option. At higher likelihoods, patients should be treated with the antiviral drug under evaluation (Vidarabine, in this case) without doing the biopsy. Three, 10 and 42% likelihood levels are toss up points between options as illustrated. Symbolically speaking, this is how decision analysts expose their decision trees to changes of seasons and weather when examining how they survive and towards which side they will lean.

13.3.2 Chagrin analysis

Even when based only on 'pruned' decision trees, decision analysis may be a cumbersome process for many. Are there other ways to simplify it? In 'classical' decision analysis as described above, competing decisions and all their relevant outcomes are analyzed. However, most outcomes, whether good or bad, are inevitable in given circumstances. Clinicians can do nothing about these outcomes. On the other hand, mistakes must be avoided. Mistakes lead to regrets, which the French language expresses as 'chagrin'. Feinstein adopted this term in his proposal to reduce decision analysis to chagrin analysis[64].

The concept of chagrin analysis may be best illustrated by the following example: A 60-year-old man

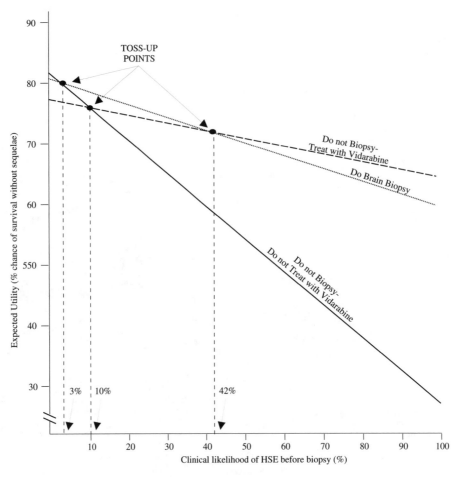

3%, 10%, 42% likelihoods indicate various toss-up points as equal alternatives to diagnose, to treat, or not, in different combinations

Figure 13.6 Sensitivity analysis results of diagnostic and therapeutic approaches to herpes simplex encephalitis. Toss-up points. Source: Ref. 61, redrawn with modifications and reproduced with permission of the American College of Physicians (*Ann Intern Med*)

goes on a week-long car trip with a physician friend. The man complains of pain in the left shoulder radiating to the left arm. The journey is long, and the man complains of sudden fatigue and sweating. Knowing that his friend suffers from angina, the physician might suspect a myocardial infarction, and might try to get his friend to the nearest hospital as fast as possible. He might also dismiss this episode as a simple spell of fatigue due to hot weather, with radicular pain caused by the long drive. Figure 13.7 illustrates the physician's two options and their consequences:

1. Upon arrival at the hospital, his friend will or will not be diagnosed as suffering a myocardial

infarction. Under proper care, he will or will not survive. If he is sent home from the emergency room after a myocardial infarction has been ruled out, the physician friend will be 'chagrined' for bringing him to the hospital 'for nothing'. If he were to die of the infarction, then if whatever could and should have been done was done, there would be no regret or 'chagrin'.

2. The physician friend may dismiss this episode as minor and suggest continuing on so as not to spoil the trip. A minor problem will resolve itself. However, if his friend were to suffer an infarction, he may or may not survive it without proper early care. If he were to survive, the physician friend would not be 'chagrined' despite having made a

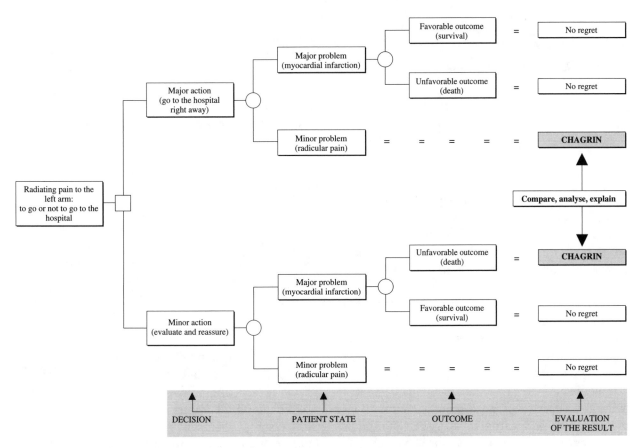

Figure 13.7 Example of chagrin analysis

wrong decision by not sending him to the hospital right away. If his friend were to die of myocardial infarction, he would regret his decision 'not to do anything'.

Hence, only two paths and their outcomes are worth comparing: the decision to undertake a major action for nothing (sending a healthy individual for advanced care); and the decision to do nothing, leading to the patient's death. Obviously, the option avoiding the most important 'chagrin' will be chosen as the best decision in the circumstances. For Brody and Thompson[65], Feinstein's strategy is essentially a 'maximin' strategy, as commented earlier in this chapter (i.e. to choose the lesser of two evils). Such an 'extremely pruned' decision analysis is known, for example, to obstetricians, who must choose between a natural birth with inherent risks for mother and child in a given clinical condition, and a maximum use of technology and/or surgery to minimize or avoid the potential greatest risk to the mother and

child's health. This is one reason why physicians may be biased in favor of the more frequent use of new and advanced technologies[65].

13.3.3 Threshold approach to clinical decisions

Based on several components of the Bayesian approach to diagnostic decision-making (see Chapter 6) and the assessment of risks, Pauker and Kassirer propose another decision tool called the **threshold approach to clinical decision-making**[66]. No diagnostic procedure (no matter how expensive), especially if it results from new technologies in medicine, is without risk. A cardiac catheterization, for example, is an invasive diagnostic method. A cardiac patient's condition may worsen during a stress test. An exploratory laparoscopy may infect the operative site. Consequently, a conservative thinking clinician will want to be as certain as possible about which one of these three options to adopt:

- Not to perform a risky test and not treat the disease under consideration;
- To perform the test and decide to treat on the basis of the test result; or
- Not to perform the risky test and treat right away on the basis of the diagnostic information already available.

Similar questions often arise when 'old' problems are to be solved, such as in this chapter's previous example of the patient presenting with a sore throat: not to treat; treat after the test results come back; or treat with antibiotics without further testing.

The principle of threshold assessment is the comparison of the best possible likelihood that the patient has the disease before further testing and/or treatment is considered (for example, a predictive value of a positive result of clinical or paraclinical assessment, adjusted or not by a pre-work-up likelihood of disease, such as its prevalence in the patient's community) with two decision thresholds. On a scale of probability of disease from 0.0 to 1.0, two thresholds are calculated – the **testing threshold** and the **test–treatment threshold**. The basic computational formulas for these thresholds are[66]:

$$\text{Testing threshold }(T_t) = \frac{(P_{pos/nd}) \times (R_{rx}) + R_t}{(P_{pos/nd}) \times (R_{rx}) + (P_{pos/d}) \times (B_{rx})}$$

$$\text{Test-treatment threshold }(T_{rxt}) = \frac{(P_{neg/nd}) \times (R_{rx}) + R_t}{(P_{neg/nd}) \times (R_{rx}) + (P_{neg/d}) \times (B_{rx})}$$

Where:

P: Probability of disease before testing

$P_{pos/d}$: Probability of a positive result in patients with disease

$P_{neg/d}$: Probability of a negative result in patients with disease

$P_{pos/nd}$: Probability of a positive result in patients without disease

$P_{neg/nd}$: Probability of a negative result in patients without disease

B_{rx}: Benefit of treatment in patients with disease

R_{rx}: Risk of treatment in patients without disease

R_t: Risk of diagnostic test

T_t: Testing threshold

T_{trx}: Test–treatment threshold

Figure 13.8 illustrates that both thresholds divide the probability range into three zones. The segment between both thresholds (the middle one) will be proportionate to other ones in the case of the reference test, disproportionately wide in the case of a test with greater accuracy or lower risk, and very narrow in the case of a test with lower accuracy or greater risk[66] (NB The term 'risk' denotes the probability of complications or undesirable effects, or outcomes of testing itself, and/or of disease itself). The deciding physician must assess the probability that the patient

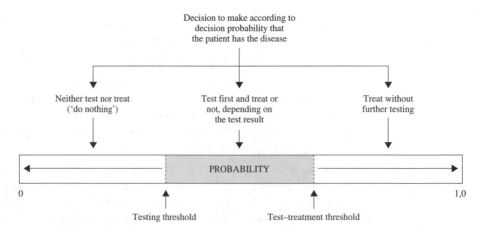

Figure 13.8 Testing and treatment thresholds in clinical decision-making. Source: Ref. 66, redrawn and reproduced with permission from the Massachusetts Medical Society (*N Engl J Med*)

has the disease (based on the best positive predictive value of the previous diagnostic process), and decide into which 'likelihood segment' of Figure 13.8 such a value will fall. Under the 'test threshold' value, the physician will do nothing. Between the 'test threshold' and 'test–treatment threshold' values, the physician will test and treat accordingly, and if estimation of likelihood of the disease is superior to the 'test–treatment threshold' value, treatment will occur without further new testing. Furthermore, expected utilities for each procedure (doing nothing, testing and treating, treating without further testing) at each level of pre-test clinical likelihood may be established and the physician may decide, at each level of likelihood of disease, what is the best option[66].

13.3.4 Cost-benefit analysis in therapeutic decision-making

Many physicians still dislike taking costs into consideration. However, every clinical decision has its price, not only in monetary terms, but also in complications, incapacity, handicaps, etc. A full-scale **cost–benefit analysis** is an **economic** analysis *in which the economic and social costs of medical care and the benefits of reduced loss of net earnings due to preventing premature death or disability are considered*[12]. A **cost-effectiveness analysis** *seeks to determine the costs and effectiveness of an activity, or to compare similar alternative activities to determine the relative degree to which they will obtain the desired objectives and outcomes*[12]. On the other hand, a **cost–utility analysis** is an *economic analysis in which outcomes are measured in terms of their social value*. A widely used utility-based measure is *quality-adjusted life years*[12]. Such a full-scale three-dimensional economic analysis is beyond the scope of this chapter. Other overviews of this methodology may be found elsewhere[67–70], along with several examples of its application to specific topics, such as immunization[71], secondary and tertiary prevention of cancer[72], the control of renovascular disease[73], and others. According to Eisenberg, the economic evaluation of medical care assesses four aspects of care with the following specific questions in mind[69]:

○ **Efficacy:** can it work?

○ **Effectiveness:** does it work?
○ **Efficiency:** what does it cost for what it gives?
○ **Equity:** how are costs and benefits distributed?

In **clinical decision analysis,** as covered in this chapter, the **cost–benefit approach** is a 'scaled down and reoriented analysis' in accordance to the definition above. Monetary values are often replaced by clinically important 'costs', such as operative case fatality, case fatality in treated and untreated individuals in the general population, occurrence of side effects of diagnosis and/or treatment, occurrence of co-morbidity and its impact. Survival or any other measure of 'positive' impact is used as an indicator of 'benefit'. The subject of evaluation is **efficiency** from the four aspects of evaluation quoted above, and based on the question 'What does it cost, and of what value is it?' **in clinical terms.** Monetary values can be taken into consideration, but they are not the principal focus of analysis. Rather, they are integrated into a larger frame of clinical considerations.

Cost–benefit analysis has the following prerequisites:

- Only one disease is under consideration (present or absent);
- An efficient treatment exists and is available;
- The clinician's decision is made in a situation of uncertainty;
- Serious consequences would appear if disease sufferers were not treated; and
- Equally serious, if not worse, consequences would appear if persons not suffering from the disease (healthy individuals or patients suffering from other health problems) were subjected to the treatment modality under consideration.

Such considerations and prerequisites apply to many surgical interventions or cancer treatments.

Pauker and Kassirer[74] propose the following practical example, which illustrates cost–benefit analysis in clinical decision-making. Figure 13.9 shows a basic structure (decision tree) whose analysis should answer the question of whether or not to operate for suspected appendicitis. An adolescent male complains of abdominal pain. The physical and laboratory findings in the emergency room are inconclusive, giving a probability of 0.3 for acute

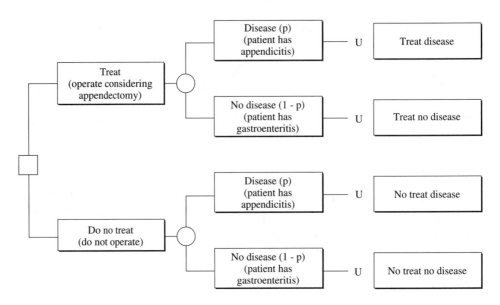

Figure 13.9 Utilities from a decision tree for cost/benefit analysis. Source: Ref. 74, redrawn and reproduced with permission from the Massachusetts Medical Society (*N Engl J Med*)

appendicitis and 0.7 for acute gastroenteritis. What cost–benefit ratio would lead to the best decision in this case? The following steps of cost–benefit analysis were followed:

1. The question of which cost–benefit analysis answer is required was formulated:

Given the state of the patient (abdominal pain, etc.)
— operate for appendicitis
— do not operate

2. Indicators of cost and benefit (utilities) were defined as follows:
Cost (in clinical terms): risk of death (case fatality rate).
Benefit (in clinical terms): probability of survival.

3. Options (chances following decisions) were listed:
   - Operate on a patient with appendicitis ($U_{treat\ dis}$);
   - Operate on a patient with gastroenteritis ($U_{treat\ no\ dis}$), i.e. who does not have appendicitis;
   - Do not operate on a patient who needs it ($U_{no\ treat\ dis}$) (appendicitis sufferer);
   - Do not operate on a patient who does not need it ($U_{no\ treat\ no\ dis}$) (gastroenteritis sufferer who does not have appendicitis).

4. Values for utilities were determined from clinical experience and the literature as follows: operative mortality (operated case fatality rate) is 0.1%; in other terms, survival for surgery is 99.9%; case fatality rate associated with delaying necessary surgery is 1% (i.e. survival of 99%). Benefits and costs were calculated as follows:

$$\text{Benefit (B)} = U_{treat\ dis} - U_{no\ treat\ dis} = 99.9\% - 99\%$$
$$= 0.9\%$$

$$\text{Cost(C)} = U_{no\ treat\ no\ dis} - U_{treat\ no\ dis} =$$
$$= 100\% - 99.9\% = 0.1\%$$

Giving a benefit/cost ratio (B/C) of 9.0

A threshold probability for B/C ratio (T) is calculated as follows:

Test–treatment (T) by definition =

$$\frac{1}{\dfrac{B}{C}+1} = \frac{1}{9+1} = 0.1$$

5. The probability of appendicitis is compared to the threshold probability and a decision is made on

this basis: in this example, the probability of appendicitis (i.e. 0.3) is higher than the threshold value (0.1), indicating that immediate operation is the preferred choice in this given situation.

NB Other benefits, besides the avoidance of deaths, may be taken into consideration according to the authors: avoidance of adhesions, abscesses, sepsis. Pain and/or a variety of medical and surgical complications represent alternative costs for such a type of cost–benefit analysis[74].

13.3.5 Desirable components and attributes of clinical decision analysis

Several basic elements contribute to good decision analysis, leading to clinically useful results and bringing relevant answers:

1. The question to be answered by clinical decision analysis needs to be clearly stated.
2. The problem must be clearly formulated in terms of a good decision tree (if this approach is used). Its quality will depend on several ingredients ('fertilizers' of the tree), such as knowledge of:
   - The general and clinical epidemiology of the problem under study (occurrence, course, risk and prognostic characteristics and their probabilities);
   - The validity of the diagnostic methods;
   - The spectrum of outcomes of clinical interest;
   - Other diseases and their treatments, associated with the problem under study;
   - All relevant competing clinical interventions (diagnostic and therapeutic maneuvers, both radical and conservative, their risks, advantages, disadvantages, and costs); and
   - The utility of various outcomes, varying from one disease and individual to another. Therefore, one must have the aptitude to evaluate them.
3. The logic of the architecture of the decision tree (and the relevance of its components).
4. The quality of analysis of the decision tree.
5. The richness of information produced by such an analysis.
6. Proposed solutions apply equally well to the disease (clinical problem) in general as to an individual patient, who should benefit from a correct decision to test and treat problem(s).
7. This type of decision analysis gives better results than any other competing method of decision-making.

Consequently, good decision analyses and decision-making are sizeable intellectual and professional challenges. It is also easier to calculate and compute them than to conceive, carry and deliver them, be it in surgery[75,76], medicine[77,78] or public health[79].

13.3.6 Advantages and limitations of decision analysis

Even a well-performed clinical decision analysis has its own inherent advantages and disadvantages.

The advantages are:

1. It is much less costly than the search for the best decision through experimental research, which is often sophisticated in design and complex in execution and analysis.
2. It can be easily translated into clinical decisions and public health policies.
3. It is an important tool in medical education. It allows students to better structure their thinking and to navigate the maze of decision-making.

The disadvantages are:

1. It is less valuable if clinical data and information are of poor quality and/or uncertain.
2. It may take up precious time in emergency situations, especially in the hands of a less-experienced decision analyst.
3. Utilities may have different values and weights in different individuals, be they patients, doctors, or community decision-makers (administrators, politicians, economists, etc.) or those of individual patients versus their community.

Obviously, all the above apply if (and only if) decision analysis is used to solve real problems, and not merely as an intellectual exercise.

13.4 Direction-giving tools in decision-making

Once the best option (evidence) is obtained either through decision analysis, clinical trial, consensus or other means, directions for decisions may be established. Such directions may have a tactical or strategic character. **Tactical tools** (in military arts, 'the tools needed to win the battle') focus on specific objects, solving an important part of the problem – for example, a diagnostic work-up of breast cancer or diabetes. *Clinical algorithms* belong to this category. **Strategic tools** (in military arts, 'the tools needed to win the war') try to give the best directions (management skills) in a broader context. What to do when taking care of breast cancer patients from diagnosis and treatment to follow-up? How to care for patients suspected of having diabetes? *Clinical practice guidelines* are a good example of strategic tools in medicine. Only these two tools will be discussed here.

As seen in the previous section, important progress has been made regarding the best way to navigate the mazes of possible decision options, which appear in diagnosing and treating health problems. Once these best ways (and decisions) are found, they should be organized in an ensemble of optimal steps leading to the best result and benefit for the patient, or for the community if disease control is in question. Such a 'best kit' must be based on the best available evidence, from whatever source it may come: decision analysis as described above; original clinical and community research studies; meta-analysis of the best clinical and epidemiological experience of the deciding physician; or the physician's careful assessment of the specific situation relative to the patient or community.

13.4.1 Tactical tools: clinical algorithms and decision tables

Clinical algorithms and decision tables are offered in increasing numbers to the practicing community to fill a need for easy-to-use and practical guides to clinical decisions. Experienced clinicians may be tempted to draw up graphical guides in a flow and chain of decision. Others draw colored 'quick fixes' for subsidized, mostly advertising-oriented periodicals for practitioners, and call them 'continuing education'.

There is a better way to develop and use clinical algorithms.

Clinical algorithms are *step-by-step written protocols for health management*[80]. **They consist of** *an explicit description of steps to be taken in patient care in specified circumstances*[12]. What diagnostic and therapeutic steps should be taken to properly treat a sore throat? How should a case of multiple trauma in (and en route to) an emergency room be managed? Clinical algorithms are a specific category of algorithms in general. Algorithm is defined as 'an alteration'. It is derived from **arithmetic**, and **algorism**, from edictal Latin **algorismus**, the latter derived from the Arabic Al-Khuwarizmi, system of numerals, identified by the name of Al-Khuwarizmi, a ninth-century Persian mathematician[81]. It is '*a set of rules for approaching the solution to a complex problem by setting down individual steps and delineating how each step follows from the preceding one*'[82]. Its character as a 'uniform procedure'[82] and a 'finite number of steps' for a solution of a given specific problem[83] are usually stressed. An algorithm, or a process that is 'in one's head', may be made concrete through different forms: algebraic notation, computer program, or graphical form. The two most widely used graphical forms of algorithms are flow charts and decision tables. The term 'algorithm' will be used here to refer to its flow chart form, which is best known to non-mathematical minds.

13.4.1.1 Algorithms as flow charts

Given its visual impact, the graphical form is the one most widely used in medicine. An algorithm in its most well known graphical form is a kind of flow chart. By definition, a flow chart is a graphical representation of the progress of a system for the definition, analysis, or solution of a data processing (or manufacturing) problem in which symbols are used to represent operations and data (or material flow and equipment), and lines and arrows represent inter-relationships among the components. (Syn. control diagram; flow diagram; flow sheet)[83]. Decision trees and algorithms are flow charts as well. The fundamental difference between the two is that a decision tree portrays the choices available to those responsible for patient care and the probabilities and values of each possible outcome that will follow a particular strategy in patient or community care. It is an open system, like a menu in a restaurant. Algorithms are a closed system; they are orders reflecting what should be eaten, starting with an appetizer and working through the '*pièce de résistance*' to dessert. Clinical algorithms have often proven useful in almost all medical specialties and fields of practice. However, as a medical tool, like any diagnostic or therapeutic method, technique or instrument, they must have a well-structured and understandable form, a reason for their creation and use, and they must be evaluated for their advantages and weaknesses in their use and impact. Consider these important aspects of 'evidence-based' algorithms.

Architecture of algorithms

Figure 13.10 illustrates an algorithm for the clinical work-up and management of a stab wound of the abdomen[84] (see also Chapter 6, Figure 6.3), presented here in the standardized fashion. It guides the practitioner from an initial evaluation of the patient by successive steps, represented alternatively by clinical findings and actions to be taken. An action may be either a final diagnosis or a surgical or medical procedure to correct the situation. This sequence progresses to the exit point from the algorithm, usually the resolution of the clinical problem, depending on the type of action points. Algorithms may be purely diagnostic (no treatment

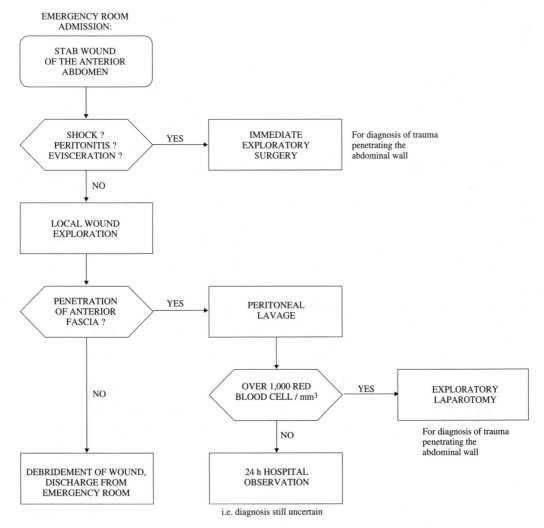

Figure 13.10 Algorithm for a stab wound of the anterior abdomen evaluation and management. Source: Ref. 84, redrawn and reorganized into standard algorithm form

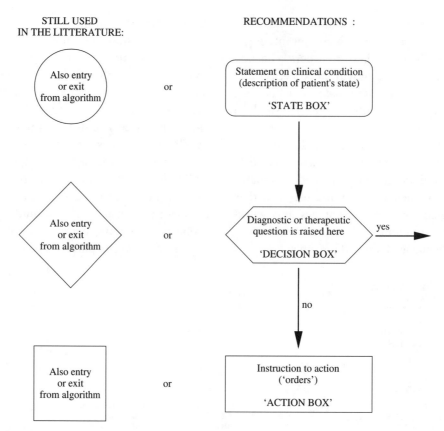

STILL USED
IN THE LITTERATURE:

RECOMMENDATIONS :

Also entry
or exit
from algorithm

or

Statement on clinical condition
(description of patient's state)

'STATE BOX'

Also entry
or exit
from algorithm

or

Diagnostic or therapeutic
question is raised here

'DECISION BOX'

yes

no

Also entry
or exit
from algorithm

or

Instruction to action
('orders')

'ACTION BOX'

Figure 13.11   Graphical components of algorithms. Based on recommendations from references 89 and 90

indicated), purely interventional, or a mixture of both.

Diagnostic work-ups of a fever of unknown origin[85], physical disease in psychiatric patients[86], anemia[87], or heart disease in neonates[88] are examples of diagnostic algorithms. They consume too much space to be reproduced here. Graphical symbols and components of algorithms as represented in Figure 13.10 are not random. Standards for clinical algorithms have been recently worked up and proposed for general use[89,90].

An algorithm's basic components have specific meaning as represented in Figure 13.11. However, some variations may still be found in the literature. Clinical boxes (rounded rectangles), decision boxes (hexagons), action boxes (rectangles), and link boxes (small ovals) are put in a sequence flowing from top to bottom and from left to right. Arrows, never intersecting if possible, are unobstructed by writing except in decision boxes, 'yes' arrows pointing right, 'no' arrows pointing down. Sequential numbering of boxes

in the above-mentioned directions is suitable, with the whole algorithm preferably covering a single page. Annotations are suitable and abbreviations are not[90].

Criteria for construction and use of clinical algorithms

An algorithm approach is indicated in specific clinical conditions, states of knowledge, or for particular users and working environments.

1. The clinical problem should be controversial and subject to uncertainty[91].
2. In practice, the problem is approached by diverse means, with such variations being hard to explain. It is felt that anarchy at the workplace should be replaced by a logical procedure that is well organized in time.
3. The problem should be common, and a frequent subject in the workload of the organization (e.g. rapid diagnosis of infections, acute surgical and gyneco-obstetrical cases (ectopic pregnancy), multiple trauma emergency cases, causes leading

to resuscitation, long and complicated diagnostic work-ups in internal medicine, etc.).

4. Clinical problems that are handled in extreme work conditions, such as intensive and emergency care.

5. Clinical problems that must be handled by less qualified, trained, and/or experienced personnel[92] – for example, in peripheral areas in the Canadian North, or elsewhere such as deserts or mountain regions, often where few physicians are available, so that diagnostic and therapeutic tasks must be conferred on nurses, midwives, paramedics, community elders, or educated people such as teachers or priests, etc.

6. Clinical care that must be provided by paramedics or laypeople before patients get to the clinic or the hospital.

7. There is a need to offer the best possible care to as many people as possible, especially when human and material resources are limited, such as in many developing countries. Here, the application of the algorithmic approach may be useful for more common and less sophisticated problems.

8. Algorithms may represent a reference point in the assessment of the quality of medical, nursing, and other professional care (process review and medical audit[93–95]).

9. Algorithms may be used as a training tool in teaching medical students; in this situation, they represent an introduction to organized and structured thinking and not a 'recipe on how to prepare the patient'.

10. Algorithms may be useful for pre-selected groups with limited access to medical care, such as company and government employees in isolated locations, people who work at sea, aboriginals and natives on their ancestral lands, etc.

To respond adequately to these tasks and expectations, algorithms must be correctly built and tested, and finally their use must be evaluated.

Steps in the construction of evidence-based clinical algorithms

The construction of clinical algorithms should follow these clearly defined steps:

1. The clinical problem to be solved by the algorithm must be well formulated and defined[96] (diagnostic, occurrence, target population, users, expected results, etc.). Current practice must be described.

2. Expected results of algorithm use must be specified (gains for practice, economy, patient, physician workload, etc.). 'Discriminators'[97], i.e. points in clinical work-up leading to a suggested action, are well defined and described in explicit terms.

3. Clear indications are given as to when, where, and by whom the algorithm is supposed to be used and what kind of patients it should be applied to:
   - Patients eligible for the algorithmic approach must be well defined (target population for use of the algorithm);
   - Situations in which algorithms should be used must be defined;
   - Users of algorithms must be identified.

4. The clinical situation statement → diagnostic statement → therapeutic and/or diagnostic options must be clearly defined in a realistic time-and-space relationship.

5. Enough data must be retrieved from the literature, original studies, data analysis, clinical trials, consensus studies, medical audits, or personal and other clinical experience, or simple 'gut feelings' or 'flair' to justify each step of the algorithm. It must be clear, from the description of the proposed algorithm, which of the above-mentioned elements was used in its construction and justification. This what makes an algorithm 'evidence-based'.

6. Entry and exit points of the algorithm need to be defined.

7. Diagnostic steps must be organized in order of their decreasing severity.

8. Therapeutic steps are organized either in order of their lifesaving importance (the worst first) or in order of their increasing cost and complexity (from the cheapest to the most expensive).

9. All indications in boxes (graphical components of the algorithm) are clear, explicit and as complete as necessary.

10. The algorithm should be drawn in a conventional, consistent manner that is understandable to the user.

If an algorithm respecting the above-mentioned rules is put into practice, its performance and effect must be evaluated.

Evaluation of clinical algorithms

An algorithm and its use is a type of clinical maneuver like any other (diagnostic or therapeutic); its process (use) and impact must be evaluated, its weaknesses and strengths known.

Subjects of **process evaluations** usually include:

- The security and appropriateness of the algorithm;
- 'Accidents' related to its use, such as errors, which might harm the patient ('patient friendliness');
- Whether using the algorithm promotes the full use of knowledge and skills of its users;
- The economy of its use; and
- How comfortable physicians are using it ('user friendliness').

Several topics are of interest when **evaluating the impact** of algorithm use:

- Does it correctly evaluate the patient's state?
- Does it produce errors leading to undesirable effects, even if properly used?
- Does it cover an important proportion and spectrum of daily cases? For example, 10 pediatric algorithms for primary pediatric care from the University of Kansas would cover 75 to 80% of primary care cases[97] – work-up of fever, cough, vomiting, diarrhea, skin rash, dysuria, headache, abdominal pain, earache, and child health assessment;
- Most importantly, does its use improve a patient's state more than any alternative approach in diagnosis and therapeutic decision-making[3]?

Observational studies are usually used in process assessment. Sauer and Rodi[91] evaluated the utility of an algorithm in diagnosing ectopic pregnancy this way.

An algorithmic approach proves useful in the assessment of new technologies. In diabetes research, algorithms were developed for glucose infusion to maintain glycemic homeostasis at different levels of insulinemia, either by a 'manual method' or with a closed-loop delivery system known as the 'artificial pancreas'. Campostano et al[98] studied the safety and stability of such an algorithm. Algorithms may also be used to tell new technologies how to function. Linear and non-linear algorithms for the QT sensing rate of adaptive cardiac pacemakers were evaluated for their impact by Baig et al[99] in a randomized, double-blind, crossover clinical trial. Controlled clinical trials, although the golden standard in treatment impact (effect) assessment, remain rarely used in the evaluation of the use of algorithms. They should become standard. Beyond the above-mentioned examples, the evaluation of algorithms across the literature focuses mainly on 'process' evaluation. The 'effect' evaluation is often more difficult.

13.4.1.2 Algorithms as decision tables

Algorithms may also be presented in a tabular form, less common than flow charts, but more appropriate in some situations. **A decision table is** *'a tabular array of sets of conditions, and of the decisions selected as a response to each set of conditions'*[100]. Figure 13.12 illustrates such a decision table for use by nurses at pediatric outpatient and emergency departments to assess children presenting with a complaint of diarrhea[97]. Each decision table contains four parts or components:

1. The **condition stub section**. It enumerates manifestations and observations of interest for decision-making. In this example, characteristics of the child, selected information from the patient's history, and clinical findings are listed.
2. The **condition entry** section, where a yes or no (dot or blank in this example) indicates the presence or absence of each required finding.
3. The **action stub**, listing possible actions or decisions that are offered to the user. In this example, it is a two-stage choice: first, paraclinical examinations are offered to complete the picture from the patient's history and physical examination; and finally second-stage decisions are listed, such as calling the physician or performing subsequent appropriate flow charts to complete the patient's assessment and make decisions about cure and care. In this example, 17 situations or combinations of findings are displayed. A combination of findings in a patient is compared to the 17 arrays in order to situate it within them, and decisions are indicated in the fourth section of the decision table.

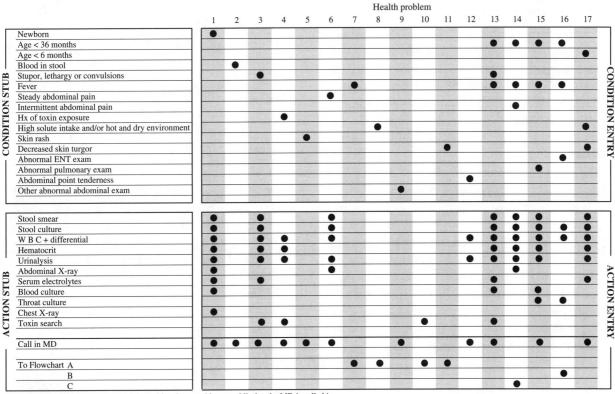

N.B. If a test marked with an asterisk is positive, i.e., outside normal limits, the MD is called in.
* **Diarrhea is defined as** :
  Patient age ≥ 6 months : ≥ 8 watery stools in 24 h
  Patient age < 6 months : ≥ 6 watery stools in 24 h
           OR   ≥ 3 watery stools in 4 h

Figure 13.12 Example of a decision table· Source: Reworked from Ref. 97 and 104, reproduced with permission from *Clinical Pediatrics* and Westminister Publications

4. The **action entry,** gives the user exact indications of what to do given that the findings match with one of the condition entry configurations. Consider column 1 of this example: if a newborn is brought to the hospital with diarrhea, a full paraclinical work-up except throat culture and toxin search is mandatory, and the nurse is required to call the attending physician right away without proceeding to any subsequent flow charts.

While a flow chart algorithm explains the decision-making path more explicitly, a decision table better portrays clinical conditions in which decisions depend on a wider array of necessary findings to arrive at the best conclusion regarding the action to take[101]. Decision tables originate in industry. General Electric and Sutherland developed this tool to better describe the increasingly complex manufacturing processes at the end of the fifties[102]. The first monograph appeared[103], and Feinstein[100] and Holland[102] introduced decisions tables to physicians. More recently, in the surgical approach to metastatic liver cancer, Schwarz et al[104] developed a computer-based decision support system in the form of decision tables. Decision table techniques were also used to improve clinical practice guidelines (*vide infra*) for the prevention of perinatal transmission of hepatitis B by immunization[105]. At present, decision tables have made only a discrete entry in the field of clinical decision-making. Their advantages and complementarity with flow chart algorithms are worth further study, use, and evaluation.

13.4.1.3 Advantages and limitations of clinical algorithms

As with any other clinical tool, clinical algorithms have both desirable and undesirable characteristics.

Desirable characteristics:

- The algorithm builder chooses a desired sequence of steps according to what is considered a priority;
- The algorithm is a closed system, defined and unequivocal, instructing the user what to do;
- The algorithm contains clear definitions and criteria for each step, such as results of paraclinical tests replacing clinical 'impressions' of the 'patient appears ill' type;
- Each step is supported by the best available evidence that this is a preferred option;
- Orders are clear, enabling more precise work from the supporting staff;
- Algorithms allow a systematic acquisition of clinical and paraclinical data, their retrieval from data banks, and interpretation;
- Algorithms help organize a clinician's thinking; and
- Algorithms represent a straightforward and economic approach to intellectual work.

Undesirable characteristics:

- Different people may have difficulty using algorithms, at different places and when treating different patients than at their origin. An algorithm (like decision analysis) often does not 'travel well';
- Algorithms must be used very often to justify all the effort put into their development;
- Algorithms cannot be used without precise indications and criteria;
- Algorithms may be blindly overused by supporting staff;
- An algorithm is costly to build well, i.e. to give all desirable characteristics;
- Algorithms are often too complex, such as in references 73 and 76;
- Any algorithms which are poorly validated, if at all; and
- No valid information on their use (instructions) is available[106,107].

Clinical algorithms should be based on more than just their author's knowledge and judgment. However good they might be, they remain unknown to potential users (i.e. readers of the paper). Usually, clinical algorithms lack detailed instructions. So, the fault lies not with the algorithms themselves, but with their proponents and authors. Until now, algorithms were developed and used mainly in the fields of diagnosis and treatment. They should also be expanded into prognosis[100] and risk assessments and may also be used advantageously in the evaluation of the quality of clinical care[101,108]. What are algorithms worth? Komaroff[109] will answer this question as a conclusion to this section:

'...*While algorithms may continue to play a role in medical decision-making, it is unlikely that they will find any role in the two other critically important aspects of caring for the patient: ... listening to the patient for what is said, how it is said, and what is not said; and explaining, providing reassurance, and showing that one cares. Algorithms are no substitute for experience, sensitivity, or compassion ... In our view, algorithms can help us to articulate how we make decisions, to clarify our knowledge and to recognize our ignorance. They can help us to demystify the practice of medicine, and to demonstrate that much of what we call the* 'art' *of medicine is really a scientific process, a science which is waiting to be articulated ...*'

There is a big difference between an 'impressionist' and an 'evidence-based' algorithm.

13.4.2 Strategic tools for right decisions: clinical practice guidelines

Preoccupations with the best possible quality of care and cost containment lead health administration and professional institutions, at various local and international levels, to develop and implement clinical practice guidelines. How to care for cancer patients after surgery? How to care for diabetics or hypertensive patients? What is the best long-term care for arthritis? **Clinical practice guidelines (CPG)** should respond to such a need. Clinical practice guidelines have been **defined** as '*systematically developed statements to assist practitioner and patient decisions about appropriate health care for specific clinical circumstances*'[110]. More precisely, **good CPGs should**[111]:

- Limit variations in practice;

- Reduce necessary costs;
- Give a scientific direction to care;
- Provide useable summaries of the best evidence-based practices;
- Have an educational value of risks and benefits of medical interventions and care.

CPGs should be valid, reliable, reproducible, clear, flexible and applicable in various settings of care[111]. The methodology of their development should be clearly defined. There are several ways to develop CPGs. On one hand, there is expert opinion and consensus; on the other, 'evidence-based guidelines' as preferred today[112–117].

How are CPGs developed[118,119]?

- A clinical problem is formulated;
- The best evidence is drawn from the literature and past experience;
- A systematic review of evidence is done as a basis for draft practice guidelines;
- Draft practice is put to a test use in the practicing community;
- Feedback is integrated into the final version of CPGs; and
- CPGs are approved and disseminated.

A clinical sequence is usually reproduced in CPGs. For cancers, as well as for many other diseases, guidelines **cover**[120] diagnostic work-up, primary treatment, adjuvant treatment, surveillance and follow-up, salvage therapy, and supportive care. CPGs have to be **reported in a standard form**[121], which includes (with some modifications):

- Definition of the *problem* and description of the *present practice* and situation.
- *Objective* of the proposed CPGs.
- *Options* (the maze through CPGs guide the clinician) with supporting evidence.
- *Outcomes* (health and economic).
- *Evidence* about all major aspects of the problem and how it was obtained, synthesized and graded.
- *Benefits*, *harms*, and *costs*.
- *Values* of potential outcomes (for clinicians and their patients as well).
- Summary of *recommendations*.
- *Validation* of CPGs themselves.
- *Sponsors* (authors of CPGs, providers of funding, endorsers and other important stakeholders).

Examples of current guidelines abound[120,122]. They have been developed for all major cancers (breast, colon, rectal, lung, ovarian, prostate, leukemia), ischemic heart disease, back pain, diabetes, pneumonia, schizophrenia, stroke, myocardial infarction, biliary tract disease, depression, pre-term birth, acute pain and many others. **CPGs may take the form** of structured narrative directions to follow or an algorithm[123]. Figure 13.13 is an example of algorithmic guidelines for the management of dyspepsia.

An evidence-based narrative form may be also considered, as Wright's guidelines for the management of elevated blood pressure[124]. Developing evidence-based guidelines is not a quick and easy task. Diagnostic and treatment options, as well as their validity, effectiveness and desirable and adverse outcomes, must be ideally endorsed by the best available evidence, which should also be explained to CPG users. Guidelines focusing on the process of care cannot always be founded on evidence. Such a consensus development may yield excellent results, such as guidelines for pre-hospital[125] and in-hospital[126] cardiopulmonary resuscitation, published by several leading medical journals and currently in field use.

Finally, CPGs have **two additional challenges:**

- Their implementation and evaluation of use[127,128]; and
- Evaluation of their effectiveness[129].

Good guidelines have to be used, but they must yield better results than unguided heterogeneous practices and care. Quality of guidelines, their use, and effectiveness evaluation should facilitate the controlling of 'guidelinitis'[130] and spreading of such a new 'syndrome'.

Several competing guidelines may be developed for the management of the same problem. For example, Cornwall and Scott[131] noted five guidelines for the management of depression as worthy of overview. Systematic reviews of such decision-making tools may become more frequent in the forthcoming times if guidelines will proliferate to such a threshold for meta-analysis. Fletcher[132] stresses rightly, that CPGs are just recommendations for the evidence-based care of **average** patients, not rules for **all** patients. '. . . *Although guidelines may point out the best research evidence to guide the care of average*

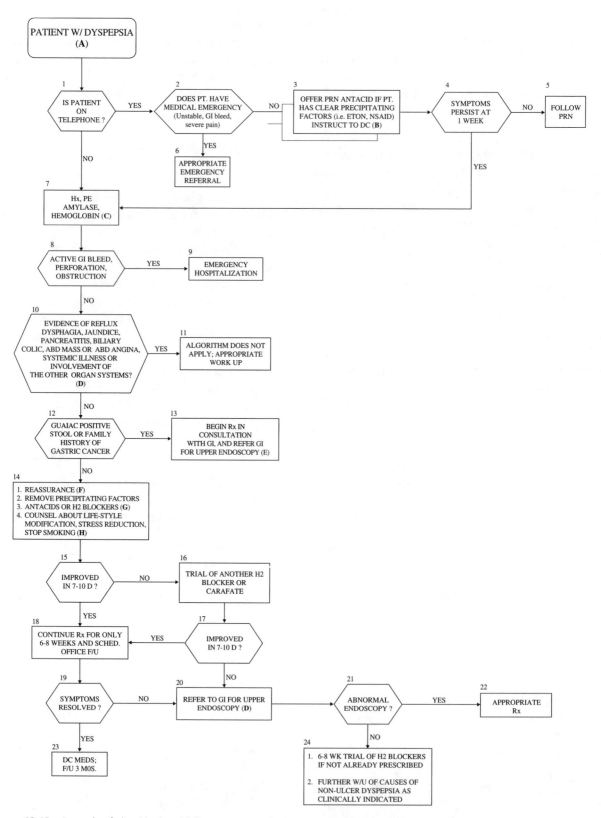

Figure 13.13 Example of algorithmic guidelines. Source: Ref. 123, reproduced with permission

patients, they are not the substitute for clinical judgment, which should be applied to each individual patient[131]. Hence, **CPGs in the framework of evidence-based medicine** are an important part of a longer process. For Lilford and Braunholtz[133-modified], in the case of a novel treatment:

- **Clinical trials** show its effectiveness;
- **Meta-analyses** confirm it;
- **Decision analysis** weights costs and benefits in favor of treatment;
- This preferred treatment option is made part of **clinical practice guidelines**;
- The impact of guidelines is evaluated by **clinical audit**;
- Implementation is handled by managerial action like **clinical governance**;
- All of the above represent **evidence-based care**.

Some of these other sources and/or uses of evidence in this chain of events, such as clinical audit, clinical governance or a less traditional research action, merit at least basic definitions here because uses of evidence, including those produced by decision analysis, are crucial to their functioning. Evidence gives meaning to these mostly managerial concepts which lie, however, beyond the scope of this reading. It also gives them some reference points. A **clinical audit** is essentially any type of regular review or monitoring of the quality of medical practice[134]. It is '*an examination or review that establishes the extent to which a condition, process, or performance conforms to predetermined standards or criteria. Assessment or review of any aspect of health care to determine its quality. . . .*'[12]. Its considerations, conclusions and recommendations rely greatly on the best evidence available (including standards).

Clinical governance is a managerial concept of health care, launched and defined in 1998 by the British National Health Service (NHS) as a '*. . . framework through which all NHS organizations are accountable for continuously improving the quality of their services and safeguarding high standards of care by creating an environment in which excellence in clinical care will flourish*'[135]. This kind of corporate accountability for clinical performance also requires evidence as a reference point and direction-giving tool, as illustrated in Figure

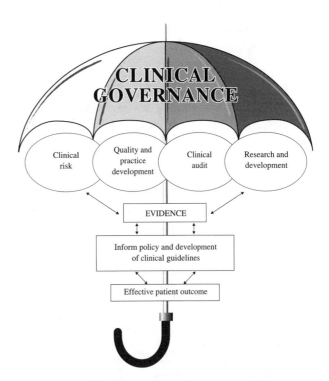

Figure 13.14 Proposed framework outlining clinical governance. Source: Ref. 136, reproduced with permission of the *British Journal of Nursing*

13.14[136]. The clinical governance concept encompasses clinical performance, leadership, audit, risk management, complaints, continuing health assessment, changing practices through evidence, continuing education, culture of excellence and clear accountability[137]. The role of its principal players and stakeholders is also defined[138]. Still in its first years of existence, clinical governance has its rightful critics and room for further development and improvements[139].

Evidence-based health care (or practice) is '*an approach to decision-making in which the clinician uses the best evidence available, in consultation with the patient, to decide upon the option which suits the patient best*'[140]. It means producing evidence – making evidence available – using evidence (getting research into practice) when caring for individual patients, groups of patients and populations[140]. It should integrate all of the above. In conclusion, patient- or management-centered decision-making both require sound *a priori* decision analysis as discussed in this chapter.

13.5 Decisions and decision-making in community medicine and public health

There are not many decision trees, flow chart algorithms, or decision tables in community medicine and public health. Decision analyses have been attempted *ad hoc* (e.g. for solving problems in fighting malaria[34] or considering immunizations[33,36,71]); currently, however, decisions are essentially made on the basis of several component considerations. Usually, when health programs such as immunization programs are under consideration, the completeness and relevance of information on the topic is assessed and decisions are taken according to:

- The occurrence (importance) of the health problem;

- The efficacy and safety of an intervention modality;
- The feasibility of the strategy to make the intervention work; and
- The evaluability of the intervention program under consideration.

White and Mathias[141] propose these considerations and apply them to immunization programs in Canada. Table 13.2 illustrates their approach.

All of the above-mentioned approaches to clinical decision-making are structured and pragmatic paths to the best possible result in terms of benefits for the patient, ease of structured work for the health professional, and satisfaction for a health economist, planner, and community decision-maker. Decision-making in community medicine and public

---

Table 13.2   Outline for the planning and evaluation of immunization programs. An example of the foundation for decision-making in public health

A.   Definition of the problem

1. What disease is to be prevented or controlled?
2. What is the evidence concerning the incidence of infection, disease, and complication by age, sex, and regional distribution?
3. What is the quality of that evidence?
4. What is the economic and social impact of the disease?

B.   Assessment of the immunizing agent

1. What are the characteristics of the immunizing agent? (e.g. live attenuated, killed, absorbed/non-absorbed, viral or bacterial product, etc.)
2. What is the evidence of short-term and long-term efficacy?
3. What is the evidence of vaccine safety? (e.g. in the laboratory, in field trials, under wide-spread use, short-term, long-term, minor and major reactions, etc.)

C.   Identification of strategies

1. What are the alternative objectives?
2. What are the alternative strategies available for meeting alternative objectives?
3. What are the alternative target groups?
4. What is the evidence concerning the short-term and long-term effectiveness of alternative strategies?
5. What is the quality of that evidence?
6. What are the underlying assumptions (e.g. probable need for booster immunizations, effect on duration of maternal antibody, etc.)?

D.   Assessment of feasibility of strategy

1. How acceptable will the chosen alternative be to the target group, and to the population at large? What levels of compliance are expected?
2. What would be the costs (vaccine and administration) of implementing and maintaining each strategy at various levels of compliance?
3. What is the availability of the vaccine, or desired vaccine combinations, in Canada?
4. What are the opportunity costs of alternative strategies?
5. What are the results of cost/benefit analysis for each strategy, and how rigorous were those analyses?
6. Are the resources available?

E.   Evaluability

1. Is evaluation an important component of the proposed program?
2. What tools are available for monitoring incidence of infection, disease and complications by age, sex, and geographical distribution?
3. How reliable are those tools?
4. Is baseline data currently available, and, if not, can it be developed?
5. If implemented, can a reliable evaluation component (A to E) be built into the program?

Source: Ref. 132, reproduced with permission of the Canadian Public Health Association

health is a separate field[142], and is beyond the methodology explained above and the scope of this reading.

13.6 Conclusions

Decision analysis is still a developing field with regard to its understanding, organization, effective use and evaluation. It is about 25 years old. Breakthroughs have been made, but much still needs to be refined. Decision analysis continues to occupy a progressively important place in literature, research and practice. It deserves to be properly understood in all its facets.

13.6.1 *Pros and cons of decision analysis*

The forces for and against decision analysis, like the yin and yang of problems in Oriental philosophy, both have serious arguments to offer. **On the 'yin' or 'nay' side:** One important argument is that a considerable gap still exists between decision analysis models and clinical practice in its reality when dealing with specific characteristics of a particular patient to whom decision analysis and its result should apply. For this reason, Detsky et al[143] propose that decision analysis should target more policymakers, textbook writers, and 'role model' clinicians, rather than a broader clinical audience. This chapter illustrates these authors' feelings of how formidable a task it is to cultivate the audience of textbook writers and role model clinicians so as to demonstrate the benefits of decision analysis for patients through formal evaluation research. This remains a challenge for the future.

Another problem is that **decision analyses and their products, like algorithms** (with their other components such as research, experience or meta-analysis), **often do not travel well.** On one hand, they are badly needed in certain environments given incomplete and imperfect data and information for straightforward matters, and/or the proliferation of new medical technologies, such as diagnostic methods and treatments in medicine and surgery. On the other hand, according to Balla et al[144], biases exist between expert and novice users (expert decision analysis belongs to expert people). Diagnostic

(base rate) errors abound. Variable meaning is attributed to findings (representativity). Variable use of relevant findings exists. Unequal weight is given by different clinicians in their working, and decisions to different findings (anchoring) and even wording of problems (framing) may affect the decision process and its result. It appears from these authors' comments, as well as from other experiences, that reluctance to use decision analysis does not focus on its substance, intellectual quality or scientific acceptability. Its greatest challenge is that it is somewhat inflexible and not adaptive enough for ever-changing daily life in different clinical environments and community health fields. These authors[144] conclude: '. . . *We are not suggesting that it is neither feasible or necessary to apply decision analytic methods to every clinical situation. Yet the insights into decision processes provided by the theory and the discrepancies between clinical intuition and formal theories should become part of the background and understanding of every clinician'.*

Are alternative approaches possible to overcome the critiques of decision analysis? Dolan[145], for example, suggests that decision analysis often does not take into account enough considerations, especially enough of its objectives. Dolan's figure (Figure 13.15) illustrates that the choice of treatment may not only depend on one desirable effect, but that a clinician often chooses a treatment that will maximize effectiveness and minimize side effects, all at a minimum cost. The choice of the best treatment in

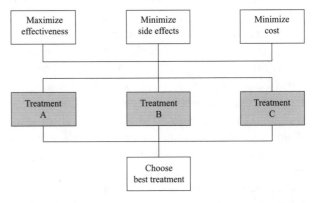

Figure 13.15 Graphic representation of an 'analytical hierachy process' in clinical decision analysis. Source: Ref. 145, reproduced with permission from Elsevier Science (*J Clin Epidemiol*)

such a situation requires innovative approaches, such as this author's 'analytic hierarchy process', which still requires further testing. The usefulness of such an approach may be illustrated in the field of the assessment of 'toss-up' situations. Adding potentially important factors should not change decisions. A significant change in the result, such as resolution of the toss-up, would indicate, according to this author[145], that the decision model did not properly reflect the clinical situation under study.

On the 'yang' or 'yea' side: Among the first reactions from the outside world of decision analysts, a cautious 'yes, but' was proposed by Ransohoff and Feinstein[146]. Quality components of the decision analysis process and a proper assessment of utilities are particularly important for these authors, if decision analysis is meant to succeed. Does decision analysis really produce better results than expert clinicians' opinions? It certainly depends on the type of problem to be solved. An overall response based on the evaluation of major clinical practices and problem solving still needs to be done. However, this kind of evaluative study exists. For example, Manu and Runge[147] compared results of threshold analysis and expert opinions of experienced cardiologists as to whether, after use of a non-invasive method (stress test), an invasive one (angiography) should be added when considering surgery for patients with stable angina pectoris. From a total of 61 experts, 37 (or 60.6%) suggested adding coronary angiography if the stress test were positive. The same was suggested by threshold analysis. These authors conclude that other cardiologists might benefit from the additional insight produced by threshold analysis. They also found that these experts as a group showed a fairly inaccurate knowledge of the probabilities necessary for decision-making, and tended to under-use coronary angiography and over-use radionuclide exercise imaging. They recognized the absence of an existing diagnostic mode among the group. The latter was replaced by the cognitive abilities of each group member. Decision analysis may prove useful in such instances to improve clinicians' performance, not by telling them what to do, but by giving them clearer directions based on organized thinking and problem handling.

Elstein et al[148] studied decisions regarding replacement estrogen therapy for menopausal women. Decisions of 50 physicians from 12 cases were compared to formal decision analysis. Physicians tended not to treat, whereas decision analysis suggested treatment or toss-up. Decision analysis took into consideration more elements, such as an increased probability of cancer detection in regular follow-up. It also showed that vasomotor symptom relief is not the issue, but that estrogen therapy should be given because of the lower fracture risk. The same authors felt that decision analysis would be further enhanced if other important, but less traditional utilities were studied, such as responsibility or anticipation of regret. Decision analysis was also found to be preferable to second opinions for surgical decisions[149]. Decision analysis, like meta-analysis (as mentioned in Chapter 11), may represent an alternative and/or complement to controlled clinical trials, whenever they are costly and/or ethically unacceptable. On the basis of Wong et al's study[150] of percutaneous transluminal coronary angioplasty being a reasonable alternative to coronary bypass surgery, Gunnar[151] stresses that decision analysis is only as good as its data base. Dolan[152] calls for a kind of 'expiration date' for the use of decision analysis results.

There is no procedure or method without shortcomings and limitations. Despite this, decision analysis is gaining ground and refinements. Kassirer et al's[42] review of its recent applications is impressive in its scope and diversity. Two main trends appear: either common strategies are researched to solve a problem concerning the disease as a whole, as in Wong et al's[150] study quoted above; or, decision analysis focuses more and more on individual clinical cases[153], as Tufts University Clinical Decision Unit has not only professed, but also practiced for many years. There are two levels of analyses[154]: **Policy level analyses** focusing on the disease or health problem as a whole and **patient specific decision analyses**[154-156], which are highly dependent on specific medical scenarios, patients' clinical and other characteristics as well as on further improvements in information technology (supporting software)[157]. Bedside use of decision analysis is most probably the essence of clinical experience.

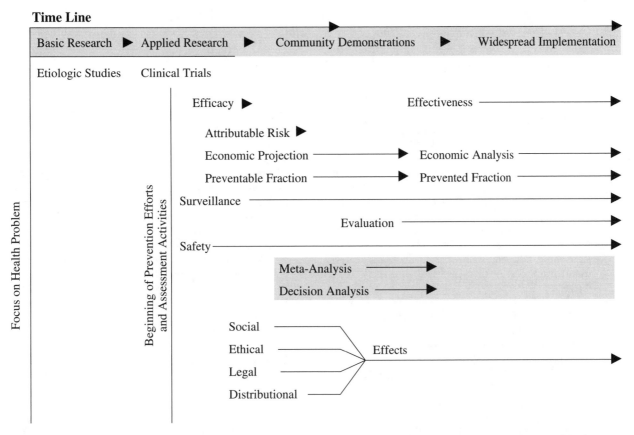

Figure 13.16   Place of decision analysis and meta-analysis in the implementation of health programs. Source: Ref. 159, public domain

Decision analysis has its own risks and costs. Pauker and Kassirer[158] believe, that the strength of decision analysis is that it forces clinicians to consider the risks and costs in obtaining desired information. Despite all inherent limitations, decision analysis as well as meta-analysis is becoming an uncontested part of the decision process in health sciences. Figure 13.16 illustrates the position of decision analysis and meta-analysis in working up strategies towards problem solving in health fields[159] such as injury prevention.

13.6.2   The future of research in clinical decision-making

In addition to further refinements in the quantitative methodology of decision analysis[160–162], the evaluation of its results, considerations of human values, and the assessment of human weaknesses in clinical

practice are necessary ingredients for the improvement of decision-making in clinical practice, community health, and medical research. This would probably explain why the results of clinical decision analyses may at times appear more counterintuitive than they really are. For Meyer et al[163], medical errors are preventable. Understanding and improving medical decision-making is one way to make the 'epidemiology of medical errors'[163] easier. Emerson concludes[164]:' . . . *Human beings are incredibly efficient at pattern recognition; computers are very bad at it and no mathematical theory as yet helps. Mathematical theories can, however, make diagnoses and decisions by logical inference . . . we do not know, and our textbooks do not tell us the conditional probabilities of symptoms, signs and positive test results being found when different disorders are present or absent . . . Next to the dusty volumes in the College's library, with their loving descriptions of common, not uncommon, not so rare and rare disorders, will be the crisp new books that list the prior and the conditional probabilities and the* utilities (values) of different states of health and illness. We need these books . . .'. This reading aspires to be one of them.

REFERENCES

1. Schoolman HM. The role of the physician as a patient advocate. *N Engl J Med*, 1997;**296**:103–5
2. Spindel E, Harty RF, Leibach JR, McGuigan JE. Decisional analysis in evaluation of hyper-gastrinemia. *Am J Med*, 1986;**80**:11–7
3. Murphy EA. *The Logic of Medicine*. Baltimore: The Johns Hopkins University Press, 1976
4. Sox Jr. JC. Decision analysis: A basic clinical skill? *N Engl J Med*, 1987;**316**:271–2
5. Ransohoff DF, Feinstein AR. Is decision analysis useful in clinical medicine? *Yale J Biol Med*, 1976; **49**:165–8
6. Zarin DA, Pauker SG. Decision analysis as a basis for medical decision-making: The tree of Hippocrates. *J Med Phil*, 1984;**9**:181–213
7. Iseman MD, Sarbaro JA. Consensus statements. *Arch Intern Med*, 1985;**145**:630–1
8. Park RE, Fink A, Brook HR, Chassin MR, et al. Physician ratings of appropriate indications for six medical and surgical procedures. *Am J Public Health*, 1986;**76**:766–72
9. Kunz JC, Shortliffe EH, Buchanan BG, Feigenbaum EA. Computer-assisted decision-making in medicine. *J Med Phil*, 1984;**9**:135–60
10. Pauker SG, Gorry GA, Kassirer JP, Schwartz WB. Towards the simulation of clinical cognition. Taking a present illness by computer. *Am J Med*, 1976;**60**: 981–96
11. Raiffa H. *Decision analysis: Introductory Lectures on Choices Under Uncertainty*. Reading: Addison-Wesley, 1968
12. Last JM (ed.). *A Dictionary of Epidemiology*. 4th Edition. New York: Oxford University Press, 2001
13. Einhorn HJ and Hogarth RM. *Decision-making: Going forward in reverse*. *Harvard Business Review*, 1987;**65**:66–70
14. Decision analysis in medicine. In: Bursztajn H, Feinbloom RI, Hamm RM, Brodsky A. *Medical Choices, Medical Chances. How Patients, Families, and Physicians Can Cope with Uncertainty*. New York: Dell Publishing Co., 1981:117–73
15. Kassirer JP. The principles of clinical decision-making: An introduction to decision analysis. *Yale J Biol Med*, 1976;**49**:149–64
16. Decision theory in clinical medicine. Thematic portion of Issue No.4 (Series of articles). *J Roy Coll Physic London*, 1979;**13**:183–220
17. Thornton JG, Lilford RJ, Johnson N. Decision analysis in medicine. *Br Med J*, 1992;**304**:1099–103
18. Detsky AS, Naglie G, Krahn MD, et al. Primer on medical decision analysis. Part 1 – Getting started. *Med Decis Making*, 1997;**17**:123–5
19. Detsky AS, Naglie G, Krahn MD, et al. Primer on medical decision-making. Part 2 – Building a tree. *Med Decis Making*, 1997;**17**:126–35
20. Naglie G, Krahn MD, Naimark D, et al. Primer on medical decision-making. Part 3 – Estimating probabilities and utilities. *Med Decis Making*, 1997;**17**: 136–41
21. Krahn MD, Naglie G, Naimark D, et al. Primer on medical decision-making. Part 4 – Analyzing the model and interpreting the results. *Med Decis Making*, 1997;**17**:142–51
22. Naimark D, Krahn MD, Naglie G, et al. Primer on medical decision-making. Part 5 – Working with Markov processes. *Med Decis Making*, 1997; **17**:152–9
23. Eiseman B, Anderson B (eds). Progress Symposium. Surgical Decision Making. *World J Surg*, 1989; **13**:239–99
24. Birkmeyer JD, Birkmeyer NO. Decision analysis in surgery. *Surgery*, 1996;**120**:7–15
25. Birkmeyer JD, Weich HG. A reader's guide to surgical decision analysis. *J Am Coll Surg*, 1997;**184**: 589–95
26. Kucey DS. Decision analysis for the surgeon. *World J Surg*, 1999;**23**:1227–31
27. Pauker SP, Pauker SG. Prenatal diagnosis: a directive approach to genetic counselling using decision analysis. Yale J Biol Med, 1977;**50**:275–89
28. Pauker SP, Pauker SG. The amniocentesis decision: An explicit guide for parents. Birth Defects: Original Article Series,1979;**XV** (No 5C):289–324
29. Twiggs LB, Potish RA. Decision theory analysis of the enteric morbidity and surgical staging in the treatment of advanced cervical cancer. *Am J Obstet Gynecol*, 1984;**148**:134–40
30. Bergman DA, Pantell RH. The art and science of medical decision-making. *J Pediat*, 1984;**104**:649–56
31. Kovacs G, Croskerry P. Clinical decision making: an emergency medicine perspective. *Acad Emerg Med*, 1999;**6**:947–52
32. Allen UD. Medical decision analysis in infectious diseases. *Can J Infect Dis*, 2000;**11**:317–21

33. Koplan JP, Schoenbaum SC, Weinstein MC, Fraser DW. Pertussis vaccine and analysis of benefits, risks and costs. *N Engl J Med*, 1979;**301**:906–11

34. Peto TEA, Gilks CF. Strategies for the prevention of malaria in travellers: Comparison of drug regimens by means of risk-benefit analysis. *Lancet*, 1986;**1**:1256–61

35. Colice GL. Decision analysis, public health policy, and isoniazid chemoprophylaxis for young adult tuberculin skin reactors. *Arch Intern Med*, 1990;**150**:2517–22

36. Stevens JP, Daniel TM. Bacille Calmette Guérin immunization of health care workers exposed to multidrug-resistant tuberculosis. A decision analysis. *Tuber Lung Dis*, 1996;**77**:315–21

37. Coleman RL. The use of decision analysis in quality assessment. *QRB*, 1989;**15**:383–91

38. Phelps CE, Mushlin AI. Focusing technology assessment using medical decision theory. *Med Decis Making*, 1988;**8**:279–89

39. Harbison J. Clinical decision-making in nursing. *J Adv Nursing*, 1991;**16**:404–7

40. McCreery AM, Truelove E. Decision-making in dentistry. Part I. A historical and methodological overview. *J Prosthet Dent*, 1991;**65**:447–51. Part II. Clinical applications of decision methods. *Idem*: 575–85

41. Ngategize PK, Kaneene JB, Harsh SB, et al. Decision analysis in animal health programs: Merits and limitations. *Prev Vet Med*, 1986;**4**:187–97

42. Kassirer JP, Moskowitz AJ, Lau J, Pauker SG. Decision analysis: A progress report. *Ann Intern Med*, 1987;**106**:275–91

43. Patrick EA. *Decision analysis in Medicine. Methods and Applications*. Boca Raton: CRC Press, 1979

44. Weinstein MC, Fineberg HV, Elstein AS, et al. *Clinical Decision Analysis*. Philadelphia: WB Saunders, 1980

45. Sox JC Jr, Blatt MA, Higgins MC, Morton KI. *Medical Decision Making*. Boston: Butterworths, 1988

46. Cebul RD, Beck LH (eds). *Teaching Clinical Decision Making*. New York: Praeger, 1985

47. Elstein AS. Decision analysis in surgical education. *World J Surg*, 1989;**13**:287–91

48. Balla JI. Teaching clinical decision analysis: Implications for nutritional assessment management. *Med J Aust*, 1989;**151**(Suppl):S32–S36

49. Shamian J. Effect of teaching decision analysis on student nurses' clinical intervention decision-making. *Res Nurs Health*, 1991;**14**:59–66

50. McNeil BJ, Pauker SG, Sox HC Jr. The patient's role in assessing the value of diagnostic tests. *Radiology*, 1979;**132**:605–10

51. Pauker SG, Kassirer JP. Clinical decision analysis by personal computer. *Arch Intern Med*, 1981;**141**:1831–7

52. Plante DA, Kassirer JP, Zarin DA, Pauker SG. Clinical decision consultation service. *Am J Med*, 1986;**80**:246–58

53. Glasziou P, Irwing LM. An evidence-based approach to individualizing treatment. *Br Med J*, 1995;**311**:1356–9

54. Glasziou P, Guyatt GH, Dans AL, et al. Applying the results of trials and systematic reviews to individual patients. *ACP J Club*, 1998(Nov-Dec);**129**:A17–A18

55. Tom E, Schulman KA. Mathematical models in decision analysis. *Infect Control Hosp Epidemiol*, 1997;**18**:65–73

56. Sulkes J, Fields S, Gabbay U, et al. Path analysis on the risk of mortality in very low birth weight infants. *Eur J Epidemiol*, 2000;**16**:337–41

57. West DC, Pomeroy JR, Park JK, et al. Critical thinking in graduate medical education. A role for concept mapping assessment? *JAMA*, 2000;**284**:1105–10

58. Pauker SG, Kassirer JP. Clinical application of decision analysis: a detailed illustration. *Semin Nucl Med*, 1978;**8**:324–35

59. Eisenberg JM. Clinical decision analysis: An introduction. In: Asawapokee N, Lilasarami A eds. *Symposium on Clinical Decision Analysis and Clinical Economics*, Pattaya, March 11–13, 1987. Bangkok: Medical Media Press, 1987:5–37

60. Sisson JC, Schoomaker EB, Ross JC. Clinical decision analysis. The hazard of using additional data. *JAMA*, 1976;**236**:1259–63

61. Barza M, Pauker SG. The decision to biopsy, treat, or wait in suspected herpes encephalitis. *Ann Intern Med*, 1980;**92**:641–9

62. Carpenter TE, Epidemiologic programs for computers and calculators. Decision-tree analysis using a microcomputer. *Am J Epidemiol*, 1986;**124**:843–50

63. Kassirer JP, Pauker SG. The toss-up. (Editorial) *N Engl J Med*, 1981;**305**:1267–9

64. Feinstein AR. The 'chagrin factor' and quantitative decision analysis. *Arch Intern Med*, 1985;**145**:1257–9

65. Brody H, Thompson JR. The 'chagrin factor' in obstetrics. *Arch Intern Med*, 1986;**146**:201

66. Pauker SG, Kassirer JP. The threshold approach to clinical decision-making. *N Engl J Med*, 1980;**320**:1109–17

67. Weinstein MC, Stasson WB. Foundations of cost-effectiveness analysis for health and medical practices. *N Engl J Med*, 1977;**296**:716–21

68. Department of Clinical Epidemiology and Biostatistics, McMaster University Health Centre

(Stoddart GL, Drummond MF). How to read clinical journals: VII. To understand an economic evaluation (part A). *Can Med Assoc J*, 1984;**130**:1428–32, and 1434. (part B): *Idem*:1542–9

69. Eisenberg JM, Clinical economics: Economic analysis in medical care. In: Asawapokee N, Lilasarami A eds. *Symposium on Clinical Decision Analysis and Clinical Economics*, Pattaya, March 11–13, 1987. Bangkok: Medical Media Press, 1987:78–120

70. Eisenberg JM. Cost-benefit and cost-effectiveness analysis. In: Cebul RD, Beck L eds. *Teaching Clinical Decision Making*. New York: Praeger Publishing Co., 1985:97–114

71. Mulley AG, Siverstein MD, Dienstag JL. Indications for use of hepatitis B vaccine, based on cost-effectiveness analysis. *N Engl J Med*, 1982;**307**: 644–52

72. Levine MN, Drummond MF, Labelle RJ. Cost-effectiveness in the diagnosis and treatment of carcinoma of unknown primary origin. *Can Med Assoc J*, 1985;**133**:977–87

73. McNeil BJ, Adelstein SJ. Measures of clinical efficacy. The value of case finding in hypertensive renovascular disease. *N Engl J Med*, 1975;**293**: 221–6

74. Pauker SG, Kassirer JP. Therapeutic decision-making: A cost-benefit analysis. *N Engl J Med*, 1975; **293**: 229–34

75. Clarke JR. Decision making in surgical practice. *World J Surg*, 1989;**13**:245–51

76. Greep JM, Siezenis LMLC. Methods of decision analysis: Protocols, decision trees, and algorithms in medicine. *World J Surg*, 1989;**13**:240–4

77. Rose DN. Short-course prophylaxis against tuberculosis in HIV-infected persons. A decision and cost-effectiveness analysis. *Ann Intern Med*, 1998; **129**:779–86

78. Burman WJ, Dalton CB, Cohn DL, et al. A cost-effectiveness analysis of directly observed therapy vs self-administered therapy for treatment of tuberculosis. *Chest*, 1997;**112**:63–70

79. Sterling TR, Brehm WT, Moore RD, Chiasson RE. Tuberculosis vaccination versus isoniazid preventive therapy: a decision analysis to determine the preferred strategy of tuberculosis prevention in HIV-infected adults in the developing world. *Int J Tuberc Lung Dis*, 1999;**3**:248–54

80. Hensyl W (ed.). *Stedman's Medical Dictionary*. 25th Edition. Baltimore: Williams & Wilkins, 1990

81. Landau SI (ed.). *International Dictionary of Medicine and Biology*. New York: John Wiley, 1986

82. *Encyclopaedia Britannica*. Chicago: William Benton Publisher, 1968

83. Parker SP (ed.). *McGraw-Hill Dictionary of Scientific and Technical Terms*. 4th Edition. New York: McGraw-Hill, 1989

84. Oreskovich MR, Carrico CJ. Stab wounds of the anterior abdomen. Analysis of a management plan using local wound exploration and quantitative peritoneal lavage. *Ann Surg*, 1983;**198**:411–9

85. Vickery DM, Quinnell RK. Fever of unknown origin. An algorithmic approach. *JAMA*, 1977;**238**: 2183–8

86. Sox HC Jr, Koran LM, Sox CH, et al. A medical algorithm for detecting physical disease in psychiatric patients. *Hosp Commun Psychiatry*, 1989;**40**: 1270–6

87. Djulbegovic B, Hadley T, Pasic R. A new algorithm for diagnosing anaemia. *Postgrad Med*, 1989;**85**: 119–30

88. Franklin RCG, Spiegelhalter DJ, McCartney FJ, Bull K. Evaluation of a diagnostic algorithm for heart disease in neonates. *Br Med J*, 1991;**302**:935–9

89. Pearson SD, Margolis CZ, Davis S, et al. The clinical algorithm nosology: A method for comparing algorithmic guidelines. *Med Decis Making*, 1992;**12**: 123–31

90. Society for Medical Decision Making Committee on Standardization of Clinical Algorithms. Proposal for clinical algorithm standards. *Med Decis Making*, 1992;**12**:149–54

91. Sauer MV, Rodi IA. Utility of algorithms to diagnose ectopic pregnancy. *Int J Gynecol Obstet*, 1990;**31**: 29–34

92. Sox Jr HC, Sox CH, Tompkins RK. The training of physician's assistants. The use of a clinical algorithm system for patient care, audit of performance and education. *N Engl J Med*, 1973;**288**:818–24

93. Gottlieb LK, Margolis CZ, Schoenbaum SC. Clinical practice guidelines at an HMO: Development and implementation in a quality improvement model. *Qual Rev Bull*, 1990;**2**:8–6

94. Wilkin A, McColl I. Surgical audit: The clinician's view. *Theor Surg*, 1987;**1**:195–206

95. Selbman HK. Quality assurance of medical information processing: The statistician's view. Examples taken form a surgical survey with 184 participating hospitals and from other health care trials. *Theor Surg*, 1987;**1**:201–13

96. Hansen DT. Development and use of clinical algorithms in chiropractic. *J Manipul Physiol Ther*, 1991;**14**:478–82

97. Green G, Defoe EC Jr. What is a clinical algorithm? *Clin Pediatr*, 1978;**17**:457–63

98. Campostano A, Altomonte F, Bessarione D, et al. A new glucose clamp algorithm: clinical validation. *Int J Artif Organs*, 1991;**14**:441–7

99. Baig MW, Green A, Wade G, et al. A randomized double-blind, cross-over study of linear and non-linear algorithms for the QT sensing rate adaptive pacemaker. *PACE*, 1990;**12**:1082–8

100. Feinstein AR. An analysis of diagnostic reasoning. III. The construction of clinical algorithms. *Yale J Biol Med*, 1974;**1**:5–32

101. Schoenbaum SC, Gottlieb LK. Algorithm based improvement of clinical quality. *Br Med J*, 1990;**301**: 1374–6

102. Holland RR. Decision tables. Their use for the presentation of clinical algorithms. *JAMA*, 1975;**233**: 455–7

103. Pollack SL, Hicks HT, Harrison WJ. *Decision Tables: Theory and Practice*. New York: Wiley Interscience, 1971

104. Schwarz V, Hohenberger P, Kohler CO, Schlag P. Setting up a decision support system with decision tables. *Meth Inf Med*, 1989;**28**:126–32

105. Shiffman RN, Greenes RA. Improving clinical guidelines with logic and decision-table techniques: Application to hepatitis immunization recommendations. *Med Decis Making*, 1994;**14**:245–54

106. Margolis CZ. Pediatric algorithms. *J Pediatr*, 1987; **110**:417–8

107. Kassirer JP, Kopelman RI. Diagnosis and decisions by algorithms. *Hosp Pract*, 1990;(March 15):23–31

108. Richardson FM. Methodological development of a system of medical audit. *Med Care*, 1972;**10**:451–62

109. Komaroff AL. Algorithms and the 'art' of medicine. *Am J Public Health*, 1982;**72**:10–1

110. Field MJ, Lohr KN (eds). *Guidelines For Clinical Practice: From Development to Use*. Washington: National Academy Press, 1992

111. Veale B, Weller D, Silagy C. Clinical practice guidelines and Australian general practice. *Aust Fam Physician*, 1999;**28**:744–9

112. Heffner JE. Does evidence-based medicine help the development of clinical practice guidelines? *Chest*, 1998;**113**(Suppl.3):172S-178S

113. Greengold NL, Weingarten SR. Developing evidence-based practice guidelines and pathways: The experience at the local hospital level. *Joint Commission J Qual Improv*, 1996;**22**:391–402

114. Hirst GH, Ward JE. Clinical practice guidelines: reality bites. *MJA*, 2000;**172**:287–91

115. Worrall G. Clinical practice guidelines: Questions family physicians should ask themselves. *Compr Ther*, 1999;**25**:46–9

116. Cook DJ, Greengold NL, Elrodt G, Weingarten SR. The relation between systematic reviews and practice guidelines. *Ann Intern Med*, 1997;**127**:210–6

117. Eccles M, Freemantle N, Mason J. North of England evidence-based guidelines development project: methods of developing guidelines for efficient drug use in primary care. *Br Med J*, 1998;**316**:1232–5

118. Brouwers MC, Browman GP. Development of clinical practice guidelines: surgical perspective. *World J Surg*, 1999;**23**:1236–41

119. Browman GP, Levine MN, Mohide EA, et al. The practice guidelines development cycle: a conceptual tool for practice guidelines development and implementation. *J Clin Oncol*, 1995:**13**:502–1

120. Winn RJ, Botnick W, Dozier N. The NCCN guidelines development program. *Oncology* (Huntingt), 1996;**10**(Suppl 11):23–8

121. Hayward RSA, Wilson MC, Tunis SR, et al. More informative abstracts of articles describing clinical practice guidelines. *Ann Intern Med*, 1993;**118**: 731–7

122. Smallwood RA, Lapsley HM. Clinical practice guidelines: to what end? *MJA*, 1997;**166**:592–5

123. Pearson SD, Margolis CZ, Davis S, et al. Is consensus reproducible? A study of an algorithmic guidelines development process. *Med Care*, 1995;**33**:643–60

124. Wright JM. Choosing a first-line drug in the management of elevated blood pressure: What is the evidence? 1:Thiazide diuretics. *CMAJ*, 2000; **163**:57–60. 2: Beta-blockers. Idem:188–92. 3: Angiotensin-converting-enzyme inhibitors. Idem: 293–6

125. Cummins RO, Chamberlain DA, Abramson NS, et al. Recommended guidelines for uniform reporting of data from out-of-hospital cardiac arrest: The Utstein Style. *Ann Emerg Med*, 1991;**20**:861–74

126. Cummins RO, Chamberlain D D, Hazinski MF, et al. Recommended guidelines for reviewing, reporting, and conducting research on in-hospital resuscitation: the in-hospital 'Utstein style'. A statement for Healthcare Professionals From the American Heart Association, the European Resuscitation Council, the Heart and Stroke Foundation of Canada, the Australian Resuscitation Council, and the Resuscitation Councils of Southern Africa. *Resuscitation*, 1997;**34**:151–83

127. Davis DA, Taylor-Vaisey A. Translating guidelines into practice. A systematic review of theoretic concepts, practical experience and research evidence in the adoption of clinical practice guidelines. *Can Med Assoc J*, 1997;**157**:408–16

128. Hayward RSA, Guyatt GH, Moore K-A, et al. Canadian physicians' attitudes about preferences regarding clinical practice guidelines. *Can Med Assoc J*, 1997;**156**:1715–23

129. Worrall G, Chaulk P, Freake D. The effects of clinical practice guidelines on patient outcomes in primary care: a systematic review. *Can Med Assoc J*, 1997;**156**:1705–12

130. Johnston BL. Guidelinitis: A new syndrome? *Can J Infect Dis*, 2000;**11**:299–303

131. Cornwall PL, Scott J. Which clinical practice guidelines for depression? An overview for busy practitioners. *Br J Gen Pract*, 2000;**50**:908–11

132. Fletcher RH. Practice guidelines and the practice of medicine: Is it the end of clinical judgment and expertise? *Schweiz Med Wochenschr*, 1998; **128**:1883–8

133. Lilford RJ, Braunholtz D. Who's afraid of Thomas Bayes? *J Epidemiol Community Health*, 2000;**54**: 731–9

134. Crinson I. Clinical governance: the new NHS, new responsibilities? *Br J Nurs*, 1999;**8**:449–53

135. Gilmore I. Clinical governance: what it is, what it isn't and what it should be. *Hosp Med*, 2000;**61**: 51–3

136. McSherry R, Haddock J. Evidence-based health care: its place within clinical governance. *Br J Nurs*, 1999;**8**:113–7

137. Heard S. Educating towards clinical governance. *Hosp Med*, 1998;**59**:728–9

138. Lugon M, Secker-Walker J (eds). *Advancing Clinical Governance*. London: RSM Press, 2000

139. Goodman NW. Clinical governance. *Br Med J*, 1998;**317**:1725–7

140. Muir Gray JA. *Evidence-based Healthcare. How to Make Health Policy and Management Decisions*. New York and Edinburgh: Churchill Livingstone, 1997

141. White FFM, Mathias RG. Immunization program planning in Canada. *Can J Public Health*, 1982;**73**: 167–71

142. Dever GEA, Champagne F. *Epidemiology in Health Services Management*. Royal Tunbridge Wells, Rockville: Aspen Publications, 1984

143. Detsky AS, Redelman D, Abrams HB. What's wrong with decision analysis? Can the left brain influence the right? *J Chron Dis*, 1987;**40**:831–6

144. Balla JI, Elstein AS, Christensen C. Obstacles to acceptance of clinical decision analysis. *Br Med J*, 1989;**298**:579–82

145. Dolan JG. Can decision analysis adequately represent clinical problems? *J Clin Epidemiol*, 1990; **43**:277–84

146. Ransohoff DF, Feinstein AR. Is decision analysis useful in clinical medicine? *Yale J Biol Med*, 1976; **49**:165–8

147. Manu P, Runge LA. Testing stable angina. Expert opinion versus decision analysis. *Medical Care*, 1985;**23**:1381–90

148. Elstein AS, Holzman GB, Ravitch MM, et al. Comparison of physicians' decisions regarding estrogen replacement therapy for menopausal women and decisions derived from a decision analytic model. *Am J Med*, 1986;**80**:246–58

149. Clarke JR. A comparison of decision analysis and second opinions for surgical decisions. *Arch Surg*, 1985;**120**:844–7

150. Wong JB, Sonnenberg FA, Salem DN, Pauker SG. Myocardial revascularization for chronic stable angina. Analysis of the role of percutaneous transluminal coronary angioplasty based on data available in 1989. *Ann Intern Med*, 1990;**113**:852–71

151. Gunnar RM. Decision analysis in the evaluation of revascularization. *Ann Intern Med*, 1990;**113**:817–8

152. Dolan JG. Clinical decision analysis (Editorial). *Med Decis Making*, 2001;**21**:150–1

153. Beck JR. Decision-making studies in patient management: Twenty years later. *Med Decis Making*, 1991;**11**:112–5

154. Eckman MH. Patient-centered decision-making: A view of the past and a look toward the future. *Med Decis Making*, 2001;**21**:241–7

155. Elwyn G, Edwards A, Eccles M, Rovner D. Decision analysis in patient care. *Lancet*, 2001:**358**:571–4

156. Naylor CD. Clinical decisions: from art to science and back again. *Lancet*, 2001;**358**:523–4

157. Helfand M. Review of DATATM, Software for Decision Analysis. *Med Decis Making*, 1997;**17**: 237–8

158. Pauker SG, Kassirer JP. Marchiafava-Bignami disease among academicians in Toronto: Can decision analysis help? *J Chron Dis*, 1987;**40**:837–8

159. Teutsch SM. A framework for assessing the effectiveness of disease and injury revention. *MMWR. Recommendations and Reports*, 1992;**41**(RR-3): 1–12

160. Fryback DG. Reflections on the beginnings and future of medical decision making. *Med Decis Making*, 2001;**21**:71–3.

161. Beck JR. Medical decision making: 20 years of advancing the field. *Med Decis Making*, 2001;**21**: 73–5

162. Habbema JDF, Bossuyt PMM, Dippel DWJ, et al. Analyzing clinical decision analyses. *Stat Med*, 1990; **9**:1229–42

163. Meyer G, Lewin DI, Eisenberg J. To err is preventable: Medical errors and academic medicine. *Am J Med*, 2001;**110**:597–603

164. Emerson PA. Clinical decisions. *J Roy Coll Physic London*, 1979;**13**:185

Epilogue
Widening horizons, staying in touch

Evidence transforms us
from practitioners of the art of medicine
into well-informed Boeotians

In God we trust (motto on US banknotes) . . .
everything else needs evidence
Paraphrasing Hui Lee, 2002

So this, Dear Reader, is the end of your journey through this book. However, it is not the end of the entire journey in medicine across epidemiology, logic and evidence-based medicine. In your future career, you will choose one of two paths offered to you.

You may will choose the **practice of medicine**. During your training and practice, you will become a skillful assessor and user of valid evidence in medical literature. *Users' Guides to the Medical Literature*[1] and many other excellent books on evidence-based medicine in various specialties and clinical areas as partially quoted in this book may be expanded readings for you. They will enhance the understanding and practical skills required to use the essentials in this book in your daily activities or at least in some critical moments of decision when tackling particularly challenging problems. Your teachers of clinical and community medicine will offer you their experience and guide you through additional training. This reading should help you understand the reasoning and recommendations of your more experienced colleagues, role models, and mentors.

You will no longer take medical articles at face value and you will be able to distinguish the best ones from those that are not as good. You will also recognize the ones that apply the most to your patient and practice setting. The task will not be easy. Haines[2] concludes from various sources that there are over 20,000 medical periodicals throughout the world today, producing about two millions articles each year, hence a general practitioner wanting to keep up with the pace of essential information should read about 19 original articles each day. To stay abreast of the exponentially growing flood of information, you may be interested to learn the easiest ways to access information on the medical Internet[3,4] through computerized data banks like *Medline*, *Infotrieve*, *Medweb*, *PubMed* and others. Several highly readable and practical introductory papers[5–17] and Ann McKibbon's guide[18] will tell you how and where to find evidence you need. Handheld computers[19] also provide an almost ubiquitous access to information.

To further help practitioners, experts in evidence-based medicine within the Cochrane Collaboration and elsewhere are continuously producing critically assessed original studies and their systematic reviews. Periodicals like *Evidence-Based Medicine* or *ACP Journal Club* are valuable models of such endeavors. Libraries on disk have also been produced by the American College of Physicians (custserv@ mail.acponline.org). An expanding number of web sites are now available on the Internet. Some of these were summarized by the Cochrane Collaboration[20]:

CANADIAN

British Columbia Council on Clinical Practice Guidelines – **http://www.hlth.gov.bc.ca/msp/infoprac/protoguides/cpgpro.html**

British Columbia Office of Health Technology Assessment – **http://www.chspr.ubc.ca/bcohta/**

Canadian Cochrane Centre – **http://hiru.mcmaster.ca/cochrane/centres/canadian/**

Canadian Coordinating Office for Health Technology Assessment (CCOHTA) – **http://www.ccohta.ca**

Canadian Health Services Research Foundation – **http://www.chsrf.ca**

Canadian Institute for Health Information (CIHI) – **http://www.cihi.ca/index.html**

Canadian Policy Research Networks – **http://www.cprn.com/cprn.html**

Canadian Task Force on Preventive Health Care – **http://www.ctfphc.org/**

Cancer Care Ontario Program in Evidence-Based Care – **http://hiru.mcmaster.ca/ccopgi/**

Centre for Evaluation of Medicines – **http://www.thecem.net/**

Centre for Health Economics and Policy Analysis (CHEPA) – **http://hiru.mcmaster.ca /chepa/**

Centre for Research and Evaluation in Diagnostics (CRED) – **http://www.crc.cuse.usherb.ca/cred**

Clinical Research and Development Program (CRDP) – **http://www.medi-fax.com/rhd/crdp/**

Conseil d'Évaluation des Technologies de la Santé du Québec – **http://www.msss.gouv.qc.ca/cets/**

Health Evidence Application and Linkage Network (HEAL*Net*) – **http://healnet.mcmaster.ca/nce**

Health Information Research Unit (HiRU) – **http://hiru.mcmaster.ca/**

Health Services Utilization and Research Commission – **http://www.sdh.sk.ca/hsurc/**

Infoward – **http://www.infoward.com**

Institute for Clinical Evaluative Sciences (ICES) – **http://www.ices.on.ca/**

Institute for Health and Outcomes Research – **http://www.usask.ca/medicine/ihor/**

Institute for Work & Health – **http://www.iwh.on.ca/**

Manitoba Centre for Health Policy & Evaluation – **http://www.umanitoba.ca/centres/mchpe/1mchpe.htm**

McMaster Evidence-Based Practice Center – **http://hiru.mcmaster.ca/epc/**

Networks of Centres of Excellence – **http://nce.nserc.ca**

Prairie Region Health Promotion Research Centre – **http://www.usask.ca/healthsci/che/prhprc**

INTERNATIONAL

Agency for Health Care Policy and Research (AHCPR) – **http://www.ahcpr.gov/**

American College of Physicians:

  – ACP Journal Club – **http://www.acponline.org/journals/acpjc/jcmenu.htm**

  – Best Evidence – **http://www.acponline.org/catalog/cbi/best_evidence.htm**

  – Evidence–Based Medicine – **http://www.acponline.org/journals/ebm/ebmmenu.htm**

Bandolier – **http://www.jr2.ox.ac.uk/Bandolier/**

BioMedNet – **http://biomednet.com** (free registration)

Centre for Evidence-Based Child Health – **http://www.ich.bpmf.ac.uk/ebm/ebm.htm**

Centre for Evidence-Based Dentistry – **http://www.ihs.ox.ac.uk/cebd/**

Centre for Evidence-Based Medicine – **http://cebm.jr2.ox.ac.uk**

Centre for Evidence-Based Mental Health – **http://www.psychiatry.ox.ac.uk/cebmh/**

Centre for Evidence-Based Nursing – **http://www.york.ac.uk/depts/hstd/centres/evidence/ev-intro.htm**

Centre for Evidence-Based Pathology – **http://www.ccc.nottingham.ac.uk/~mpzjlowe/evcent.html**

Cochrane Collaboration – **http://hiru.mcmaster.ca/cochrane/**

Critical Appraisal Skills Programme – **http://www.ihs.ox.ac.uk/casp/**

Guide to Best Practices – **http://www.futurehealthcare.com/pages/guidetobestpractices.htm**

International Society of Technology Assessment in Health Care – **http://www.istahc.org/**

Medical Technology and Practice Patterns Institute – **http://www.mtppi.org**

NHS Centre for Reviews and Dissemination (NHS CRD) – **http://www.york.ac.uk/inst/crd/**

National Guideline Clearinghouse – **http://www.guideline.gov**

The ScHARR Guide – Netting the Evidence – **http://www.med.unr.edu/medlib/netting.html**

Swedish Council on Technology Assessment in Health Care (SBU) – **http://www.sbu.se/**

Turning Research Into Practice – **http://www.gwent.nhs.gov.uk/trip/**

U.S. Preventive Services Task Force – **http://www.ahcpr.gov/clinic/uspsfact.htm**

The Unit for Evidence-Based Practice and Policy – **http://www.ucl.ac.uk/primcare-popsci/uebpp/uebpp.htm**

An increasing number of sites produced by various academic institutions, professional bodies, governments or research groups should be also considered. Their list goes well beyond the scope of this message.

Alternatively, you might follow the path of **fundamental** or **bedside, decision-oriented medical research** or **community medicine and public health**. If this is the case, you will feel that this reading has just opened your mind to further training and to a better and more complete understanding of biostatistics, fundamental and clinical epidemiology, health administration, health economics, qualitative research as well as related methodology in social sciences and politics. Graduate programs in clinical research methodology like the *Robert Wood Johnson Clinical Scholar Programs* in the United States, or graduate programs in general and community medicine health research methodology are now available nationally and internationally at practically all major medical training institutions around the world. Sometimes, some of these graduate programs and degrees are offered in pair with basic medical training or within residency programs and training in various clinical specialties.

Whatever your choice in the maze of further training and fields of practice, let it be the wisest and the best for your personal fulfillment and for the benefit of your patients. To conclude, let us quote Frank Davidoff[21]:

'. . . Evidence-based medicine, like any other medical technique, does not provide magic solutions; that it was never meant in any sense to 'replace' clinical experience. On the contrary, clinical experience is what provides the context and gives meaning to the 'evidence' . . . which . . . can inform, refine, sharpen, enrich, and enhance clinical experience. . . . Perhaps the ultimate criterion for judging the contribution of evidence-based medicine, however, is for each of us to consider what we will want for ourselves when we get sick. . . . It is only fair, therefore, to ask why we should settle for anything less in making clinical decisions for, and with, the patients under our care.'

EBM has still a way to go! If evidence-based medicine means for some a new paradigm, its achievements must prove unprecedented enough to attract an enduring group of adherents away from competing modes of activity and it should be open-ended enough to allow its practitioners all sorts of problems to resolve[22]. It looks that it does. And what about this book and many others? Our own judgment counts a lot. T.S. Kuhn reminds us, that 'it is a poor carpenter who blames his tools' and adds: '. . . the man who reads a science text can easily take applications to be the evidence for the theory, the reasons why it ought to be believed. But science students accept theories on the authority of teacher and text, not because of evidence. What alternative have they and what competence? The applications given in the texts are not there as evidence but because learning them is part of learning the paradigm at the base of current practice . . .' [22]. Reading and learning from this book and any book in medicine should go then well beyond that.

May this book help open just a little bit more the door to your future enlightened decisions and choices!

REFERENCES

1. Guyatt G, Rennie D (eds). *Users' Guides to the Medical Literature. A Manual for Evidence-Based Practice.* Chicago: American Medical Association Press, 2002

2. Haines A. The science of perpetual change. *Br J Gen Pract*, 1996;**46**:115–9

3. Doyle DJ, Ruskin KJ, Engel TP. The Internet and medicine: Past, present, and future. *Yale J Biol Med*, 1996;**69**:429–37

4. Ruskin KJ, Doyle DJ, Engel TP. Development of an academic Internet resource. *Yale J Biol Med*, 1996;**69**:439–44

5. Akatsu H, Kuffner J. Medicine and the Internet. *West J Med*, 1998;**169**:311–17

6. Hunt DL, Jaeschke R, McKibbon KA for the Evidence-Based Medicine Working Group. Users' Guides to the Medical Literature. XXI. Using electronic health information resources in evidence-based practice. *JAMA*, 2000;**283**:1875–9

7. Jadad AR, Haynes RB, Hunt D, Browman GP. The Internet and evidence-based decision-making: a needed synergy for efficient knowledge management in health care. *CMAJ*, 2000;**162**:362–5

8. McCombs B. Out behind the barn. *Can J Rural Med*, 1999;**4**:245–6

9. Stewart A. Creating your own medical Internet library. *CMAJ*, 1999;**161**:1155–60

10. McCombs B. Literature searches on Internet. *Can J Rural Med*, 2000;**5**:158–60

11. Indrajit IK. Medline. *Nat Med J India*, 2001;**14**:50–3

12. McCombs B. Spotlight on Google. *Can J Rural Med*, 2001;**6**:211–2

13. Kiley R. Finding health information on the Internet: health professionals. *Hosp Med*, 2000;**61**:736–8

14. McCombs B. New Canadian Internet resources. *Can J Rural Med*, 2001;**6**:57–8

15. McCombs B. Obstetrics on the Web. *Can J Rural Med*, 2000;**5**:233–5

16. Conly J. *Can J Infect Dis*, 1999;**10**:329–30
17. Kiley R. Evidence-based medicine and Internet. *J Roy Soc Med*, 1998;**91**:74–5
18. McKibbon A, Eady A, Marks S. *PDQ Evidence-Based Principles and Practice*. Hamilton, London, St. Louis: BC Decker Inc., 1999
19. McCombs B. Handheld computers. *Can J Rural Med*, 2001;**6**:138–40
20. Oliver T. *Evidence-Based Health Care Organizations*. Information sheet. Hamilton: Canadian Cochrane Centre, 2000
21. Davidoff F. In the teeth of the evidence: The curious case of Evidence-Based Medicine. *Mount Sinai J Med*, 1999;**66**:75–83
22. Kuhn TS. *The Structure of Scientific Revolutions*. 3rd edition. Chicago and London: The University of Chicago Press, 1996

Index

Numbers in bold indicate pages where fundamental definitions of terms can be found.